Disorders of the Heel, Rearfoot, and Ankle

Disorders of the Heel, Rearfoot, and Ankle

Chitranjan S. Ranawat, MD

Director
Department of Orthopedic Surgery
Ranawat Orthopedic Institute and Center for Total Joint Replacement
Lenox Hill Hospital
New York, New York

Attending Orthopedic Surgeon
Hospital for Special Surgery
New York, New York

Professor of Orthopedic Surgery
Cornell University Medical College
New York, New York

Rock G. Positano, MSc, MPH, DPM

Director
Practice for Disorders of the Heel and Rearfoot
Hospital for Special Surgery
New York, New York

Foot and Ankle Division
The Combined Orthopedic Trauma and Fracture Service
New York Presbyterian Hospital/Hospital for Special Surgery
New York, New York

Department of Orthopedic Surgery
Foot and Ankle Division
Lenox Hill Hospital
New York, New York

Professor
The Institute for Orthopedic and Sports Engineering
The Cooper Union for the Advancement of Science and Art
Albert Nerken School of Engineering
New York, New York

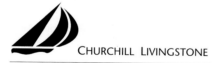

CHURCHILL LIVINGSTONE

A Division of Harcourt Brace & Company
New York, Edinburgh, London, Philadelphia, San Francisco

CHURCHILL LIVINGSTONE
A Division of Harcourt Brace & Company

The Curtis Center
Independence Square West
Philadelphia, Pennsylvania 19106

Library of Congress Cataloging-in-Publication Data

Disorders of the heel, rearfoot, and ankle / [edited by] Chitranjan S. Ranawat and
Rock G. Positano.—1st ed.

p.   cm.

ISBN 0–443–07838–6

1. Foot—Abnormalities.   2. Foot—Diseases.   3. Heel bone—Abnormalities.
4. Heel bone—Diseases.   5. Ankle—Abnormalities.   6. Ankle—Diseases.
I. Ranawat, Chitranjan S.   II. Positano, Rock G. [DNLM: 1. Foot Diseases.
2. Foot Injuries.   3. Heel—Injuries.   4. Ankle Injuries.   WE 880 D612
1999]

RD781.D57 1999   617.5′85—dc21

DNLM/DLC   98–54193

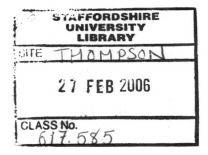
DISORDERS OF THE HEEL, REARFOOT, AND ANKLE   ISBN 0–443–07838–6

Printed in the United States of America.

Last digit is the print number: 9   8   7   6   5   4   3   2   1

05021850

Dedicated to the memory of
Senator Abraham A. Ribicoff
Gentleman, Humanitarian, Scholar

"I must have confidence and I must be worthy of the great DiMaggio who does all things perfectly even with the pain of the bone spur in his heel. . . . Do you believe the great DiMaggio would stay with a fish as long as I will stay with this one? . . . I am sure he would and more since he is young and strong. Also, his father was a fisherman. But would the bone spur hurt him too much?

The Old Man and The Sea
Ernest Hemingway—1952

Contributors

Sherry I. Backus, MA, PT

Senior Research Physical Therapist, Motion Analysis Laboratory, Department of Biomechanics and Biomaterials, Hospital for Special Surgery, New York, New York
The Foot and Ankle During Gait

Robert L. Bard, MD

Director, New York Trauma Imaging, New York, New York
Ultrasound Imaging of the Ankle and Rearfoot

Craig S. Bartlett III, MD

Fellow in Traumatology, Orthopedic Trauma Service, Hospital for Special Surgery, New York, New York
Calcaneal Fractures: Etiology, Diagnosis, and Classification; Calcaneal Fractures: Conservative and Surgical Treatment; Fractures of the Ankle; Pilon Fractures: Classification, Diagnosis, and Treatment

Helen Bateman, MD

Rheumatology Fellow, Department of Medicine, Hospital For Special Surgery, New York, New York
Heel Pain in the Setting of Metabolic, Infiltrative, and Bone Disorders; Heel Pain and Achilles Pain Associated with Rheumatoid Arthritis and Seronegative Spondyloarthropathies

Finn Bojsen-Møller, MD, PhD

Professor of Anatomy, Department of Medical Anatomy, University of Copenhagen, Copenhagen, Denmark
Biomechanics of the Heel Pad and Plantar Aponeurosis

Jeffrey S. Borer, MD

Gladys and Roland Harriman Professor of Cardiovascular Medicine, Professor of Cardiovascular Medicine in Radiology, Professor of Cardiovascular Medicine in Cardiothoracic Surgery, Chief, Division of Cardiovascular Pathophysiology, Cornell University Medical College, New York; Attending Physician, New York Presbyterian Hospital, New York, New York
Edema and Foot Injuries: Pathophysiology and Differential Diagnosis

Michael J. Brunetti, DPM

Department of Orthopedic Surgery, Lenox Hill Hospital, New York, New York
Heel Pain Syndrome: Etiology, Diagnosis, and Conservative Treatment

Lisa R. Callahan, MD

Assistant Professor, Department of Medicine, Cornell University Medical College, New York; Assistant Attending Physician, Hospital for Special Surgery, New York; Medical Director, Women's Sports Medicine Program, New York, New York
Stress Fractures of the Rearfoot, Midfoot, Distal Tibia, and Fibula

Mark A. Caselli, DPM

Professor, Department of Orthopedics, The New York College of Podiatric Medicine, New York, New York
Orthotic Therapy in the Treatment of Heel, Achilles Tendon, and Ankle Injuries

Heber C. Crockett, MD

Resident in Orthopedic Surgery, Hospital for Special Surgery, New York, New York
Achilles Tendon Injuries

Thomas M. DeLauro, DPM

Professor, Division of Medical Sciences, Division of Surgical Sciences, The New York College of Podiatric Medicine, New York, New York
Surgical Correction of Heel Spur and Plantar Fascia Tears

David M. Dines, MD

Chairman, Department of Orthopedic Surgery, Long Island Jewish Medical Center, New York; Associate Professor of Orthopedic Surgery, Albert Einstein College of Medicine, New York; Assistant Attending Orthopedic Surgeon, Hospital for Special Surgery, New York, New York
Heel Pain Syndrome: Etiology, Diagnosis, and Conservative Treatment

Jordan Ditchek, MD

Resident in Radiology, Cornell University Medical College, Hospital for Special Surgery, New York, New York
Imaging of the Hindfoot and Ankle

John J. Doolan, DPM

Podiatric Medicine and Surgery Resident, Cabrini Medical Center, New York, New York
Heel Pain Syndrome: Etiology, Diagnosis, and Conservative Treatment

Daria Dykyj, PhD

Professor and Chairman, Department of Morphological Sciences, New York College of Podiatric Medicine, New York, New York
Anatomy of the Heel and Rearfoot

Carl Heise, MD

Associate Attending in Neurology, Cornell University Medical College, New York; Medical Director, The Clinical Neurophysiology Laboratory, Hospital for Special Surgery, New York, New York
Electrodiagnosis in Heel and Foot Disorders

David L. Helfet, MD

Professor of Orthopedic Surgery, Cornell University Medical College, New York; Director, Combined Orthopedic Trauma Service, Hospital for Special Surgery, New York Presbyterian Hospital, New York, New York
Calcaneal Fractures: Etiology, Diagnosis, and Classification; Calcaneal Fractures: Conservative and Surgical Management; Fractures of the Ankle; Pilon Fractures: Classification, Diagnosis, and Treatment

Stuart D. Katchis, MD

Chief, Section of Foot and Ankle, Department of Orthopedic Surgery, Lenox Hill Hospital, New York; Orthopedic Foot and Ankle Consultant, New York Islanders
Tarsal Tunnel Syndrome; Peroneal Tendon Disorders; Posterior Tibial Tendon Dysfunction

Gerrit J. Kleinrensink, PhD

Senior Lecturer, Department of Anatomy, Erasmus University, Rotterdam, The Netherlands
The Chronically Unstable Ankle: Anatomic, Biomechanical, and Neurologic Considerations

David S. Levine, MD

Instructor in Surgery (Orthopedics), Cornell University Medical College, New York; Assistant Attending Orthopedic Surgeon, Hospital for Special Surgery, New York Presbyterian Hospital, New York, New York
Chronic Compartment Syndrome and Shin Splints

Michael Levinson, PT

Adjunct Instructor, Hunter College, New York; Long Island University, Brooklyn; Columbia University, New York; Clinical Director, Sports Medicine Performance and Research Center, Hospital for Special Surgery, New York, New York; Team Physical Therapist, New York Mets
Physical Therapy for Ankle and Rearfoot Disorders

Eric J. Lindberg, MD

Denver Orthopedic Specialists, Denver, Colorado
Peroneal Tendon Disorders

Steven S. Louis, MD

Director, Orthopedic Trauma, Good Samaritan Hospital, Downers Grove, Illinois
Calcaneal Fractures: Etiology, Diagnosis, and Classification; Calcaneal Fractures: Conservative and Surgical Management

Jan Willem K. Louwerens, MD, PhD

Surgeon, Department of Orthopedic Surgery, Academic Hospital Utrecht, Utrecht, The Netherlands
Lateral Ankle Instability: An Overview

Steven K. Magid, MD

Associate Professor, Department of Medicine, Cornell University Medical College, New York; Associate Attending Physician, Hospital for Special Surgery, New York, New York
Rheumatology Laboratory Evaluation

Ralph C. Marcove, MD

Clinical Professor of Orthopedic Surgery, Columbia Presbyterian Medical Center of New York; Associate Professor of Orthopedic Surgery, Cornell University Medical College, New York, New York
Treatment of Bone and Soft Tissue Tumors of the Ankle and Foot

Joseph A. Markenson, MD

Professor of Clinical Medicine, Cornell University Medical College, New York; Attending Physician, Hospital for Special Surgery and New York Presbyterian Hospital, New York, New York
Heel Pain in the Setting of Metabolic, Infiltrative, and Bone Disorders; Heel Pain and Achilles Pain Associated with Rheumatoid Arthritis and Seronegative Spondyloarthropathies

Joseph Moreira, MD

Fellow in Neurology, Cornell University Medical College, New York; Fellow in Neuromuscular Disease and Neurophysiology, Hospital for Special Surgery, New York, New York
Electrodiagnosis in Heel and Foot Disorders

Jeffrey Y. F. Ngeow, MD

Associate Professor, Department of Anesthesiology, Cornell University Medical College, New York; Associate Attending Anesthesiologist, Hospital for Special Surgery, New York, New York
Reflex Sympathetic Dystrophy: Complex Regional Pain Syndrome of the Ankle and Foot

Stephen J. O'Brien, MD

Associate Professor of Orthopedic Surgery, Cornell University Medical College, New York; Associate Attending Orthopedic Surgeon, Hospital for Special Surgery, New York, New York; Assistant Team Physician, New York Giants
Chronic Compartment Syndrome and Shin Splints

Stephen A. Paget, MD

Professor of Medicine, New York Presbyterian Hospital, Cornell University Medical College, New York; Physician-in-Chief, Hospital for Special Surgery, New York, New York
Heel Pain in the Setting of Metabolic, Infiltrative, and Bone Disorders; Heel Pain and Achilles Pain Associated with Rheumatoid Arthritis and Seronegative Spondyloarthropathies

Dipak V. Patel, MD, MSOrth

Fellow in Sports Medicine, Hospital for Special Surgery, New York, New York
Ankle Sprain: Clinical Evaluation and Current Treatment Concepts

Helene Pavlov, MD

Professor of Radiology, Cornell University Medical College, New York; Radiologist-in-Chief, Department of Radiology and Imaging, Hospital for Special Surgery, New York, New York
Imaging of the Hindfoot and Ankle

Rock G. Positano, MSc, MPH, DPM

Director, Practice for Disorders of the Heel and Rearfoot, Hospital for Special Surgery, New York; Foot and Ankle Division, The Combined Orthopedic Trauma and Fracture Service, New York Presbyterian Hospital/ Hospital for Special Surgery, New York; Department of Orthopedic Surgery, Foot and Ankle Division, Lenox Hill Hospital, New York; Professor, The Institute for Orthopedic and Sports Engineering, The Cooper Union for the Advancement of Science and Art, Albert Nerken School of Engineering, New York, New York
Heel Pain Syndrome: Etiology, Diagnosis, and Conservative Treatment; Surgical Correction of Heel Spur and Plantar Fascia

Tears; Orthotic Therapy in the Treatment of Heel, Achilles Tendon, and Ankle Injuries

Hollis G. Potter, MD

Associate Professor of Radiology, Cornell University Medical College, New York; Chief, Magnetic Resonance Imaging, Department of Radiology and Imaging, Hospital for Special Surgery, New York, New York
Imaging of the Hindfoot and Ankle

Cathleen L. Raggio, MD

Assistant Attending Orthopedic Surgeon, Hospital for Special Surgery, New York, New York
Heel and Hindfoot Pain in the Pediatric and Adolescent Patient

Raymond D. Reiter, MD

Assistant Clinical Instructor, Department of Physical Medicine and Rehabilitation, Cornell University Medical College, New York; Assistant Attending Physician, Hospital for Special Surgery, New York, New York; Team Physician, New Jersey Nets
Achilles Tendinitis

Michael Rubin, MD, FRCP(C)

Associate Attending in Neurology and Neuroscience; Director, Electromyography Laboratory, Cornell University Medical College, New York; New York Presbyterian Hospital, New York, New York
Electrodiagnosis in Heel and Foot Disorders

Robert Schneider, MD

Associate Professor of Radiology, Cornell University Medical College, New York; Attending Radiologist, Hospital for Special Surgery, New York, New York
Imaging of the Hindfoot and Ankle

Gary Sclar, MD, PhD

Assistant Professor, Director, EMG Laboratory, Department of Neurosciences, University of Medicine and Dentistry of New Jersey, Newark; Attending Neurologist, University Hospital, Newark, New Jersey
Electrodiagnosis in Heel and Foot Disorders

Brian Shaffer, BA

Second Year Medical Student, Hahnemann School of Medicine, Philadelphia, Pennsylvania
Edema and Foot Injuries: Pathophysiology and Differential Diagnosis

Peter T. Simonian, MD

Associate Professor, Chief, Sports Medicine Clinic, Director, Sports Medicine Research, University of Washington, Department of Orthopedic Surgery, Seattle, Washington
Knee Pathology and Pain Related to Rearfoot and Heel Dysfunction

Chris J. Snijders, PhD

Professor and Chairman, Department of Biomedical Physics and Technology, Faculty of Medicine and Allied Health Science, Erasmus University, Rotterdam, The Netherlands; Professor, Industrial Design Engineering, Delft University of Technology, Delft, The Netherlands
Plantar Fascia: Mechanical and Clinical Perspectives; Lateral Ankle Instability: An Overview; The Chronically Unstable Ankle: Anatomic, Biomechanical, and Neurologic Considerations

Ellen Sobel, DPM, PhD

Associate Professor, Department of Orthopedics, The New York College of Podiatric Medicine, New York, New York
Orthotic Therapy in the Treatment of Heel, Achilles Tendon, and Ankle Injuries

Ely L. Steinberg, MD

Fellow in Traumatology, Orthopedic Trauma Service, Hospital for Special Surgery/New York Presbyterian Hospital, New York, New York
Fractures of the Ankle

Rob Stoeckart, PhD

Senior Lecturer, Department of Anatomy, Erasmus University, Rotterdam, The Netherlands
The Chronically Unstable Ankle: Anatomic, Biomechanical, and Neurologic Considerations

Vijay B. Vad, MD

Assistant Professor, Department of Physical Medicine and Rehabilitation, Cornell University Medical College, New York; Assistant Attending Physician, Hospital for Special Surgery, New York, New York
Achilles Tendinitis

David M. Wallach, MD

Chief Resident, Department of Orthopedic Surgery, Lenox Hill Hospital, New York, New York
Tarsal Tunnel Syndrome

David Y. Wang, MD

Fellow, Department of Anesthesiology, Hospital for Special Surgery, New York, New York
Reflex Sympathetic Dystrophy: Complex Regional Pain Syndrome of the Ankle and Foot

Russell F. Warren, MD

Surgeon-in-Chief, Attending Orthopedic Surgeon, Hospital for Special Surgery, New York; Professor of Orthopedic Surgery, Cornell University Medical College, New York, New York; Head Team Physician, New York Giants
Ankle Sprain: Clinical Evaluation and Current Treatment Concepts

Andrew J. Weiland, MD

Professor of Orthopedic and Plastic Surgery, Cornell University Medical College, New York; Attending Orthopedic Surgeon, Hospital for Special Surgery, New York, New York

Achilles Tendon Injuries

Geoffrey H. Westrich, MD

Instructor in Surgery (Orthopedic), Assistant Clinical Professor in Surgery, Cornell University Medical College, New York; Assistant Attending Orthopedic Surgeon, Hospital for Special Surgery, New York, New York
Thrombophlebitis as a Cause of Heel and Rearfoot Pain

Thomas L. Wickiewicz, MD

Associate Professor of Orthopedic Surgery, Cornell University Medical College, New York; Chief, Sports Medicine and Shoulder Service, Hospital for Special Surgery, New York, New York
Knee Pathology and Pain Related to Rearfoot and Heel Dysfunction

John M. Wright, MD

Resident in Orthopedic Surgery, Hospital for Special Surgery, New York, New York
Achilles Tendon Injuries

L. Ricardo Zuniga-Montes, MD

Rheumatology Fellow, Department of Medicine, Hospital for Special Surgery, New York, New York
Heel Pain in the Setting of Metabolic, Infiltrative, and Bone Disorders; Heel Pain and Achilles Pain Associated with Rheumatoid Arthritis and Seronegative Spondyloarthropathies

Foreword

Disorders of the Heel, Rearfoot, and Ankle, co-edited by Chitranjan S. Ranawat and Rock G. Positano, is a unique text, which for the first time presents a comprehensive approach to the treatment of specific foot disorders that affect approximately one third of all Americans.

The book focuses on anatomy, imaging techniques, rheumatologic evaluation, and electrodiagnostic techniques prior to discussion of specific clinical entities. Various topics are covered in depth and provide the practitioner with pertinent information regarding the diagnosis, possible systemic causes of the pathology, and most impor-

tantly, an algorithm for treatment which incorporates both conservative and possible surgical approaches.

The editors are to be congratulated for bringing together contributions from leading practitioners in several fields, all of which deal with disorders of the heel, rearfoot, and ankle. These specialists include orthopedic surgeons, rheumatologists, podiatrists, radiologists, sports medicine and physical medicine.

The editors are to be applauded for providing to practitioners this much needed information in one text.

Andrew J. Weiland, MD
Professor of Orthopedic Surgery and
 Plastic Surgery
Cornell University Medical College

President
American Orthopedic Association
American Board of Orthopedic Surgery

Preface

This volume presents an exhaustive, yet readable, exploration of that which has been only tangentially covered in the past: the heel, the rearfoot, and the ankle. Never before has there been a perceptive examination of the interplay between these areas of the lower extremity and systemic disease.

This text brings together the leading experts in the disciplines of orthopedics, neurology, biomechanics, physical rehabilitation, rheumatology, sports medicine, and podiatric medicine and orthopedics.

Each chapter stands alone as the most recent and definitive in that one field, but it is also interwoven with the other specialties. Presented in detail are the treatment protocols for heel, rearfoot, and ankle disorders that most commonly present in the foot and ankle practice. The clear text is supplemented with the very latest research and the most advanced imaging and diagnostic techniques.

New ground is broken for the discernment of systemic disease that is reflected in the foot and ankle. While the topic has been covered elsewhere, nowhere is it covered in such detail and with such authority.

Clinical gait analysis and neurophysiologic testing round out the array of the medical text. The text then augmented by an extensive coverage of rearfoot traumatology, fractures, ankle disorder diagnosis, lateral ankle instability, sprains, surgical options, and conservative treatment of maladies.

Sports medicine, orthopedic, podiatric, rheumatology, rehabilitation, and neurology specialists would benefit greatly from this resource. It will prove of great value for attendings in these fields as well. Last, but not least, medical students in all fields will find the information of great importance not merely in study but also in practice.

Chitranjan S. Ranawat, MD
Rock G. Positano, MSc, MPH, DPM

Contents

1 Anatomy of the Heel and Rearfoot

Daria Dykyj

Anatomically, the limbs represent two similar musculoskeletal packages designed to transport the trunk and head. In human anatomy, upright stance and bipedal gait have liberated the upper extremity from regular weight-bearing gait function, but the common anatomic design precedes the evolution of bipedalism. The arrangement of bones, muscles, and neurovascular trunks is similarly laid down in development before the unique functions of each extremity determine the further growth and development of each structure in specific detail. In the hand the wrist bones remain small and the digits relatively long for maximizing manipulative ability, whereas in the foot the tarsal bones, especially those of the rearfoot, are greatly enlarged and the toes are relatively shortened to transform the extremity into a mobile gait pedestal.

Unlike the hand, the position of the foot to the leg is distinguished by its fixed hyperextended position, limiting flexion of the foot in relation to the long axis of the extremity. As a result, one is intuitively inclined to refer to a fully plantar flexed foot as an "extended" foot: even at its most flexed, it does not form a visibly "reduced angle" at the joint but rather a fully opened joint with no angular acuity, as in elbow and knee extension. The massive posterior projection of the calcaneus, forming the heel, is an anatomic requirement for bipedal stance, which checks the range of motion of the foot in a posterior direction.

SKELETAL ANATOMY

The calcaneus and talus are the largest tarsal bones, each responsible for transmitting the entire force of body weight. In normal anatomic position, the calcaneus supports the talus with an anterior elevation, or pitch, of about 15° from the transverse plane. This elevation ensures that the strongest part of the calcaneus, the tuber or calcaneal process, hits the ground first, and is an important skeletal character defining both longitudinal arches. When loaded in gait, the pitched calcaneus, with its associated ligaments and tendons, is believed to provide elastic recoil in the arch system.[1]

For purposes of visualizing the important soft tissue arrangements around the lower posterior leg and heel, the skeletal framework is best viewed as an arrangement of the talocrural and talocalcaneal joints together. In its descent to the heel, all body weight carried by the tibia from the knee is almost entirely transmitted through the wide tibial roof (plafond) of the ankle joint directly to the body of the talus. From here, most of this force is transmitted directly to the calcaneus through the posterior facets of the talocalcaneal (subtalar) joint.

Calcaneus

The superior, or dorsal, surface of the calcaneus shares three sets of smooth articular facets with the talus; all three form the functionally designated "subtalar joint," although anatomically only the large posterior facets are known by that name because they are entirely enclosed by a separate joint capsule. The posterior pair of talocalcaneal facets has the most direct anatomic and functional relationship to the heel. The large posterior talar facet is securely placed in the center of the bone's superior surface; directly inferior to this facet, the cancellous trabeculae within the bone radiate from this area of force concentration toward the calcaneal tuber. The anterior and middle facets of the talar head are located on the anterior third of the superior calcaneal surface and are separated from the posterior facet by the calcaneal sulcus.

The posterior third of the calcaneus has no articular facets; it provides attachment for soft tissue and ends in the massive tuber, or calcaneal process. In addition to its rugosity, the posterior section is elongated between the posterior talar facet and the calcaneal (Achilles) tendon insertion at the very end of the bone. The distance between

1

the ankle joint axis of rotation and the insertion of the tendon, approximately 6 to 7 cm, is the tendon moment arm at the joint, its increased length increasing the tendon's mechanical efficiency. The development of the posterior end of the bone is one of the best examples in the body of an "apophysis," a secondary ossification center at a tendon insertion. The relatively great force generated by the gastrocnemius-soleus ("triceps surae") muscle group on the very end of growing calcaneus requires a firm anchorage, and the formation of a secondary osseous center at the tendon insertion provides a more secure insertion in the immature bone.

The posterior surface of the calcaneus is anatomically described as having three transverse levels. The calcaneal tendon inserts transversely in a thick band across the middle part of this surface; the slender plantaris tendon inserts at the most medial point on this site. The superior third is tilted up and anteriorly away from the calcaneal tendon, forming a space that is occupied by the retrocalcaneal bursa. The inferior third of the posterior surface is the tuber; it divides inferiorly to form the medial and lateral calcaneal processes, which provide attachment for the plantar deep fascia and for origins of the first layer of intrinsic plantar muscles.

The medial process is approximately 1.5 to 2 cm in diameter with a wide and often sharp anterior edge, a frequent site of heel spur formation, whereas the lateral process is smaller, approximately 1 cm in diameter. The calcaneal inferior, or plantar, surface also includes an anterior tubercle, which marks the attachment of the short plantar (plantar calcaneocuboid) ligament. This is one of three ligaments that help to maintain the calcaneal pitch and inferiorly support the midtarsal joint (Fig. 1–1). Medial to the short plantar ligament, the spring ligament (plantar calcaneonavicular) is attached to the anterior edge of the sustentaculum tali and radiates over most of the inferior surface of the navicular bone. Providing additional support laterally, the long plantar ligament forms a thick strap under the lateral longitudinal arch and short plantar ligament, with its posterior attachment on the broad inferior calcaneal surface and its anterior attachments on the cuboid and metatarsal bases.

Projecting medially from the calcaneus,

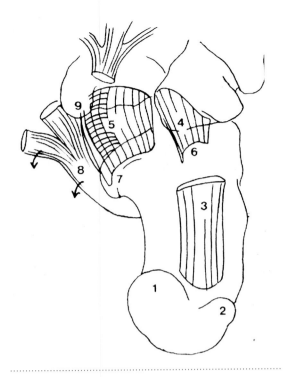

Figure 1–1. Inferior aspect of calcaneus with ligament attachments: 1 = medial calcaneal process; 2 = lateral calcaneal process; 3 = long plantar ligament (severed); 4 = short plantar ligament (plantar clacaneocuboid); 5 = spring ligament (plantar calcaneonavicular) with hatched area indicating groove for tibialis posterior tendon; 6 = anterior calcaneal tubercle; 7 = sustentaculum tali; 8 = tendon of tibialis posterior (reflected medially); 9 = navicular tuberosity.

and continuous with its superior surface, is the sustentaculum tali, approximately 1 cm in width and 2.5 cm in anteroposterior length. This prominent shelf of bone "sustains the talus," or talar head, at the medial junction of the subtalar and midtarsal joints; its superior aspect bears the smooth middle talar facet, which articulates with the talar head. Immediately posterior to the sustentaculum tali is the narrow medial end of the calcaneal sulcus; the corresponding sulci of the articulated talus and calcaneus form the narrow, medial ("tarsal canal") outlet of the sinus tarsi.

The sustentaculum tali is situated within a nest of ligaments whose fibers merge, forming a thick ligamentous wall that medially supports the ankle, subtalar, and midtarsal joints. The main component of this "compound ligament" is the "deltoid," which is itself composed of the four medial collateral ligaments of the ankle joint. All the deltoid components are attached superiorly to the medial malleolus and spread out widely inferiorly in an anteroposterior triangular array, which includes the tibionavicular, anterior tibiotalar (shorter and more deeply positioned than the other deltoid components), tibiocalcaneal, and posterior tibiotalar ligaments. Deeper than the deltoid group is the medial talocalcaneal ligament, a medial capsular ligament of the subtalar joint. Anterior and inferior to this group is the spring ligament, a ligament supporting and enclosing the talar head within the talocalcaneonavicular joint capsule (Fig. 1–2).

Wrapping around the sustentaculum tali with its extensive ligamentous strapping are the three deep muscle tendons from the posterior compartment of the leg, passing posteromedially to the ankle joint and into the plantar foot. The tibialis posterior tendon passes above the level of the sustentaculum tali as it approaches its insertion to the navicular tuberosity, the flexor digitorum longus tendon passes directly around the medial edge of the sustentaculum, and the flexor hallucis longus passes under the sustentaculum tali (which has a groove for this tendon on its inferior surface), against which it is secured by an osseofibrous tunnel fixed to the bone.

On its lateral aspect, the calcaneus bears a fibular (peroneal) tubercle or trochlea, an enlargement of highly variable size and shape.* In spite of its morphologic variability,[2] it represents the site where the central slip of the inferior fibular retinaculum is attached, dividing the fibularis (peroneus) longus and fibularis (peroneus) brevis tendons in their course along the lateral side of the foot. The bone is usually grooved, at least for the fibularis longus tendon, and these tendon grooves, together with the tubercle in between, create a "trochlea" or pulley-shaped form. Posterior to the tubercle, the calcaneus usually exhibits a slight bulge, the retrocalcaneal eminence, which is related to the trabecular arrangement within the bone.

Talus

The talus forms the centerpiece of the rearfoot joint complex, linking three articular entities: the talocrural (ankle), talocalcaneal (subtalar), and talonavicular (midtarsal) joints. It is not surprising that three fifths of its surface is articular, thus inaccessible to direct vascularization, and all but its posterior process and neck are enclosed inside joint capsules. The inferior surface of the bone is entirely articular except for the deep sulcus tali along the talar neck, which, when articulated with the sulcus calcanei, forms the sinus tarsi between the two bones.

The posterior calcaneal facet of the talus occupies the entire inferior aspect of the talar body directly under the trochlea of the ankle joint; its large surface area and its position above the heel are indicative of the large forces transmitted from the leg at that site. The anterior and middle talar facets of the calcaneus, together with the broad,

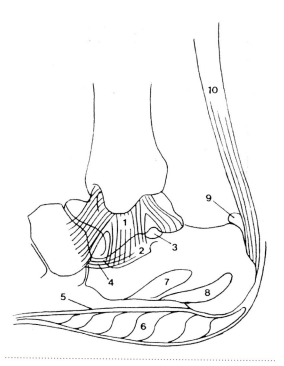

Figure 1–2. Medial aspect of ankle and heel: 1 = deltoid ligament; 2 = sustentaculum tali; 3 = medial opening ("canalis") of sinus tarsi; 4 = spring ligament; 5 = deep plantar fascia; 6 = heel pad; 7 = origin of medial part of flexor accessorius; 8 = origin of abductor hallucis; 9 = retrocalcaneal bursa; 10 = calcaneal (Achilles) tendon.

---

*"Fibular"/"fibularis" replace "peroneal"/"peroneus" in current anatomic usage; the change is applied to the appropriate terms in this chapter; the previous usage is indicated in parentheses only in the first reference to a structure.

concave talar facet of the navicular bone, are enclosed within a capsule that envelops the entire talar head, forming the anatomically distinct talocalcaneonavicular joint. Against the main action between the posterior talocalcaneal facets, the anteromedially projecting talar head is supported by the anterior talar facet of the calcaneus when the joint is supinated and by the middle talar facet when it is pronated.

Superiorly, the talar body is very securely positioned within the ankle mortise formed by the tibia and fibula. The superior surface of the body forms the "trochlea," shaped with a slight sagittal indentation to resist transverse motion. The trochlea and the matching tibial plafond represent the main force transmission surfaces of the ankle joint. The medial and lateral sides of the talar body articulate with the malleoli as gliding support surfaces of the joint and the sites of supporting collateral ligament attachments. On the medial side, the articulation with the medial malleolus is relatively small, and the medial surface itself is slightly concave. The lateral surface of the body is broad, projects laterally as the "lateral process" of the body of the talus, and bears a large triangular facet for the lateral malleolus.

Like most hinge joints, the ankle needs only collateral ligaments to suspend the talus on both sides. The medial collateral ligaments form a dense interconnected "deltoid" ligament group (see previous discussion); two of its components, the anterior and posterior tibiotalar ligaments, connect the medial malleolus to the talar body and to the medial talar tubercle, respectively. The three lateral collateral ligaments, anterior and posterior talofibular and calcaneofibular, are each anatomically distinct and more likely to rupture individually (Fig. 1–3). Two of these ligaments, the anterior and posterior talofibular, are also attached to the talus.

The anterior talofibular ligament forms a broad, flat band attached anteriorly to the lateral malleolus and to the talar neck; it is the most isolated of the seven collaterals and ruptures most frequently, poorly protecting the ankle against excessive forces tending to open the joint in inversion. The calcaneofibular ligament is attached from the lateral malleolus to the lateral surface of the calcaneus. It passes somewhat obliquely and posteriorly to the calcaneus

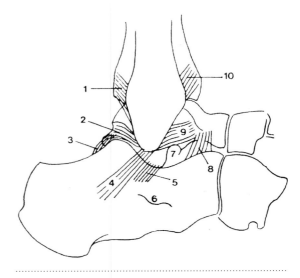

Figure 1–3. Lateral aspect of ankle and heel: 1 = posterior tibiofibular ligament; 2 = posterior talofibular ligament; 3 = posterior talocalcaneal ligament; 4 = calcaneofibular ligament; 5 = lateral talocalcaneal ligament; 6 = fibular (peroneal) trochlea; 7 = sinus tarsi; 8 = cervical ligament; 9 = anterior talofibular ligament; 10 = anterior tibiofibular ligament.

and is the only one of the seven collateral ligaments that is anatomically distinct from the ankle joint capsule. Deep to this ligament, and also obliquely oriented, is the lateral talocalcaneal ligament, attached to the tip of the lateral process of the talar body and to the lateral surface of the calcaneus. The third of the lateral collateral ligaments of the ankle, the posterior talofibular ligament, is the strongest, deeply attached to the malleolar fossa of the lateral malleolus and to the lateral talar tubercle.

The posterior slope of the talar trochlea ends above the posterior process, which provides attachment for numerous ligaments and fasciae in the rearfoot. The posterior process is a horizontal shelf of bone centrally divided by a groove into two tubercles. When observed in its articulated position, the posterior process of the talus is oriented posteromedially, forming a boundary of the deep lateral space of the tarsal tunnel. The groove and tubercle arrangement creates a secure position for the passage of the flexor hallucis longus tendon and provides attachment for the superior end of the osseofibrous tunnel through which the tendon travels into the foot. Both tubercles are inferiorly continuous with the posterior facet of the talus, thus forming part of the posterior articular facet of the subtalar joint. Of the two talar tubercles, the lateral is usually the larger ("Stieda's process," when unusually enlarged). Its position immediately posterior to the talar trochlea, especially when enlarged, makes it vulnerable to fracture. It is also one of the most frequent sites of accessory ossicles, the os trigonum. When this ossicle is present, it has a fibrous attachment to the lateral tubercle, which is variably reduced in size but still present.

The talar tubercles provide important ligament anchorage for the ankle and subtalar joints (Fig. 1–4). Each tubercle provides attachment for a posterior collateral ligament of the ankle connecting a malleolus with a talar tubercle on each side: the posterior tibiotalar ligament attaching to the medial tubercle and the posterior talofibular ligament to the lateral tubercle. Immediately below, the posterior talocalcaneal ligament spans the posterior facets of the subtalar joint, with its talar attachment mainly to the lateral talar tubercle. Fibers of this ligament also reach across the flexor hallucis longus tendon to the medial tubercle, thus reinforcing the superior edge of the osseofibrous tunnel of the tendon.

The posterior talocalcaneal ligament is one of four ligaments that connect only the talus and calcaneus and prevent the talus from literally shearing off the calcaneus in weight bearing. They are located posteriorly, medially, laterally, and anteriorly to the large posterior talocalcaneal facets. The medial and lateral talocalcaneal ligaments are both (see previous discussion) located deep to collateral ligaments of the ankle. Of the four talocalcaneal ligaments, the interosseous talocalcaneal, with its lateral extension, the cervical ligament, is the strongest. Situated within the sinus tarsi, this tough ligament, formed by two overlapping bands, controls the position of the talus on the calcaneus, allowing only a limited range of supination and pronation between them. The presence of the ligament separates the posterior talocalcaneal facets from the anterior and middle facets, reinforcing the separation of the two joint capsules, and separates the body of the talus from the head.

Tibia and Fibula

The distal ends of the tibia and fibula not only form the upper part of the ankle joint,

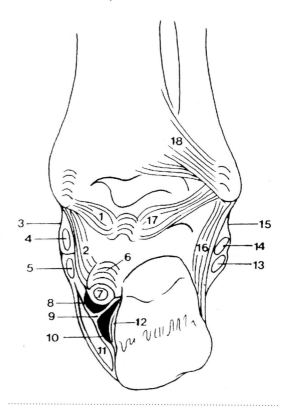

Figure 1–4. Posterior aspect of ankle and heel: 1 = attachment of posterior tibiotalar ligament to medial talar tubercle; 2 = tibiocalcaneal ligament; 3 = flexor retinaculum (deep fascia); 4 = tendon of tibialis posterior; 5 = tendon of flexor digitorum longus; 6 = sustentaculum tali (inferior surface); 7 = tendon of flexor hallucis longus; 8 = "upper calcaneal chamber"; 9 = fascial septum between abductor hallucis fascia and sustentaculum tali; 10 = "lower calcaneal chamber"; 11 = abductor hallucis; 12 = flexor accessorius (medial origin); 13 = tendon of fibularis (peroneus) longus; 14 = tendon of fibularis (peroneus) brevis; 15 = inferior fibular (peroneal) retinaculum; 16 = calcaneofibular ligament; 17 = attachment of posterior talofibular ligament to lateral talar tubercle; 18 = posterior tibiofibular ligament.

but their collateral ligaments contribute greatly to the stability of the rearfoot. The two malleoli are of different lengths: the shorter medial malleolus allows freer inversion and the tendons from the posterior compartment pass around it at a higher level relative to the foot, whereas the lateral malleolus is inferiorly elongated, close to the calcaneus in eversion and the tendons passing around it from the leg must take more of an acute bend as they enter the foot. On its posterior inferior edge, the tibia may form a slight eminence (with the tendon of flexor hallucis longus passing along its surface), which is clinically distinctive as the third part of a characteristic ("trimalleolar") ankle joint fracture. The label indicates something about the nature of the fracture and that the site is clinically important enough to warrant a designation. However, the term can only refer to its clinical state, when fractured, because it is hardly perceptible as a morphologic feature in the normal bone.

The same site on the tibia is better known anatomically for often having a groove for the flexor hallucis longus tendon as it approaches the talus. The position of this tendon (and both its tibial and the talar grooves) is midway between the medial and lateral malleoli. These structures are also directly anterior to the position of the calcaneal tendon. The posterior surface of the medial malleolus is more clearly and usually grooved by the malleolar sulcus, against which the tibialis posterior tendon rests. The posterior surface of the lateral malleolus may also bear a groove for the fibular tendons, but the groove is in fact usually very poorly marked, if present at all[3]; thus the fibula is not considered to have its own malleolar sulcus in the usual case.

The ankle joint mortise is itself very tightly fixed by close adherence of the distal ends of the tibia and fibula with the help of the anterior and posterior inferior tibiofibular ligaments and interosseous tibiofibular ligament. The anterior and posterior ligaments are both broad and transversely attached to the two bones at their extreme ends. The orientation of both is somewhat inclined inferiorly from the tibia to the fibula, corresponding to the orientation of the interosseous membrane between the tibial and fibular shafts. The inferior fibers ("transverse") of the posterior tibiofibular ligament extend below the actual edge of the tibia to reinforce the posterior wall of the ankle joint capsule, and this segment is on its internal aspect (facing the joint) covered with fibrocartilage. The strongest connection between the two bones distally, however, is the interosseous tibiofibular ligament, situated deeply between the two bones inferior to the interosseous membrane. The presence of this deep ligament in the absence of smooth, cartilage-covered articular facets, synovial membrane, or enclosing joint capsule defines this joint as a syndesmosis, as opposed to a "diarthrosis"

or synovial joint such as the ankle joint immediately below.

Against this firm osseoligamentous framework, the soft tissue anatomy of the heel and surrounding areas consists of (1) subcutaneous structures surrounding the area, (2) the calcaneal tendon directly posterior to the heel, (3) structures descending from the posterior compartment of the leg and passing medial to the heel and (4) those passing into the plantar foot, and (5) structures descending from the lateral compartment of the leg and passing lateral to the heel.

SUPERFICIAL FASCIA AND NERVES

The superficial fascia of the heel and rearfoot forms an enlarged and specialized fat pad. Continuous with the superficial fascia of the medial and lateral surfaces of the heel, the heel pad is anchored to the plantar skin of the heel and is innervated by the medial and lateral calcaneal nerves. Posteriorly, its deep surface is directly related to periosteum and bone of the calcaneal tuber and medial and lateral calcaneal processes. Inferiorly, a subcalcaneal bursa has been identified between the heel pad and the medial process and associated with heel pain, but its presence is highly variable.[4, 5] Anteriorly, the deep surface of the pad is related to the deep plantar fascia and its deeper plantar muscles, nerves, and vessels.

The subcutaneous fibrous-fatty fascia of the heel is similar to that of other weight-bearing parts of the volar skin in the hands and feet, but is the largest and best developed of these. Its importance in shock absorption of the heel during gait has made it the focus of years of study.[6–11] The adipose tissue contained within the pad is arranged in vertical chambers separated by fibrous septa. The septa form a spiral-like pattern and are attached superficially to the skin and deeply to the calcaneus itself, thus securing the position of the pad against shearing forces between the skin, fascia, and bone during weight-bearing motion. Contrary to earlier assumptions of gradual structural and mechanical degeneration of the heel pad through the cumulative effects of wear, more recent research suggests that its structure, shock-absorbing capacity, thickness, and compressibility are surprisingly resistant to amount of applied force, cumulative applied force, or increasing age.[7, 8]

Innervation of the skin and superficial fascia surrounding the posterior aspect of the lower leg is derived from overlapping nerve branches of the sural, lateral sural, and saphenous nerves. The sural nerve begins as the medial sural cutaneous branch of the tibial nerve in the popliteal fossa. It usually receives a smaller contribution from the common fibular (peroneal) nerve, thus jointly forming the complete sural nerve. This nerve descends between two gastrocnemius heads, pierces the deep fascia in the upper half of the leg, and joins the medial side of the small saphenous vein. At midcalf, this superficial neurovenous couple is located directly posterior to the gastrocnemius muscle mass, but gradually shifts laterally and descends along the lateral border of the calcaneal tendon toward the lateral malleolus (Fig. 1–5).

Approaching the lateral malleolus, the sural nerve gives its lateral calcaneal branch, whereas the rest of the nerve continues along the lateral surface of the foot. This nerve branch is accompanied by the lateral calcaneal artery and vein, which are derived from the fibular (peroneal) artery and vein in the posterior compartment of the leg. Together they supply the lateral side of the heel and a relatively small plantar area of the skin and heel pad. These short branches first split off the sural nerve 5 cm above the lateral malleolar apex. In its descent around the ankle, the sural nerve passes approximately 1.5 cm posterior and inferior to the malleolus,[12] thus clearing both the fibular and calcaneal tendons in its path. Once on the lateral side of the foot, where it is also known as the lateral dorsal cutaneous nerve, the nerve travels superficially against the fibular tendons and is separated from them by deep fascia.

As the leg narrows toward the ankle, the probability increases of functional overlap among the surrounding cutaneous nerves. A branch of the common fibular, the lateral sural nerve, descends laterally from its origin in the popliteal fossa, supplying the skin of the lateral aspect of the leg as far as the ankle. Thus, the skin covering the lateral malleolus itself may be innervated by three overlapping nerves: sural, lateral sural, and the superficial fibular. Medially, the sural nerve overlaps the saphenous nerve, the only nerve of the leg and foot not derived

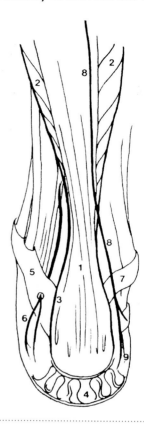

Figure 1–5. Posterior aspect of leg and heel: 1 = calcaneal tendon; 2 = soleus muscle; 3 = tendon of plantaris; 4 = heel pad; 5 = flexor retinaculum; 6 = medial calcaneal nerve; 7 = superior fibular (peroneal) retinaculum; 8 = sural nerve; 9 = lateral calcaneal nerve.

from the sciatic nerve. The saphenous nerve covers the anteromedial surface of the leg, ankle, and medial border of the foot.

Posteromedial and inferior to the ankle joint, the medial calcaneal nerve, artery, and vein enter the subcutaneous fascia by piercing the flexor retinaculum. This nerve is the last branch of the tibial nerve before its bifurcation; however, the site of its separation from the tibial nerve is quite variable.[13] Its superior area of innervation, between the malleolus and the calcaneal tendon, overlaps with the saphenous nerve and the sural nerve. Inferiorly, the nerve innervates the greater area of skin and superficial fascia of the plantar aspect of the heel. Because the heel pad is thick and adheres closely to the medial calcaneal process, branches of the medial calcaneal nerve closely approach the attachment of the plantar deep fascia in the same area.

SUPERFICIAL VEINS

The heel, ankle, and lower leg represent an important transition area for blood return. Here the venous blood collected in the foot initiates its vertical ascent along both superficial and deep veins. Like the rungs of a ladder, perforating veins and valves are built into the veins to facilitate the ascent[14]; it is around the ankle that the first (following the direction of blood flow) regularly occurring sites of valves have been clearly mapped.[15]

The superficial venous flow begins dorsally where the dorsal venous arch collects blood from the toes and adjacent superficial areas of the foot as well as from deep areas of the forefoot through perforating veins. At its medial and lateral ends, the arch is joined by the veins from the border of the hallux and fifth toe, respectively. From this junction to the malleolus on the same side, the vessel continues as a medial or lateral marginal vein. The marginal veins receive numerous plantar superficial tributaries wrapping around the border of the foot in a parallel arrangement. These small veins pick up much of the blood from both the deep and superficial areas of the plantar foot.[16] Deep venous drainage of the plantar compartments of the foot is carried by the medial and lateral plantar veins (thus passing through the tarsal tunnel and superiorly carried by the posterior tibial veins).[17, 18]

The incidence of (both superficial and deep) venous valves in the foot is much more variable than in the leg (demonstrating less than 50% average frequency in perforating veins),[15] and when visualized, the valves appear to be oriented in reverse to those of the leg, directing blood flow from the deep veins into the superficial veins. When valves are not present in pedal veins, the blood flow is bidirectional between deep and superficial veins.

The saphenous veins are continuous with the marginal veins and at the ankle form a malleolar set of perforating veins that communicate with deep veins of the leg (Fig. 1–6). Anterior and inferior to the medial malleolar apex, the "anterior medial malleolar vein" perforates the deep fascia, connecting the great saphenous and anterior tibial

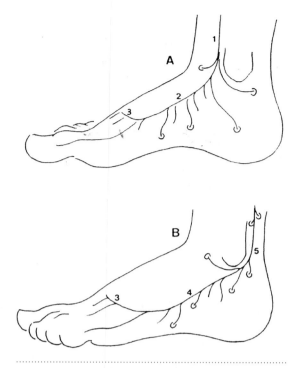

Figure 1–6. Superficial and perforating veins of the *(A)* medial and *(B)* lateral aspect of the foot: 1 = great saphenous vein; 2 = medial marginal vein; 3 = dorsal venous arch; 4 = lateral marginal vein; 5 = small saphenous vein.

veins (the venae comitantes or doubled veins, which usually accompany arteries in the upper and lower extremities). This perforator has no valve itself but marks a level above which all valves are directed from superficial to deep and below which they are directed from deep to superficial, thereby demarcating the separation between the leg and foot as anatomic regions with distinct venous patterns. At this same location, a short but wide tributary of the great saphenous vein passes just inferior and posterior to the malleolar apex, where it perforates the deep fascia and joins the posterior tibial or plantar veins within the tarsal tunnel. On the lateral side, as the small saphenous vein passes behind the lateral malleolus, a less consistently present set of perforating veins pierce the deep fascia and connect it to the terminal branches of the fibular veins in the posterior compartment of the leg.

Skin and superficial fascia of the heel are drained via the medial and lateral calcaneal veins, tributaries of the posterior tibial and the fibular (peroneal) veins, respectively. Calcaneal branches of both the arteries and veins to the plantar skin and fat pad form a dense concentration of vessels in parallel rows closely adhering to the skin and following the dense collagenous fiber arrangement between the skin and the fascia. More deeply, within the heel pad itself, the veins follow the arrangement of septa and anastomose with deep veins through perforating veins. Compression of the pad in weight bearing promotes drainage of the tissue superficially toward the marginal and saphenous veins instead of the deep veins.[4]

Both deep and superficial veins transmit blood mainly into the posterior compartment, the deep veins passing through the tarsal tunnel and into the posterior tibial and fibular veins. The saphenous veins distribute much of their blood through the many perforating veins alongside the soleus-gastrocnemius muscle mass. The soleus is informally but widely designated as the "calf pump" because of its close anatomic relationship to the superficial venous trunks and associated chains of perforators as well as two sets of deep veins in the posterior compartment. Unlike its partner in the "triceps surae," the gastrocnemius, the soleus originates within the leg, with its total mass available for direct penetration by perforating veins and its contractions providing direct access to deep veins. The large muscle bellies of the gastrocnemius are also capable of providing "pumping" action on perforating veins but are anatomically distant from the deep veins of the leg. Blood supply to the medial and lateral heads of the muscle is almost entirely derived from branches of the popliteal artery posterior to the knee, and most drainage is returned through corresponding tributaries of the popliteal vein. Thus, the gastrocnemius muscle bypasses the deep veins of the leg but is directly connected to the larger vein of the lower extremity above the leg.

POSTERIOR ANATOMY: CALCANEAL (ACHILLES) TENDON

The posterior aspect of the heel and lower leg is defined by the descent and insertion of the calcaneal tendon; it (and the plantaris tendon) does not pass through a retinaculum and has no synovial sheath. The tendon

is formed by two heads of the gastrocnemius and the one large muscle belly of the soleus, hence "triceps surae," or "three-headed calf muscle." Unlike the other extrinsic tendons passing the ankle joint into the foot, the course of the calcaneal tendon is direct from its superior origins to its calcaneal insertion and thus has no need for restraint to maintain its position in relation to the joint. The position of the tendon, posteriorly separated by a considerable space from the actual joint, is also far removed from the retinacular attachments (described below) on the medial and lateral sides of the joint.

When the deep fascia of the leg is incised along the tendon, it is observed to be wrapped in a clear connective tissue: the paratenon. In the absence of a synovial tendon sheath, which in other tendons transmits neurovascular supply to tendons in their retinacular compartments, the calcaneal tendon is chronically at risk of vascular insufficiency. The paratenon has no synovial component and is merely a continuation of the connective tissue that fills the intermuscular spaces of this and other musculoskeletal compartments of the upper and lower extremities. It is specially named in relation to the calcaneal tendon because of the isolated position of the tendon from other tendons in the leg and its complete investment by this connective fascia. It is by way of this paratenon investment that the nonmuscular part of the tendon derives much of its blood supply; the musculotendinous and osseotendinous junctions are too distant from each other to alone ensure adequate vascularization of this massive tendon. Indeed, the area of the tendon 2 to 5 cm above the insertion that most frequently ruptures is the area farthest from muscle fiber attachments and from the tendon insertion and is the least well vascularized.[19, 20]

The course and insertion of the plantaris muscle, a small third muscle in the superficial subcompartment of the posterior leg, are usually independent of the formation of the calcaneal tendon, and this muscle is usually not included in the triceps surae designation. The small and variable plantaris muscle belly originates on the femur adjacent to the origin of the lateral head of the gastrocnemius and forms a narrow, flat tendon while still in the popliteal fossa. The tendon then descends between the medial head of the gastrocnemius and the soleus muscle bellies. In the lowest third of the leg, the plantaris tendon slips medially from between these two muscular parts of the "triceps" and inserts directly medial to the insertion of the calcaneal tendon on the posterior surface of the calcaneus. The presence, course, and insertion of this narrow tendon are quite variable, and its insertion may be expected to include other areas such as the deep surface of the calcaneal tendon, the flexor retinaculum, and the medial surface of the heel.[21]

At midleg, the gastrocnemius has formed a broad aponeurosis. Deep to this tendinous sheet, the soleus muscle belly is wide, but its posterior fibers already also contain a large proportion of tendon fibers. The inferior extent of the muscular part of soleus is highly variable and contributes to the shape of the lower part of the leg. Its deep adherence to the gastrocnemius portion of the tendon is important in the vascularity available to the tendon in its lowermost course. The soleus muscle fibers are gradually replaced by tendon, and when complete, the tendon fibers of the calcaneal tendon can be observed to be oblique, or to twist, in their descent to insertion. This fiber rotation about the long axis of the tendon is variable; 13 to 52% of its fibers spiral in an inferolateral direction,[21] and the degree of torsion is between 11 to 65°; the torsion does not occur until about age 10.[22] This course brings the fibers from the medial head of the gastrocnemius to a more lateral position within the tendon at its calcaneal insertion. It may, therefore, affect any differential function of the two gastrocnemius heads on the foot, more so at the subtalar joint than at the ankle joint, because the medial and lateral ends of the tendon insertion may be differently related to the subtalar joint axis.

The extreme rugosity of the bone at the insertion demonstrates the strength of the tendon; its thickness, which may vary by as much as 25% in individuals,[23] may transmit four times the power of any of the other crural tendons. Beyond the strength of the tendon owing to its size (as much as 2.5 cm in width, 17 cm in length, and 5–7 mm in thickness[21–23]) and its large muscle mass, its strength is further relatively increased by a 7-cm length of its moment arm at the ankle joint. Each of the other tendons acting on the ankle joint adhere closely to the joint in their course, thereby having short moment arms as well as comparatively small muscle mass for each tendon.

The calcaneal tendon has been known to have some continuity with the plantar fascia, whose thick, tendon-like, central "aponeurosis" is posteriorly attached to the medial calcaneal process. However, a 1985 study[24] showed that although such a continuity occurs in infancy, it is progressively reduced during growth and is virtually eliminated by early adulthood. In early childhood the tuber itself is cartilaginous and attenuated; thus the growing tendon has a poorly defined insertion site until the 6th to 8th year, when the calcaneal apophysis begins to ossify. Its presence in association with the posterior insertion of the calcaneus suggests that the tendon is anatomically intended to terminate on the posterior rather than inferior surface of the calcaneus.

Two bursae are associated with the calcaneal tendon. The retrocalcaneal ("behind the calcaneus") bursa is a standard part of the heel anatomy. It is located deeply between the upper third of the posterior surface of the calcaneus and the calcaneal tendon. In this position, the bursa is precisely situated where the tendon rubs against the upper edge of the bone in acute ankle dorsiflexion. The superficial, or subcutaneous, calcaneal bursa is adventitial, developed as required by excessive shearing forces and develops posteriorly between the skin and the point of insertion of the calcaneal tendon. This is the most posterior point of the foot and that area of the heel that is the most compressed by an irritating heel counter. The retrocalcaneal and subcutaneous calcaneal bursae are thus anatomically separated by the tendon.

MEDIAL ANATOMY: TARSAL TUNNEL

The deep fascia of the leg surrounds the ankle and forms five retaining bands, or retinacula, which restrain the extrinsic tendons passing out of the three compartments of the leg and into the foot. Because of their strong attachment to subcutaneous bone, these retinacula were previously known as "annular ligaments." They are, however, no more than parallel fiber arrangements of deep fascia, which itself is normally attached to subcutaneous bone. To ensure that exactly the right tendon position is maintained at all times, most tendons have fixed tracks or compartments within the retinacula and are invested with protective synovial tendon sheaths as they pass through.

The flexor retinaculum ("laciniate ligament") retains the tendons of the three muscles of the deep subcompartment of the leg as they pass posteromedially around the ankle joint and into the plantar compartments of the foot. The retinaculum is anteriorly attached to the medial malleolus and posteriorly to the medial surface of the calcaneal tuber. The space thus enclosed is wide next to the retinaculum and narrows laterally in a cone or funnel shape; its deepest and most lateral point is at the lateral tubercle of the talus. An additional layer of deep fascia inside the tunnel ("deep part" of the retinaculum) is the inferior end of the "transverse" intermuscular septum of the leg. This septum separates the three superficial muscles (gastrocnemius, soleus, and plantaris) from the three deep muscles (flexor digitorum longus, flexor hallucis longus, and tibialis posterior) in the posterior crural compartment. It adheres to the origins of the two long flexors as they descend the leg and inferiorly contributes to the containment of the tendons, particularly that of the flexor hallucis longus, against the ankle joint (see Fig. 1–6). The superior osseous framework ("retromalleolar level")[4] of the tunnel includes the posterior border of the medial malleolus and inferior end of the tibial shaft and the posterior process of the talus with its medial and lateral tubercles. Inferiorly ("talocalcaneal level") the osseous landmarks include the sustentaculum tali and medial surface of the calcaneus.

The tibialis posterior is the deepest of the muscles at its origin on the interosseous membrane, but inferiorly its tendon lies medially and slips out from its deep space to lie directly posterior to the medial malleolus. There it rests against the malleolar sulcus. The flexor digitorum longus originates posteromedially on the tibial shaft, and its tendon follows close behind that of the tibialis posterior. These two tendons have separate retinacular compartments against the medial malleolus and maintain their position when the retinaculum is incised posteriorly. The flexor hallucis longus originates posteriorly on the fibular shaft and is, therefore, the most laterally positioned of the three tendons in the tarsal tunnel. Because it inserts most medially on the foot, it has the most deviated course from its origin and requires more control in its course around

the rearfoot than do the other tendons. This muscle may have a large muscular belly as far inferiorly as the talar tubercles, where its tendon passes in the groove between them. The flexor hallucis longus lies directly anterior to the calcaneal tendon and is separated only by a fat-filled space, sometimes noted radiographically as the "calcaneal triangle." This anatomic proximity is one factor in consideration of the flexor hallucis longus as a tendon replacement for the calcaneal tendon, as is the close proximity of the flexor digitorum longus in similar consideration for the tibialis posterior tendon.[25]

Adhering to both long flexor muscles in the leg, the transverse intermuscular septum ends posterior to the ankle by attaching to the medial and lateral talar tubercles and contributing to the formation of an "osseofibrous tunnel" for the flexor hallucis longus. The enclosure of the tendon against the tubercles is further reinforced by the attachment of the posterior talocalcaneal ligament. This tendon tunnel is merely an osseous groove closed by thick fascia, which securely guides the flexor hallucis longus tendon around the osseous grooves in the talus and calcaneus. The osseofibrous tunnel begins superiorly between the talar tubercles and ends inferiorly, attached along the groove on the inferior surface of the sustentaculum tali.

In learning the anatomy of this area, a medical student memorizes the sequence of the contents of this space: tibialis anterior, flexor digitorum longus, posterior tibial artery and veins, tibial nerve, and flexor hallucis longus. The line-up of these structures is neither directly anteroposterior nor mediolateral; instead, the sequence forms an arc from the most medial position behind the medial malleolus, at which the tibialis posterior and flexor digitorum are so close together as to be hardly distinguishable, to a most lateral, deep, and posterior position at the talar tubercles for the tendon of flexor hallucis longus. Compared with the tight retinacular compartments for each of the three tendons, the space between the two flexors is large and less confining; it represents the neurovascular compartment of the tarsal tunnel. The space is wide enough to avoid constricting the nerves and vessels under normal functional conditions and provides a plug of fatty tissue to cushion these structures.

Superiorly, the neurovascular compartment of the tarsal tunnel contains the posterior tibial artery, its venae comitantes, and the tibial nerve with its medial calcaneal branch. The vessels (the artery is larger and always in between its two veins) enter the tarsal tunnel medial to the tibial nerve and are, therefore, directly under the deep fascia. The tibial nerve is more lateral than the vessels, deeper within the space and closer to the tendon of the flexor hallucis longus. (The tibial nerve requires no "posterior" designation because the nerve trunk descends without division from its formation in the sacral plexus. The anatomically specific term for the "anterior tibial nerve" is deep fibular.) Inferiorly, these trunks have bifurcated into two neurovascular groups.[4, 26, 27]

Before its bifurcation, the tibial nerve gives its last branch, the medial calcaneal nerve, which typically pierces the flexor retinaculum midway between the medial malleolus and calcaneal tuber to reach the skin and superficial fascia of the heel. This is a constant nerve usually branching from the tibial by 2 to 7 cm above the medial malleolus.[13, 28] The bifurcation pattern of the tibial nerve in the tarsal tunnel is variable; sometimes the two terminal branches join with the medial calcaneal and form a trifurcation. In most cases, the tibial nerve bifurcation occurs either with the vascular bifurcation at the "malleolar-calcaneal axis" (an imaginary midline through the flexor retinaculum from its malleolar to calcaneal attachments) or 1 to 2 cm above this axis but still within the tunnel.[27–30]

Immediately upon bifurcating, the lateral plantar nerve gives a branch that descends on its own course around the medial and lateral calcaneal processes to innervate the abductor digiti minimi muscle in the first layer of plantar muscles. This nerve is variously designated as the "first branch" (FB) of the lateral plantar nerve, the nerve to the abductor digiti minimi, or the inferior calcaneal nerve. As a small branch appearing deep to the flexor retinaculum, it may be confused with the medial calcaneal nerve, but its course is directed deeply and inferiorly toward the abductor hallucis and calcaneus rather than superficially and medially toward the skin. The proximity of the course of this nerve to the medial tubercle and its myofascial attachments has implicated this nerve as a cause of chronic heel pain.[27, 28, 31, 32]

The branches of the posterior tibial ar-

tery in the tarsal tunnel are more numerous than those of the tibial nerve. Before its bifurcation, the artery with accompanying veins gives a communicating branch to the fibular artery across the posterior surface of the ankle joint and through the fatty tissue of the "calcaneal triangle." It also gives a medial calcaneal branch that joins the medial calcaneal nerve, a posterior medial malleolar branch that passes around the posterior tibial and flexor digitorum tendons to join the ankle anastomosis, and a combined deltoid artery and artery to the tarsal canal. At this superior, or retromalleolar, level, the tibial nerve may already be bifurcated, while the artery and its veins bifurcate at or below the malleolar-calcaneal axis. Inferiorly, the nerves and vessels are arranged in two bundles: the medial plantar anteriorly and the lateral plantar posteriorly, each having a nerve, one artery, and two veins (the inferior calcaneal nerve together with the lateral plantar group). The medial calcaneal nerve exits the tunnel more proximally to supply the superficial fascia and skin.

The inferior boundary of the tarsal tunnel is marked by the abductor hallucis muscle, which originates on the medial and inferior border of the medial calcaneal process and forms a potential barrier to continuity of the structures out of the tarsal tunnel. The outlet of the nerves and vessels is formed between this muscle and the calcaneus, a hiatus formerly termed *porta pedis*. Medial to the muscle is the calcaneus and the upper medial part of the origin of the flexor accessorius (quadratus plantae), a muscle of the second plantar layer. Between the two muscles is part of the calcaneal attachment of the medial intermuscular septum of the foot. At the level of the sustentaculum tali, the medial and lateral plantar neurovascular bundles are separated by a fascial septum (Fig. 1–7).[4]

The tendons and neurovascular structures each have a different means of leaving the tarsal tunnel and entering the plantar region. If the sustentaculum tali may be said to represent a bony landmark at the end of the tunnel, the three tendons each have a unique relationship to it. The tibialis posterior passes superior to the sustentaculum tali toward the talar head, entirely without involvement with the neurovascular contents of the tunnel. The flexor digitorum longus passes directly medial to the sustentaculum tali, then passes deep to the

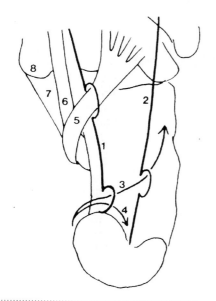

Figure 1–7. Plantar intermuscular septae: 1 = medial intermuscular septum; 2 = lateral intermuscular septum; 3 = course of lateral plantar nerve and vessels; 4 = course of "inferior calcaneal" nerve; 5 = tendon of flexor digitorum longus; 6 = tendon of flexor hallucis longus; 7 = inserting tendon of tibialis posterior; 8 = navicular tuberosity.

abductor hallucis and through an opening in the medial intermuscular septum to gain entrance into the central compartment of the foot. The flexor hallucis longus completes its course through its unique osseofibrous tunnel as it passes under the sustentaculum tali and then enters the medial plantar compartment of the foot.

The medial plantar and lateral plantar neurovascular bundles exit the tunnel separately, each through a myofascial opening formed by a fascial slip attached to the sustentaculum tali and the abductor hallucis muscle fascia. The borders of these openings, particularly of the lower calcaneal chamber, are reinforced by the deep aponeurosis of the abductor hallucis muscle and the medial intermuscular septum.[4] The medial plantar nerve and vessels pass through the upper calcaneal chamber or tunnel and follow the flexor hallucis tendon toward the medial compartment. The lateral plantar nerves and vessels, which are potentially larger in diameter as they supply and drain the greater portion of plantar structures, pass through the lower calcaneal chamber, a potentially more confining opening, possibly leading to nerve and vascular compression.[33]

PLANTAR ANATOMY

The deep fascia of the plantar surface is continuous with the dorsal deep fascia of the foot and with the fascia, including retinacula, surrounding the ankle joint. As in the palmar surface of the hand, the plantar deep fascia forms a central band of highly concentrated fibers that are tightly adherent to the skin and radiate distally toward each of the five digits. In the hand, this central band, or central aponeurosis, is continuous with the palmaris longus tendon, which enters the hand superficial to the carpal tunnel. Although the plantar aponeurosis does not demonstrate such a functional continuity with the plantaris muscle (pedal homologue to palmaris longus), a continuity of calcaneal tendon fibers can be seen in the early growth of the foot.[24] Here the posterior enlargement and projection of the heel for weight support may indeed have interrupted a homologous prenatal continuity. Posteriorly, the central band of deep fascia is firmly anchored to the edge of the medial calcaneal process. Anteriorly, at the level of the metatarsal bases, the central band separates into five slips, each terminating at a metatarsophalangeal joint where its complex attachment includes the skin, superficial fat pad, and joint capsular structures.

The lateral band of the plantar fascia is also dense and fibrous and usually forms a cordlike longitudinal thickening attached to the lateral calcaneal process and to the fifth metatarsal base. The medial band of plantar fascia resembles deep fascia elsewhere, having no thick fibrous concentration as in the other two parts. It is, however, posteriorly continuous with the flexor retinaculum, which encloses the tarsal tunnel and covers the abductor hallucis muscle.

The three longitudinal bands of the deep plantar fascia form a connective tissue sheet covering the three muscles in the first plantar muscle layer: abductor hallucis, flexor digitorum brevis, and abductor digiti minimi. Each band adheres intimately to its underlying muscle, providing an inner surface for muscle fiber origin. Between the muscles, the deep fascia projects medial and lateral intermuscular septa to deep attachments on bone and ligament, thereby creating three long muscle compartments. The medial septum is attached to the medial surface of the calcaneus, where it is reinforced by fascial and myotendinous fibers of the abductor hallucis origin and which is perforated by an opening for transmission of the lateral plantar neurovascular bundle out of the tarsal tunnel. The tendon of the flexor digitorum longus pierces the medial septum more distally as it courses toward the central compartment and second layer of plantar muscles. The septum is distally attached to the navicular, medial cuneiform, and first metatarsal.

The lateral septum is attached to the lateral edge of the medial calcaneal process and to the inferior calcaneal ligaments as well as distally to the fifth metatarsal. Like the medial septum, it is perforated by the lateral plantar neurovascular structures on their course toward the forefoot. Both septae are perforated by branches of nerves and vessels distributing within the forefoot; thus, the intermuscular septae provide only a partial separation of the medial, lateral, and central compartments.

All three muscles of the first plantar muscle layer originate on the calcaneus and on adjacent deep fascia of the medial, central, or lateral band and medial or lateral intermuscular septa. More specifically, all three muscles originate along the anterior border of the medial calcaneal process. On the medial and lateral sides are the abductors of the first and fifth toes, abductor hallucis, and abductor digiti minimi; in the center is the short flexor to the middle three or four toes: flexor digitorum brevis.

The layer designation may erroneously suggest a flat transverse plane arrangement of these three muscles, but in reality the muscle mass of abductor hallucis and the medial origin of flexor accessorius are positioned more medially on the calcaneus than on its inferior aspect. In this way the abductor hallucis is situated as the inferomedial boundary of the tarsal tunnel, and forms a landmark on the medial side of the heel for surgical approach to the plantar fascia and medial calcaneal process.

As the first plantar layer muscle in the central compartment, the flexor digitorum longus is situated in a fascial "box" with the plantar aponeurosis superficially, the medial and lateral intermuscular septa on the sides, and an intermuscular fascia between itself and the second layer muscle, the flexor accessorius. It originates on the anterior border of the medial process and also on the aponeurosis and both septa. Directly supe-

rior and deep, the flexor accessorius originates in two wide bands on medial and lateral areas of the inferior surface of the calcaneus (but not to the calcaneal processes); the deeper calcaneal attachment of the long plantar ligament is visible in between. These two bands converge anteriorly to insert on the tendon of the flexor digitorum longus as it enters the central compartment and separates into its four digital tendons. Because of this insertion, the flexor accessorius is aptly named for its function as accessory to the long digital flexor. The most lateral muscle in the first muscle layer, abductor digiti minimi, originates from both the medial and lateral calcaneal processes and from adjacent deep fascia and lateral intermuscular septum.

Once past the abductor hallucis opening, the lateral plantar nerve and vessels travel laterally and anteriorly in the potential space between the flexor digitorum brevis and the flexor accessorius. Initially, the neurovascular bundle passes close to the anterior border of the medial calcaneal process; the artery and its venae comitantes are closer (than the nerve) to the bone. Thus, the lateral plantar nerves and vessels are anatomically closely related to the medial calcaneal process but at a deeper level than the attachments of the plantar fascia and the first layer muscles. Their passage through this confined space around a bony shelf with dense myofascial attachments may provide potential compressive forces on dilated vessels.

The inferior calcaneal (or first) branch of the lateral plantar nerve is the most closely related of the neurovascular structures to both the medial and lateral calcaneal processes as it winds around them in its approach to the abductor digiti minimi. It arises as the first branch of the lateral plantar nerve between the origin of abductor hallucis medially and the medial band of the flexor accessorius on its lateral side. It then breaks up into an array of small branches as it passes beneath the flexor accessorius, of which some may include periosteal or calcaneal branches.[28, 31, 32]

LATERAL ANATOMY: LATERAL HEEL AND ANKLE

The lateral side of the heel is marked by the fibularis longus and fibularis brevis tendons as they descend from the lateral compartment of the leg and enter the lateral border of the foot. The osseous landmarks include the lateral malleolus and fibular trochlea, against which the tendons are anchored by retinacula. The superior fibular retinaculum is superiorly attached to the lateral malleolus and inferiorly to the posterolateral surface of the calcaneal tuber; the tendons are arranged anterior (fibularis brevis) and posterior (fibularis longus) to each other. The combined power of the tendons against the malleolus, especially in eversion when their tendons are prominently palpable, indicates the need for a secure retaining band in this position. Like the flexor retinaculum on the medial side, the orientation of the fibers is oblique; from the lateral malleolus above, the fibers course inferior and posterior. Unlike the medial malleolus, which always bears a posterior groove for its tendons, the lateral malleolus may have only a shallow groove or none at all for the fibular tendons.[3] The periosteum is thickened by fibrocartilage, which creates, or deepens, a groove against the bone.

The inferior fibular retinaculum is located on the lateral surface of the calcaneus, where the tendons are arranged superior (fibularis brevis) and inferior (fibularis longus) to each other. The superior attachment of this retinaculum interdigitates with the lateral attachment of the stem of the inferior extensor retinaculum, which encloses the tendons coming out of the anterior compartment of the leg: flexor digitorum longus and fibularis tertius. The precise area of fiber merging is directly anterior to the malleolus and, because it separates two groups of strapped tendons, forms a hollow; this is normally filled by a plug of fatty superficial fascia. The middle attachment is to the fibular trochlea, by which the two tendons are separated into separate retinacular tunnels. The bone above and below the trochlea may be grooved by the tendons, and is also covered by periosteum thickened with fibrocartilage, forming secure indentations for the movement of the tendons. Thus, the inferior fibular and inferior extensor retinacula form a continuous band of tendon restraint across the dorsum of the foot at the ankle. The communication between these retinacula forms an important link between the sinus tarsi and the fibular tendons with their tendon sheaths.[34]

The fibularis longus originates on the head, neck, and superior half of the lateral surface of the fibula, whereas the fibularis brevis originates inferiorly on the lower half of the lateral fibular surface. In their descent, the fibularis longus lies posterior to fibularis brevis as far as the the lateral malleolus, where they share a single synovial tendon sheath within their superior retinaculum. As the tendons pass inferior to the malleolus, the synovial sheath divides, forming a separate sheath for each tendon as it passes through its own compartment in the inferior fibular retinaculum. Out of the retinaculum, the fibularis brevis tendon travels briefly to its broad insertion on the tuberosity (styloid process) of the fifth metatarsal base, whereas the fibularis longus continues toward the cuboid notch, where it takes another acute turn into the plantar aspect of the foot.

From their position behind the ankle joint, the tendons pass directly superficial to two of the three lateral ankle ligaments and one talocalcaneal ligament. In their course posterior to the lateral malleolus, the tendons are directly posterior and lateral to the posterior talofibular ligament. As they round the apex of the malleolus, the tendons pass directly across and bisect the calcaneofibular ligament and the deeper lateral talocalcaneal ligament. The tendons have no direct relationship to the anterior talofibular ligament, which is situated well above them and above the sinus tarsi; the ligament is attached to the lateral side of the neck of the talus where it joins the talar body, whereas the tendons pass below the sinus and along the lateral side of the calcaneus.

Between the anterior talofibular ligament and the fibular tendons is the lateral opening of the sinus tarsi (see Fig. 1–4). It represents a complex area both in its many attachments and in its relationship to subtalar joint mechanics. Like other anatomic spaces in the body, the sinus tarsi on its wider, lateral end contains a fatty plug, which helps to secure the course of small vessels and nerves passing through. These include the artery of the sinus tarsi, formed anteriorly by anastomosing branches of the dorsalis pedis, lateral tarsal, and perforating branch of the fibular artery as well as branches of the deep fibular nerve. Deeper within the sinus, this branch anastomoses with the artery of the tarsal canal, a branch of the posterior tibial artery that enters the sinus from the tarsal tunnel.

One of the attachments at the lateral end of the sinus tarsi is a band of deep fibers of the inferior extensor retinaculum ("frondiform" or "fundiform" ligament), which helps to keep the flexor digitorum longus tendons in position and reinforces the interosseous talocalcaneal ligament within the sinus. In close lateral proximity to both structures is the cervical ligament, attached as an almost vertical strip of ligament to the lateral side of the talar neck and to the calcaneus below. Once considered to be the lateral extension of the interosseous ligament, it now frequently receives separate reference. In either case, the interosseous and cervical ligaments, with the deep fibers of the retinaculum, form an apparently continuous wall of dense ligamentous fibers from within the sinus tarsi through to its lateral outlet. Finally, the floor of the sinus tarsi outlet is covered by the origin of the extensor digitorum (and hallucis) brevis muscle. The close communication between these fibers, the sinus tarsi vasculature, the interdigitation of the stem of the retinaculum with the upper fibers of the superior fibular retinaculum, and the fibular tendon sheaths within provide pathways for the spread of fluids in lateral ankle and heel injuries.[34]

REFERENCES

1. Simkin A, Leichter I. Role of calcaneal inclination in the energy storage capacity of the human foot—a biomechanical model. Med Biol Eng Comput 28:149, 1990.
2. Ruiz JR, Christman RA, Hillstrom HJ. Anatomical considerations of the peroneal tubercle. J Am Podiatr Med Assoc 83:563, 1993.
3. Hanam SR, Dale SJ. Subluxation of the peroneal tendons: a report of two cases. J Am Podiatr Med Assoc 76:286, 1986.
4. Sarrafian SK. Anatomy of the Foot and Ankle, ed 2. Philadelphia: J. B. Lippincott, 1993.
5. Barrett SL, Day SV, Pignetti TT, Egly BR. Endoscopic heel anatomy. Analysis of 200 fresh frozen specimens. J Foot Ankle Surg 34:51, 1995.
6. Aerts P, Ker RF, DeClerq D, et al. The mechanical properties of the human heel pad: a paradox resolved. J Biomech 28:1299, 1995.
7. Prichasuk S, Mulpruek P, Siriwongpairat P. The heel pad compressibility. Clin Orthop 300:197, 1994.
8. Kinoshita H, Ogawa T, Kuzuhara K, Ikuta K. In vivo examination of the dynamic properties of the human heel pad. Int Sports Med 14:312, 1993.
9. Levy AS, Berkowitz R, Franklin P, et al. Magnetic resonance imaging evaluation of calcaneal fat pads in patients with os calcis fractures. Foot Ankle 13:57, 1992.
10. Jorgensen U, Bojsen-Møller F. The shock absorbency of factors in the shoe/heel interaction with special focus on the role of the heel pad. Foot Ankle 9:294, 1989.
11. Miller E. The heel pad. Am J Sports Med 10:19, 1982.
12. Lawrence SJ, Botte MJ. The sural nerve in the foot and ankle: an anatomic study with clinical and surgical implications. Foot Ankle Int 15:490, 1994.
13. Didia BC, Horsefall AU. Medial calcaneal nerve: an anatomical study. J Am Podiatr Med Assoc 80:115, 1990.
14. Staubesand J, Hachlander A. Topography of the perforating veins on the medial side of the leg (Cockett's veins). Clin Anat 8:399, 1995.
15. Lofgren EP, Myers TT, Lofgren KA, Kuster G. The venous valves of the foot and ankle. Surg Gynecol Obstet 127:289, 1968.
16. Kuster G, Lofgren EP, Hollinshead WH. Anatomy of the veins of the foot. Surg Gynecol Obstet 127:817, 1968.
17. White JV, Katz ML, Cisek P, Kreithen J. Venous outflow of the leg: anatomy and physiologic mechanism of the plantar venous plexus. J Vasc Surg 24:819, 1996.
18. Sukovatykh BS, Nazarenko PM, Belikov LN. [Patterns in the spread of the vertical blood reflux in the musculo-venous "pump" of the foot in varicose disease]. Vestn Khir Im I I Grek 154:34, 1995.
19. Carr AJ. The blood supply of the calcaneal tendon. J Bone Joint Surg Br 71:100, 1989.
20. Bouche RT. Chronic compartment syndrome of the leg. J Am Podiatr Med Assoc 80:633, 1990.
21. Cummins JE, Anson JB, Carr WB, et al. The structure of the calcaneal tendon (of Achilles) in relation to orthopedic surgery with additional observations on the plantaris muscle. Surg Gynecol Obstet 83:197, 1946.
22. Van Gils CC, Steed RH, Page JC. Torsion of the human Achilles tendon. J Foot Ankle Surg 35:41, 1996.
23. Koivunen-Niemela T, Parkkola K. Anatomy of the Achilles tendon (tendo calcaneus) with respect to tendon thickness and measurements. Surg Radiol Anat 17:263, 1995.
24. Snow SW, Bohne WHO, CiCarlo E, Chang VK. Anatomy of the Achilles tendon and plantar fascia in relation to the calcaneus in various age groups. Foot Ankle Int 16:418, 1985.
25. Wapner KL, Hecht PJ, Shea JR, Allardyce TJ. Anatomy of the second muscular layer in the foot: considerations for tendon selection in transfer for Achilles and posterior tibial tendon reconstruction. Foot Ankle Int 15:42, 1994.
26. Frey C, Kerr R. Magnetic resonance imaging and the evaluation of tarsal tunnel syndrome. Foot Ankle 14:159, 1993.
27. Schon LC. Nerve entrapment, neuropathy, and nerve dysfunction in athletes. Orthop Clin North Am 25:47, 1994.
28. Davis TJ, Schon LC. Branches of the tibial nerve: anatomic variations. Foot Ankle Int 16:21, 1995.
29. Havel PE, Ebraheim NA, Clark S, et al. Tibial nerve branching in the tarsal tunnel. Foot Ankle 9:117, 1988.
30. Pace N, Serafini P, LoTacono E, et al. The tarsal

tunnel and calcaneal tunnel syndromes. Ital J Orthop Traumatol 17:247, 1991.

31. Baxter DE, Thigpen CM. Heel pain—operative results. Foot Ankle 5:16, 1984.

32. Arenson DJ, Cosentino GL, Suran SM. The inferior calcaneal nerve. J Am Podiatr Med Assoc 70:552, 1980.

33. Carrel JM, Davidson DM, Golstein KT. Observations on 200 surgical cases of tarsal tunnel syndrome. Clin Podiatr Med Surg 11:609, 1994.

34. Klein SN, Oloff LM, Jacobs AM. Functional and surgical anatomy of the lateral ankle. J Foot Surg 20:170, 1981.

2 Imaging of the Hindfoot and Ankle

Helene Pavlov
Jordan Ditchek

Hollis G. Potter
Robert Schneider

Hindfoot or ankle pain or both is a clinical and radiographic challenge because symptoms are often vague and difficult to localize specifically to either the hindfoot or the ankle.[1] All the imaging modalities—plain radiographs, radionuclide bone scan, tomography (routine and computed [CT]), arthrography, ultrasonography, and magnetic resonance imaging (MRI)—have a role in evaluating hindfoot and ankle complaints. Clinical information regarding the suspected abnormality is essential to maximize diagnostic yield for several reasons. First, the anticipated pathology is necessary to determine the appropriate imaging modality. Second, the location of the suspected abnormality helps to determine the correct positioning for the plain radiographs or the tomographic examination and the proper selection of coil, determination of correct coil placement, and appropriate sequences for the MRI examination.

The routine plain roentgenogram is the appropriate initial imaging examination for a hindfoot or ankle complaint in both acute trauma and chronic pain.[2] The standard foot series includes a standing anteroposterior (AP) and lateral view and a non–weight-bearing oblique view. The standard ankle series consists of a weight-bearing AP and lateral view and an internal oblique (mortise) projection. The axial calcaneal view provides an excellent view of the calcaneus and the posterior subtalar and sustentacular joints. In specific clinical scenarios, such as suspected osteomyelitis, and to confirm or exclude a suspected injury or localize the site of abnormality, a radionuclide bone scan is useful. A CT examination can provide detailed cross-sectional demonstration of the osseous structures and can detect subtle soft tissue calcifications or osseous fragments.[3] Arthrography and ultrasonography for intra-articular and tendon pathology, respectively, can be very diagnostic but are dependent on examiner experience. MRI, because of its multiplanar capabilities, superior soft tissue contrast, and lack of ioniz-

ing radiation, is an excellent method to evaluate superficial soft tissues, muscles, tendons, ligaments, articular cartilage, the synovial joint lining, and occult osseous disease. The presence of a joint effusion further enhances demonstration of intra-articular structures but is not necessary to visualize articular cartilage adequately.[4] The information provided by MRI can affect both the treatment plan and the surgical approach.[5]

In this discussion we focus on the appropriate imaging for both general and nonspecific hindfoot and ankle symptoms, including fractures and dislocations, osteochondral injuries, strains and sprains, arthritic and synovial abnormalities, infection and tumors, and localized or specific presenting symptoms.

GENERAL OR NONSPECIFIC SYMPTOMS

Fractures and Dislocations

In the acute setting of suspected fracture, the initial evaluation is the standard plain radiographic series (e.g., AP, oblique, lateral). Radiographs are indicated in a patient with an inability to bear weight or with tenderness to palpation.[6] Gross dislocations of the foot or ankle are rare and are easily diagnosed clinically and radiographically (Fig. 2–1A, B). A fracture of the tibia, fibula, talus, or calcaneus can be readily diagnosed on the routine lateral view of the ankle. In cortical bone, fractures manifest radiographically as a cortical discontinuity with a radiolucent line. In cancellous bone, a fracture is manifest as a radiopacity secondary to overlap of impacted cancellous bone and healing endosteal callus. Additionally, fractures may present as a small, separate bony fragment secondary to avulsion.[7] On plain films, soft tissue abnormalities, such as obliteration of normal fat planes, may be the only indication of a fracture.[8] The presence of an ankle effusion is highly sug-

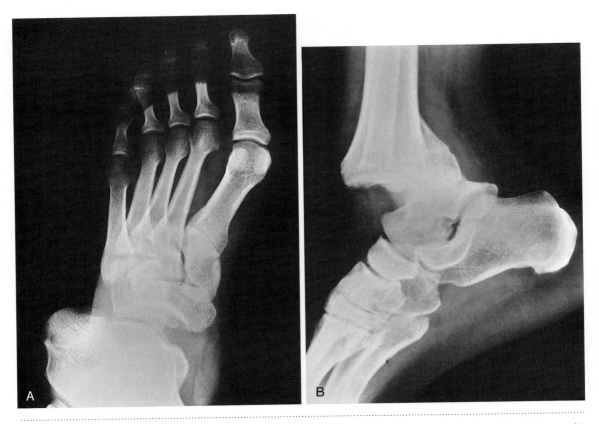

Figure 2–1. *A,* Frontal view of the right foot demonstrates a talonavicular and calcaneocuboid (Chopart's) dislocation. *B,* Lateral view of the foot demonstrates a posterior tibiotalar dislocation.

gestive of an occult fracture.[9, 10] Plain radiographs can assess angulation or displacement of fracture fragments and intra-articular extension. In the clinical setting of suspected fracture and normal plain radiographs, radionuclide bone scanning, CT, or MRI can confirm the presence of a subtle fracture.[11] The radionuclide bone scan can confirm or exclude a suspected fracture. When an area of augmented isotope is demonstrated, a CT scan provides greater osseous detail than plain films and can identify a subtle fracture as well as demonstrate the position and rotation of a fracture fragment in complex fracture deformities.[12, 13] On MRI, an occult intraosseous injury, or "bone bruise," is identified as a geographic, nonlinear area of bone marrow edema.[3]

Calcaneal and Talar Fractures

The calcaneus is the most commonly fractured tarsal bone, being subjected to a variety of mechanisms of injury including

compression, avulsion, and stress or insufficiency.[14] The Boehler angle, as measured on the lateral radiograph, identifies the height of the posterior facet of the subtalar joint and is a useful radiographic measurement in the evaluation of a subtle calcaneal compression injury (Fig. 2–2A, B). The normal angle is between 20° and 40°, and if reduced, a compression fracture is highly suspect. Intra-articular fractures typically occur with axial loading (e.g., a fall from a height).[15] Vertical calcaneal fractures may not be apparent on the lateral view. In suspected calcaneal injury, an axial view of the hindfoot should be obtained in addition to the standard projections (Fig. 2–3). CT provides greater osseous detail and allows for direct comparison, if necessary, with the contralateral uninjured foot. CT is especially sensitive for certain findings with significant prognostic implications, such as comminution and intra-articular fracture extension, which may be suggested on plain films, but the extent of injury is unclear

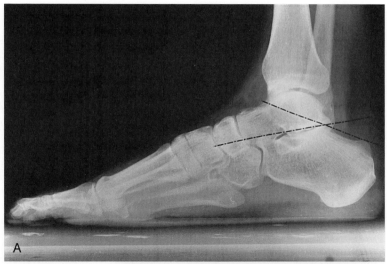

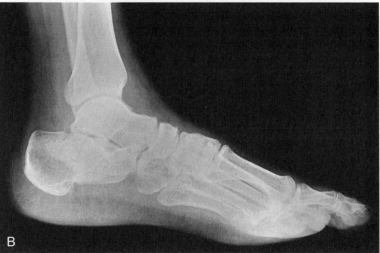

Figure 2–2. *A,* Boehler angle is the angle between a line tangent to the talar articulation and the posterior calcaneal bursal projection and a line tangent to the anterosuperior spine of the calcaneus and the talar articulation. The normal angle measures 20° to 40°. *B,* Lateral view of the foot demonstrates a comminuted compression fracture of the calcaneus. The radiolucent fracture line is noted, interrupting the superior cortex, and there is loss of the normal contour of the calcaneus. Boehler angle is approximately 0°.

(Fig. 2–4*A, B*). Thin CT sections through an area of interest minimize volume averaging artifact and enable reformatting of images in additional desired planes.

The talus is the second most common site of fracture in the hindfoot. In addition to a variety of avulsion fractures, the talus is prone to vertically oriented fractures through the neck or body, often associated with subtalar dislocations. Vertical fractures of the talus typically result from a force from below, driving the talus against the tibia, originally termed aviator's astragalus.[16] Vertical fractures through the talar neck must be distinguished from those through the body,[17] a distinction that can be reliably made on plain radiographs.[18] Talar neck fractures, which are extra-articular,

jeopardize the blood supply of the talus and may cause avascular necrosis of the bone (Fig. 2–5*A, B*). Fractures through the body of the talus are intra-articular and may predispose the patient to osteoarthritis. As with calcaneal fractures, CT is useful in fully characterizing the fracture pattern and facilitates management of these injuries.[19] The posterior talar tubercle is injured by severe plantar flexion. This injury must be differentiated from an accessory ossicle, the os trigonum, and is further discussed in the section on Posterior Symptoms.

Avulsion Fractures

Several avulsion injuries of the foot present clinically as ankle pain. One of these injur-

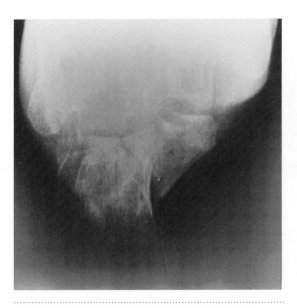

Figure 2–3. Axial view of the heel demonstrates a comminuted intra-articular fracture of the calcaneus interrupting the sustentacular and posterior subtalar joint articular surfaces.

ies is at the anterosuperior spine of the calcaneus, which results from foot inversion (Fig. 2–6A, B).[2, 7, 20] This is the site of origin of the bifurcate ligament. The avulsed frac-

ture fragment is identified on lateral or oblique views of the hindfoot or ankle. The acute fracture is differentiated from an os calcaneus secondarious (a normal juxta-articular ossicle) by the marginal contour; the margins of an acute fracture are jagged and fit together, whereas those of an os calcaneus secondarious or an old fracture are smooth and round. Diagnosis on plain films of an acute diastasis of either an old fracture fragment or juxta-articular ossicle is usually equivocal at best. Confirmation of the diagnosis is usually dependent on localized augmented isotope uptake on a radionuclide bone scan or on MRI by diminished signal in the normally hyperintense fatty marrow (see Fig. 2–6B), with increased signal, secondary to bone marrow edema, on long echo time fast-spin echo (FSE) sequence performed with fat suppression.

Another avulsion fracture in this category occurs at the origin of the extensor digitorum brevis at the lateral anterior aspect of the distal calcaneus. Diagnosis of this injury on plain films is contingent on proper radiographic penetration of the anterolateral aspect of the calcaneus on the AP view of the hindfoot and inclusion of the calcaneus on the AP view of the ankle to identify the localized soft tissue swelling and bone changes (Fig. 2–7A, B).

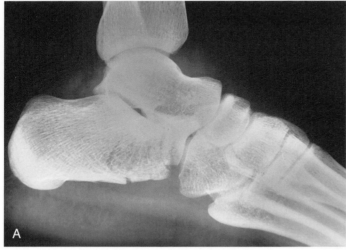

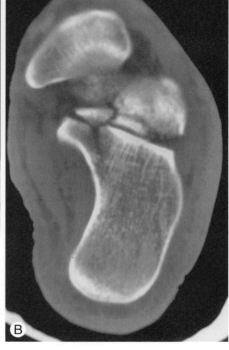

Figure 2–4. Lateral plain radiographic view *(A)* and axial computed tomographic (CT) image *(B)* through the calcaneus demonstrate a comminuted intra-articular fracture. The degree of comminution is best evident on the CT examination.

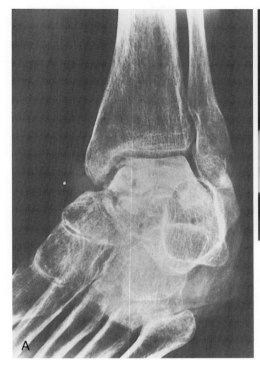

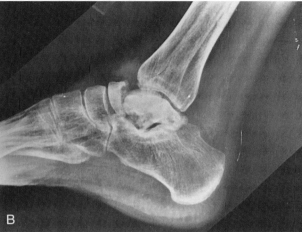

Figure 2–5. Mortise *(A)* and lateral *(B)* views demonstrate a fracture through the neck of the talus with increased radiodensity of the middle and posterior aspect of the talus, consistent with avascular necrosis and collapse. The ankle mortise is preserved.

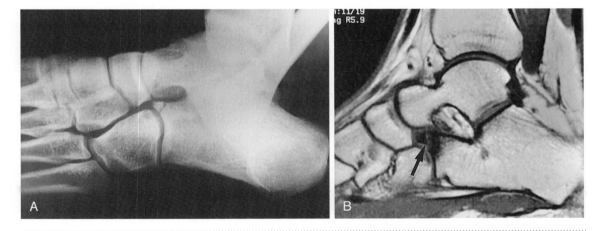

Figure 2–6. An oblique view of the hindfoot *(A)* demonstrates a radiolucent fracture line through the anterosuperior process of the calcaneus. The fracture margins are sharp, and the fracture fragments fit together, indicating an acute injury. Sagittal T1-weighted magnetic resonance sequence *(B)* in a different patient demonstrates hypointense marrow at the anterior process of the calcaneus *(arrow)* resulting from a radiographically occult anterior process fracture.

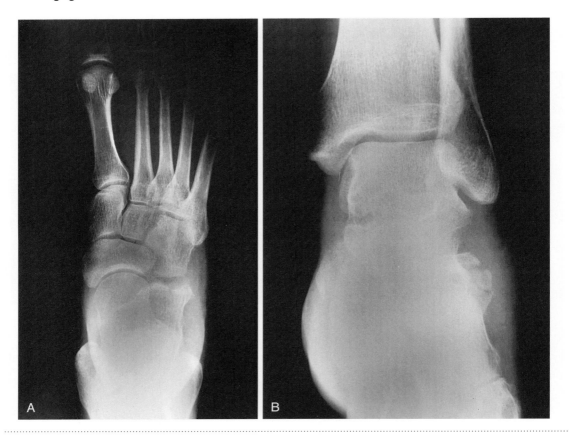

Figure 2–7. Frontal view of the foot penetrated to visualize the hindfoot optimally *(A)* and a frontal view of the ankle, including the osseous and soft tissue structures distal to the fibula *(B)*, demonstrate a comminuted avulsion fracture of the anterolateral aspect of the distal calcaneus at the origin of the digitorum brevis.

The last avulsion injury in this category occurs at the base of the fifth metatarsal, involving either the tuberosity (Fig. 2–8*A*) or the metatarsal shaft, distal to the tuberosity (Fig. 2–8*B*). Both injuries are associated with basketball and running. The prognoses of these two fractures differ; the fracture through the tuberosity usually heals without incident, whereas the fracture distal to the tuberosity (Jones fracture) has a high propensity for healing complications (delayed union, nonunion, and refracture).[21–24] Delayed union is diagnosed radiographically by the presence of sclerosis partially obliterating the medullary cavity along the fracture margins; a nonunion is diagnosed by the presence of complete medullary sclerosis bordering the fracture margins. In children, the normal apophysis is oriented parallel to the long axis of the metatarsal base, and an avulsion of the apophysis at the base of the fifth metatarsal

can be diagnosed by distraction of the ossification center and associated soft tissue swelling. A fracture through the tuberosity is horizontal (perpendicular to the long axis of the metatarsal) and can extend through the apophysis. Diagnosis is evident on lateral, frontal, and oblique views of the foot or the ankle, and the base of the fifth metatarsal should always be included on the oblique and lateral views of the ankle.

Stress Fractures

A stress fracture results from repetitive prolonged muscular force on the bone.[1] Compressive fractures are more common in cancellous bone, whereas distraction fractures are more common in cortical bone.[25] The early signs of cortical stress fracture on plain radiographs include medullary sclerosis, cortical hyperostosis with periosteal and endosteal irregularity, and intracortical lin-

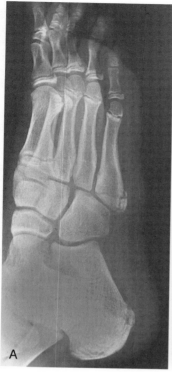
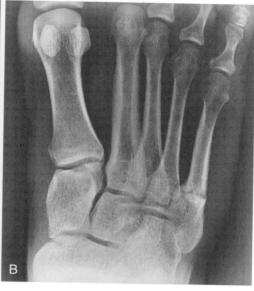

Figure 2–8. *A,* An oblique view of the foot demonstrates a horizontal radiolucent line at the base of the fifth metatarsal, extending through the tuberosity and the apophysis. The apophysis is oriented parallel to the long axis of the bone. *B,* A fracture of the metatarsal shaft distal to the tuberosity, a Jones fracture, is evident, with sclerosis partially obliterating the fracture margin, consistent with delayed union.

ear radiolucency (Fig. 2–9).[21, 26] In cancellous bone, linear sclerosis oriented perpendicular to the longitudinal axis of the trabeculae secondary to endosteal healing and remodeling is typical; however, it is not usually radiographically evident until 3 to 4 weeks after the acute event (Fig. 2–10*A*–*C*).[8, 26, 27] For a timely diagnosis of stress injuries in cases of clinical suspicion and normal plain radiographs, other imaging modalities are indicated.[28] Radionuclide bone scan demonstrates focal increased radiotracer uptake at the location of a stress fracture weeks before an abnormality is evident on plain films (Fig. 2–10*D*). Although the radionuclide bone scan is sensitive, it is limited by its poor specificity and has essentially been replaced by MRI imaging on which findings reflect the evolution of pathologic changes in the natural course of stress injury. Early findings of a stress fracture on MRI include marrow edema with decreased signal on T1-weighted sequences (Fig. 2–10*E*) and hyperintensity on long TE

FSE sequences with fat suppression or short inversion time recovery (STIR) images. The fracture itself may be seen as an irregular linear area of low signal on all pulse sequences. Periosteal reaction may be seen as a rim of high signal around the cortex in 7 to 10 days, which enhances with contrast administration.[29–31]

Stress fractures of the tibia, fibula, calcaneus, and talus occur in both athletic and osteopenic patients. Both the fatigue and insufficiency types of stress fracture occur in predictable locations. In the distal tibia, the typical cortical stress fracture (e.g., a linear lucency within a focal area of cortical hyperostosis) occurs in the posterior tibial cortex at the junction of the middle and distal thirds.[1] A less frequent site for tibial stress fractures is the base of the medial malleolus. The typical site for a tibial cancellous stress fracture (e.g., a linear area of increased radiopacity oriented perpendicular to the flow, or trabeculae) occurs proximal and parallel to the plafond (Fig. 2–10*A,*

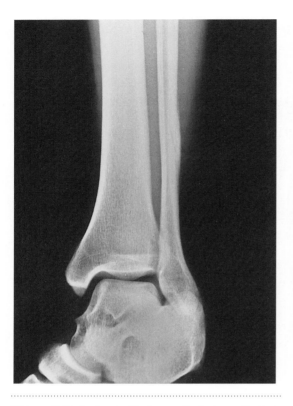

Figure 2–9. A classic fibular cortical stress fracture is evident within the lateral fibular cortex at the juncture of the middle and distal thirds. The radiolucent fracture line is located within a focal area of cortical hyperostosis.

B). In the distal fibula, both cancellous and cortical stress fractures occur; cancellous fractures occur more distally (see Figs. 2–9 and 2–10*A*). In the calcaneus, vertically oriented cancellous stress fractures occur posteriorly (Fig. 2–10*C*). In the talus, stress fractures may be typical or atypical.[32] Typical stress fractures are vertically oriented at the talar neck, parallel to the talonavicular joint (Fig. 2–11*A*, *B*); atypical talar stress fractures are horizontally oriented in the talar body or horizontally or vertically oriented in the posteromedial talus (Fig. 2–11*C*). Atypical talar stress fractures are primarily insufficiency fractures and occur in females. MRI imaging demonstrates the location and orientation of talar stress fractures and also helps to identify unsuspected concomitant fractures.

Osteochondral Injuries

Osteochondral fractures and osteochondritis dissecans may be associated with loose bod-ies and are responsible for chronic ankle pain, decreased range of motion, locking, and disability. Osseous, osteochondral, and chondral fractures of the talar dome typically result from shearing, rotatory, or impaction forces that act tangentially to the joint surface and are difficult to detect radiographically.[33–36] Although these findings are typically best seen on the routine frontal or mortise views, the defect should also be looked for on the lateral view (Fig. 2–12*A*, *B*). An osteochondral injury in the lateral talar dome usually results from plantar flexion and foot inversion followed by tibial rotation on the talus, resulting in a "gouging out" of an osteochondral talar fragment.

Osteochondritis dissecans of the talar dome is common at the medial talar dome and is more common than osteonecrosis of the talus (Fig. 2–13*A*, *B*). Both an MRI examination and a tomograph (CT or routine) after an arthrogram are appropriate methods to demonstrate the cartilaginous component of an osteochondral injury and to determine whether there is a loose fragment (Fig. 2–14*A*, *B*).[37] Although most chondral or osteochondral fragments attach to the synovium or are resorbed, if the fragment remains loose, it may result in locking and degenerative osteoarthritis.[35, 36] In chronic cases with minimal joint fluid, it has been reported that evaluation of the articular cartilage may benefit from the intra-articular injection of gadolinium, although newer sequences are being developed to visualize the cartilage directly.[38]

Osteonecrosis of the talus is not uncommon, especially after trauma. The body of the talus is more prone to osteonecrosis than the talar head or neck. Osteonecrosis is diagnosed on plain films by increased radiodensity, articular surface collapse, and bony fragmentation (see Fig. 2–5*A*, *B*). MRI is extremely sensitive for detecting osteonecrosis and is usually diagnostic before plain film evidence.

Sprains and Strains

In the adult, localized soft tissue swelling around the ankle after a twisting injury, without evidence of fracture, suggests a ligament or tendon injury. In the skeletally immature patient, soft tissue swelling after a twisting injury of the ankle, even without an obvious fracture, is highly suspect for a

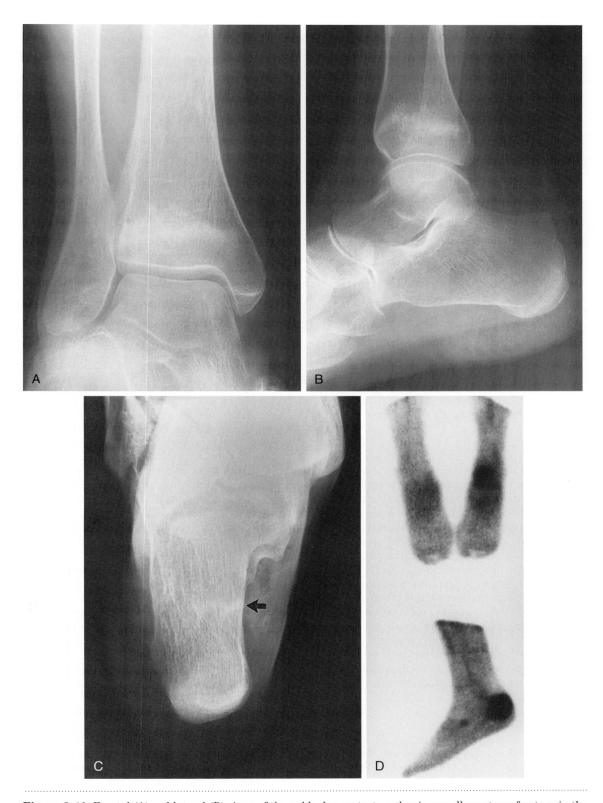

Figure 2–10. Frontal *(A)* and lateral *(B)* views of the ankle demonstrate a classic cancellous stress fracture in the distal tibia identified as a horizontal linear area of radiodensity. *C,* A classic cancellous stress fracture *(arrow)* is identified on the axial view of the calcaneus. The horizontal linear sclerosis is oriented perpendicular to the long axis of the trabeculae. *D,* Radionuclide bone scan of a calcaneal stress fracture demonstrated by a focal area of augmented isotope uptake.

Illustration continued on following page

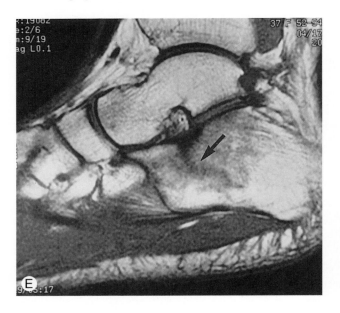

Figure 2–10 *Continued. E*, Sagittal T1-weighted magnetic resonance sequence through the hindfoot of a 37-year-old female competitive runner demonstrates a linear focus of diminished signal intensity *(arrow)* surrounded by ill-defined marrow edema resulting from a calcaneal stress fracture.

Salter fracture.[2] Common sites for Salter injuries include the distal tibia and fibula and the base of the fifth metatarsal (Fig. 2–15).

The routine series of ankle radiographs is often insufficient to evaluate ankle sprains and instability.[39] Stress views of the ankle have been reported to demonstrate ligamentous disruption and instability; however, because there is a wide normal range, radiographs of the uninjured side are needed for comparison. Unfortunately, stress views are often nondiagnostic because of guarding and pain.[8]

On MRI, normal tendons and ligaments have homogeneous low signal intensity (Fig. 2–16A, B).[3, 40] Ligamentous and tendinous injuries are diagnosed by increased signal and abnormal morphology, including thickening, thinning, disruption, and irregularity.[41–44] Discontinuity is seen in complete ligamentous and tendinous disruption.[45]

Ligament Sprains

Partial and complete ruptures of the ligaments on the lateral aspect of the ankle are common. Eighty-five percent of ankle sprains, especially in athletes, involve the lateral collateral ligamentous complex. The lateral collateral ligamentous complex is composed of the anterior and posterior talofibular ligaments and the calcaneofibular ligament. The sequence of ruptures is predictable.[46, 47] Inversion of a plantar-flexed foot results initially in rupture of the anterior talofibular ligament (see Fig. 2–16A), followed by associated rupture of the calcaneofibular ligament (see Fig. 2–16B). Because the calcaneofibular ligament is in close apposition to the inner aspect of the peroneal tendon sheath, the sheath usually ruptures. An isolated posterior talofibular ligament rupture is not typical but may rupture in conjunction with tears of the anterior talofibular and calcaneofibular ligaments.

Injuries of the tarsal sinus and tarsal canal are often associated with lateral collateral ligamentous injury secondary to inversion.[48] The tarsal sinus and canal form an anatomic space between the posterior subtalar joint and the talocalcaneonavicular joint, medial and posterior to the sustentaculum tali. The ligaments within the canal maintain alignment between the talus and calcaneus. The sinus tarsi syndrome is discussed later under synovial abnormalities.

There is one strong ligament medially, the deltoid ligament, which is a triangular structure that extends from the medial malleolus to the talus; there are three superficial and two deep layers. Deltoid injuries occur secondary to eversion and lateral rotation and are usually confined to the anterior portion; a complete rupture is uncommon.

The tibia and fibula are connected by a tibiofibular syndesmosis. The distal tibio-

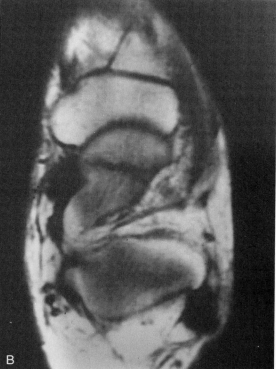

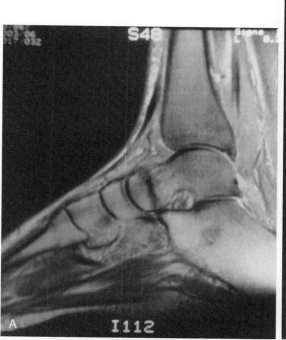

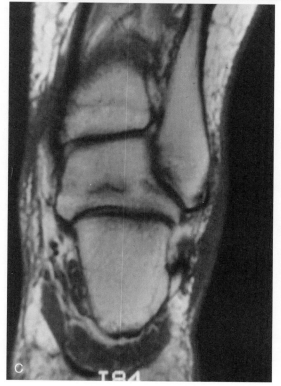

Figure 2–11. Sagittal fast-spin echo long TR–short TE-weighted sequence *(A)* demonstrates a typical talar stress fracture. There is a linear area of low signal intensity through the talar neck surrounded by ill-defined high signal intensity representing a fracture with associated marrow edema. On an axial T1-weighted spin echo sequence *(B)*, the linear fracture of low signal intensity is readily evident in the talar neck. *C,* Coronal T1-weighted spin echo magnetic resonance image demonstrates a horizontally oriented linear fracture of low signal intensity in the posteromedial talus, which represents an atypical orientation and location of an insufficiency fracture in the talus.

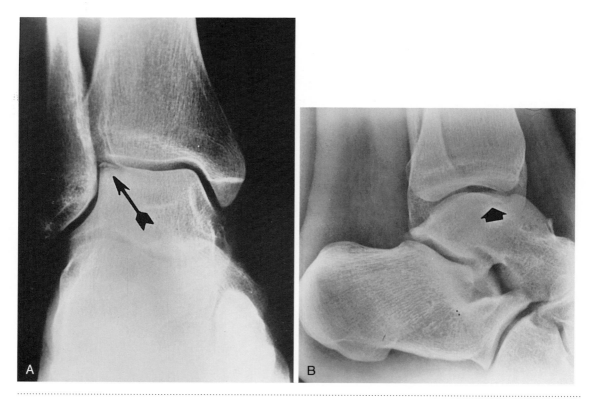

Figure 2–12. *A*, Frontal view demonstrates an osteochondral fracture of the superolateral aspect of the talar dome *(arrow)*. *B*, Lateral view shows depression of the fracture *(arrowhead)*. The ankle mortise is preserved.

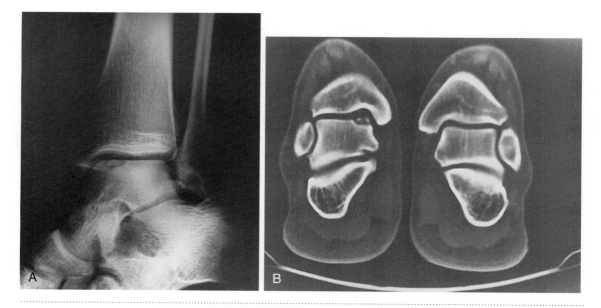

Figure 2–13. *A*, Mortise view demonstrates an osteochondral lesion consistent with osteochondritis dissecans at the superomedial talar dome. The ankle mortise is preserved. *B*, On coronal computed tomographic images through the ankle mortise, an osteochondral defect on the right medial talar dome is identified.

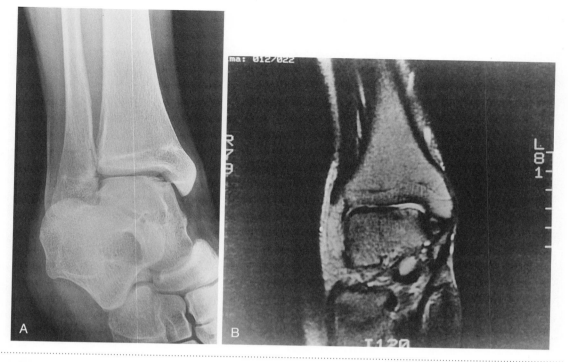

Figure 2–14. *A,* Ankle mortise demonstrates an osteochondral lesion at the superomedial aspect of the talar dome with suggestion of collapse of the articular cartilage and loose fragment. *B,* On a T2-weighted magnetic resonance image in another patient, there is absence of cartilage and bone over an area of marrow edema within the superomedial aspect of the talus, loss of overlying articular surface, and small joint effusion. A definitive loose body is not identified.

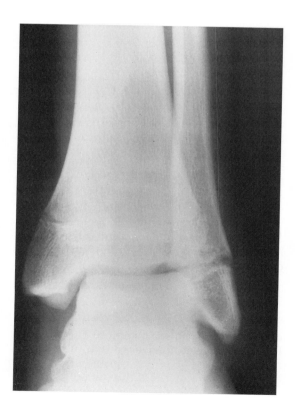

Figure 2–15. Frontal view of the ankle obtained 10 days after initial injury demonstrates periosteal bone formation along the distal lateral fibular cortex secondary to a healing Salter I fracture. There is widening of the fibular physis laterally.

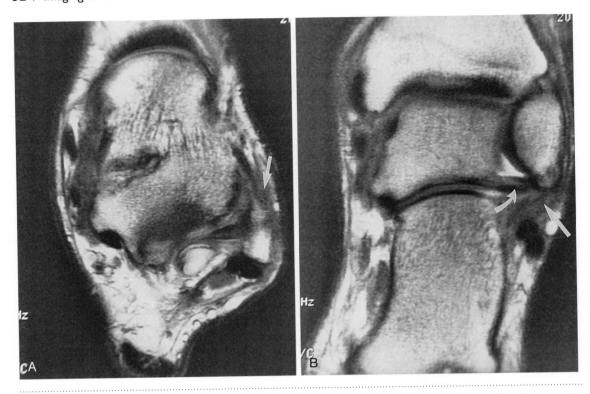

Figure 2–16. A 20-year-old patient status post inversion injury with lateral pain. Axial fast-spin echo magnetic resonance (MR) image *(A)* demonstrates normal peroneal longus and brevis tendons identified as round and void of signal inferior to the fibula. There is increased signal intensity in the anterior talofibular ligament *(arrow)* resulting from prior partial tear at the fibular insertion. Coronal fast-spin echo MR image *(B)* demonstrates signal hyperintensity and abnormal morphology in the calcaneofibular ligament *(straight arrow)* as a result of partial tear. Note the intact posterior talofibular ligament *(curved arrow)*.

fibular syndesmotic complex is composed of an anterior and a posterior tibiofibular ligament, the inferior transverse ligament, and the interosseous ligament[49]; the distal fascia of the anterior ligament is implicated in talar impingement syndrome.[50] The syndesmosis is commonly disrupted secondary to a twisting injury and is usually associated with a rupture of the deltoid ligament or with stress fractures of the tibia or fibula. Heterotopic ossification and interosseous bridging can follow tibiofibular syndesmosis disruption (Fig. 2–17).

Tendon Strains

Tendon injuries include tendinosis, tenosynovitis, and partial or complete rupture. Before MRI, these injuries were an underdiagnosed cause of acute pain or chronic disability around the ankle or both. Tenography for evaluation of the peroneal tendon sheaths and the posterior tibial tendon sheaths is invasive and difficult to perform (Fig. 2–18).[51, 52] On CT, a normal tendon is diagnosed as a homogeneous, well-circumscribed round density of higher attenuation value than muscle, highlighted by surrounding fat; a partial tendon rupture is diagnosed by an increase in tendon girth and intratendinous radiolucency; a complete rupture is identified by absence of the tendon.[2] Posttraumatic or postsurgical tenosynovitis is diagnosed by increased density relative to fat obliteration of the normal fat around the tendon secondary to synovial proliferation and scar tissue.

On MRI, normal tendons are identified as low signal, homogeneously black structures on all pulse sequences.[53–55] Tendon rupture is diagnosed by high signal intensity within the tendon substance on the T2-weighted, long TE images. The percentage of tendon abnormality can be determined on

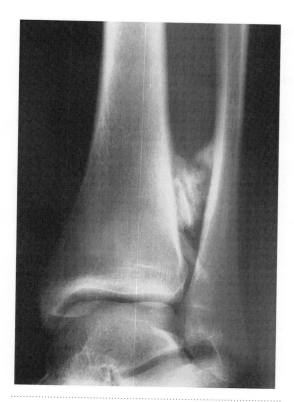

Figure 2–17. Oblique view of the ankle demonstrates attempted interosseous bridging of the distal-most aspect of the interosseous membrane secondary to prior injury.

image planes obtained at 90° to each other (e.g., axial and sagittal).[3, 56, 57] A complete tendon rupture is detected as a focal gap in the course of the tendon often with an empty fluid distended sheath.[55]

There are several potential pitfalls in MRI evaluation of the hindfoot and ankle tendons. The synovial sheath around a tendon cannot be visually separated from the tendon substance unless there is synovial fluid distention of the sheath.[54] Fluid in a shared peroneal tendon sheath is normal and not to be confused with a longitudinal tendon tear.[44] The flexor hallucis longus tendon sheath communicates with the ankle joint in 20% of patients, and fluid within the sheath is usually physiologic.[58] Long TE–weighted images help differentiate intratendinous signal in the peroneus longus or brevis tendons as a result of "magic angle" artifact from true pathology.[59] A heterogeneous signal in the posterior tibial tendon as it inserts on the navicular is normal.[44, 57, 60]

Arthritis and Synovial Abnormalities

A joint effusion in the ankle is identified on the routine lateral view as a teardrop-shaped radiopacity anterior to the tibial talar articulation. Acute causes of a joint effusion include fracture, capsular rupture, and articular cartilage injury; chronic causes include synovitis, intra-articular loose bodies, synovial abnormalities, and arthritis. Anatomically, the synovial lining of the ankle joint is smooth with redundancy in the anterior and posterior compartments. The joint extends between the tibia and fibula 1 to 2.5 cm proximally from the talus. In 10% of patients, the ankle joint communicates with the posterior subtalar joint.[61] The synovium is optimally evaluated on arthrography or on MRI.

Sinus Tarsi Syndrome

The sinus tarsi syndrome is characterized by pain at the lateral aspect of the foot associated with a sensation of hindfoot in-

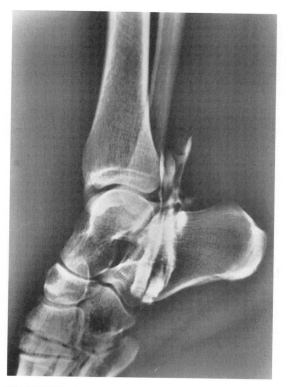

Figure 2–18. After intratendinous sheath injection of contrast, the normal tendon can be identified within the tendon sheaths.

stability.[62–64] The sinus tarsi is an anatomic space below the medial malleolus, anterior to the posterior subtalar joint and posterior to the talocalcaneal navicular joint and medial and posterior to sustentacular tali. Symptoms in 70% of cases follow a severe inversion injury and in 30% are associated with inflammatory arthritis. The sinus tarsi syndrome is diagnosed on MRI by loss of fat in the sinus tarsi, with poor definition of the cervical and talocalcaneal ligaments secondary to fibrosis or edema. Abnormalities on MRI include chronic synovitis and synovial cysts (increased T2-weighted signal intensity, decreased T1-weighted signal intensity) and fibrosis (decreased signal intensity on both T1- and T2-weighted sequences), which have been shown to correlate well both with the patient's symptoms and with pathologic findings at surgery.[63]

Tarsal Tunnel Syndrome

The tarsal tunnel is a fibro-osseous channel extending from the medial malleolus to the navicular, lateral to the flexor retinaculum, the long flexor tendons, and the posterior tibial neurovascular bundle. Tarsal tunnel syndrome results from compression of the posterior tibial nerve and branches within this fibro-osseous "tunnel."[65–68] Symptoms vary depending on the level of compression, the duration and extent of compression, and the individual nerve component damaged. Symptom onset is usually insidious, consisting of tingling, burning, sharp pain, and either hypo- or hyperesthesia on the sole of the foot, which extends to the great toe medially and spares the heel pad. Pain is usually increased with activity, and Tinel's sign reproduces the pain. In chronic cases, toe flexion at the metatarsophalangeal joint may be weak secondary to atrophy of the abductor hallucis. MRI can diagnose this entity and reliably distinguish between the variety of causes of posterior tibial nerve compression, including fractures, and soft tissue injuries, varicosities, mass lesions, scar tissue, and tenosynovitis.[69] Pathologic entities seen on MRI include neurilemomas, tenosynovitis, ganglion cysts, post-traumatic fibrosis or neuroma, lipomas, and varicosities in the region of the posterior tibial nerve.[67–69] MRI is useful both to monitor conservative treatment and for surgical planning.

Degenerative Osteoarthritis

On plain films, degenerative osteoarthritis is diagnosed by joint space narrowing, sclerosis of the subchondral bone, subchondral cysts, and proliferative hypertrophic osteophytes. Degenerative arthritis may result from unbalanced forces or secondary to trauma. Degenerative arthritis in the hindfoot may affect the talotibial, sustentacular portion of the subtalar, posterior subtalar, or talonavicular joints (Fig. 2–19). MRI further demonstrates the presence of intra-articular fluid, synovial hypertrophy, and cartilage loss.[70, 71] MRI can demonstrate cartilage changes before joint space narrowing is radiographically evident and can also demonstrate bone marrow edema and soft tissue changes secondary to osteophyte impingement.

Psoriatic Arthritis

Psoriatic arthritis occurs in 5 to 7% of patients with psoriasis. The typical radiographic findings of psoriatic arthritis in the hands and feet consist of joint space narrowing, articular erosions with a "mouse ear" contour, fluffy periostitis, and soft tissue swelling. Psoriatic arthritis in the foot typically affects the distal interphalangeal joints and the undersurface of the calca-

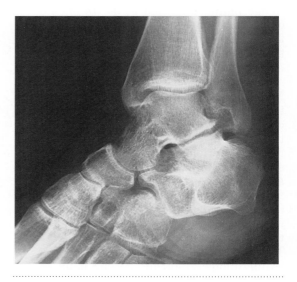

Figure 2–19. Oblique view of the hindfoot demonstrates isolated degenerative osteoarthritic changes involving the posterior subtalar joint with joint space narrowing, proliferative osteophytic spurs, and sclerosis bordering the joint margin.

neus. The calcaneal findings include a broad-based osteophyte on the plantar surface, the presence of erosions, and fluffy periostitis.

Septic Arthritis

Septic arthritis is diagnosed on plain films by a joint effusion, diffuse joint space narrowing, and subchondral bony erosions.[72, 73] On arthrography, an infectious or inflammatory synovitis may manifest with fuzzy synovial coating and contrast uptake within the lymphatics. On MRI, hypertrophic synovium proliferation or edematous synovium has a lobulated, nodular, or thickened contour. Synovial hypertrophy may be further demonstrated on MRI with intravenous gadolinium-diethylenetriamine-penta-acetic acid (Gd-DTPA).

Adhesive Capsulitis

Posttraumatic adhesive capsulitis is diagnosed on arthrography or MRI by a decrease in the size of the joint capsule and obliteration of the normal anterior and posterior recesses.[74]

Neuropathic Joint

A neuropathic ankle or hindfoot is usually the result of diabetes or syphilis. Radiographically, the diagnosis is made by multiple fracture fragments, dislocations and subluxations, soft tissue swelling, and normal mineralization. The bony mineralization is normal because the patient continues to use the body part, despite the serious injuries, as a result of decreased or absent pain sensation (Fig. 2–20A, B).

Reflex Sympathetic Dystrophy

Reflex sympathetic dystrophy syndrome (RSDS)[75] was originally described in 1864[76] and is clinically referred to by many names, including causalgia,[77] Sudeck's atrophy or osteodystrophy,[78] post-traumatic osteoporosis,[79] reflex dystrophy of the extremities,[80] and others.[81, 82] The diagnosis of RSDS depends on clinical as well as radiographic findings of soft tissue swelling and regional osteoporosis. Resorption of metaphyseal cancellous or trabecular bone results in bandlike periarticular osteoporosis. There is preservation of the joint space. Radionuclide bone scintigraphy is more sensitive than radiographs to these changes, demonstrating

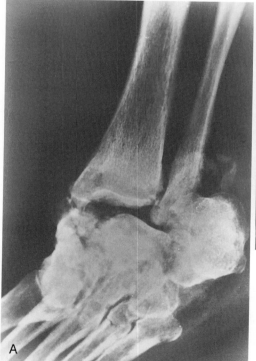

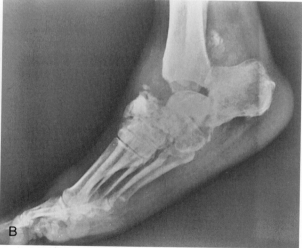

Figure 2–20. Mortise *(A)* and lateral *(B)* views demonstrate a classic neuropathic joint with fracture dislocation of the tibiotalar joint, multiple osseous fragments, and normal mineralization.

increased periarticular augmentation presumably secondary to increased vascularity (Fig. 2–21A, B).[81–83]

Infection and Tumors

An elaborate discussion of the imaging methods for evaluation of infection and tumors of the foot and ankle is beyond the scope of this chapter. The foot is a common site for infection, especially in the diabetic patient. In general, infection can be suspected on plain film by periosteal new bone formation, sequestrum, involucrum, and sinusoidal tracks. On MRI, infected bone marrow has a low signal intensity on T1-weighted images and a high signal intensity on long-TE–weighted images secondary to increased edema, exudate, hyperemia, and ischemia. Bone erosions identified on plain film indicate infection, tumor, or inflammatory arthritis and may require an MRI for further evaluation (Fig. 2–22A–D).

Calcifications within the soft tissues in the hindfoot on plain radiographs, not associated with calcific tendinitis, are highly suspect for synovial sarcoma and must be further investigated. Calcifications within tumor or adjacent soft tissues are best detected by CT. As elsewhere in the musculoskeletal body system, MRI is excellent for identifying an osseous or soft tissue tumor as well as the proximity of the tumor to the neurovascular structures and joints. Although MRI provides superior sensitivity, the differentiation of benign from malignant may be limited, depending on the pulse sequences used, the tumor characteristics, and the experience of the radiologist.[84–86]

LOCALIZED SPECIFIC SYMPTOMS

Rigid Flatfoot Deformity

A common cause of a rigid flatfoot deformity is a tarsal coalition.[87] Coalitions may be fi-

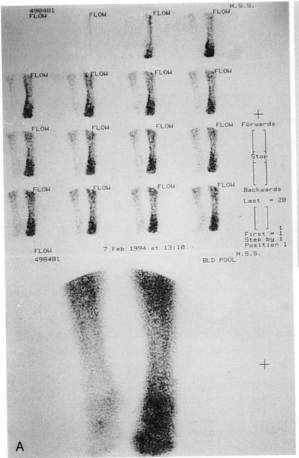

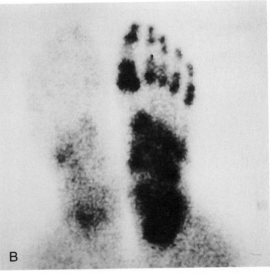

Figure 2–21. Reflex sympathetic dystrophy syndrome demonstrated on radionuclide bone scan. On dynamic flow and blood pulse scans (A), there is diffuse increased vascularity in the left ankle and foot. On delayed static images (B), there is diffuse uptake in the left foot, most prominent around the joints.

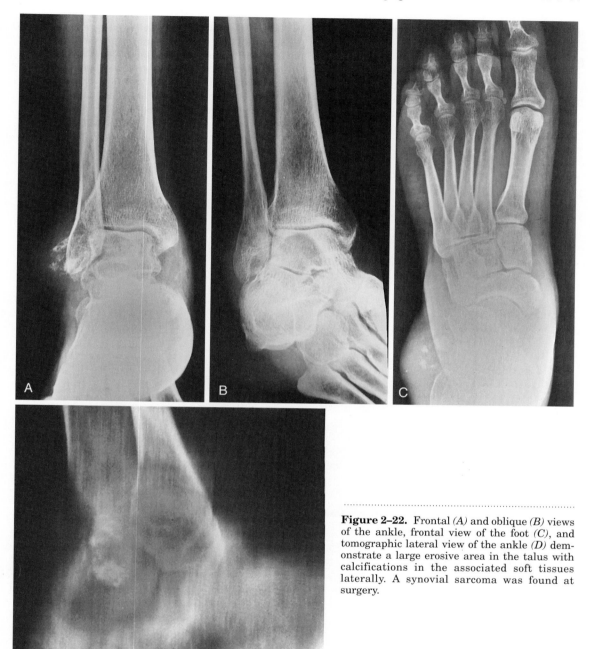

Figure 2–22. Frontal *(A)* and oblique *(B)* views of the ankle, frontal view of the foot *(C)*, and tomographic lateral view of the ankle *(D)* demonstrate a large erosive area in the talus with calcifications in the associated soft tissues laterally. A synovial sarcoma was found at surgery.

brous, cartilaginous, or osseous and may be asymptomatic, presenting as an incidental finding. Approximately 30% of coalitions involve the calcaneonavicular joint and 60% involve the sustentacular subtalar joint.[88-90] Calcaneonavicular coalitions occur equally in both sexes and present at 8 to 12 years of age; 60% are bilateral. Sustentacular co-

alitions are three to four times more common in boys than girls and present at 12 to 16 years of age; 50% are bilateral.

When a tarsal coalition is clinically suspected, multiple projections of the ankle or foot are necessary to evaluate optimally each of the potentially fused joint spaces. An osseous calcaneonavicular joint coalition is diagnosed on the routine oblique view of the foot by an elongation of the anterior process of the calcaneus and attempted or complete bony bar.[91] A sustentacular coalition is suspected on the routine lateral view by a talar beak, which is an osseous protuberance arising from the distal dorsal talus (Fig. 2–23A). This projection must be distinguished from a normal talar variation, a traction exostosis, or a juxta-articular ossicle (see Fig. 2–25B). The C sign, a C-shaped line formed by the medial outline of the talar dome and the inferior outline of the sustentaculum tali, is another indicator of subtalar coalition that may be seen on the lateral view.[92] A poorly positioned radiograph may cause artifactual overlap of the tarsal bones, resulting in a tarsal "pseudocoalition," or false-positive findings.[93] Angulation of the x-ray beam must be along the

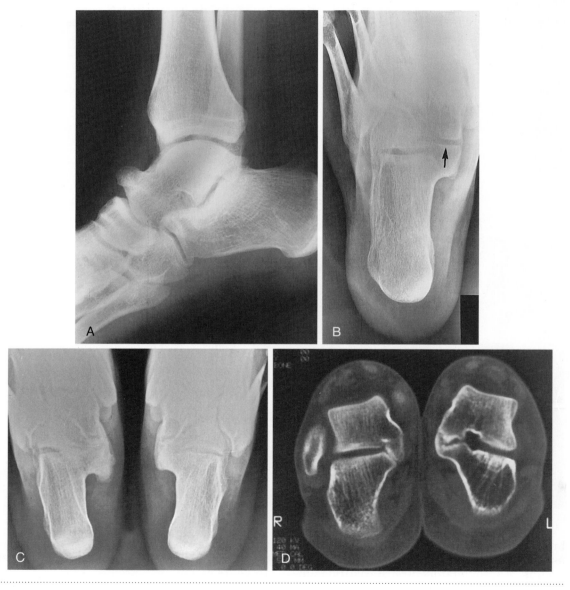

Figure 2–23. *A,* Lateral view of the foot demonstrates a large anterosuperior process or calcaneal beak, suggesting an abnormal talar calcaneal coalition. *B,* Axial view demonstrates the normal sustentacular *(arrow)* and subtalar joints. The joint spaces are normally oriented parallel to one another and uniform in width. *C,* Bilateral axial views demonstrate bilateral osseous sustentacular joint coalitions. *D,* On coronal computed tomographic images, sustentacular coalitions are present bilaterally with a continuous osseous bar on the left.

axis of the joint space in question, and this parameter is subject to considerable normal variation. The middle and posterior facets of the subtalar joint are usually visible on the lateral view of the foot; the anterior subtalar facet is seen on the oblique view, and the posterior and sustentacular joints are optimally seen on the Harris view or axial (CT or MRI) images. Normally, the posterior and sustentacular subtalar joints are uniform in width and parallel to each other (Fig. 2–23B). A coalition is diagnosed radiographically by an osseous bar crossing

the joint or by irregularity of the articular surfaces, joint space narrowing, or abnormal orientation (Fig. 2–23C, D).[89] Proper technique is crucial for the evaluation of a suspected tarsal coalition, and alternative imaging modalities play significant roles in the evaluation of tarsal coalition. Radionuclide bone scanning has been proposed as a screening procedure for diagnosing a subtalar coalition.[94] Increased radiotracer uptake in the region of the posterior subtalar joint and at the superior surface of the talus indicates abnormal mechanical forces caused by

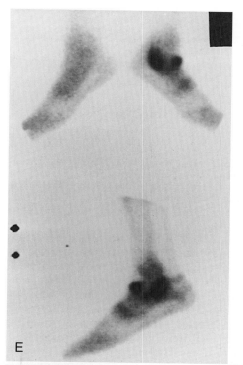

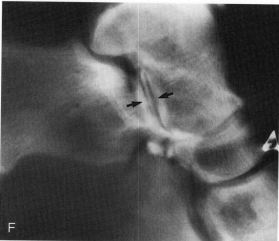

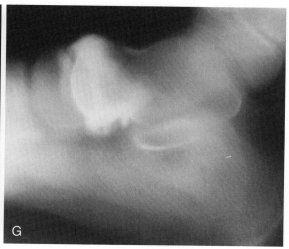

Figure 2–23 *Continued. E,* Radionuclide bone scan (in same patient as in Figure 2–23A) demonstrates augmented isotope uptake in the region of the anterosuperior talar beak and in the posterior subtalar joint characteristic of a sustentacular coalition. *F,* Talonavicular arthrogram demonstrates contrast communicating normally in the sustentacular joint *(arrows),* eliminating the possibility of a coalition. *G,* A lateral tomographic section through the sustentacular joint after contrast injection into the talonavicular joint demonstrates absence of contrast within the sustentacular portion of the subtalar joint, confirming a coalition.

Illustration continued on following page

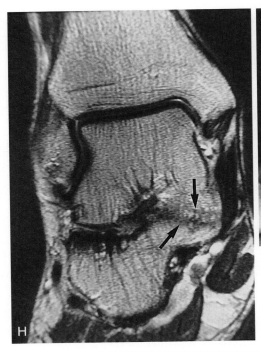
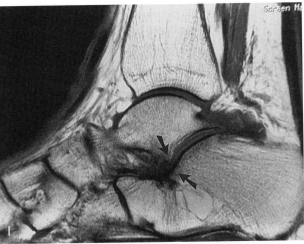

Figure 2–23 *Continued.* Coronal fast-spin echo magnetic resonance (MR) image *(H)* through the hindfoot demonstrates the presence of the fibrous coalition through the medial facet of the subtalar joint *(arrows)*. Sagittal T1-weighted MR sequence *(I)* demonstrates subchondral sclerosis at the anterior margin of the posterior facet of the subtalar joint *(arrows)* attributed to altered weight-bearing stresses in the presence of the coalition.

the sustentacular coalition (Fig. 2–23E). CT is excellent for demonstrating this osseous anatomy and is helpful in surgical planning and postsurgical assessment, but has limited sensitivity for detection of fibrous coalitions. Arthrography can be used to confirm or exclude a coalition. A talonavicular injection of contrast normally communicates with the sustentacular joint (Fig. 2–23F); if a coalition is present, the contrast will be confined to the talonavicular joint. (Fig. 2–23G) MRI can detect osseous, fibrous, and cartilaginous coalitions and can demonstrate marrow edema caused by the altered axis of weight bearing (Fig. 2–23H, I).[95, 96]

Anterior Symptoms

Symptoms at the anterior aspect of the ankle are usually associated with flexion. A traction exostosis on the dorsal mid-talus can form secondary to microtrauma at the capsular insertion (Fig. 2–24A). Focal soft tissue irritation may result when there is also a proliferative osteophyte on the anterior lip of the tibia (Fig. 2–24B).[21] Occasion-

ally, one or both of these proliferative osteophytes may fracture. Avulsion injuries at the dorsal talus or navicular or juxta-articular ossicles (os supratalare or os supranaviculare) are all potential sources of pain or injury (Fig. 2–25A, B).

Four anterior tendons (anterior tibialis, extensor hallucis longus, extensor digitorum longus, and peroneus tertius) are maintained in place by the superior and inferior extensor retinacula: isolated anterior tibial tendon injury can present as anterior soft tissue pain and swelling. MRI provides specific detail regarding the regional soft tissues as well as the bones.

Posterior Symptoms

Os Trigonum Syndrome

Pain in the posterior aspect of the ankle is usually associated with forced plantar flexion (e.g., deep knee bend performed on the ball of the foot, plié in ballet, or "duck walk" exercises). The posterior aspect of the talus is anatomically variable, having either a blunted or a long process (Stieda's process)

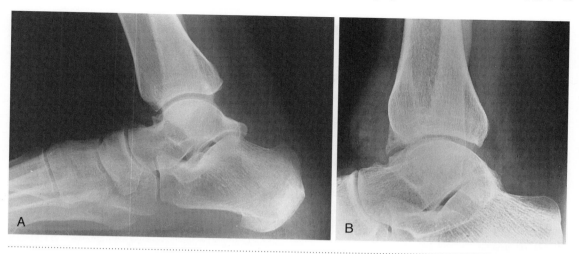

Figure 2–24. *A,* Lateral views of the ankle demonstrate a traction spur at the anterior midportion of the dorsal talus. *B,* There is a large anterior proliferative osteoarthritic spur at the anterior lip of the tibia with a corresponding small spur at the dorsal midtalus with associated soft tissue swelling.

(Fig. 2–26*A*). The os trigonum is a secondary ossification center posterior to the talus, which usually fuses with the talus to form Stieda's process (Fig. 2–26*B*). In 7 to 14% of patients, the os trigonum remains as a separate ossicle and is often bilateral.[97] Pain and swelling in the posterior ankle secondary to repetitive microtrauma result when the posterior aspect of the talus or the os trigonum or both is crushed between the tibia and calcaneus.[98] These injuries typically recur if the patient resumes the aggravating activity unless the osseous fragment is removed.[2] A fracture of the posterior aspect of the talus or the os trigonum can usually be diagnosed on the routine lateral view of the ankle. A chronic injury may be manifest by irregularity or sclerosis along

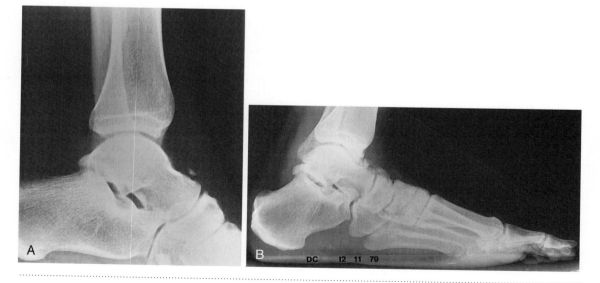

Figure 2–25. *A,* An avulsion fracture is present at the anterior dorsal aspect of the distal talus. *B,* There is an os supratalare and a large proliferative spur at the proximal dorsal aspect of the talonavicular joint.

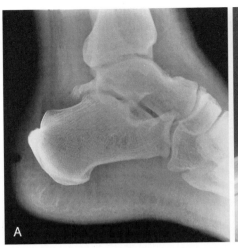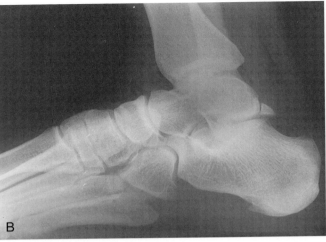

Figure 2–26. *A,* There is a long posterior process of the talus consistent with Stieda's process. In addition, there is an os trigonum. *B,* There is a classic os trigonum at the posterior aspect of the talus. The soft tissues are normal.

the margins of the os trigonum and talus. CT scanning can further differentiate this condition.[99] A normal radionuclide bone scan or MRI virtually excludes this diagnosis.[100]

Achilles Tendon Injuries

The Achilles tendon is the largest and strongest tendon in the ankle and foot. It is a common site of injury, secondary to trauma in middle-aged (third to fifth decade) male athletes.[101] Although an Achilles tendon injury can be diagnosed by physical examination and clinical history, plain films are indicated to exclude related osseous injuries such as an avulsion of the calcaneal insertion, a finding that would affect management decisions. On the routine lateral view of the ankle, the normal Achilles tendon measures approximately 4 to 9 mm with a defined anterior interface with the pre-Achilles fat pad (Fig. 2–27A). An Achilles tendon rupture usually occurs secondary to pre-existing degenerative changes. Most commonly, the rupture is located in the region of poorest blood supply, 2 to 6 cm proximal to the calcaneal insertion.[102] On the routine lateral ankle, an increase or decrease in thickness, a focal fusiform thickening 2.5 cm proximal to its insertion site, or complete absence of the tendon is highly suspect for an Achilles tendon rupture (Fig. 2–27B). Loss of a sharp interface between the tendon and the pre-Achilles fat pad suggests

tendinitis. Calcification in the Achilles tendon 2.5 cm above the calcaneus indicates an old chronic rupture. Discrete calcification at the insertion site of the tendon is a common condition and is usually asymptomatic (Fig. 2–27C). Linear-oriented calcifications in the distal portion of the Achilles tendon indicate calcific tendinitis (Fig. 2–27D).

Sonography of the Achilles tendon and the adjacent bursae has been reported to define the internal anatomy of the tendon better than roentgenograms or xeroradiography.[103–106] As with other modalities, user experience is directly proportional to accuracy.

The Achilles tendon is the only ankle tendon without a sheath and is surrounded by a peritenon.[107] On MRI, an acute injury can be distinguished from a chronic injury, and injuries can be graded.[108] Tendons composed of type I collagen have homogeneously low signal on all MRI pulse sequences. Chronic tendinosis may be seen on MRI as morphologic changes, such as focal thickening or enlargement, or longitudinal signal abnormalities indicating interstitial tears.[31] Increased intratendinous signal with horizontal orientation indicates a partial tear. A complete rupture is diagnosed by discontinuity and high signal interposition between the tendon fragments. The distance between the tendon fragments in a complete rupture can accurately be assessed with MRI (Fig. 2–28A, B). MRI can also be helpful in evaluating for other pertinent associated find-

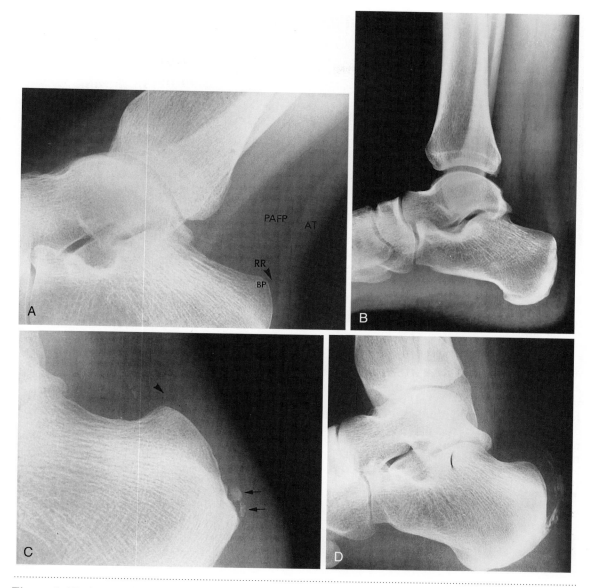

Figure 2–27. *A,* Lateral view of the hindfoot demonstrates normal soft tissues. The Achilles tendon (AT) is sharply delineated against the pre-Achilles fat pad (PAFP). The retrocalcaneal recess (RR) is identified as a 2-mm radiolucency between the Achilles tendon and the posterosuperior aspect of the calcaneus (the bursal projection [BP]). *B,* An acute rupture of the Achilles tendon in the classic location for injury approximately 2.5 cm proximal to the insertion. The tear is identified by loss of the sharply delineated tendon morphology. *C,* Small corticated osseous bodies *(arrows)* at the insertion of the Achilles tendon are typically not associated with symptoms. Note that the retrocalcaneal recess between the bursal projection and the insertion of the Achilles tendon *(arrowhead)* is normal. *D,* Elongated calcification within the tendon is consistent with calcific tendinitis.

ings, such as hemorrhage or edema.[109] In chronic cases, MRI may demonstrate atrophy in the soleus or gastrocnemius, in which case tendon reconstruction rather than repair, is usually considered.

Accessory Muscles Syndrome

An accessory muscle may present as a painful mass in the region of the Achilles tendon after exercise if the muscle becomes sore

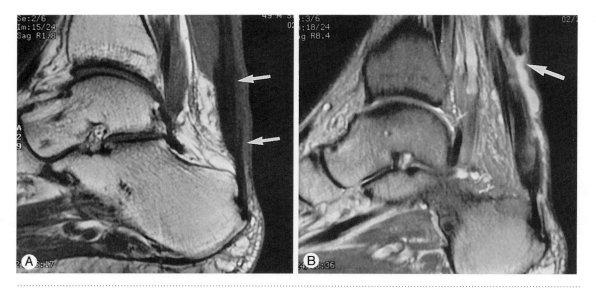

Figure 2–28. Sagittal T1-weighted magnetic resonance image *(A)* through the hindfoot demonstrates an enlargement and inhomogeneity in the Achilles tendon *(arrows)*. Sagittal long-TR/short-TE sequence with fat suppression *(B)* yields superior soft tissue contrast such that an obliquely oriented complete tear of the Achilles tendon is evident *(arrow)*.

and swollen (Fig. 2–29A, B).[110] The accessory soleus muscle inserts on the medial posterior calcaneus. A plantar tendon is found in 90% of individuals and inserts medial to the Achilles tendon onto the calcaneus, the Achilles tendon, or the flexor retinaculum.

Bursitis

Retrocalcaneal Bursitis

On the routine lateral radiograph of the hindfoot, a normal 2-mm radiolucent retrocalcaneal recess is present at the inferior extent of the pre-Achilles fat pad, extending

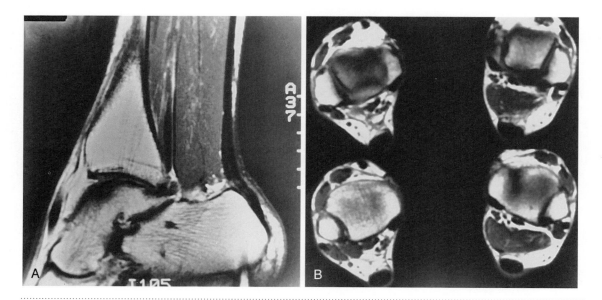

Figure 2–29. Sagittal T1-weighted magnetic resonance sequence *(A)* through the hindfoot demonstrates muscle replacing the pre-Achilles fat pad. Axial T1-weighted image *(B)* confirms the accessory soleus muscle anterior to the Achilles tendon on the left compared with the normal pre-Achilles fat on the right.

between the Achilles tendon insertion and the posterior aspect of the calcaneus (see Fig. 2–27A). Loss of this radiolucency indicates edema, hemorrhage, or inflammation of the retrocalcaneal bursa (Fig. 2–30A). On MRI, retrocalcaneal bursitis is diagnosed by localized increased signal on long-TE–weighted or T2-weighted sequences (Fig. 2–30B, C).

Superficial Tendo-Achilles Bursitis

The superficial tendo-Achilles bursa is an adventitious bursa, which on the routine lateral view of the hindfoot, is a concavity posterior to the Achilles tendon insertion. An isolated inflammation of this bursa occurs secondary to focal irritation by the posterior shoe counter, and superficial tendo-

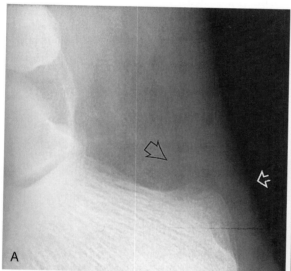

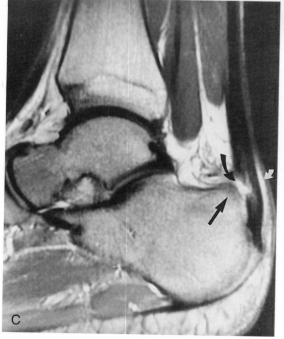

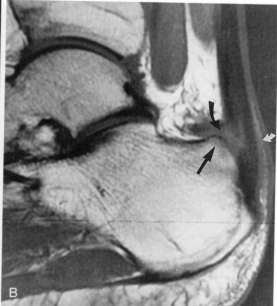

Figure 2–30. *A,* Retrocalcaneal bursitis is demonstrated by a loss of the normal radiolucent retrocalcaneal recess *(open black arrow)* between the bursal-calcaneal projection and the Achilles tendon. There is a normal superficial tendo-Achilles bursa *(open white arrow)*. Sagittal T1-weighted image through the hindfoot *(B)* demonstrates retrocalcaneal bursitis *(curved black arrow)* as well as superficial tendo-Achilles bursitis *(curved white arrow)*. Note the bony excrescence at the posterosuperior aspect of the calcaneus *(straight black arrow)*, indicating a prominent bursal projection. On the T2-weighted long TE magnetic resonance image *(C)*, the presence of fluid in the retrocalcaneal and superficial tendo-Achilles bursae is accentuated.

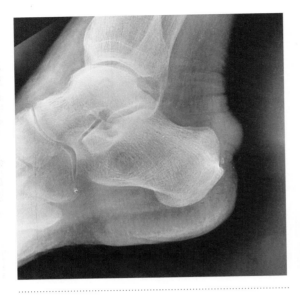

Figure 2–31. Lateral view of the hindfoot demonstrates an isolated superficial tendo-Achilles bursitis. The Achilles tendon and the retrocalcaneal recess are normal.

Achilles bursitis is diagnosed on the routine lateral view as a soft tissue convexity posterior to the Achilles tendon insertion (Fig. 2–31) and on MRI by localized increased signal in this area on the long-TE–weighted sequences.

Haglund's Disease Complex

A focal soft tissue swelling, a "pump bump" in the region of the Achilles tendon inser-tion, occurs in runners, tennis players, and golfers secondary to Achilles tendinitis, ret-rocalcaneal bursitis, or superficial tendo-Achilles bursitis. Each of these conditions can exist as an isolated condition or in com-bination. Haglund's disease is a complex of findings, including retrocalcaneal bursitis, superficial tendo-Achilles bursitis, Achilles tendinitis, and a prominent bursal-calca-neal projection (Fig. 2–32).[111, 112] The bursal-calcaneal projection refers to the postero-superior portion of the calcaneus, which, when prominent, contributes to irritation of the retrocalcaneal soft tissues as they are squeezed against the posterior shoe counter. A large medial plantar calcaneal tuberosity increases the calcaneal pitch and effective prominence of the calcaneal projection. Sev-eral radiographic measurements of the post-erosuperior calcaneus have been described, including the parallel pitch lines,[112] the su-perior calcaneal angle,[113] and other angles measured on a weight-bearing lateral radio-graph.[114, 115] The parallel pitch lines are two lines: a plantar base line drawn tangent to the medial and anterior tuberosities of the calcaneus and a second line drawn parallel to this base line at the perpendicular dis-tance of the talar articulation. The normal bursal-calcaneal projection lies below the top parallel pitch line; a prominent or clini-cally relevant bony projection extends above the top line (Fig. 2–33). Conservative treat-ment for Haglund's disease complex is a shoe wedge to decrease the calcaneal pitch and effective prominence of the bony projec-

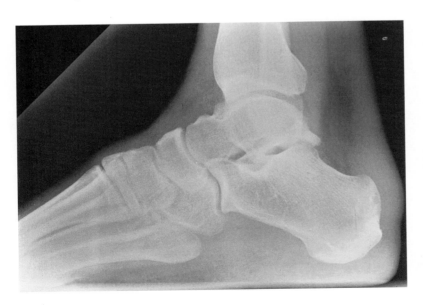

Figure 2–32. Lateral view of the hindfoot demonstrates clas-sic Haglund's disease complex with superficial tendo-Achilles bursitis identified by convexity of the soft tissue superficial to the Achilles tendon, loss of the normal radiolucent retrocalca-neal recess consistent with ret-rocalcaneal bursitis, thickening of the Achilles tendon, and a prominent bursal projection.

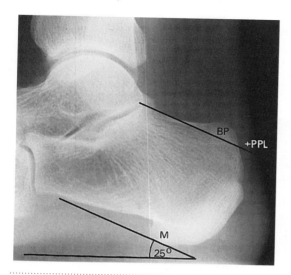

Figure 2–33. Parallel pitch lines (PPL) identify a prominent bursal projection. The lines are drawn as a baseline along the plantar aspect of the foot tangential to the medial (M) and anterior tuberosities and a second line drawn parallel to the baseline at the perpendicular distance at the talar articulation. The bursal projection (BP) is prominent, projecting above the top line.

tion. When conservative treatment is ineffective, the bony bursal projection is removed. The absence of calcaneal abnormalities in a patient with retrocalcaneal soft tissue findings is more suggestive of a systemic inflammatory disease such as rheumatoid arthritis or Reiter's syndrome.[112] In children, retrocalcaneal bursitis can present as localized pain characterized radiographically with increased calcaneal apophysis radiopacity and possible fragmentation and loss of definition of the retrocalcaneal recess without associated superficial soft tissue swelling or Achilles tendon thickening. These findings characterize localized retrocalcaneal bursitis; the increased radiopacity of the calcaneal apophysis is normal, indicates normal ambulation, and should not be misdiagnosed as bone necrosis.[116]

Plantar Lateral Symptoms

Os Peroneum Syndrome

The os peroneum is a sesamoid in the peroneus longus tendon. The painful os peroneum syndrome identifies a spectrum of plantar lateral mid- to hindfoot pain, including an acute os peroneum fracture or diasta-

sis, partial or complete rupture, or attrition of the peroneus longus tendon.[117] Injuries to the peroneus longus tendon or a fracture of the os peroneum or cuboid injury may present with pain or a sensation of walking on a pea (Fig. 2–34A, B). Elongation of the os peroneum suggests an old peroneus longus tendon injury (Fig. 2–34C).[117] Evaluation of patients with plantar lateral foot pain should include an oblique radiograph of the foot to best visualize the os peroneum and cuboid. Radionuclide bone scan, with a plantar image, may be useful in acute injury to document isotope uptake in the os peroneum versus the cuboid. An enlarged calcaneal peroneal tubercle can cause entrapment of the os peroneum or the peroneus longus tendon and may contribute to attrition of the tendon. The calcaneal peroneal tubercle can be assessed on the Harris (axial) view of the calcaneus, CT, or MRI (Fig. 2–34D, E). The tendons are best assessed on MRI (see Fig. 2–16A). In addition to attrition or disruption, the peroneal tendons may dislocate anteriorly with avulsion of the overlying peroneal retinaculum. Given the clinical setting of plantar lateral pain, an MRI evaluation is indicated.[117]

Medial Symptoms

Posterior Tibial Tendon Injuries

Rupture of the posterial tibial tendon presents with pain and swelling along the course of the tendon from the medial malleolus to the navicular bone. The posterior tibial tendon is subject to chronic mechanical pressure in runners, skaters, and skiers secondary to excessive pronation. Chronic ruptures of the posterial tibial tendon occur primarily in the middle-aged to elderly (fifth to the sixth decade) female patient and is associated with complaints of progressive painful flatfoot and hindfoot valgus.[52, 108–122] Acute onset of symptoms usually occurs in younger individuals and is associated with seronegative inflammatory disease.[121]

The most common site for rupture of the posterior tibial tendon is the level of the medial malleolus, where forces are exerted to maintain the longitudinal arch during walking, and just distal to the medial malleolus, where there is hypovascularity predisposing the tendon to injury. Diagnosis can be suggested on both radionuclide bone scan and MRI (Fig. 2–35A–D). On MRI there is

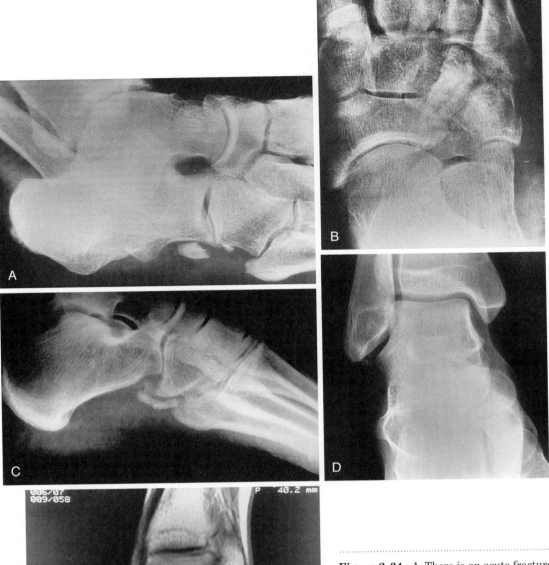

Figure 2–34. *A,* There is an acute fracture with distraction of the os peroneum. *B,* Comminuted fracture of the cuboid. *C,* There is elongation of the os peroneum attributed to chronic attrition of the peroneus longus tendon. *D,* Frontal view of the hindfoot and ankle demonstrates a prominent peroneal tubercle. *E,* Coronal magnetic resonance image through the calcaneus demonstrates a prominent peroneal bursal projection *(arrow)* as it abuts the peroneal tendons.

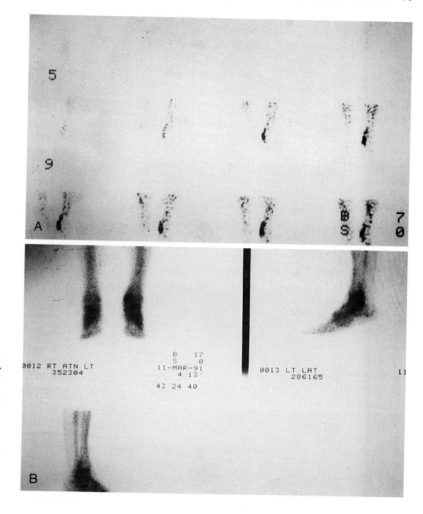

Figure 2–35. A partial tear of the posterior tibial tendon is diagnosed on radionuclide bone scan and magnetic resonance (MR) image. Dynamic flow sequences *(A)* and blood flow scans *(B)* demonstrate increased vascularity in the medial aspect of the left ankle.

Illustration continued on following page

a normal heterogeneous signal at the insertion of the tendon on the navicular bone.[44, 57, 59, 60] An abnormal tendon may be thickened and round instead of oval secondary to edema, hemorrhage, and scarring and may also have increased signal secondary to longitudinal splits or edema. Fluid within the tendon sheath suggests a partial tear (see Fig. 2–35D). A thick tendon with increased signal is usually seen after years of symptoms and tendon discontinuity; retraction is seen with a complete tear.[122]

Plantar Symptoms

Calcaneal Stress Fracture

Calcaneal stress fractures frequently occur in military recruits and in basketball players and other athletes involved in jumping sports.[123] The classic cancellous stress frac-

ture (linear radiopacity oriented perpendicular to the trabeculae) is diagnosed on plain films and even earlier on MRI by a linear signal void with surrounding edema (see Fig. 2–10C–E).[1, 30, 123, 124]

Calcaneal Spur and Plantar Fasciitis

The plantar fascia is a fibrous aponeurosis that stretches when the toes are extended. Plantar fasciitis is an inflammation or degeneration of the plantar fascia at its attachment to the medial calcaneal tuberosity, which produces exquisite pain during heel strike and occurs secondary to repetitive stress and trauma (e.g., in runners, tennis players, basketball players, and dancers).[125–128] A lateral routine radiograph of the foot may demonstrate distortion of soft tissue planes or periostitis.[8] In chronic cases, a traction exostosis of the medial

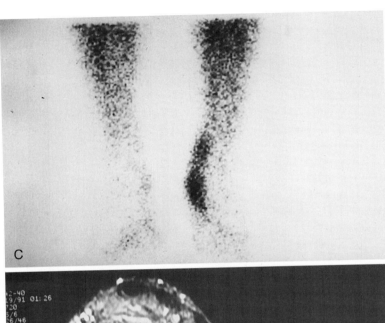

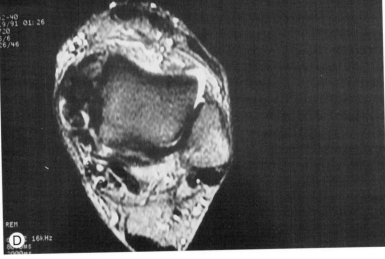

Figure 2–35 *Continued.* Delayed static scan *(C)* shows mild increased uptake in the medial aspect of the right ankle. The MR axial T2-weighted image *(D)* demonstrates increased signal in the posterior tibial tendon with fluid in the tendon sheath consistent with a partial tear.

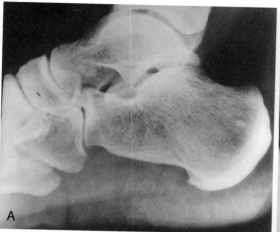

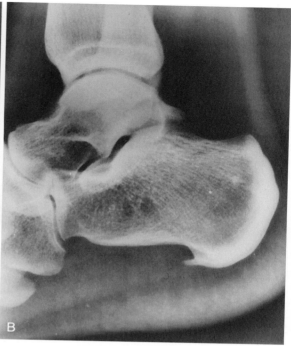

Figure 2–36. Lateral view of the foot *(A)* demonstrates a small plantar spur *B,* Same patient 5 years later demonstrates elongation of the plantar spur secondary to traction of the plantar aponeurosis on the medial tuberosity.

calcaneal tuberosity, a plantar spur, may form, which is evident on plain films (Fig. 2–36*A, B*). The plantar spur can fracture (Fig. 2–37).[2] The soft tissues inferior to the medial tuberosity or calcaneal spur when thickened and inflamed are typically responsible for the patient's pain. Calcification within the fascia or in the soft tissues infe-

rior to the spur are also associated with symptoms (Fig. 2–38*A, B*).

A three-phase radionuclide bone scan has been shown to be useful in diagnosing plantar fasciitis and in distinguishing this entity from other causes of heel pain.[129] Classically, blood pool images will demonstrate a linear focus of increased radiotracer uptake in the medial plantar aspect of the calcaneus. On static images, a more focal area of increased activity is seen on the inferior surface of the calcaneus anteriorly (Fig. 2–39*A–C*).[2] On MRI, the normal fascia has low signal intensity and measures 2 to 4 mm in sagittal and coronal planes; fasciitis is diagnosed by intermediate signal with increased fusiform girth of 6 to 10 mm (Fig. 2–40).[125]

Fluffy proliferative changes on the plantar spur or medial tuberosity are often associated with diffuse idiopathic skeletal hyperostosis or with Reiter's syndrome and occurs in younger individuals and is usually bilateral.

Plantar fibromatosis or benign fibrotic proliferation in the plantar fascia is nodular and has no communication to the calcaneus.[130] Plantar fibromatosis will be seen as nodular areas within the fascia, isointense to muscle on MR imaging.[130]

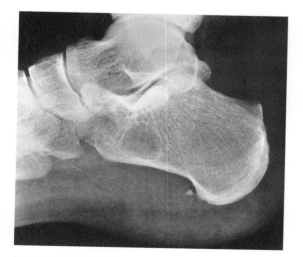

Figure 2–37. Lateral view of the calcaneus demonstrates a fracture of the plantar spur.

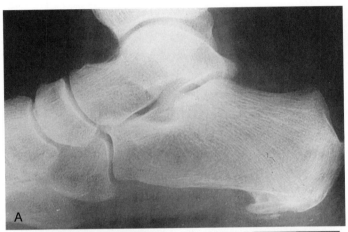

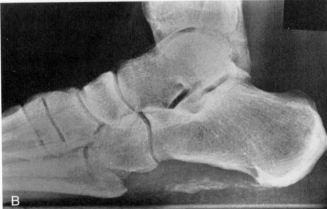

Figure 2–38. *A,* Lateral view of the hindfoot demonstrates a large plantar spur with calcification of soft tissues inferior to the plantar spur. *B,* There is extensive calcification in the plantar aponeurosis as it attaches to the medial tuberosity of the calcaneus.

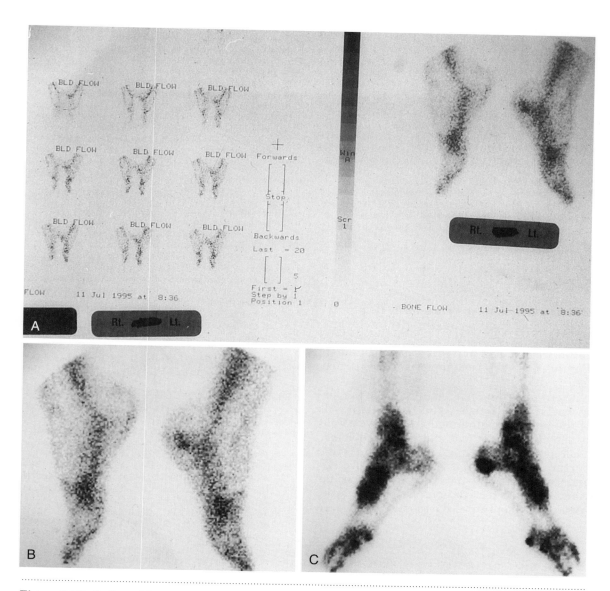

Figure 2–39. Radionuclide demonstration of plantar fasciitis as identified on dynamic flow *(A)* and blood flow *(B)* scans by increased vascularity in the plantar aspect of the calcaneus. On the delayed static images *(C)*, there is high uptake in the plantar aspect of the calcaneus on the left.

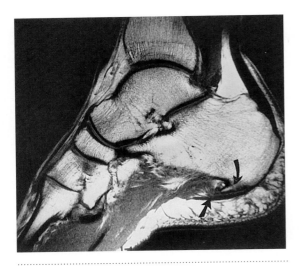

Figure 2–40. Sagittal T1-weighted magnetic resonance image demonstrates a plantar calcaneal spur *(curved arrow)* and thickening and increased signal at the insertion of the plantar fascia *(straight arrow)*, indicating plantar fasciitis.

SUMMARY

The foot and ankle are constantly being subjected to trauma, ranging from normal walking activities to the excessive forces encountered in the active sport enthusiast. Painful feet can be temporarily or permanently disabling. Early, expedited, and cost-efficient diagnosis is a challenge for the clinician, the radiologist, and the patient. All of the major imaging modalities have a role in the diagnosis of foot and ankle problems. The suspected clinical diagnosis is important to determine the appropriate sequence of imaging modalities, the specific views, and correct patient positioning and sequences to optimize diagnostic yield.

REFERENCES

1. Daffner R, Pavlov H. Stress fracture: current concepts. AJR Am J Roentgenol 159:245, 1992.
2. Pavlov H. Imaging of the foot and ankle. Radiol Clin North Am 28:991, 1990.
3. Kier R, McCarthy S, Dietz MJ, et al. MR appearance of painful conditions of the ankle. Radiographics 11:401, 1991.
4. Beltran J, Noto AM, Herman LG, et al. Joint effusions: MR imaging. Radiology 158:133, 1986.
5. Anzilotti K, Schweitzer ME, Hecht P, et al. Effect of foot and ankle MR imaging on clinical decision making. Radiology 201:515, 1996.
6. Rubin A, Sallis R. Evaluation and diagnosis of ankle injuries. Am Fam Physician 54:1609, 1996.
7. Norfray LF, Rogers LF, Adams GP, et al. Common calcaneal avulsion fracture. AJR Am J Roentgenol 134:119, 1980.
8. Byers GE, Benquist T. Radiology of sports related injuries. Curr Probl Diagn Radiol 25:1, 1996.
9. Clark TWI, Janzen DL, Ho K, et al. Detection of radiographically occult ankle fractures following acute trauma: positive predictive value of ankle effusion. Am J Radiol 164:1185, 1985.
10. Clark TW, Janzen DL, Logan PM, et al. Improving the detection of radiographically occult ankle fractures: positive predictive value of an ankle joint effusion. Clin Radiol 51:632, 1996.
11. Moss EH, Carty H. Scintigraphy in the diagnosis of occult fractures of the calcaneus. Skeletal Radiol 19:575, 1990.
12. Zeiss J, Ebraheim N, Rusin J, Coombs RJ. MR imaging of the calcaneus: normal anatomy and application in calcaneal fractures. Foot Ankle Int 11:264, 1991.
13. Crosby LA, Fitzgibbons T. CT scanning of acute intra-articular fractures of the calcaneus. J Bone Joint Surg Am 72:852, 1990.
14. Cave EF. Fractures of the os calcis—the problem in general. Clin Orthop 30:64, 1963.
15. Lowery RB, Calhoun J. Fractures of the calcaneus. Part I: Anatomy, injury mechanism, and classification. Foot Ankle Int 17:230, 1996.
16. Canale ST, Kelly FB. Fractures of the neck of the talus. J Bone Joint Surg Am 60:143, 1978.
17. Inokuchi SI, Ogasawa K, Usami N, Hashimoto T. Long-term follow up of the talus fractures. Orthopaedics 19:477, 1996.
18. Inokuchi SI, Ogasawa K, Usami N. Classification of fractures of the talus: clear differentiation between neck and body fractures. Foot Ankle Int 17:758, 1996.
19. Frawley P, Hart J, Young D. Treatment outcome of major fractures of the talus. Foot Ankle Int 16:339, 1995.
20. Renfrew DL, El-Khoury GY. Anterior process fractures of the calcaneous. Skeletal Radiol 14:121, 1985.
21. Jones R. Fracture of the base of the 5th metatarsal bone by indirect violence. Am Surg 35:697, 1902.
22. Zelko RR, Torg JS, Rachun A. Proximal diaphyseal fractures of the 5th metatarsal: treatment of the fractures and their complications in athletes. Am J Sports Med 7:95, 1979.
23. Torg JS, Balduini FC, Zelko RR, et al. Fractures of the base of the 5th metatarsal distal to the tuberosity. J Bone Joint Surg Am 66:209, 1984.
24. Lehman RC, Torg JS, Pavlov H, et al. Fractures of the base of the 5th metatarsal distal to the tuberosity: a review. Foot Ankle Int 7:245, 1987.
25. Devas M. Stress Fractures. New York: Churchill Livingstone, 1975.
26. Savoca CJ. Stress fractures: a classification of the earliest radiographic signs. Radiology 100:519, 1971.
27. Sweet DE, Allman RM. RPC of the month from the AFIP: stress fracture. Radiology 99:687, 1971.
28. Umans H, Pavlov H. Stress fractures of the lower extremities. Semin Roentgenol 29:176, 1994.
29. Stafford SA. MRI in stress fracture. AJR Am J Roentgenol 147:533, 1986.
30. Kier R. MR imaging of foot and ankle tumors. Magn Reson Imaging 11:149, 1993.

31. Schweitzer ME, Karasick D. MRI of the ankle and hindfoot. Semin Ultrasound CT MR 15:410, 1994.
32. Umans H, Pavlov H. Insufficiency fractures of the talus: diagnosis with MR imaging. Radiology 197:437, 1995.
33. Berndt AL, Harty M: Transchondral fractures (osteochondritis dissecans) of the talus. J Bone Joint Surg Am 41:988, 1959.
34. Newberg AH. Osteochondral fractures of the dome of the talus. Br J Radiol 52:105, 1979.
35. Milgram JW. Injury to articular cartilage joint surfaces: displaced fractures of underlying bone. Clin Orthop 206:236, 1986.
36. Milgram JW, Rodgers LS, Miller JW. Osteochondral fractures: mechanism of injury and fate of fragments. AJR Am J Roentgenol 130:651, 1978.
37. De Smet A, Fisher DR, Burnstein MI, et al. Value of MR imaging in staging osteochondral lesions of the talus (osteochondritis dissecans). AJR Am J Roentgenol 154:555, 1990.
38. Koenig SH, Sauter R, Deimling M, et al. Cartilage disorders: comparison of spin echo, CHESS and FLASH sequences MR images. Radiology 164:753, 1987.
39. Cass JR, Murray B. Ankle instability: current concepts, diagnosis, and treatment. Mayo Clin Proc 59:154, 1984.
40. Klein MA. MR imaging of the ankle: normal and abnormal findings in the medial collateral ligament. AJR Am J Roentgenol 162:377, 1994.
41. Beltran J, Munchow AM, Khabiri Hoonen K, et al. Ligaments of the lateral aspect of the ankle and sinus tarsi: an MR imaging study. Radiology 177:455, 1990.
42. Mesgarzadeh M. MRI of the ankle ligaments: emphasis on anatomy and injuries to lateral collateral ligaments. J Magn Reson Imaging 2:39, 1994.
43. Schneck CD, Mesgarzadeh M, Bonakdarpour A, et al. MR imaging of the most commonly injured ankle ligaments. Part 1. Normal anatomy. Radiology 184:499, 1992.
44. Noto AM, Cheun Y, Rosenberg ZS, et al. MR imaging of the ankle: normal variants. Radiology 170:121, 1989.
45. Candone BW, Erickson SJ, Den Hartog BD, et al. MRI of injury to lateral collateral ligamentous complex of the ankle. J Comput Assist Tomogr 17:102, 1993.
46. Kaye JJ. The ankle. In Freiberger RH, Kaye JJ, eds. Arthrography. New York: Appleton-Century-Crofts, 1979, p 237.
47. Erickson SJ, Smith JW, Ruiz ME, et al. MR imaging of the lateral collateral ligament of the ankle. AJR Am J Roentgenol 156:131, 1991.
48. Meyer JM, Garcia J, Hoffmeier P, et al. The subtalar sprain: a roentgenographic study. Clin Orthop 226:169, 1988.
49. Henry HJ, Anderson J, Cothren CC. Tibiofibular synostosis in professional basketball players. Am J Sports Med 21:619, 1993.
50. Bassett FH, Gates HS, Billys JB, et al. Talar impingement by the anterior inferior tibiofibular ligament. J Bone Joint Surg Am 72:55, 1990.
51. Gilula LA, Plo HL, Casuti RL, et al. Ankle tenography: a key for unexplained symptomatology: II. Diagnosis of chronic tendon disabilities. Radiology 151:581, 1984.
52. Jahss MH. Spontaneous rupture of the tibialis posterior tendon: clinical findings, tenographic studies, and a new technique of repair. Foot Ankle Int 3:158, 1982.
53. Kneeland JB, Macrander SJ, Middleton WD, et al. MR imaging of the normal ankle: correlation with anatomic sections. AJR Am J Roentgenol 151:117, 1988.
54. Beltran J, Noto AM, Herman LF, et al. Tendons: highfield strength, surface coil MR imaging. Radiology 162:735, 1987.
55. Daffner RH, Reimer BL, Lupetin AR, et al. Magnetic resonance imaging in acute tendon ruptures. Skeletal Radiol 15:619, 1986.
56. Alexander IJ, Johnson KA, Berquist TH. Magnetic resonance imaging in the diagnosis of disruption of the posterior tibial tendon. Foot Ankle Int 8:144, 1987.
57. Schweitzer ME, Caccese R, Karasick D, et al. Posterior tibial tendon tears: utility of secondary signs for MRI diagnosis. Radiology 188:655, 1993.
58. Schweitzer ME, van Leersum M, Ehrlich SS, et al. Fluid in normal and abnormal ankle joints: amount and distribution as seen on MR images. AJR Am J Roentgenol 162:111, 1994.
59. Erickson SJ, Cox IH, Hyde JS, et al. Effect of tendon orientation on MR imaging signal intensity: a manifestation of the "magic" angle phenomenon. Radiology 181:389, 1991.
60. Link SC, Erickson SJ, Timins ME. MR imaging of the ankle and foot: normal structures and anatomic variants that may simulate disease. AJR Am J Roentgenol 161:607, 1993.
61. Pavlov H. Ankle and subtalar arthrography. Clin Sports Med 1:47, 1982.
62. O'Connor DL. Sinus tarsi syndrome: a clinical entity. J Bone Joint Surg Am 40:720, 1958.
63. Klein MA, Spreitzer AM. MR imaging of the tarsal sinus and canal: normal anatomy, pathologic finds and features of the sinus tarsal syndrome. Radiology 186:233, 1993.
64. Taillard W, Meyer JM, Farcia J, et al. The sinus tarsi syndrome. J Orthop 5:117, 1981.
65. Finkel JE. Tarsal tunnel syndrome. Magn Reson Imaging Clin North Am 2:67, 1994.
66. Keck CL. The tarsal tunnel syndrome. J Bone Joint Surg Am 44:180, 1962.
67. Lam SJS. A tarsal tunnel syndrome. Lancet 2:1354, 1962.
68. Myerson M, Soffer S. Lipoma as an etiology of the tarsal tunnel syndrome: a report of two cases. Foot Ankle Int 10:176, 1990.
69. Kerr R, Frey C. MR imaging in tarsal tunnel syndrome. J Comput Assist Tomogr 15:280, 1991.
70. Kulkarni MV, Drolshagen LF, Kaye JJ, et al. MR imaging of hemophilic arthropathy. J Comput Assist Tomogr 10:449, 1986.
71. Yulish BS, Lieberman SM, Strandjord SE. Hemophilic arthropathy: assessment with MR imaging. Radiology 164:759, 1987.
72. Thould AK, Simon G. Assessment of radiological changes in hands and feet in rheumatoid arthritis. Ann Rheum Dis 25:220, 1966.
73. Tang JSH, Gold RH, Bassett LW, et al. Musculoskeletal infections of the extremities: evaluation with MR imaging. Radiology 166:205, 1988.
74. Goldman AB, Katz MC, Freiberger FH. Post-traumatic adhesive capsulitis of the ankle. Arthrographic diagnosis. AJR Am J Roentgenol 127:535, 1976.
75. Evans JA. Reflex sympathetic dystrophy: a report of 57 cases. Ann Intern Med 26:417, 1947.

76. Mitchell SW, Morehouse JR, Keen WW. Gunshot Wounds and Other Injuries of Nerves. Philadelphia: J. B. Lippincott, 1864.

77. Mitchell SW. Injuries of Nerves and Their Consequences. Philadelphia: J. B. Lippincott, 1872.

78. Lenggenhager K. Sudeck's osteodystrophy: its pathogenesis, prophylaxis and therapy. Minn Med 54:967, 1971.

79. Fontaine R, Hermann L. Post traumatic painful osteoporosis. Ann Surg 97:26, 1933.

80. DeTakats G. Reflex dystrophy of the extremeties. Arch Surg 34:939, 1937.

81. Kozin F, Genant H, Bekerman C, McCarty DJ. The reflex sympathetic dystrophy syndrome. Roentgenographic and scintigraphic evidence of bilateral and of peri-articular accentuation. Am J Med 60:332, 1976.

82. Genant HK, Kozin F, Bekerman C, McCarty DJ, Sims J. The reflex sympathetic dystrophy syndrome. A comprehensive analysis using fine-detail radiography, photon absorptometry and bone and joint scintigraphy. Radiology 117:21, 1975.

83. Simoi H, Carlson DH. The use of bone scanning in the diagnosis of reflex sympathetic dystrophy. Clin Nucl Med 5:116, 1980.

84. Kransdorf JD, Jelinek JS, Moser RP Jr, et al. Soft-tissue masses: diagnosis using MR imaging. AJR Am J Roentgenol 153:541, 1989.

85. Berquist TH, Ehman RL, King BF, et al. Value of MR imaging in differentiating benign from malignant soft-tissue masses: study of 95 lesions. AJR Am J Roentgenol 155:1251, 1990.

86. Crim JR, Seeger LL, Yao L, et al. Diagnosis of soft-tissue masses with MR imaging: can benign masses be differentiated from malignant ones. Radiology 185:581, 1992.

87. Ehrlich MG, Elmer EB. Tarsal coalition. In Jahss M, ed. Disorders of the Foot and Ankle, ed 2. Philadelphia: W. B. Saunders, 1991:921.

88. Lee MS, Harcke HT, Kumar SJ, et al. Subtalar joint coalition in children: new observations. Radiology 172:635, 1989.

89. Beckley DE, Anderson PW, Pedegana LR. The radiology of the subtalar joint with special reference to talocalcaneal coalition. Clin Radiol 26:333, 1975.

90. Cowell HR, Elener V. Rigid painful flatfoot secondary to tarsal coalition. Clin Orthop 177:54, 1983.

91. Oestreich AE, Mize WA, Crawford AH, Morgan RC. The "anteater nose": a direct sign of calcaneonavicular coalition on the lateral radiograph. J Pediatr Orthop 7:709, 1987.

92. Lateur LM, Van Hoe LR, Van Ghillewe KV, et al. Subtalar coalition: diagnosis with the C sign on lateral radiograph of the ankle. Radiology 193:847, 1994.

93. Shaffer HA, Harrison RB. Tarsal pseudo-coalition—a positional artifact. J Can Assoc Radiol 31:236, 1980.

94. Goldman AB, Pavlov H, Schneider R. Radionuclide bone scanning in subtalar coalitions: differential considerations. AJR Am J Roentgenol 138:427, 1982.

95. Wechsler RJ, Schweitzer ME, Deely DM, et al. Tarsal coalition: depiction and characterization with CT and MR imaging. Radiology 193:447, 1994.

96. Kulik SA, Clanton TO. Tarsal coalition. Foot Ankle Int 17:286, 1996.

97. Lawson JP. Clinically significant radiologic anatomic variants of the skeleton. AJR Am J Roentgen 163:249, 1994.

98. Johnson RP, Collier BD, Carrera GF. Os trigonum syndrome: use of bone scan in the diagnosis. J Trauma 24:761, 1984.

99. Karasick D, Schweitzer ME. The os trigonum syndrome: imaging features. AJR Am J Roentgenol 166:125, 1996.

100. Wakeley CJ, Johnson DP, Watt I. The value of MR imaging in diagnosis of os trigonum syndrome. Skeletal Radiol 25:133, 1996.

101. Quinn SF, Murray WT, Clark RA, et al. Achilles tendon: MR imaging at 1.5T. Radiology 164:767, 1987.

102. Marcus DS, Reider MA, Kellerhouse LE. Achilles tendon injuries: the role of MR imaging. J Comput Assist Tomogr 13:480, 1989.

103. Biel CL, Nirsche RP, Grant EG. Achilles tendon: US diagnosis of pathologic conditions. Radiology 159:765, 1986.

104. Fornage BD. Achilles tendon examination: US examination. Radiology 159:759, 1986.

105. Mathieson JR, Connell DG, Cooperberg PL, et al. Sonography of the Achilles tendon and adjacent bursae. AJR Am J Roentgenol 151:127, 1988.

106. Leekram RN, Salsberg BB, Bogoch E, et al. Sonographic diagnosis of partial Achilles tendon rupture and healing. J Ultrasound Med 5:115, 1986.

107. Kirsch MD, Erickson SJ. Normal magnetic resonance imaging of the ankle and foot. Magn Reson Imaging Clin North Am 2:1, 1994.

108. Rosenberg ZS, Cheung Y, Jahss MH. Computed tomography scan overview. Foot Ankle Int 8:297, 1988.

109. Chandani VP, Bradley YC. Achilles tendon and miscellaneous tendon lesions. Magn Reson Imaging Clin North Am 2:89, 1994.

110. Ekstrom JE, Shuman WP, Mack LA. MR imaging of accessory soleus muscle. J Comput Assist Tomogr 14:239, 1990.

111. Haglund P. Beitrag zur Klinik der Achillessehne. Z Orthop Chir 49:49, 1927.

112. Pavlov H, Heneghan MA, Hersh A, et al. Haglund's deformity: diagnosis and differential diagnosis of posterior heel pain. Radiology 144:83, 1982.

113. Stephens M. Haglund's deformity and retrocalcaneal bursitis. Orthop Clin North Am 25:41, 1994.

114. Fowler A, Philip JF. Abnormality of the calcaneus as a cause of painful heel: its diagnosis and operative treatment. Br J Surg 32:494, 1945.

115. Chauveaux D, Liet P, et al. A new radiologic measurement for diagnosis of Haglund's deformity. Surg Radiol Anat 13:39, 1991.

116. Heneghan MA, Wallace T. Heel pain due to retrocalcaneal bursitis: radiographic diagnosis. Pediatr Radiol 15:119, 1985.

117. Sobel M, Pavlov H, Geppert MD, et al. Painful os peroneum syndrome: a spectrum of post traumatic conditions responsible for plantar lateral foot pain. Foot Ankle Int 15:112, 1994.

118. Funk DA, Cass JR, Johnson KA. Acquired adult flat foot secondary to posterior tibial tendon pathology. J Bone Joint Surg Am 68:95, 1986.

119. Rosenberg ZS, Cheung Y, Jahss MH, et al. Rupture of posterior tibial tendon: CT and MR imaging with surgical correlation. Radiology 169:229, 1988.

120. Monto RR, Moorman CT, Mallon WJ, et al. Rupture of the posterior tibial tendon associated with closed ankle fracture. Foot Ankle Int 11:400, 1991.
121. Woods L, Leach RE. Posterior tibial tendon rupture in athletic people. Am J Sports Med 19:495, 1991.
122. Rosenberg ZS. Chronic rupture of posterior tibial tendon. Magn Reson Imag Clin North Am 2:79, 1994.
123. Hullinger CW. Insufficiency fracture of the calcaneus. J Bone Joint Surg Am 26:751, 1944.
124. Erickson SJ, Quinn SF, Kneeland JB, et al. MR imaging of the tarsal tunnel and related spaces. Normal and abnormal findings with anatomic correlation. AJR Am J Roentgenol 155:323, 1990.
125. Berkowitz JF, Kier R, Rudicel S. Plantar fasciitis: MR imaging. Radiology 179:665, 1991.
126. Kwong PK, Kay D, Voner RT. Plantar fasciitis: mechanics and pathomechanics of treatment. Foot and ankle injuries. Clin Sports Med 7:119, 1988.
127. Leach R, Jones R, Silva T. Rupture of the plantar fascia in athletes. J Bone Joint Surg Am 60:537, 1978.
128. Furey JG. Plantar fasciitis: the painful heel syndrome. J Bone Joint Surg Am 57:672, 1975.
129. Intenzo CM, Wapner KL, Park CH, et al. Evaluation of plantar faciitis by three phase bone scintigraphy. Clin Nucl Med 16:325, 1991.
130. Lee JK, Yao L. Stress fractures: MR imaging. Radiology 169:217, 1988.

3 Ultrasound Imaging of the Ankle and Rearfoot

Robert L. Bard

ULTRASOUND SCANNING PRINCIPLES

State-of-the-art musculoskeletal ultrasound imaging requires frequencies at least 5 MHz and specially designed and focused linear array transducers. The small anatomic ankle and foot structures and superficial locations are best examined with probes greater than 10 MHz in frequency. The higher the scanning frequency, the poorer is the sound penetration. This results in improved resolution, but loss of distal information may occur when scanning deeper structures such as the bursae subtendinea and the triceps surae muscle when examining the Achilles tendon in the standard ultrasound scanning planes. Linear probes, as contrasted with sector scanners, better outline the course of tendons, which are most often aligned in straight paths. Also, sector scanners produce bright echoes at the center of the image and fewer echoes at the periphery. A stand-off pad may sometimes be used to insonate the subcutaneous structures. Comparison with the opposite side is possible and usually helpful in diagnosis. Cysts or fluid-filled areas are without internal echoes and are called echo free. Solid regions have internal echoes and are classified as echo poor or hypoechoic if there are few internal echoes. The term echogenic or hyperechoic is used if there are many internal echoes. The skin of the foot appears highly echogenic as do the bony structures. Bone, air, foreign bodies, and calcification stop the transmission of sound waves, producing a "sonic shadow," which is a dark region distal to the echogenic obstructing region. The term *acoustical shadowing* is also used to describe the low or absent echoes associated with these lesions. *Acoustic window* refers to an optimal placing of the transducers so that the areas of interest are clearly imaged.

COMPARISON WITH COMPUTED TOMOGRAPHY AND MAGNETIC RESONANCE IMAGING

As with any imaging modality, transverse and longitudinal scans or any set of orthogonal planes are obtained to produce a three-dimensional representation of abnormalities. Sonography is a dynamic study permitting physiologic real-time observation of an anatomic region. Subluxations of peroneal tendons may be diagnosed dynamically. Unlike with computed tomography (CT) and magnetic resonance imaging (MRI), metal prostheses and postsurgical metallic clips are not a major hindrance, because alternative scan planes can be used to look for these devices. The magic angle effect noted in curving tendons is not present. Haziness from vaguely increased signal as a result of the specific MRI partial volume effect of the surrounding fat is common in the peroneal tendons. In particular, the partial volume effect of the cortical bone of the malleolus may make imaging of the more anteriorly located peroneus brevis more difficult. Likewise, the dark bands of MRI signal-less retinacula may be inseparable from tendon with MRI, although the retinaculum is an echogenic structure with ultrasound and readily separable during scanning.[1] Similarly, peritendineum of the Achilles tendon that appears as an echo-poor or echo-free space on sonography cannot be distinguished on the MRI scan as a distinct structure.[2] Intra-articular loose bodies have various MRI signals. Mature marrow fat will have high signal. Heavily calcified bodies are often dark on all imaging sequences. Chondral and soft tissue areas often have intermediate signals.[3] Ultrasound distinguishes easily between calcific and non-calcific regions because of the bright signals produced by the highly reflective calcium and bony entity. Errors resulting from MRI and CT positioning may also be avoided by sonography. For example, a low-lying belly of the muscular peroneus brevis so that it lies within the fibular groove is said to increase the risk of peroneus brevis tendon rupture or dislocation. A 1997 report shows that this anatomic occurrence may occur in dorsiflexion of the foot during examination.[4] The dynamic nature of sonograms often prevents misinterpretation as a result of anatomic positioning. Additionally, sonography by its real-time dynamic nature permits full-length imaging of the posterior tibial tendon, peroneal tendons, and fibulocalcaneal ligament, which are difficult to visualize in total course by standard MRI sequences and planes.[5]

However, use of ultra-high-frequency probes limits penetration of the sound beam. Examination of a pathologically enlarged Achilles tendon with a 12- to 15-MHz probe may result in poor penetration of the sound waves to the deeper pre-Achilles fat pad, the bursae subtendinea, and the triceps surae muscle.[2] Likewise, a lower extremity that is edematous as a result of lymphedema, heart failure, and similar causes of limb swelling could limit tendon imaging (Fig. 3–1). In these cases, MRI examination provides better anatomic detail. MRI also affords a panoramic view, which is easier for the surgeon to use. The deeper structures or superficial regions that lie deep to the skin surface as a result of overlying edema, tumor, or hematoma may be imaged with lower frequency transducers offering greater penetration of the sound beams. Imaging from the side that is closer

to the structure of interest is also possible to avoid degradation of the high-frequency images as a result of excessive distance parameters.

The examiner should look for normal variants and other pathologic processes associated with any abnormal finding. For example, in tears of the peroneus brevis tendon, ruptures of the lateral collateral ligaments, stripping of the superior peroneal retinaculum, peroneal longus subluxations, and low-lying muscle bellies of the peroneus brevis and peroneus quartus may be concomitantly identified. Bony pathologies such as abnormally curved surfaces or osteophytes and avulsion-type microfractures may similarly be discovered. Patient comfort is another important consideration that makes sonograms preferable as a diagnostic procedure. Infants or uncooperative patients may be accurately scanned with real-time units, providing instantaneous data. Indeed, children may be held in their mother's arms. If necessary, portable equipment may be brought to the bedside or nursing home. Because scan times with low-strength MRI units may exceed one-half hour, the rapidity of ultrasound examination for the elderly provides a significant positive patient compliance factor. Claustrophobia does not occur as a problem either. Other imaging methods are cited here for completeness. Tenography[6] technique is highly examiner dependent and is so specialized that it does not fall within the scope of this chapter. Light scanning, also known as fiberoptic transillumination or diaphanography, is discussed later.[7–10]

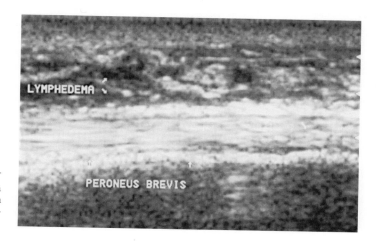

Figure 3–1. Increased distance from skin to peroneus brevis tendon resulting from lymphedema could decrease high-frequency sound penetration.

SONOGRAPHY OF TENDONS

Normal Anatomy

The imaged anatomy of normal tendons depends on the frequency and angulation of the transducer applied to the structure. The probes from 5 to 10 MHz usually show internal linear echogenic bands regularly alternating with echo-poor areas within the tendon, whereas higher frequency probes (11–20 MHz) will demonstrate many more and thinner echogenic bandlike regions. These correspond to the parallel alignment of the regularly arranged collagen fiber bundles. Angulation of the probe to an oblique incidence of the sound beam will cause the tendon to lose the internal echogenic step-ladder architecture and appear echo free in certain cases. This is due to the normal anisotropic nature of sound in tendon. This seeming artifact is used to diagnostic advantage when examining pathology that may simulate a tendon. The absence of disappearance of internal echoes during angulation maneuvers suggests that the structure is other than tendinous in nature[11] (Fig. 3–2).

Achilles Tendon

The Achilles tendon is a confluence of the individual tendons of the gastrocnemius and the soleus muscles. In the ankle, the tendon lies immediately beneath the skin and subcutaneous tissues. The most common variety of formation is two thirds from

Table 3–1. Table of Normal Values (Greatest Anteroposterior Diameter)

Structure	Males (mm)	Females (mm)
Achilles tendon	6.9	5.2
Posterior tibial tendon	3.7	3.7
Flexor digitorum longus tendon	4.8	4.8
Flexor hallucis longus tendon	4.9	4.9
Anterior tibial tendon	5.1	5.0
Peroneus brevis tendon	3.9	3.9
Peroneus longus tendon	4.1	4.1
Plantar fascia	4.0	4.0

the gastrocnemius and one third from the soleus. The fibers twist about 6 cm proximal to the calcaneal insertion, which is also a hypovascular region, accounting for the majority of ruptures at this anatomic site. The anteroposterior (AP) diameter of the tendon is less than 6.9 mm in normal males and less than 5.2 mm in normal females (Table 3–1). The distal surface is flat to slightly concave anteriorly, although the distal tendon near its calcaneal insertion assumes a more ovoid and anteriorly flattened shape, assuming a width that is twice the size of the AP diameter. The edges are rounded, and the tendon is 10 to 15 cm in length. The muscle fibers at the musculotendinous junction appear linear and hypoechoic and must be distinguished from a tear. Dorsal to the tendon is the hypoechoic Kager's fat (Fig. 3–3). Deeper yet is the flexor hallucis longus muscle. Pathology in both these

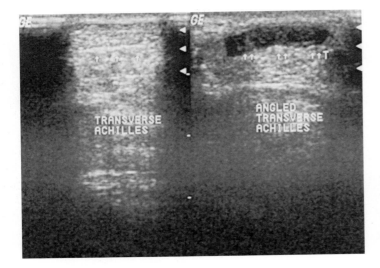

Figure 3–2. *Left,* Transverse scan of Achilles tendon *(arrows)*; perpendicular scan plane shows echogenic nature of fibrillar structure. *Right,* Cephalic angulation shows echo-poor echo pattern indicative of anisotropic effect of scanning *(double arrows).*

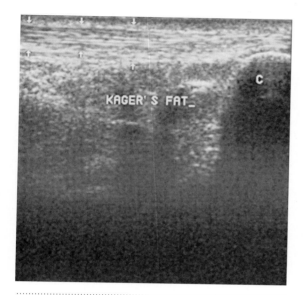

Figure 3–3. Longitudinal scan of Achilles tendon *(arrows)* showing calcaneus (C) at end. Kager's fat pad is less echogenic than tendon structure.

structures may be elicited at the time of examination of the Achilles tendon. The patient is scanned prone with the feet hanging over the table edge. Dynamic dorsal and plantar flexion positioning are performed. The diagnosis of tendon rupture is easily made by ultrasound, usually with the tear located at the level of the posterior malleolus and the defect in the echogenic tendon filled with anechoic blood or fluid. Retraction of the proximal and distal edges may be better observed during dorsiflexion and plantar flexion maneuvers. Longitudinal partial tears may be imaged similarly and the presence of peritendon fluid or Achilles bursal fluid documented. Chronic tears may lose the tendon-fluid interface, and even the disrupted tendons may be quite difficult to image (Fig. 3–4). Tendinitis is diagnosed when the distance between the tendon bundles increase and there is a 2-mm increase in AP diameter of the entire tendon compared with the normal contralateral side. Xanthomas of the Achilles tendon are the most characteristic location for heterozygous familial hypercholesterolemia. These appear as a speckled or reticulated pattern within the tendon, although focal nodules are also found. Because of the exquisite sensitivity of ultrasonic findings, it has been suggested that sonography be part of the work-up of suspected patients.[12] Although there is no tendon sheath, fluid may be found in the adjacent bursae. A finding associated with both tendinitis and tears is increased echogenicity of the subjacent fat pad. This is due to decreased tissue or in-

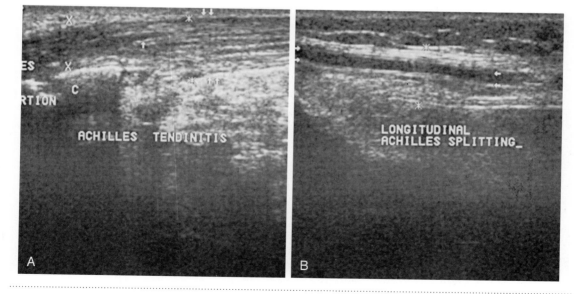

Figure 3–4. *A,* Acute longitudinal tear of Achilles tendon. Insertion of tendon at calcaneus (C) is enlarged and echo poor. Linear fissuring *(arrow)* in supracalcaneal tendon is echo free. Note widening and echo-poor nature of tendon. *B,* Chronic longitudinal tear of Achilles tendon. Fluid in split-tendon substance *(arrows* mark beginning and end) appears as echo-free regions in supracalcaneal tendon.

creased fluid in the region of the normal tendon, allowing better sonic penetration. Healing of the tendon may be followed by serial ultrasound scans. The differential diagnosis of accessory soleus muscle may be easily made because of the characteristic appearance of the muscle fibers in the supracalcaneal region.

Posterior Tibial Tendon

The posterior tibial muscle-tendon junction arises several centimeters above the medial malleolus. It then turns under the malleolus to fan out in its insertion on the navicular, cuneiformis, and bases of the second through fourth metatarsal bones.

The normal supramalleolar tendon is hyperechoic and oval shaped, having an AP diameter ranging from 4 to 6 mm. At the level of the medial malleolus, the average tendon diameters are 7.8 × 3.7 mm. A thin hypoechoic tendon sheath surrounds the tendon and may contain a thin layer of fluid (Fig. 3–5A, B). The posterior tibial tendon usually tears longitudinally and demonstrates an internal cleft oriented in a cephalocaudal direction (Fig. 3–6A, B). Associated swelling of the tendon is noted, and the presence of transverse tears must be evalu-

ated and look similar to Achilles tendon tears with the ruptured tendon straddling the hematoma. In transverse scanning, the supramalleolar groove will appear empty (Fig. 3–7). In longitudinal images, the ruptured ends may have a wavy fibrillar appearance that results from absence of tendon tension. In chronic and late-stage injuries, fluid may be absent, and the retracted tendon ends may be sonographically invisible. MRI examination of this tendon has difficulty distinguishing between tendinitis and early tendon rupture.[13] Tenosynovitis of this tendon presents with hypoechoic features and enlargement. The hypoechoic rim of the peritendon fluid is larger than the contralateral side. This appears as a target sign in cross-section with the echogenic centrally located tendon surrounded by the echo-poor or echo-free fluid.[14] Irregularity of the tendon contour may be noted. A technical reminder is that the flexor digitorum longus may simulate a normal posterior tibial tendon in the longitudinal scan plane. This error is identified by careful correlative imaging in the transverse plane (Fig. 3–8).

Peroneal Tendons

The peroneus longus tendon arises from the tibia, fibula head, and intermuscular sep-

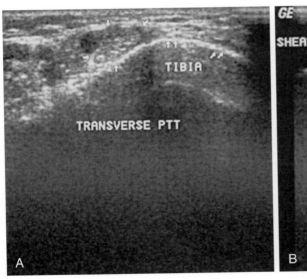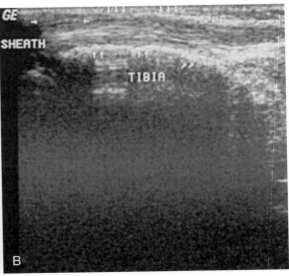

Figure 3–5. *A,* Normal posterior tibial tendon. Transverse sonogram through supramalleolar tendon (PTT) shows oval shape *(arrows).* The adjacent tibia is brightly echogenic *(double arrows). B,* Longitudinal scan in perpendicular plane shows stepladder pattern of tendon *(triple arrows)* and thin hypoechoic tendon sheath *(opposing single arrows).*

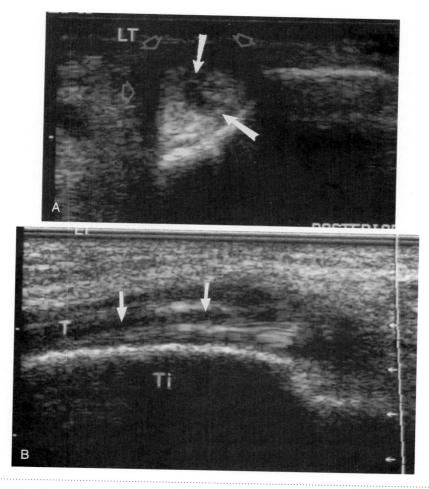

Figure 3–6. *A,* Tear of posterior tibial tendon. Transverse sonogram shows a cleft *(arrows)* in the posterior tibial tendon and a fluid-filled tendon sheath *(open arrows)* in a patient with a surgically proven split in the posterior tibial tendon. *B,* Longitudinal sonogram shows a longitudinal cleft *(arrows)* that follows the long axis of the tendon (T). Ti = medial tibia. (Figure 3–6 *A, B* from Fornage BD. Musculoskeletal Ultrasound. New York: Churchill Livingstone, 1995. Reprinted with permission of Churchill Livingstone.)

tum. The peroneus brevis tendon originates from the lower fibula and intermuscular septum somewhat anteriorly to the longus, and both are bound in their common synovial sheath by a fibrous superior and inferior retinaculum. The peroneal tendons lie in a tunnel that is formed by the malleolus in front, the superior peroneal retinaculum posteriorly and laterally, and the posterior talofibular and calcaneofibular ligaments medially.[15] Distal to the malleolus, the peroneus brevis and longus tendons diverge and have separate tendon sheaths (Fig. 3–9).

The peroneal tendons are almost round in transverse scans and nearly equal in size. A tendon sheath is present for both, although it may be larger in the peroneus longus. Small amounts of fluid are seen in asymptomatic patients. Large volumes or proximally located fluid is considered abnormal. The normal peroneus quartus tendon or muscle lies medial to the peroneus longus tendon. It should not be confused with splitting-type deformity of the peroneus brevis tendon. Hypertrophy of the peroneus longus may be noted in conjunction with hypertrophy of the peroneal tubercle. It appears with the normal striated echo pattern and is increased in size. Like the posterior tibial tendon, ultrasound may differentiate between intrasubstance tears and full-thickness ruptures. The peroneal tendons usually tear in a longitudinal plane. Tears of the longitudinal type usually center at the retromalleolar

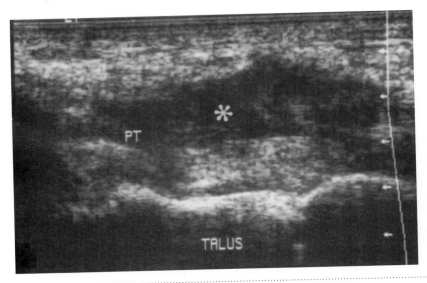

Figure 3–7. Torn, retracted posterior tibial tendon (PT) with an empty tendon sheath *(asterisk)*. Compare with sonogram of normal tendon shown in Figure 3–5A. (From Fornage BD. Musculoskeletal Ultrasound. New York: Churchill Livingstone, 1995. Reprinted with permission from Churchill Livingstone.)

groove in the case of the peroneus brevis tendon and show a characteristic wrapping around the peroneus longus tendon. In one series of peroneus brevis tears, there was a 29% incidence of concomitant tears in the peroneus longus tendon.[16] Peroneal tenosynovitis accompanies rupture of the superior peroneal retinaculum with associated subluxation of the peroneal brevis and longus tendons out of the bony groove behind the lateral malleolus (Fig. 3–10). Partial loss

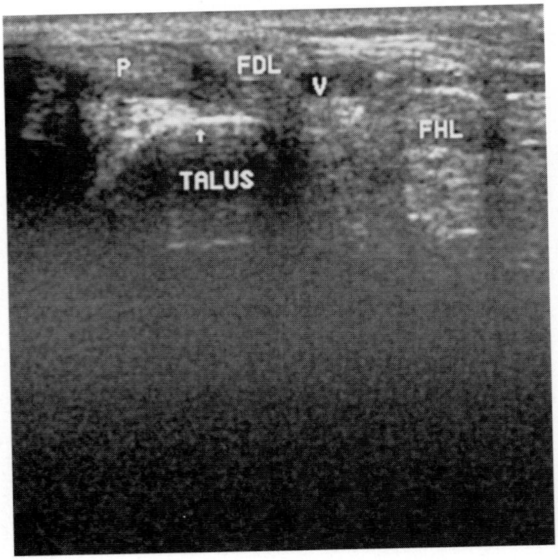

Figure 3–8. Transverse scan of medial talar tendons. Note that alignment of tendons and vascular bundle is similar to that seen on magnetic resonance imaging. Posterior tibial tendon (P), flexor digitorum longus (FDL), vascular bundle (V) consisting of artery and veins, and flexor hallucis longus (FHL) line up from left to right.

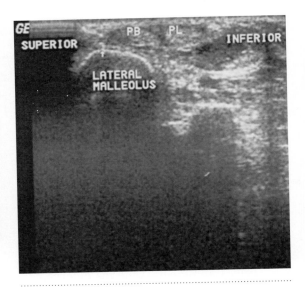

Figure 3–9. Normal peroneal tendons. Transverse scan at lateral malleolus at the superior margin of the picture shows echogenic peroneus brevis tendon (PB) with lower and more laterally situated peroneus longus tendon (PL).

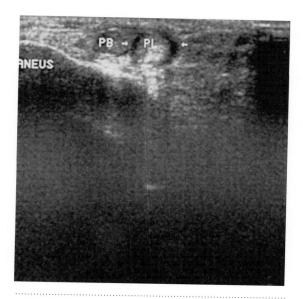

Figure 3–10. Peroneal tenosynovitis. Peroneal brevis tendon is echo poor and minimally enlarged (PB). The peroneal longus tendon is echogenic (PL) because it is surrounded by fluid *(arrows)*.

of congruity between the tendons and the peroneal groove is termed *subluxation* and appears as lateral location of the tendon with respect to the lateral margin of the fibula. Lateral malleolar bursitis or a lateral malleolar ganglion cyst must not be mis-

taken for peroneal tendon disease (Fig. 3–11).

Flexor Hallucis Longus Tendon

The flexor hallucis longus tendon arises posteriorly from the tibia and fibula. It normally runs posterolateral to the posterior tibial tendon and flexor digitorum longus tendon. The tendon then descends through a fibro-osseous tunnel on the posterior talar aspect between the medial and lateral tubercles. It is often well imaged when scanning the Achilles tendon because it lies deep to Kager's fat pad. The course of this tendon may be followed well with standard scanning planes until the level of the curve at the sustentaculum, where it is difficult to image. Tenosynovitis is common in ballet dancers in whom fluid may be found surrounding the tendon. This fluid must be differentiated from fluid arising out of communication of the tendon sheath with a large ankle joint effusion, which occurs in 20% of normal patients.[17] Chronic inflammation and hypertrophy of the musculotendinous unit may lead to stenosing tenosynovitis. The operative treatment of dancer's tendinitis in the absence of commonly associated posterior impingement syndrome uses a medial approach. If ultrasound can rule out flexor hallucis longus disease (Fig. 3–12),

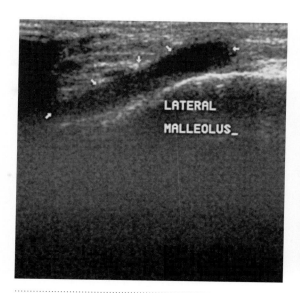

Figure 3–11. Lateral malleolar bursitis. Echo-free fluid *(arrows)* lies adjacent to the lateral malleolus, causing pain.

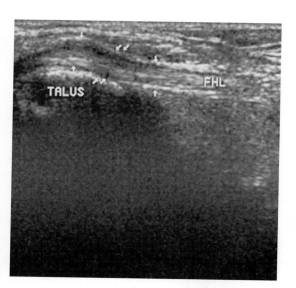

Figure 3–12. Normal flexor hallucis longus (FHL) is outlined by *arrows*. The tendon is echo poor *(double arrows)* because of a change in course, producing the anisotropic effect.

then a lateral approach is surgically preferable for posterior impingement syndrome therapy.[18] The distal tendon may be imaged with a stand-off pad or large amounts of gel on the skin as it courses along the plantar aspect of the foot to its insertion into the great toe.

Anterior Tibial Tendon

The anterior tibial muscle becomes tendinous at the level of the distal tibial metaphysis (Fig. 3–13). More distally, it acquires a synovial sheath where it attaches into the first cuneiform and first metatarsal base. Tears of the tendon occur between the superior and inferior retinacula that hold the tendon in its normal position. Tears may be partial, complete, or longitudinal in nature. Tendinitis in this tendon is similar to others already discussed. This tendon has a tendon sheath so that fluid collections resulting from trauma or rheumatoid disease are easily imaged (Fig. 3–14). Inflammatory synovium may be identified. Infection resulting from foreign bodies in this superficial structure may be diagnosed by peritendon fluid, and the foreign body itself is often identified.

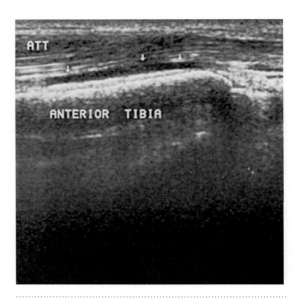

Figure 3–14. Anterior tibial tendon tenosynovitis. The proximal tendon (ATT) is echo poor and enlarged, and demonstrates distal fluid *(arrows)*. More proximal fluid is displaced by transducer pressure.

SONOGRAPHY OF LIGAMENTS

The anterior tibiofibular ligament is imaged as an echogenic band between the tibia and fibula and is evaluated by scanning anteriorly. Also noted at this time is the anterior tibiotalar recess and the echo-poor hyaline cartilage covering the talar dome. Lateral scanning at the malleolus demonstrates the echogenic anterior tibiofibular and calcaneofibular ligaments. A posterior transverse approach shows the posterior tibiofibular ligament to its best advantage, because it is short and horizontal. It has been suggested that sonography may be more accurate than noncontrast MRI because of the complex orientations of ligaments.[19] The normal ligament has a similar ultrasound appearance to normal tendon substance. Trauma usually produces a hematoma in the space of the disrupted ligament, which appears as an echo-free region (Fig. 3–15A, B). In the case of the ruptured anterior tibiofibular ligament, stress on the syndesmosis may be measured ultrasonically and the degree of widening evaluated. After a week, echo-poor granulation may be noted to fill the gap in the distracted ligament. Partial tears may show as echo-free clefts paralleling the ligamentous fiber orientation.

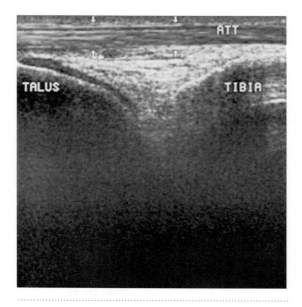

Figure 3–13. Normal anterior tibial tendon (ATT) bridging between the tibia and the talus.

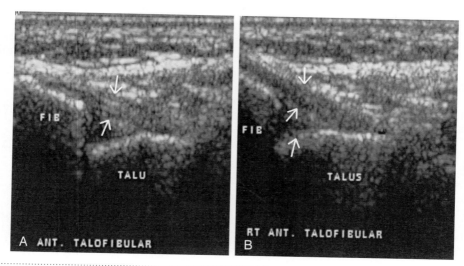

Figure 3–15. *A,* Normal anterior talofibular ligament *(arrows)* is echogenic and traverses the distal fibula to the talus anteriorly. *B,* Edema of anterior talofibular ligament *(arrows)* demonstrates lack of internal echogenic structure. FIB = fibula.

SONOGRAPHY OF SYNOVIAL DISEASES

Dynamic study of the heel and ankle for diagnosis of synovial disease of the fluid or proliferative variety includes searching for bursal fluid and abnormalities of the adjacent tendons, articular cartilage, and juxtaarticular bone. Use of power Doppler sonography aids in differentiating solid synovial hypertrophy from simple fluid collections and is covered separately at the end of the chapter. Chronic untreated bursitis may appear solid on MRI.[20] In tenosynovitis (Fig. 3–16), the complete disappearance of peritendon echo-poor areas during compression signifies that fluid was present as opposed to pannus or thickened synovial membrane. Careful search for intratendinous rheumatoid nodules as well as areas of rupture of the peroneal and posterior tibial tendons must be performed. Synovial cysts may be simply diagnosed by ultrasound. Ganglia and their possible communication with a joint or tendon sheath may be evaluated. Synovitis in rheumatoid arthritis occurs commonly in the anterior recess and may be difficult to distinguish from fluid. A rheumatoid nodule is a vasculitis that destroys by contact with adjacent structures. Power Doppler sonography shows increased flow in active synovitis and active nodules and has proven valuable in separating synovial fluid from active pannus and nodules.[21] The tibio-

talar joint is best evaluated in the longitudinal scan plane with the foot in plantar flexion. Posttraumatic fluid collections are echo free and usually resolve within a month after injury.

Because the presence of joint fluid is a natural ultrasonic window for evaluation of

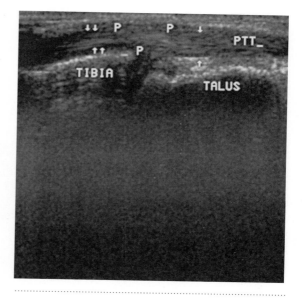

Figure 3–16. Stenosing tenosynovitis. Narrowing *(double arrows)* of the posterior tibial tendon (PTT) is due to pannus (P) that erodes the tendon near the joint and is compared with the normal sized tendon distally *(arrows).*

intra-articular lesions, small loose bodies may be readily identified as the examiner presses alternately on the lateral and medial joint recesses. Ultrasound is considered the most appropriate modality for diagnosing loose bodies in the ankle joint.[22] Unlike with MRI, debris within fluid may be classified as calcific or soft tissue. Calcific foci produce bright echoes on perpendicular scanning that cast sonic shadows in appropriate planes. Soft tissue debris parallels the specific disease as to its echo-poor or echogenic entities without the bright specular reflectors and sonic shadow signs. Free air or gaseous media within a fluid-filled joint will also cast a sonic shadow with bright echoes; however, this may be diagnosed by plain film radiographs and ultrasonic compression techniques.

Another entity capable of producing ankle symptoms and pathologic findings is Baker's cyst of the popliteal fossa associated with rheumatoid arthritis. As the cyst becomes distended with fluid and synovial proliferation, it may extend distally into the ankle. Baker's cysts developing in the framework of rheumatoid arthropathy are characterized by internal echoes within the fluid and marked irregularity of the synovium. Ultrasonically, this manifests as echogenic fluid with irregular internal walls of medium amplitude echoes. The power Doppler feature of the ultrasound unit will detect increased flows in the active pannus. Tenosynovitis with increased tendon echogenicity is an anomaly found with inflamed tendons within large fluid collections. The usual inflamed tendon is echo poor and enlarged. However, the pathologic tendon that is surrounded by water-type medium will show higher echogenicity than expected because of the greatly increased sound penetration in fluid. If possible, scanning the tendon in a path that avoids the fluid region will produce more useful information, thus avoiding the false impression of normal tendon echogenicity. Compression maneuvers to disperse the fluid away from the site under investigation may also be useful in deciding the true echogenicity of a tendon.

SONOGRAPHY OF MUSCLE

Normal muscle bundles are hypoechoic and separated by well-ordered symmetric hyperechoic bands of fibroadipose septa (Fig. 3–17). Hypertrophy, atrophy, and variations from normal are imaged. Muscle anomalies, such as the accessory soleus muscle, appear as normal muscular striations within the echo-poor background. Trauma is the most common muscular traumatic condition in the lower extremity. Muscles are best examined during rest and during contraction. Comparison with the contralateral side is often helpful. Direct trauma usually crushes muscle adjacent to underlying bone, whereas indirect trauma stretches the muscle beyond its normal limit. The most commonly injured muscle is the medial gastrocnemius, primarily a result of jumping during athletic sports. Strains produce no visible alteration of the normal oblique parallel echogenic striae. Contusions have a variety of appearances depending on the degree of focal fluid collection and the time course. Indeed, the only finding may be enlargement in the AP diameter of the muscle. Partial rupture shows disruption of the homoge-

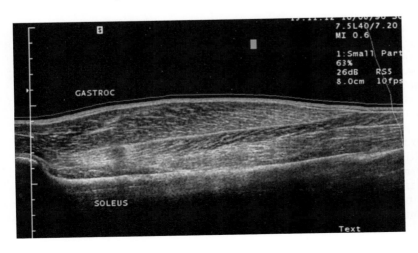

Figure 3–17. Normal muscle. Computer extension of gastrocnemius muscle permits axial imaging similar to magnetic resonance imaging. Note the orderly striations. GASTROC = gastrocnemius muscle; SOLEUS = soleus muscle.

neous striations and the presence of extracellular fluid. The gastrocnemius frequently demonstrates a detachment of the lower end of the medialis muscle fibers from the common aponeurosis of the triceps surae. Partial ruptures are shown to better advantage during the contraction phase (Fig. 3–18). Complete rupture appears as a hypoechoic hematoma with the retracted ends of the muscle noted as echogenic fragments at the border of the fluid collection, occasionally appearing as a bell clapper configuration. Early healing shows an infusion of echogenic vessels at the periphery, which is later serially followed to complete resolution. This influx of neovascularity produces a blizzard-like picture, which may mimic the "snowstorm" appearance of ruptured silicone prostheses. It may be differentiated by power Doppler exam, which literally shows the neovascularity in the healing region.[23] Cystic lesions, fibrous scars, myositis ossificans, and hernias (especially of the tibialis anterior muscle) are sequelae of incomplete healing. Fibrous scars are initially echo poor and later become echogenic.[24] Dynamic sonography may be used to document the functional damage caused by adhesions and permanent scarring (Fig. 3–19).[25]

SONOGRAPHY OF NERVES

Sonograms of peripheral nerves have become commonplace in the last few years

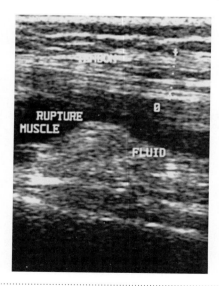

Figure 3–18. Rupture of soleus muscle at the origin of the Achilles tendon. Black fluid separates muscle structures.

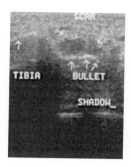

Figure 3–19. Posttraumatic scarring of muscle. A bullet is brightly echogenic in the gastrocnemius muscle and casts a black sonic shadow. Proximal to the bullet is an echo-poor mass *(arrows)* that is scar formation, which caused pain while walking as a result of abnormal muscle dynamics.

with the advent of high-frequency transducers. At 5-MHz imaging, the normal nerve fibers appear echo poor. The honeycombed internal structure is strikingly apparent at 10 to 15 MHz as the structure shows an echo-free background with internal linear echogenic fibrils, similar to those found in tendon although more widely spaced in longitudinal or axial scanning. This presents a stippled pattern in cross-section. This feature is used in documenting the digital nerve entering a neuroma or Morton's-type lesion. Inflamed nerves appear echo poor and show flow patterns on power Doppler interrogation. True nerve tumors appear echo free at 7 to 10 MHz but fill in with fine echoes at higher frequency ranges. Sonography can be completely reliable only when the tumor and the junction of the nerve of origin are simultaneously documented.[26]

SONOGRAPHY OF THE SOFT TISSUES

Ganglia

Ganglia commonly found around the ankle and dorsum of the foot are typically anechoic. The examiner may search for a neck that may enter the adjacent joint space. Aspiration may be performed under ultrasound guidance. Inflammation and infection resulting from foreign bodies may be diagnosed, and fistulous tracts may be identified. Ultrasound may be used to guide the removal of nonradiopaque objects such as

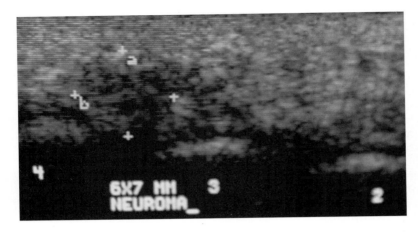

Figure 3–20. Morton's neuroma. Echo-poor mass of fibrotic tissue in the typical location between the third and fourth metatarsal heads. Neuroma measures 6 × 7 mm by calipers (a, b).

wooden splinters, tooth picks, plastic or glass fragments, and cactus spines.

Morton's Neuroma

Morton's neuroma is a fibrosing process occurring in and around the plantar digital nerve. Fibrosis on sonography is echo poor in character. The transducer is first placed transversely over the plantar region of the metatarsal heads. Any hypoechoic mass is then scanned longitudinally along the axis of the digital nerve to show a connection (Fig. 3–20). The size of this lesion may be serially monitored by sonography. Improved imaging of this disorder occurs when the examiner pushes with a finger on the dorsal web space as compression is used on the plantar positioned transducer. True plantar neuromas are composed of neural tissue and are usually echo free, simulating fluid resulting from the high homogeneity of the structure. Dynamic imaging by pressure shows true fluid to change shape, whereas compression of the tumor will cause no alteration in appearance. Alignment with the hypoechoic nerve is demonstrable as well.[27]

Plantar Fasciitis

The normal plantar fascia (Fig. 3–21) is homogeneously echogenic, measuring between 2 and 4 mm in normal patients and showing no difference in thickness between males and females. The plantar fascia is scanned transversely for overall integrity and geometry. It is then imaged longitudinally to show the total length of the fascia and its insertion site. The edges of the plantar fascia are imaged as parallel smoothly echogenic lines. The structure within is noted to be one of fine parallel echogenic lines reflecting its fibrillar organization. The thickness tends to be homogeneous along its entire length. Plantar fasciitis syndrome is characterized by heel pain at the insertion of the plantar fascia onto the medial tubercle of the calcaneus. Plantar fasciitis is noted by thickening of the structure as well as hypoechoic transformation of the area[28] (Fig. 3–22). This process may be focal or diffuse.[29] Interruption of the fascia because of partial or complete tearing may be ap-

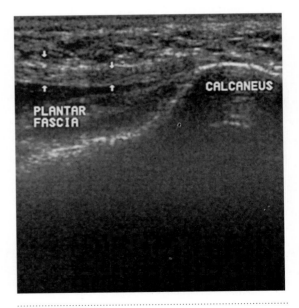

Figure 3–21. Normal plantar fascia. Homogeneously echogenic structure emanating from the plantar calcaneus (arrows).

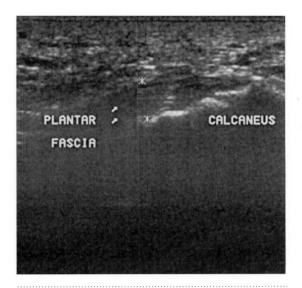

Figure 3–22. Plantar fasciitis. The enlarged plantar fascia *(double arrows)* is echo poor.

preciated. In one study, the maximal thickening occurred approximately 2 cm from the calcaneal insertion site.[30] Peri-insertion edema has also been reported.[31] De novo fluid collections may sometimes be identified. Ultrasound diagnosis is important, because the appearance of plantar calcaneal spurs has no direct relation to heel pain. Plantar fibromas appear as hypoechoic nodules with a heterogeneous echo pattern.

Tarsal Tunnel Syndrome

The neurovascular bundles of the tarsal tunnel contents are fixated by fibrous septa. Traction disorders or compression from mass lesions readily produce sensory symptoms. Ultrasonography may show a ganglion as an echo-free, focal, well-circumscribed cystic region, whereas free fluid will conform more to the anatomy of the adjacent tarsal tunnel. Peripheral nerve sheath tumors and neurilemomas are usually hypoechoic and lie in the plane of the nerve structure. Hemangiomas have various echo patterns and are thus not easily diagnosed. Indeed, Doppler flows may be high or low in these masses. Dilated or varicose veins have a wormlike appearance (Fig. 3–23). Doppler flows are quite clear as is compression venous reflux. Fibrous scars are typically echo poor and are adjacently inseparable to other anatomic structures. Hypertrophy of the abductor hallucis muscle or accessory abductor hallucis muscle appears as typical echogenic linear muscle striations and poses no diagnostic difficulty. Tenosynovitis with effusion or synovial hypertrophy may be well evaluated. Various posttraumatic causes may be noted, depending on the type of disease involved. Whereas most disorders of the tarsal tunnel are identifiable by ultrasound, pathologies of the sinus tarsi, especially of the bifurcated ligament, can be studied only by MRI.[1]

EVALUATION OF FOREIGN BODIES

Only 15% of wooden fragments are seen on plain x-ray films. Sutures (Fig. 3–24), plastic, and small glass pieces are similarly difficult to identify radiographically. Ultrasound quickly images these echogenic structures either by their bright reflections or by the associated acoustic shadowing that occurs when sound transmission is blocked.[32] Indeed, intraoperative transducers are commercially available to localize and remove foreign bodies, such as thorns and cactus needles, that may hide along fascial planes. The often associated inflammatory response may be distinguished as an echo-free region of fluid or echo-poor abscess focus that typically forms a halo around the foreign body. Metal objects have a specific comet tail artifact that is recogniz-

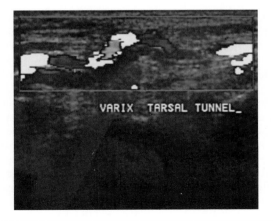

Figure 3–23. Varicosities in tarsal tunnel. There is a varix producing compression on the tunnel structures. The dilated veins are tortuous and enlarged and appear multicolored with color flow Doppler techniques.

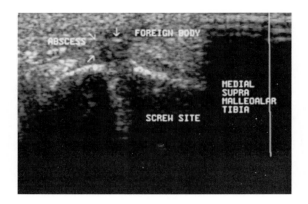

Figure 3–24. Retained suture producing abscess. Postoperative abscess *(side arrows)* is echo poor, and within this is noted an echogenic structure *(down arrow)* proven to be suture material.

able as a series of bright echoes trailing the initial bright echo. Skin lesions, free subcutaneous air, sesamoid bones, and post-inflammatory, posttraumatic, and bursal calcifications all cast acoustic shadows.

COLOR AND POWER DOPPLER APPLICATIONS

Conventional pulsed- and continuous-wave Doppler exams are used to demonstrate blood flow. However, these are time consuming and relatively insensitive. Color Doppler sonography uses computer coding to demonstrate directional blood flows in a clinically useful manner. Power Doppler sonography is a new feature of blood flow analysis that is proportional to the total number of moving scatterers. This allows low-flow states and minute vascular structures to be imaged. Potential clinical applications include determining the neovascular regions found in healing fractures, resolving hematomas, determining inflammatory tenosynovitis and acute gouty inflammation, and distinguishing synovial fluid from vascular synovium. Gouty arthritis demonstrates the highest vascular power Doppler response, and active rheumatoid synovitis is next, closely followed by the new callus of fracture healing. Evaluation of arterial and venous malformations is possible by the high sensitivity of power Doppler sonography. Abnormal pulsatility may be noted in a nonvascular region during routine scanning. Arterial occlusive disease is best examined by color

Doppler and pulsed-wave ultrasound because power Doppler sonography is nondirectional. Venous insufficiency is best studied with color Doppler and pulsed-wave sonography as well for similar reasons.

ALTERNATIVE IMAGING TECHNIQUES IN SOFT TISSUE INJURIES

Light Scanning

The oldest, fastest, and certainly the least expensive study used for centuries is light scanning. The noninvasive procedure of transillumination, clinically used for breast disease evaluation and diagnosis of scrotal disease, shows great promise in evaluating injuries. Potentially important is the role of light scanning, the current term for transillumination, in the diagnosis of the nature and extent of muscle rupture and tendon injury. Although light scanning has been used for breast cancer detection for more than 50 years[7] and scrotal hydrocele analysis for many years, its usage in musculoskeletal injury is relatively new and seemingly quite logical. Light absorption of the transilluminated area is compared with the contralateral side or with adjacent normal tissue architecture and adjusted for differences in depth. Early usage called the test diaphanography and required photographic picture acquisition and visual observation.[8] Today's interpretation is often made with a radiographic sensitometer or a low-light level closed-circuit television monitor.[9] Although not widely appreciated, it may be used to narrow the focus of other imaging modalities to a specific region and is of particular use in the younger pediatric population.

Minor trauma to a muscle belly may be accompanied by serous fluid extravasation. If this process is localized, light scanning will be unremarkable. If the leakage is accompanied by hemorrhage, light absorption will be noted, because the deoxygenated hemoglobin in the hematoma dramatically blocks light transmission as a result of absorption in proportion to the hematoma's size and borders. Light absorption is compared with that of the unaffected normal contralateral side. It is important to realize that calcification or bone does not affect the absorption of the optical transmission in the

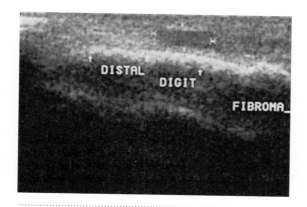

Figure 3–25. Fibroma of distal digit. Echo-poor mass in superficial location may be ideal for aspiration biopsy or therapeutic cautery because needle localization using ultrasonography is proven effective. Also, vascular and other structures may be identified before and during needle maneuvers.

way that x-rays are absorbed by calcium. A long-standing serous leakage may become secondarily infected, thus producing unilateral light absorption. Thus, trauma, blunt or penetrating, may be associated with bleeding or products of tissue inflammation that absorb light rays. Thus, normal symmetric transillumination may suggest the probability of structural intactness of the muscle. Medium degrees of transmission blockage are associated with structural failure of the muscle, and massive light absorption loss accompanies hemorrhage or infection in the muscle or its associated traumatic seroma. The tendon may be examined with simultaneous fiberoptic light scanning. Light scanning showed intratendinous hematomas larger than 1 mm. Resolution of this may be followed with this modality. Indications for transillumination are cyst diagnosis and suspected bleeding or a suspicious lesion not clearly defined by MRI or ultrasound. Certain inflammatory conditions such as peritendon exudates were imaged well by transillumination.[10]

FUTURE DEVELOPMENTS

For many years, ultrasound guidance of needle localization for masses and fine-needle aspiration biopsy has been preferred to radiographic localization both for its accuracy and speed. Therapeutic considerations of ultrasound guidance of focal injections

into muscular structures, inflamed joints, fascial planes, and tendon sheaths are feasible. Dynamic muscle testing will show decreased mobility around areas of fibrous scarring as well as absence of change and size of muscle tissue.[33] Because needling and injection infiltration is considered the most effective modality for immediate relief of pain and complete removal of disease causing pain,[34] this could be performed under ultrasound guidance to promote optimal healing in muscular ankle injuries. Indeed, cavitation ultrasound or electrocautery of peripheral tumors may be feasible (Fig. 3–25).

REFERENCES

1. Deutsch AL, Mink JH, Kerr R. MRI of the Foot and Ankle. New York: Raven Press, 1992.
2. Neuhold A, Sitskal M, Kainberger F, et al. Degenerative Achilles tendon disease: assessment by magnetic resonance and ultrasonography. Eur J Radiol 14:213, 1992.
3. Mink JH, Reicher MA, Crues JV, Deutsch AL. MRI of the Knee. New York: Raven Press, 1993.
4. Rademaker J, Rosenberg ZS, Beltran J, et al. Alterations in the distal extension of the musculus peroneus brevis with foot movement. AJR Am J Roentgenol 168:787, 1997.
5. Maldjian C, Mezgarzadeh M, Roach NA, et al. Efficacy of 3-dimensional FSE MRI of the ankle. AJR Am J Roentgenol 168:25, 1997.
6. Habra G, van Holsbeeck M. Tendon pathology: multimodality imaging. AJR Am J Roentgenol 168:205, 1997.
7. Cucin R, Bard R. False positive mammographic imaging of a breast implant. N Y State J Med 93:151–152, 1993.
8. Gunderson J, Nilsson D, Ohlsson B. Diaphanography for assessment of mammary changes. Lakartidningen 76:1425–1429, 1979.
9. Bard R. Multimodality imaging. The Female Patient 17:11, 1996.
10. Bard R. Light scanning of tendon injury. Presented at Sixth Annual Conference on Musculoskeletal Ultrasound, Montreal, 1996.
11. Van Holsbeeck M, Introcaso JH. Musculoskeletal Ultrasound. St. Louis, MO: C. V. Mosby, 1991.
12. Bureau N, Roederer G. Achilles tendon xanthoma: ultrasound vs. MRI. Presented at Sixth Annual Conference on Musculoskeletal Ultrasound, Montreal, 1996.
13. Cheung Y, Rosenberg ZS, Magee T, et al. Normal anatomy and pathologic conditions of ankle tendons: current imaging techniques. Radiographics 12:429, 1992.
14. Hsu T, Wang C, Wang T, et al. Ultrasonographic examination of the posterior tibial tendon. Foot Ankle Int 18:34, 1997.
15. Rosenberg Z, Feldman F, Singson R. Peroneal tendon injuries: CT analysis. Radiology 161:743, 1986.
16. Rosenberg ZS, Beltran J, Cheung YY, et al. MR features of longitudinal tears of the peroneus brevis tendon. AJR Am J Roentgenol 168:141, 1997.

17. Chhem RK, Beauregard G. Synovial diseases. In Fornage BD, ed. Musculoskeletal Ultrasound. New York: Churchill Livingstone, 1995:47.

18. Hamilton WG, Geppert MI, Thompson FM. Pain in the posterior aspect of the ankle in dancers. J Bone Joint Surg Am 78:1491, 1996.

19. Marcelis S, Daenen B, Ferrara MA. Peripheral Musculoskeletal Ultrasound Atlas. New York: Thieme, 1996:162.

20. Zeiss J, Coombs RJ, Booth RL, et al. Chronic bursitis presenting as a mass in the pes anserine bursae: MR diagnosis. J Comput Assist Tomogr 17:137, 1993.

21. Adler R. Power Doppler applications in musculoskeletal ultrasound. Presented at 6th Annual Conference of Musculoskeletal Ultrasound, Montreal, 1996.

22. Marcelis S, Daenen B, Ferrara MA. Peripheral Musculoskeletal Ultrasound Atlas. New York: Thieme, 1996:172.

23. Bard R. The blizzard sign of intramuscular healing hematoma. Presented at the 6th Annual Conference of Musculoskeletal Ultrasound, Montreal, 1996.

24. Letho A, Alanen A. Healing of a muscle trauma: correlation of sonographical and histological findings of an experimental study in rats. J Ultrasound Med 6:425, 1987.

25. Solbiati L, Rizzato G. Ultrasound of Superficial Structures. New York: Churchill Livingstone, 1995:324.

26. Fornage BD. Sonography of peripheral nerves of the extremities. Radiol Med 85:162, 1993.

27. Redd RA, Peters VJ, Emery SF, et al. Morton neuroma: sonographic appearance. Radiology 171:415, 1989.

28. Singer K, Jones D. Soft tissue conditions of the ankle and foot. In Nicholas J, Hershman E, eds. The Lower Extremity in Sports Medicine. St. Louis, MO: C. V. Mosby, 1986:498.

29. Frey C, Shereff M. Tendon injuries about the ankle in athletes. Clin Sport Med 7:103, 1988.

30. Wall RW, Harkness MA, Crawford A. Ultrasound diagnosis of plantar fasciitis. Foot Ankle 14:465, 1993.

31. Gibbon WW. Plantar fasciitis. Radiology 182:285, 1992.

32. Gooding GAW, Hardiman T, Sumers M, et al. Sonography of the hand and foot in foreign body detection. J Ultrasound Med 6:441, 1987.

33. Fornage B, Touche DH, Segal P, et al. Ultrasonography in the evaluation of muscular trauma. AJR Am J Roentgenol 134:375, 1980.

34. Fischer A. Local injections in pain management. Phys Med Rehabil Clin North Am 6:851, 1995.

4 Rheumatology Laboratory Evaluation

Steven K. Magid

The clinical laboratory can be of great help in the diagnosis of disorders of the foot. Although laboratory tests are often informative, they are rarely definitive or diagnostic. Laboratory examinations must be used in conjunction with a complete history and physical and radiographic examinations.

Laboratory tests may be used in a number of different ways. They may be used to diagnose a specific illness involving the foot. Examples of this include detecting the presence of intracellular urate crystals in synovial fluid aspirated from an acutely inflamed joint. This finding is diagnostic of gout. A positive Gram's stain or culture from an acutely inflamed joint is diagnostic of infection. Laboratory tests may also be used to diagnose a systemic illness (e.g., a complete blood cell count [CBC] and bone marrow examination may be diagnostic of leukemia in a patient with bone pain). The laboratory should always be used with a goal in mind: to arrive at a specific diagnosis; to provide further evidence of a suspected diagnosis, such as a positive rheumatoid factor in a patient with a systemic polyarthritis; to rule out competing diagnoses; to guide therapy; or to assess prognosis or response to treatment.

Four characteristics of diagnostic tests help determine their usefulness in evaluating patients:

1. Sensitivity, or the likelihood that a test will be positive in a person with the disease
2. Specificity, or the likelihood that a test will be a negative in a person without the disease
3. Positive predictive value, or the likelihood that a disease will be present in a person with a positive test result
4. Negative predictive value, or the likelihood that a disease will be absent in a person with a negative test result

TESTS ASSOCIATED WITH INFLAMMATION

When diagnosing a disorder, one of the most important considerations is to determine whether the cause is inflammatory (and frequently systemic) or noninflammatory.

Many metabolic changes occur in the setting of inflammatory processes. Together they are called the acute phase response. The acute phase response occurs after many events, including infections, trauma, immune diseases, crystalline diseases, and malignancy.

C Reactive Protein

C reactive protein (CRP) is composed of five identical subunits that are linked together. This protein is present in animals that trace their evolutionary origins for hundreds of millions of years (such as the horseshoe crab).

CRP is normally present in plasma in only trace amounts: approximately 0.2 mg/dL. Levels increase dramatically and quickly after a stimulus. Moderate elevations occur in most connective tissue diseases (1–10 mg/dL). Very high levels are seen in bacterial infections and systemic vasculitis (15–20 mg/dL). CRP is not thought to be altered by age or gender. CRP levels fall when inflammation subsides. Of interest, in systemic lupus erythematosus (SLE) and other connective tissue diseases, CRP levels are lower than one would expect for the amount of inflammation present.

CRP was initially identified by its ability to form a precipitin reaction with pneumococcal c polysaccharide. It is now measured by either latex agglutination or rocket electrophoresis. In contrast to the erythrocyte sedimentation rate (ESR), CRP can be assayed on specimens that have been stored by freezing. This can offer an advantage over ESR, which must be performed on fresh blood.

Erythrocyte Sedimentation Rate

Although CRP is highly associated with inflammation, ESR has been the most widely used indicator of inflammation and the acute phase response. ESR is performed by placing anticoagulated blood in a vertical glass tube and measuring the rate of red blood cell (RBC) settling. Normally, RBCs repel each other because the electrical charges on the surface of all RBCs are the same. When inflammation is present, there is an increase in the concentration of asymmetrically charged proteins that bind to the RBCs and thus prevent this repulsion. The RBCs, therefore, tend to aggregate. Aggregated clumps of cells settle more rapidly than individual cells, thus providing a higher ESR.

Fibrinogen is the protein that is most responsible for elevations in ESR in acute states of inflammation. An increase in immunoglobulin such as that seen with myeloma or monoclonal gammopathies can also lead to an ESR elevation, although such changes may not necessarily indicate an inflammatory state.

The ESR is influenced by anemia, polycythemia, and alterations in the size and shape of erythrocytes. Falsely low levels are seen in sickle cell disease, anisocytosis, spherocytosis, polycythemia, and heart failure. Prolonged storage of blood before testing or tilting of the calibrated tube will tend to increase the ESR. In addition, the ESR increases with age; thus, "normal" levels are variable. Levels up to 40 mm/hour are common in healthy elderly people.

The Westergren method is thought to be the most reliable. This method measures the fall of RBCs in millimeters per hour in a standardized tube. Normal is considered 0 to 15 for males and 0 to 20 for females. A rule of thumb is that the age-adjusted upper limit of normal of ESR is age divided by 2 for men and age plus 10 divided by 2 for women.

The ESR is probably most helpful if it is normal. Active inflammatory disorders such as acute rheumatic fever, SLE, rheumatoid arthritis (RA), temporal arteritis, and infections tend to have elevated ESRs. Although elevations of the ESR in septic arthritis and crystal-induced arthritis is the rule, a normal ESR does not completely rule out these entities. Joint aspiration is required.

From this, it is clear that the ESR and CRP are neither diagnostic nor specific. Nonetheless, they can be helpful in evaluating patients when RA or other systemic and local inflammatory conditions are being considered.

In the setting of systemic features, such as stiffness and symmetric polyarthralgias and arthritis, a connective tissue disease is more likely with an elevated, than with a normal, ESR-CRP.

Of course, one should always consider that a mechanical cause of foot pain (such as the frequently present bunion) coexists with another cause of ESR elevating inflammation (such as an infected tooth).

Rheumatoid Factor

Rheumatoid factors are autoantibodies that are directed against the Fc fragment of immunoglobulin (Ig) G. They seem to be synthesized in response to immunoglobulins that have been conformationally altered after reaction with antigen. They are most commonly associated with RA but are also found in other disorders (Table 4–1).

Historically, the test was performed by coating sheep RBCs or latex particles with human IgG and measuring the dilution of patient serum that will still aggregate the particle. Newer methods include radioimmunoassay, enzyme-linked immunoassay (ELISA), and nephelometry. These methods increase sensitivity and specificity.

The rheumatoid factor is one of the laboratory tests most frequently ordered in the evaluation of patients with joint complaints. The test is positive in 75 to 90% of patients with RA. However, these data are taken from highly selected populations and might be subject to referral bias. The high specificity that is also reported in studies from these populations may not be observed in patients who have weak indications for the test, who may be elderly, or who have other diseases that may cause a false-positive rheumatoid factor. In fact, the prevalence of false-positive rheumatoid factors in patients older than 75 years is between 2% and 25%.

Although there may be an increased likelihood of developing rheumatoid arthritis in a rheumatoid factor–positive asymptomatic

Table 4–1. Frequency of Rheumatoid Factor as Measured by Latex Agglutination in Rheumatic and Nonrheumatic Diseases

Disease	Approximate Frequency (%)
Sicca syndrome	90
Mixed cryoglubinemia	90
Rheumatoid arthritis	75
Mixed connective tissue disease	25
Polymyositis	20
Systemic lupus erythematosus	30
Systemic sclerosis (scleroderma)	20
Juvenile rheumatoid arthritis	10
Subacute bacterial endocarditis	40
Chronic interstitial pulmonary fibrosis	35
Pulmonary silicosis	30
Elderly (> 60 years)	15
Waldenström's disease (macroglobulinemia)	28
Cirrhosis	25
Infectious hepatitis	25
Leprosy	25
Tuberculosis	15
Trypanosomiasis	15
Sarcoidosis	10
Syphilis	10

From Paget S, Pellicci P, Beary JF III. Manual of Rheumatology and Outpatient Orthopedic Disorders: Diagnosis and Therapy, ed 3. Boston: Little, Brown, 1993:15.

individual, the use of the rheumatoid factor as a screening test performs poorly because of the high frequency of false-positive test results. Rheumatoid factors are most common in patients with RA, but they are also present in normal sera as well as in sera of patients with acquired immunodeficiency syndrome, hepatitis, various parasitic diseases, chronic bacterial infections such as tuberculosis and subacute bacterial endocarditis (SBE), tumors, chronic lymphocytic leukemia, and other hyperglobulinemic states such as cryoglobulinemia, chronic liver disease, sarcoidosis, and some chronic pulmonary diseases. For example, when rheumatoid factor is found in a patient with fever, arthralgia, and a heart murmur, SBE may be a more likely cause of a positive rheumatoid factor than RA.

When found in patients with RA, rheumatoid factors are usually specific for human IgG, are of high affinity, and include not only IgM rheumatoid factors but also IgG, IgA, and IgE variants.

High levels of rheumatoid factor have been associated with a worse prognosis; there tend to be more involved joints when first seen by a physician, more erosions, and greater ligamentous instability. A high level of rheumatoid factor is considered a risk factor for vasculitis.

Other laboratory findings that are common in RA include leukocytosis (usually with a normal differential), thrombocytosis, anemia (normochromic, normocytic), normal uric acid (if the patient is not taking salicylates, which can raise uric acid levels), a negative antinuclear antibody (ANA) and antideoxyribonucleic acid antibody (DNA), and normal or elevated serum complement.

Typical arthrocentesis results include straw-colored, slightly cloudy fluid, with between 5000 and 25,000 white blood cells (WBCs) per cubic millimeter. The differential demonstrates approximately 85% polymorphonuclear leukocytes (PMNs); no crystals are present, and synovial glucose may be depressed to less than 25 mg/dL. (Similar reductions may be found in the septic joint).

Antinuclear Antibodies

Lupus is another of the autoimmune diseases with major joint manifestations. It usually causes a nonerosive, nondeforming symmetric arthropathy. Multiple joints are typically involved. The ankle and foot are less commonly involved than with RA. In addition, more systemic features are more common. These include rash, fever, central nervous system involvement, renal disease, and serositis. Unlike RA, many types of autoantibodies are typically found in SLE and related syndromes.

ANAs are a hallmark of SLE. The ANA is positive in 95 to 99% of patients. The indirect immunofluorescence ANA is the method most commonly used. It is performed by diluting test sera and incubating with substrate cells. Traditionally, thin sections of frozen rat kidney or liver are used. However, cytocentrifuged preparations of cells from tissue culture such as Hep-2 can give optimal sensitivity and pattern discrimination.

Any bound ANAs are then detected by fluorescein-tagged antihuman immunoglobulin. The substrate cell is then viewed under a fluorescence microscope. ANAs are reported by either intensity of fluorescence (i.e., 1+ to 4+) or by maximal dilution of serum giving a positive result. Values of 2+

or greater or titers of 1:40 or greater are considered abnormal.

The pattern of the ANA is also reported (e.g., speckled, diffuse, rim, centromere). ANAs have different targets, and the pattern of immunofluorescence can provide differential diagnostic information. Homogenous patterns are least specific, and can be seen in up to 5% of normal patients, especially women and the elderly. In this setting, they are usually present in low titers. The rim pattern is characteristic of SLE. Nucleolar and speckled patterns are also seen and are associated with scleroderma, CREST (calcinosis, Raynaud's phenomenon, esophageal motility disorders, sclerodactyly, telangiectasia), mixed connective tissue disease (MCTD), and other diseases (Table 4–2).

Once a patient has been documented to have a positive ANA, it is usually not necessary to repeat the test unless a major change in therapy or status is detected. It should be noted that steroids and other immunosuppressant agents may lower the ANA titers.

Many diseases can produce anti–single-stranded DNA antibodies. These include liver diseases and drug-induced lupus. However, for the most part, only SLE (and MCTD) is associated with high-titer anti–double-stranded anti-DNA antibodies. These occur in nearly all SLE patients.

Antibodies to DNA are measured by many different methods. The Farr technique measures the percentage of DNA binding. This test uses radiolabeled C14. A positive Farr (> 30% binding) is usually found only in SLE or MCTD. In contradistinction to the ANA, levels of anti–double-stranded DNA antibodies are frequently used in monitoring disease activity.

Many other laboratory tests may be abnormal in SLE, and can be used in conjunction with the more specific tests for assessing disease. These include a low WBC (usually with neutropenia and lymphopenia), anemia (sometimes an autoimmune hemolytic anemia with positive Coombs'), thrombocytopenia, elevated partial thromboplastin time (PTT), false-positive Venereal Disease Research Laboratories (VDRL) and anticardiolipin antibody.

As suggested by the variety of ANA immunofluorescent patterns, ANAs may be directed against a number of different cellular constituents. Immunodiffusion and counterimmunoelectrophoresis can be performed using soluble components of cells (i.e., extractable nuclear antigens, or ENA). In addition to nucleic acids, other protein antigens from both nuclei and cytoplasm have been shown to be targets of ANAs. The antinuclear specificities that are most common with SLE are anti–double-stranded DNA

Table 4–2. Patterns of Immunofluorescence (ANA)*

Disease	Diffuse (Homogeneous)	Peripheral (Rim)	Speckled	Nucleolar	% ANA Positivity
SLE	+ +	+ +	+	0	≥90
MCTD	0	0	+ +	0	≥90
RA	+	0	0	0	30
Sicca syndrome	0	0	+ +	+	70
Scleroderma	+	0	+	+ +	≥70
Drug-induced SLE	+	+	0	0	≥90
Polymyositis	0	0	+0	0	≥70
WG†	+	0	0	0	30
PAN†	+	0	0	0	30
Elderly (> 60 years)	+0	+0	+0	+0	20
Chronic liver disease	+0	+0	+0	+0	20
Idiopathic pulmonary fibrosis	+0	+0	+0	+0	10

+ = common; + + = most common; 0 = less common; +0 = variable pattern; SLE = systemic lupus erythematosus; MCTD = mixed connective tissue disease; RA = rheumatoid arthritis; WG = Wegener's granulomatosis; PAN = polyarteritis nodosa; ANA = antinuclear antibody.

*ANA patterns may vary considerably, and different tissue or cellular substrates may give different patterns and degrees of staining.

†With conventional substrates, approximately 30% of WG and PAN is ANA positive. With neutrophils as substrate, approximately 80% of WG is positive for a finely granular cytoplasmic staining, and approximately 60% of PAN is positive for a perinuclear cytoplasmic staining.

From Paget S, Pellicci P, Beary JF III. Manual of Rheumatology and Outpatient Orthopedic Disorders: Diagnosis and Therapy, ed 3. Boston: Little, Brown, 1993:17.

and anti-Sm. Antinuclear ribonuclear protein antibodies are seen in MCTDs.

There are two subsets of anti–ANA-negative lupus patients. Some of these patients will be complement deficient; thus, a CH_{50} should be ordered. Others will have a positive anti-Ro or anti-Sm antibody.

Complement

The complement cascade contains at least 18 distinct plasma proteins. It is one of the major effector arms of the humoral immune system. Complement activation is thought to occur primarily by two mechanisms: the classic and the alternative.

In the classic activation pathway, antigen-antibody complexes act on C1 and C2 to cause cleavage of C3. In the alternative pathway, complex polysaccharides act on properdin factors d and b to cause cleavage of C3. Once C3 is cleaved, the terminal components (C5–C9) are activated. This leads to the lysis of the target cell and cellular membrane injury. Subsequently, there is generation of many mediators that trigger inflammation and anaphylaxis. Serial measurements of C3, C4, or CH_{50} are useful in monitoring disease activity (particularly renal disease) in SLE.

URIC ACID AND GOUT

Gout is one of the more common rheumatic diseases that affects the foot and ankle. In its classic, acute presentation, it is not likely to be confused with RA or SLE. However, in its chronic tophaceous form, there are many features that can mimic RA, including polyarthritis, symmetry of joint involvement, nodules, fusiform swelling, and erosions. Although gout and RA are said almost never to coexist, positive rheumatoid factors have been reported in up to 30% of patients with chronic tophaceous gout.

Conversely, a high uric acid may be seen in patients with RA for reasons unrelated to the type of arthritis present, including obesity, renal insufficiency, hypertension, alcohol intake, and genetic factors. The use of such common drugs as salicylates, in low doses, and diuretics is also a factor. It should be stressed that an elevation of serum uric acid is not sufficient for the diagnosis of gout. In fact, hyperuricemia has

been described in more than 15% of certain populations.

Further complicating the diagnosis is the fact that it is not uncommon for serum urate to be normal in the setting of gouty arthritis, particularly in chronic tophaceous gout or in alcoholics.

The diagnosis is best established by joint aspiration and evaluation with compensated polarized light microscopy. The identification of needle-shaped, negatively birefringent crystals within PMNs is diagnostic. A word of caution is necessary because it has been established that a variety of materials, including lipids and other crystals such as previously injected intra-articular steroids, can be confused with those of uric acid.

CALCIUM PYROPHOSPHATE DEPOSITION DISEASE AND LABORATORY FEATURES

Another crystal disease that can affect the foot and ankle must be distinguished from gout. That condition is calcium pyrophosphate deposition disease (CPPD). This is the arthritis associated with calcium pyrophosphate. Acute arthritis (or pseudogout) rarely affects the first metatarsophalangeal (MTP) joint the way gout does. More often, it affects the knees and wrists, but it may also involve the ankle and on occasion the first MTP.

Although most often associated with a familial predisposition or with aging, a number of other diseases have been associated with CPPD. Many of these have characteristic laboratory features, including CPPD associated with

1. Hemochromatosis (elevated iron, iron saturation, and ferritin)
2. Hyperparathyroidism (high parathyroid hormone [PTH], hypercalcemia, hyperchloremic acidosis). CPPD may be seen in 20 to 30% of patients with hyperparathyroidism
3. Hypomagnesemia
4. Hypophosphatasia

As with gout, the diagnosis of CPPD is confirmed by joint aspiration and crystal search.

DIABETES

Diabetes has been associated with CPPD, although this is thought more likely to be the chance occurrence of two common diseases. Diabetes, however, does have major manifestations in diseases of the foot. These include

1. Peripheral neuropathy
2. Diabetic ulcers with and without underlying osteomyelitis
3. Charcot joints

The laboratory diagnosis of diabetes is, therefore, germane. Screening may be performed with a fasting blood glucose. Stress testing can include 2-hour postprandial sugars or a full glucose tolerance test. Hemoglobin A1C or glycosylated hemoglobin may be useful in monitoring diabetic control in an individual patient. Usually by the time the foot complications of diabetes occur, the diagnosis is well established.

PERIPHERAL NEUROPATHY

There are many causes of peripheral neuropathy, other than diabetes, that enter the differential, including

1. Other metabolic causes (e.g., thyroid)
2. Lead poisoning and other heavy metals
3. Toxic—both drug and alcohol related
4. Various vitamin deficiencies and toxicities; pernicious anemia, in which B12 levels can be used in the diagnosis

SERONEGATIVE SPONDYLOARTHROPATHIES

Another major group of rheumatic diseases that have frequent manifestations in the ankle and foot are the seronegative spondyloarthropathies. These include psoriatic arthritis, Reiter's syndrome, ankylosing spondylitis, and the enteropathic arthritides. As with most forms of rheumatic disease, the diagnosis is made clinically.

Psoriatic arthritis has a number of different clinical presentations. These include spondylitis, rheumatoid arthritis-like, asymmetric distal arthritis, dactylitis that causes sausage digits, and arthritis mutilans. Nail changes are common. There are no diagnostic lab findings, although an elevated ESR and slight elevation of uric acid are common.

Reiter's syndrome is associated with a pauciarticular arthritis, frequently of the knees, ankles, metatarsals and toes. Conjunctivitis, urethritis, prostatitis, sacroiliitis, and a skin rash (keratoderma blennorrhagicum) are frequent clinical findings. Here too, an elevated ESR can be seen. Pyuria may also be a manifestation of Reiter's syndrome when associated with prostatitis or urethritis (which may be asymptomatic).

Probably the most important lab test when evaluating a patient with a mono- or pauciarticular arthritis, with urethritis, rash, and enteritis, is to rule out an infectious cause. Joint aspiration and culture should be performed to rule out gonorrhea as well as other organisms. When appropriate, urethral, cervical, and rectal cultures should be performed.

Chlamydia is one of the organisms thought to induce Reiter's syndrome, and an effort should be made in the lab to identify this pathogen. Cultures are not reliable. Swabs should be taken for direct fluorescent antibodies and enzyme immunoassay or preferably for polymerase chain reaction assays.

A variety of enteric pathogens such as *Salmonella, Shigella, Yersinia, and Campylobacter* can also induce Reiter's syndrome. These may be confirmed by stool culture.

Arthritis associated with Crohn's disease and with ulcerative colitis will have negative stool and synovial fluid cultures. Intestinal histopathology should be helpful in confirming clinical suspicions of an inflammatory bowel disease.

Human immunodeficiency virus (HIV) infection has also been associated with a Reiter's syndrome–like arthritis. Screening ELISA and confirmation with Western blot should be considered after appropriate history and physical examination and counseling.

It is well known that there is a relationship between HLA-B27 and ankylosing spondylitis. The sensitivity of this test is approximately 95% in ankylosing spondylitis, 80% in Reiter's syndrome, and 50% in the spondylitis associated with inflammatory bowel disease. The background prevalence of this marker (6–10% in Whites) and the fact that only a small minority of HLA-B27-positive individuals will ever experience an arthropathy make the test of limited use. According to some authors, a person with a pretest probability of 10% has only a 64% chance of having disease if HLA-

B27 is present. Thus, when the test is ordered for patients with back pain that is not clinically suggestive of sacroiliitis, the test may yield more false-positive than true-positive results.

Thus, a positive HLA-B27 may be of some value, but, as noted previously, it may result in the misclassification of diseases if it is relied on too heavily.

SYNOVIAL FLUID ANALYSIS

Synovial fluid analysis is one of the most useful lab tests that can be performed in the evaluation of arthritis. It should be performed as part of the work-up in most every patient with a joint effusion. It is particularly important in the evaluation of septic arthritis.

Even in patients with an established diagnosis, it may provide evidence about the activity of disease. Alternatively, it may demonstrate the coexistence of another disease. For example, a patient with an underlying inflammatory arthritis such as RA may also have a superimposed infection. Similarly, a patient with RA or osteoarthritis (OA) may also have gout or pseudogout.

Joint fluid has often been classified into five groups:

1. Normal: often less than 1 mL; with high viscosity, transparent, colorless or straw colored, with less than 200 WBCs and less than 25% of them PMNs and with a negative culture

2. Noninflammatory (e.g., osteoarthritis): greater than 1 mL; transparent with high viscosity, although the color may be more yellow; 50 to 1000 WBC with less than 25% PMNs; culture negative

3. Inflammatory: greater than 1 mL of fluid is present and may be greater than 1000 mL; with low viscosity, translucent but not transparent, yellow, and with cell counts of 1000 to 75,000; the percentage of PMNs are typically greater than 50%; cultures are also negative. This category includes RA, psoriatic arthritis, Reiter's syndrome, bowel-related SLE, scleroderma, Wegener's granulomatosis, Sjögren's syndrome, sarcoidosis, crystal-induced, as well as a host of others

4. Septic: greater than 1 mL of opaque fluid colored yellow to green; WBC counts often higher than 100,000 and greater than 85% are PMNs; culture is typically positive, although it is important to recognize that the Gram's stain is frequently not positive

5. Hemarthrosis: the presence of grossly and diffusely bloody fluid suggests a group of diagnoses, including trauma, pigmented villonodular synovitis (PVNS), coagulation defects, and tumors

Evaluation of the specimen under compensated polarized light microscopy is of critical importance. This is the only reliable method of diagnosing an acute attack of gout or pseudogout. Monosodium urate crystals are intensely negatively birefringent and form needles and rods. When found intracellularly, they are virtually diagnostic of gout. Calcium pyrophosphate dihydrate is weakly birefringent and often rhomboid in shape. Many other crystals have been described and include those composed of hydroxyapatite clumps, calcium oxalate, cholesterol, depot steroids (from prior joint injections), lipids, Charcot-Leyden crystals, and immunoglobulins. These crystals are found in a variety of clinical settings and may be useful in the diagnosis of many diseases.

METABOLIC BONE DISEASE

Stress fractures of the foot are common causes of foot pain. In patients with normal bone, they typically occur either after new types of exercise are performed or after more vigorous activity is undertaken than customary. A history of change in footwear or exercise pattern may be elicited. However, stress fractures may also occur with normal levels of activity.

Osteoporosis is a frequent cause of abnormal bone that can lead to stress fractures. There are many different causes and risk factors for osteoporosis. Many of them are associated with laboratory abnormalities.

For example, among the causes are

1. Drugs, such as steroids (hypokalemia)
2. Estrogen and testosterone deficiency states (measurement of specific hormone levels)
3. Renal disease (blood urea nitrogen, creatinine clearance)
4. Gastrointestinal and liver disease (liver function tests, antimitochondrial antibody, stool fat, lactose tolerance tests, and carotene)

5. Abnormalities of vitamin D, phosphate, and calcium metabolism (Ca^{++}, $PO4^{--}$, 25-OH vitamin D, 24-hour urine for calcium)

6. Hyperthyroidism and hyperparathyroidism (thyroid stimulating hormone, thyroxine [T4], T4 uptake, triiodothyronine, T7 index, PTH, electrolyte abnormalities, calcium levels, urinary calcium)

7. Marrow replacement, such as with myeloma (serum immunoelectrophoresis [SIEP], ESR, CBC) or leukemia (CBC)

8. Autoimmune diseases: not only may these illnesses cause an inflammatory arthritis that can involve the foot, but most are associated with osteoporosis

Paget's disease is another metabolic disease of bone that should be suspected as a cause of foot pain if there is an elevated alkaline phosphatase and high urinary hydroxyproline levels. Although it most often occurs in the spine, pelvis, skull, femur, and tibia, it may also occur in the small bones of the foot. Similarly, osteomalacia may also affect the lower extremity, and characteristic laboratory findings may be sought (e.g., calcium level, phosphorus, vitamin D).

INFECTION

Infections may involve the foot in a number of ways. Laboratory assessment is helpful in their identification. The most important mechanism is direct infection, such as septic arthritis. In this situation, aspiration of the joint with aseptic technique with Gram's stain and culture is of paramount importance.

Lyme disease can affect the joints of the feet, although it most often affects the knee joints. The diagnosis of Lyme disease is based primarily on the clinical history (e.g., erythema migrans, cardiac, neurologic, joint), exposure to the tick vector in an endemic area, and confirmation with lab testing.

If Lyme disease is suspected, a screening test is performed. Most often, the ELISA is used, although immunofluorescent techniques are also available. The ELISA may give false-positive results (and very rarely false-negative results); thus, a confirmatory test with Western immunoblot is required. It should be stressed that IgG Lyme titers usually stay elevated long after Lyme disease is treated. Thus, a positive IgG titer only indicates past exposure and not necessarily an active infection.

As noted previously, Reiter's syndrome frequently affects the feet. Reiter's syndrome may be triggered by a number of infections, which, of course, may have laboratory correlates. SBE will sometimes cause an immune-related arthritis, unrelated to direct infection. In the proper clinical setting (fever, heart murmur, embolic events), blood cultures are indicated.

VASCULITIS-VASCULOPATHIES

A variety of vasculitic syndromes may present with manifestations in the feet. One major mode of presentation is vascular insufficiency. This may initially cause claudication, and may later progress to pallor, cyanosis, ulceration and eventually gangrene of the toes or feet. Often, small-vessel vasculitis will present as a rash or palpable purpura. Hydrostatic forces are thought to play a role in their preferential appearance in the lower extremities. Finally, neuropathy resulting from infarction of the vasa nervorum may have major manifestations in the foot.

Immunologic causes of vasculitis often have characteristic laboratory findings. For example, active generalized Wegener's granulomatosis is highly associated with antineutrophil cytoplasmic antibodies (ANCA). These antibodies cause a characteristic pattern of cytoplasmic granular staining with immunofluorescence. The antibodies appear to be directed against proteinase 3 (PR3), a serine protease found in the primary granules of neutrophils. C-ANCA is found in 90% of cases of Wegener's granulomatosis and is usually not present in other types of vasculitis. The titers of C-ANCA parallel disease activity of Wegener's granulomatosis. They are not as commonly found in the limited forms of Wegener's granulomatosis.

Antibodies directed against myeloperoxidase produce a perinuclear pattern of staining referred to as P-ANCA. P-ANCAs are characteristic markers of systemic necrotizing vasculitis, and are seen in microscopic polyarteritis, idiopathic glomerulonephritis, and Churg-Strauss syndrome.

Atypical ANCAs directed against targets other than myeloperoxidase (MPO) and PR3 are found in a wide variety of conditions.

These include inflammatory bowel disease, liver disease, chronic infections, RA, HIV, and others. Mounting evidence directly implicates ANCAs in the pathogenesis of vasculitis.

ANTIPHOSPHOLIPID ANTIBODIES

A factor has been known to exist in the serum of some SLE patients that prolongs the PTT. This inhibitor was frequently associated with false-positive serologic tests for syphilis. The factor could be absorbed from plasma by phospholipids. This factor became known as the lupus anticoagulant, even though approximately half of the patients with this serologic abnormality do not have SLE. In addition, although the inhibitor acts as an anticoagulant in vitro, patients with the lupus anticoagulant were not prone to excess bleeding. In fact, the opposite was found: they were prone to both arterial and venous thromboses as well as thrombocytopenia and fetal loss or miscarriage.

Antiphospholipid antibodies include the lupus anticoagulant, anticardiolipin antibodies, and antibodies to other negatively charged phospholipids. Antiphospholipid antibodies may be formed directly against phospholipids or to a cofactor protein, beta-2 glycoprotein-1, that binds to phospholipid (or the antibodies may be directed against both).

Patients with these syndromes may present with ischemia, necrosis, and gangrene of the toes. Treatment with anticoagulation is usually indicated.

CRYOGLOBULINEMIA

Cryoglobulins are usually immune complexes (rarely they include other serum constituents) that precipitate at low temperatures.

1. Type I cryoglobulinemia is associated with monoclonal immunoglobulins such as those occurring in Waldenström's disease, lymphoma, or multiple myeloma
2. Type II cryoglobulinemia is composed of a monoclonal IgM-rheumatoid factor bound to autologous IgG
3. Type III cryoglobulinemia is the most common type and contains polyclonal rheumatoid factor bound to polygonal IgG

Many patients with type II or III cryoglobulins have hepatitis C infection. Thus, evaluation for hepatitis C with appropriate antibody tests is usually warranted. Hepatitis B, endocarditis, and many other infections may be associated with cryoglobulins. The typical presentation includes a palpable purpura on the lower extremities in nearly all patients. Ischemic toes may also develop.

Diagnosis requires the identification of a cryoprecipitate in the serum. Blood should be kept at body temperature (37°C) until the serum is separated. The serum is then kept at 4°C for 48 hours and examined for a precipitate. The precipitate is expressed as a percentage of the serum volume, and may be further characterized by electrophoresis and immunofixation. Complement activation may frequently be present on lab evaluation. In addition, evidence of glomerulonephritis and nephrosis may be present (e.g., active urine sediment, proteinuria, and abnormal renal function tests).

A number of hypercoagulable states may present in much the same way as the vasculitides. These include disorders of coagulation related to deficiency of factor C, factor S, and antithrombin III. Factor 5 Leyden may also lead to a hypercoagulable state. Specific coagulation assays should be performed when these conditions are suspected, particularly if there is a family history of coagulopathy.

NODULES

Tendon nodules are another common finding in clinical practice and one in which the lab may be useful in diagnosis. I have already discussed the laboratory diagnosis of a number of diseases in which nodules of the foot may occur. These include RA, SLE, gout (tophi), and rheumatic fever.

Another group of fairly common entities should also be considered in the differential diagnosis of foot and tendon nodules: the hyperlipidemias. Type II hyperlipoproteinemia may present with Achilles tendinitis and tenosynovitis. Asymmetric oligoarticular synovitis has been described in type IV hyperlipoproteinemia. Cholesterol and triglyceride profiles are useful in the evaluation of these disorders.

From this discussion, it is clear that laboratory testing is an invaluable part of the diagnostic process. However, it is best used only in a directed fashion and only as part of a complete evaluation that includes a history and physical examination.

SELECTED BIBLIOGRAPHY

ARA Glossary Committee. Dictionary of the Rheumatic diseases: Vol II: Diagnostic Testing. New York: Contact Associates, 1985.

Kelley WN, Harris ED, Ruddy S, Sledge CB, eds. Textbook of Rheumatology. Philadelphia: W. B. Saunders, 1997.

Khan MA, Kellner H. Immunogenetics of spondyloarthropathies. Rheum Dis Clin North Am 18:837, 1992.

McCarty GA. Autoantibodies and their relation to rheumatic diseases. Med Clin North Am 70:237–261, 1986.

Nolle B, Specks U, Ludermann J, et al. Anticytoplasmic autoantibodies: their immunodiagnostic value in Wegener granulomatosis. Ann Intern Med 111:28–40, 1989.

Paget S, Pellicci P, Beary JF, eds. Manual of Rheumatology and Outpatient Orthopedic Disorders. Boston: Little, Brown, 1993.

Sammaritano LR, Gharavi AE, Lockshin MD. Antiphospholipid antibody syndrome: immunologic and clinical aspects. Semin Arthritis Rheum 20:81 1990.

Schumacher HR, ed. Primer on the Rheumatic Diseases. Atlanta: Arthritis Foundation, 1993.

Schumacher HR, Reginato AJ. Atlas of Synovial Fluid Analysis and Crystal Identification. Philadelphia: Lea & Febiger, 1991.

Sox HC Jr, Liang MH. The erythrocyte sedimentation rate: guidelines for rational use. Ann Intern Med 104:515–523, 1986.

5

Electrodiagnosis in Heel and Foot Disorders

Gary Sclar
Carl Heise

Joseph Moreira
Michael Rubin

Electrodiagnostic investigations, comprising nerve conduction studies (NCSs) and electromyography (EMG), play a central role in the differential diagnosis of heel and foot pain. Radiculopathies, proximal entrapment neuropathies, and compression neuropathies affecting nerves at or distal to the ankle may be mistaken for bony or ligamentous abnormalities in the foot with unfavorable consequences if missed and left untreated. In this chapter, we review the general principles of NCS and EMG and their role in the evaluation of neurologic disorders affecting the foot.

NERVE CONDUCTION STUDIES

Motor and sensory nerves are studied individually, but the underlying principle for each is identical. A nerve is stimulated at one or more sites along its course, and a recording is made at a second site. If a motor nerve is being studied, the recording electrode is placed over any muscle that the nerve supplies, and the nerve is stimulated, usually at several points proximally along its course (Fig. 5–1). If a sensory nerve is studied, both the recording and stimulating electrodes are placed over the nerve, and the nerve is usually stimulated at only one location. This technique is used for sensory nerve studies because, unlike motor nerves, sensory nerves have no end organ from which a recording can easily be made.

The general technique is best illustrated by example (see Fig. 5–1A). The peroneal nerve has both motor and sensory branches, and separate motor and sensory responses may be studied (other nerves, such as the sural, may only have a sensory function). The motor branch of the peroneal supplies, among other muscles, the extensor digitorum brevis (EDB), which is commonly used as the "recording muscle" in tests of this nerve. To record a motor response, a pair of recording electrodes are used. One, the active electrode G1, is placed over the motor point. This is the region where the motor neuron endplates (synapses) are found, and it is generally located in most muscles midway between the muscle origin and insertion; as an approximation, a location over the main bulk of the muscle is generally used. Failure to locate the active electrode over this point accurately can result in distortion of the initial deflection of the motor response and a diminished response amplitude. Second, a reference electrode, G2, is placed distal to the active electrode, generally over the muscle's tendinous insertion. For the EDB this would be over the fifth metatarsophalangeal joint. Both electrodes are plugged into the inputs of a recording amplifier. The relative location of the two electrodes is important because recording amplifiers are generally constructed to cancel similar signals presented over the two electrodes, thereby reducing the noise in small electrical signals. If, for instance, the reference electrode is placed by accident over part of the muscle and picks up or "sees" the same motor response as the active electrode, such common mode rejection by the amplifier may cause a dramatic reduction in the amplitude of the signal of interest.

After electrode placement, the peroneal nerve is electrically stimulated at several points, usually at the distal tibia anteriorly between the malleoli, at the neck of the fibula, and behind the knee (lateral popliteal fossa). Particular care must be taken when stimulating over the popliteal fossa because the tibial nerve lies only a small distance medial to the peroneal, and current spread may activate both nerves concurrently. The reason for stimulating at multiple sites is discussed later. The response resulting from each stimulation is known as an M response (muscle response) or CMAP (compound muscle action potential). Note

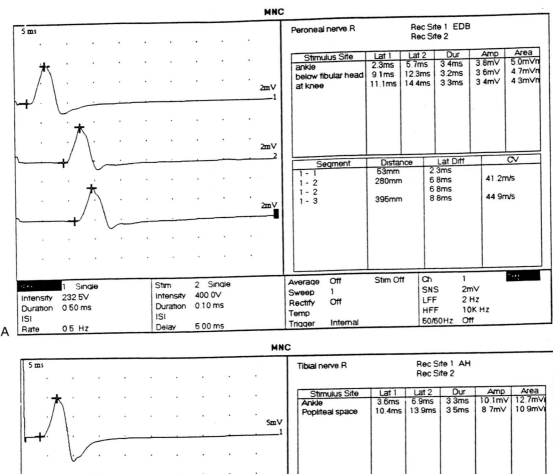

Figure 5–1 *See legend on opposite page*

that the size of the response (the evoked response amplitude) normally decreases as the distance between the stimulating and recording electrodes increases, but the drop should not exceed 10% of the CMAP obtained at the smallest distance used; a greater decrement may indicate disease. The tibial motor nerve can similarly be studied using a tibial innervated foot muscle, usually the abductor hallucis (AH) (see Fig. 5–1*B*), although the abductor digiti quinti pedis is used in special circumstances, such as in tarsal tunnel studies (see later discussion).

The technique for sensory nerve stimulation and recording is slightly different; both stimulating and recording electrodes are placed directly over the nerve of interest (Fig. 5–2). Thus, to study the sural nerve, a pair of electrodes (G1 and G2) is placed over the nerve behind the lateral malleolus, and the nerve is stimulated some distance from the recording electrodes, over the midcalf. For superficial peroneal sensory nerve study, the G1 and G2 electrodes are placed over the nerve at the ankle, and the nerve is stimulated on the lateral aspect of the lower leg. In this instance, the resulting response is known as a sensory nerve action potential (SNAP). Technique in placing the recording electrodes is important. Response amplitude will vary with the distance of the recording electrodes from the sensory branches of the nerve being tested; thus, anatomic knowledge of the course of the nerve is important. Moreover, placing the active and reference electrodes too close together can result in a diminished sensory response amplitude because of common mode rejection by the recording amplifier. Theoretic considerations suggest that the optimal interelectrode separation will vary with respect to the speed with which a sensory response is propagated (i.e., the sensory nerve conduction velocity), a parameter that can be affected by disease states and that cannot be estimated before one performs a study. An interelectrode (G1 active to G2 reference) distance of 3 cm, as found in most commonly used bar electrodes, is adequate for most studies, but whatever distance is used should be applied to all the nerves studied on a consistent basis.

The raw data obtained using these techniques (SNAPs and CMAPs) consist of biphasic negative-positive potentials. From these measurements, several parameters can be derived: nerve conduction velocity (NCV), evoked response amplitude, and distal latency. NCV, the speed with which the electrical impulse is propagated along the nerve, is derived by dividing the distance traversed by the impulse by the time taken for the impulse to travel that distance. Time is measured from the onset of the electrical stimulus to the start of the initial deflection of the recorded waveform from baseline, referred to as onset latency. Note that to derive a sensory nerve conduction velocity, it is sufficient to take the distance between the stimulating and active (G1 recording) electrodes for this purpose and divide this by the onset latency. In the case of a motor nerve conduction velocity, the nerve is stimulated at two locations; the distance between these two stimulation sites is used for the calculation of conduction velocity. This distance is then divided by the difference in onset latency obtained for the two sites. By taking the difference of the two onset latencies, neuromuscular transmission time is eliminated from the calculation. The evoked

---

Figure 5–1. Normal motor nerve conduction studies for the foot. *A,* Normal peroneal motor response. The active electrode was placed over the bulk of the extensor digitorum brevis (EDB) muscle on the dorsolateral aspect of the foot. The reference electrode was placed over the tendon of the muscle (metatarsophalangeal joint; fifth digit). The three traces correspond to (top trace) stimulation over the dorsal aspect of the ankle just lateral to the tendon of the tibialis anterior muscle (S-R distance was 53 mm), stimulation just below the fibular head (middle trace) (S-R distance was 280 mm), and stimulation over the lateral third of the popliteal fossa (S-R distance was 395 mm). Motor nerve conduction velocities were 41.2 m/s (fibular head-ankle segment) and 44.9 m/s (popliteal fossa to ankle); normal in our lab is 41–59 m/s. Evoked response amplitudes for the three locations were 3.8, 3.6, and 3.4 mV, respectively. Normal in our lab is >0.5 mV. *B,* Normal tibial motor response (different subject). The active electrode was placed 1 cm behind and 1 cm below the navicular bone, over the motor point of the abductor hallucis (AH) muscle on the medial aspect of the foot. The reference electrode was placed over the first metatarsophalangeal joint. The two traces correspond to (top trace) stimulation over the nerve, posterior to the medial malleolus and above the flexor retinaculum (S-R distance was 80 mm), and stimulation over the crease of the popliteal fossa 1/2–2/3 from the medial side. Motor nerve conduction velocity was 48.5 m/s; normal in our lab is 41–59 m/s. Evoked response amplitudes for the two locations were 10.1 and 8.7 mV, respectively. Normal in our lab is >0.5 mV. Normal distal motor latency values are available for this muscle for standard S-R distances of 80 (<4.4 ms) and 100 (< 4.8 ms) mm and are useful in tarsal tunnel studies. In this case, results for the AH are compared with those obtained from recording from the abductor digiti minimi (ADM) muscle on the lateral aspect of the foot; the same stimulating site and S-R distances are used (generally measured with a caliper); (at 80 mm, distal latency for the ADM should be <4.6 ms, at 100 mm it should be <4.9 ms). When recording from the ADM the active electrode is placed half-way between the tip of the lateral malleolus and the sole of the foot. The reference is placed as for recording from the EDB: over the metatarsophalangeal joint of the fifth digit.

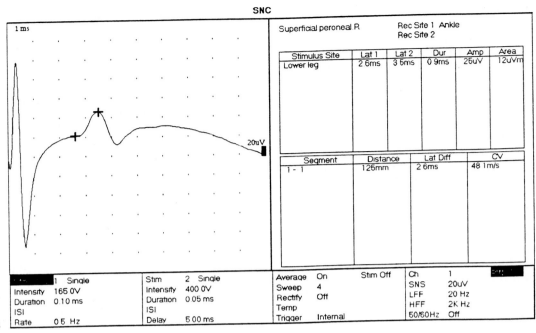

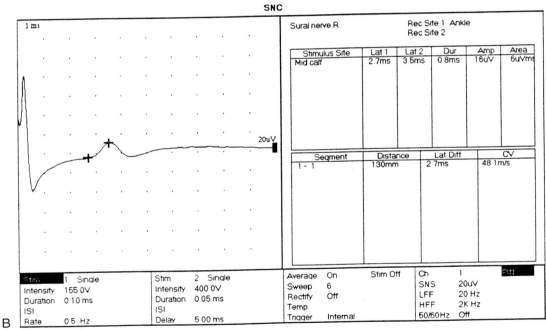

Figure 5–2. Normal sensory nerve conduction studies for the foot. *A,* Normal superficial peroneal nerve sensory response. The recording electrodes were placed on the dorsal aspect of the foot over one of the dorsal cutaneous branches of the nerve. The active electrode was located 3 cm proximal to the reference. The stimulating electrodes were placed (anode distal) over the anterolateral calf. Anode (S, stimulus) to active (R, recording) distance was 125 mm. The ground electrode was, as is usual, placed in between the stimulating and recording electrodes. Sensory nerve conduction velocity was 48 m/s (normal in our lab is 41–59 m/s); response amplitude was 25 µV (normal is >5 µV). *B,* Normal sural nerve sensory response. The recording electrodes were placed below and posterior to the lateral malleolus. The active electrode was 3 cm proximal to the reference. The stimulating electrodes were placed (anode distal) just lateral to the midline over the lower third of the posterior side of the leg. The interelectrode distance (S to R) was 130 mm. Sensory nerve conduction velocity was 48 m/s (normal in our lab is 41–59 m/s); response amplitude was 16 µV (normal is >5 µV).

response amplitude is measured as the size of the response recorded over the muscle (motor in millivolts, sensory in microvolts) and is a measure used to estimate the number of functioning fibers in the nerve. However, responses in NCSs are typically dominated by the largest fibers in the nerve. Thus, diseases that predominantly affect small fibers may, in fact, result in NCSs that are completely normal.

The distal motor latency, often of inestimable value in foot disorders, is the onset latency obtained, recording from a muscle, at the most distal site of stimulation. In entrapment neuropathies, the distal motor latency may be prolonged as a result of nerve compression and resultant demyelination (see later discussion). The same is true for the distal sensory latency, which measures the time for the stimulus to conduct along the most distal segment of nerve studied.

Late responses include F waves and H reflexes and can assist in the diagnosis of foot problems (Fig. 5–3). The F wave is a compound muscle action potential that can be obtained from most muscles by supramaximal electrical stimulation of the nerve. The F wave results from antidromic (i.e., opposite the normal direction of conduction) activation of the anterior horn cell motor neurons in the spinal cord, which then send an impulse back down the nerve orthodromically to stimulate the muscle. The F wave is of smaller amplitude than the M response, follows the M response by a variable latency, and normally varies in configuration from trial to trial. The fastest F-wave latency after a number of trials provides information regarding the entire length of the motor nerve from the anterior horn cell in the spinal cord to the muscle fibers it innervates. Thus, in the case of a radiculopathy, for instance, routine NCSs involving the below-knee nerve segment may be normal, but the F wave, as it traverses the proximal, abnormal nerve segment, may be delayed.

The H reflex is essentially limited to the tibial nerve–soleus muscle and provides information of both the afferent and efferent S1 nerve fiber. It is the electrical counterpart of the Achilles reflex and, like the F wave, may be delayed with proximal disease, even though routine NCSs are normal. It can be facilitated by asking the client to contract the gastrocnemius gently; however, too large a contraction may eradicate the

response. It is recorded over the soleus by stimulating the tibial nerve behind the knee. The impulse again travels orthodromically, this time along 1a muscle spindle (sensory) afferents to the dorsal horn, synapses on the anterior horn cell, and continues along the anterior horn cell axon (motor nerve) to the muscle. A delayed response, in the face of normal NCSs, indicates proximal, usually root, disease.

Tables of normal data for these parameters are available in textbooks of electrodiagnostic medicine.[1, 2] These typically specify the interelectrode distance (stimulating to recording electrode) and sometimes other recording conditions (such as limb temperature; see later discussion), and so data need to be collected under similar conditions to render comparison meaningful. Where data are unavailable for a particular nerve, a common practice is to make side-to-side comparisons within a single subject, supposing that one side is affected by a condition and the other is normal. Side-to-side amplitude comparisons ought not to exceed a difference of 50% within a normal subject.[3, 4] For latency, a difference greater then 10% is considered significant.

A practitioner of NCSs must be aware of several potential sources of error that can occur in making such measurements. Some, such as interelectrode separation and placement, have already been alluded to previously. Several other factors bear consideration, particularly in electrodiagnostic studies of the foot and ankle. One of the most important of these is limb temperature.

Lower limb temperatures of less than 30°C are thought to have significant effects on NCSs. Extremities with poor circulation or affected by severe muscle atrophy are particularly prone to these effects. Cooling generally results in slowing of nerve conduction velocity of approximately 2 m/s/°C. There may be a concomitant increase in onset latency and a prolongation of the waveform of the response. The response amplitude may decrease secondary to temporal dispersion; individual fibers making up the nerve may be slowed to different extents, leading their responses to arrive at the recording site at different times. These desynchronized responses may act, in part, to cancel each other out.

Another important factor is anomalous innervation patterns. In the case of the foot,

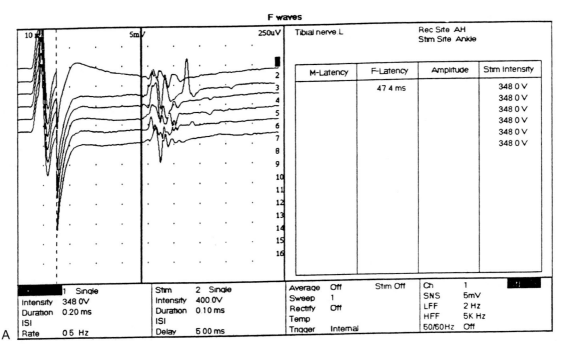

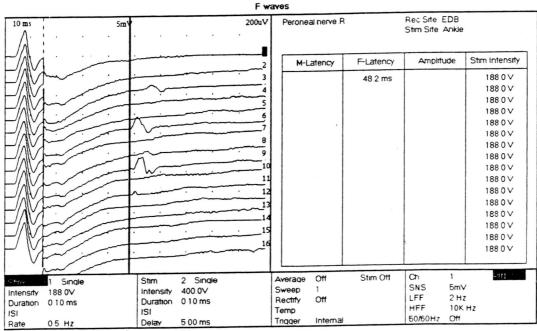

Figure 5–3. Normal late response (F-wave) studies for the foot. *A,* Normal tibial F wave. Recording electrode placement is as for the motor nerve conduction study. Stimulating electrode is placed at most distal stimulating position (medial ankle) except that the position of the anode and cathode are exchanged (i.e., anode distal). Stimulus intensity is adjusted to maximize the M response (on the left) and a series of tracings are recorded. The earliest F wave is used to derive the F-response latency. In this example it was 47.4 ms. (Normal values in our lab for both the F-extensor digitorum brevis (EDB) and F-Abductor hallucis (AH) are <56.5 ms). *B,* Normal peroneal F wave. This is the same as for Figure 5–3A except that the recording is made from the EDB, and stimulation was applied over the dorsal aspect of the ankle, as for the motor nerve conduction study for this muscle, with the anode and cathode reversed.

the EDB may infrequently receive a motor branch from the superficial peroneal nerve, which courses posterior to the lateral malleolus (accessory peroneal nerve). Typically, one may record a large CMAP by stimulating the EDB at the fibular head and a much smaller one at the ankle. Stimulation behind the lateral malleolus will make up the difference.

ELECTROMYOGRAPHY

EMG is the study of the electrical activity of muscle, performed by means of a needle electrode inserted directly into the muscle. It complements NCS, and together they can distinguish neuropathy from myopathy, localize neuropathic disorders, and quantify and provide prognostic information in many conditions causing heel and foot pain.

The muscle to be studied should be completely relaxed. Muscle activity in an unrelaxed muscle may hide abnormal activity. Specific landmarks for different muscles are available in a number of textbooks, but it is good practice to check, after the initial insertion, that one is in the correct muscle by asking the patient to perform the muscle's expected action gently. Some motor activity (recruitment) should be easily elicited. The subject is asked to relax the muscle completely, and insertions along each of several directions (through the same skin penetration) are gently undertaken. After each progression of the electrode, the examiner should stop to assess the muscle.

An EMG study involves evaluation of several different parameters: (1) insertional activity, (2) spontaneous activity, (3) motor unit potentials, and (4) interference patterns.

INSERTIONAL ACTIVITY. Inserting an electrode into a muscle at rest is associated with a brief burst of electrical activity, the result of the muscle fibers being depolarized by the physical displacement caused by the needle's movement. Insertional activity may be decreased (absent or <300 ms) in diseases that cause fibrosis or increased (when it lasts >300–500 ms) in processes causing denervation. Muscles displaying prolonged insertional activity are referred to as "irritable."

SPONTANEOUS ACTIVITY. The electrical recording of normal muscle at rest is electrical silence. Spontaneous activity is usually an abnormal finding and may be defined as electrical activity that is present while the muscle is fully relaxed. It takes several forms, the most common being fibrillation potentials and positive sharp waves, which generally occur together.

Fibrillations are brief (<5 ms) biphasic spikes. They represent the spontaneous action potential of a single muscle fiber and usually have a peak-to-peak amplitude of less than 1 mV. They may be seen in a variety of denervating disorders, muscle trauma, and destructive myopathies (myositis, muscular dystrophy). Positive sharp waves, which occur under similar conditions, are biphasic (positive-negative) potentials, are longer in duration than fibrillations, and have an amplitude of 1 mV. They tend to fire with frequencies of 1 to 50 Hz and may occur in "trains." Both fibrillation potentials and positive sharp waves tend to fire regularly but may occur irregularly. Other types of spontaneous activity may occur (i.e., complex repetitive discharges) but do so less frequently and are not discussed here.

Other forms of activity may also be recorded during needle EMG in a muscle at rest, and these must be distinguished from abnormal spontaneous activity. In part, these may result from recording near the end plate or synaptic region of a muscle. One type, referred to as *end-plate noise*, produces a "seashell" sound or roar when played over a speaker and represents low-amplitude (10–20 μV), short-duration (0.5–1 ms) monophasic potentials that likely result from miniature end-plate potentials. End-plate spikes are short (2–4 ms), moderate-sized (100–300 μV) biphasic "spikes" (negative-positive) that occur in short, irregular, high-frequency (50–100 Hz) bursts that represent single muscle fiber depolarizations and occur only near the end plate. Other less commonly encountered forms of activity include fasciculation potentials, myotonic discharges, myokymic discharges, and cramp discharges. When found, it is common to grade spontaneous activity quantitatively (Table 5–1).

MOTOR UNIT POTENTIALS. When a motor nerve (anterior horn cell) discharges, it activates all the muscle fibers innervated by that nerve, causing them to depolarize and

Table 5–1. Grading Spontaneous Activity

Grade	Criterion
0	Spontaneous activity absent
1+	Persistent activity in at least two muscle regions
2+	Moderate activity in three or more muscle regions
3+	Abundant activity in all muscle regions tested
4+	Fills the CRT screen in all regions of the muscle examined

contract. The summated electrical response of the depolarizing muscle fibers of a single motor unit is referred to as the motor unit potential (MUP). MUPs become large, polyphasic, and of increased duration in neurogenic disorders but small and of short duration in myopathies. In experienced hands, the evaluation of individual MUPs is as accurate as muscle biopsy in differentiating myopathy from neuropathy, with the advantage of being less invasive.

INTERFERENCE PATTERN. When a muscle contracts, the cumulative electrical activity of all the motor units firing is referred to as the interference pattern. A full interference pattern fills the oscilloscope screen during contraction and is present in normal muscle. In neurogenic disorders, axons degenerate, the number of motor units in an individual nerve falls, and the result is an incomplete, or decreased, interference pattern.

NEUROLOGIC CAUSES OF FOOT PAIN

The three most common neurologic causes of foot pain are entrapment neuropathies, peripheral neuropathies, and posttraumatic pain syndromes.

Entrapment Neuropathies

Tibial, Plantar, and Digital Nerves

The tibial nerve is most susceptible to entrapment as it passes under the flexor retinaculum behind the medial malleolus (i.e., the posterior tarsal tunnel). At this point, the tibial nerve branches into the medial and lateral plantar nerves, although the branching may occur proximal or distal to the tunnel.[5] The calcaneal nerve also branches from the tibial nerve in this area to supply sensation to the plantar aspect of the heel.

The (posterior) tarsal tunnel syndrome, an entrapment neuropathy of the tibial nerve or its branches at the level of the medial malleolus, usually results from trauma to the ankle such as fracture[6] or dislocation. The nerve may be externally compressed by footwear or a cast. Fibrosis, which can follow an episode of trauma by years, can also lead to compression. Within the tarsal tunnel, in addition to the nerve, typically run the tendons of three muscles: tibialis posterior, flexor digitorum longus, and flexor hallucis longus. Synovial cysts arising from these, as well as ganglia[7] or cysts[8] arising from the nerves themselves, may compromise the nerve within the tunnel. Less commonly, abnormal muscles,[9] schwannomas,[10, 11] and lipomas[12] can impact on the nerve. The syndrome has been noted as a cause of foot and ankle pain in runners.[13] Systemic causes include diabetes, hyperuricemia, alcoholism, rheumatoid arthritis,[14] and hypothyroidism.[15]

Symptoms include dull, aching, or burning pain in the ankle and foot, with paresthesia in the sole typically exacerbated by standing or walking. The intrinsic foot muscles, which receive their innervation from the plantar nerves, are usually weak, although this may be difficult to assess clinically. Although bilateral abnormalities have occasionally been demonstrated on nerve conduction studies,[16] symptoms are usually unilateral. These can often be reproduced by percussing the area of the tarsal tunnel, posterior and inferior to the medial malleolus (Tinel's sign), and by extending the great toe or everting the ankle. Sensory loss may be demonstrable over the sole of the foot or limited to the distribution of the medial or lateral plantar nerves.

The diagnosis is confirmed by nerve conduction studies demonstrating prolonged distal latencies of the lateral and medial plantar motor and sensory nerves, stimulating the tibial nerve at the medial malleolus proximal to the tarsal ligament and recording over the appropriate muscle (usually at a standard distance of 8 or 10 cm) for motor latencies or at the first and fifth toes for sensory latencies. The contralateral foot serves as the control. Although the sensory technique is the more sensitive of the two,[17] the sensory responses are small and require averaging to demonstrate clearly.[4]

Mixed NCSs (both motor and sensory), performed by stimulating the medial and lateral plantar nerves over the sole and recording from the posterior tibial nerve proximal to the flexor retinaculum (at a standard distance of 14 cm),[18] may be superior for presurgical diagnosis of tarsal tunnel[17] and are preferred by some authors.[4] Peak latencies should be less then 3.6 ms for both the lateral and medial nerve branches. This technique, however, has a number of pitfalls. It may be difficult to perform in patients with thick plantar calluses and in patients with significant ankle swelling (which can affect the size of the posterior tibial response). Some patients may not be able to tolerate the stimulus intensities required to obtain a response.

Finally, techniques for measuring the conduction of motor nerve responses across the tarsal tunnel, which may allow for differentiation of the nerves within the tunnel as opposed to distal to it (see later discussion), have been published.[19]

EMG of the symptomatic foot in tarsal tunnel syndrome may demonstrate spontaneous activity at rest with abnormalities of motor unit potential form localized to the muscles of the affected nerve.[20] However, caution is warranted because up to 11.1% of normal persons (higher in some series) may have positive waves in the pedal musculature as a result of the trauma inflicted by daily activities.[21]

Tumors of the tibial nerve in the calf region and the sciatic nerve in the thigh or Baker's cysts in the popliteal fossa may mimic tarsal tunnel syndrome.[22, 23] Knee trauma infrequently causes tibial nerve damage. NCS and EMG of the leg are essential in these instances to localize the level of mononeuropathy. Partial sciatic neuropathies, S1 radiculopathies, and polyneuropathies are also in the differential diagnosis, and NCS and EMG help distinguish between these possibilities. Interestingly, painful diabetic polyneuropathy has been reported to improve after tarsal tunnel decompression.[24]

The medial and lateral plantar nerves may be entrapped distal to the tarsal tunnel. Pain, paresthesia, and sensory loss in this case are confined to the distribution of the particular nerve involved. Sensation over the heel is usually preserved in these patients because the calcaneal nerve commonly branches off *in* the tarsal tunnel. NCSs are technically difficult in such instances but may reveal prolongation of the distal latency in the particular nerve affected. Published techniques for recording across the tarsal tunnel[19] may allow localization of nerve compression to these sites.

Baxter's nerve, the first branch of the lateral plantar nerve, runs deep to the fascia of the abductor hallucis muscle and supplies the abductor digiti quinti. This muscle may hypertrophy in runners, resulting in nerve entrapment. Thickening of the plantar fascia, chronic inflammation, or calcaneal spur may also compress the nerve. The resulting pain is similar to that of plantar fasciitis but with more of a burning quality. It may also radiate proximally up the leg. Tenderness over the course of the nerve is usual.[25, 26] Other sports such as power lifting have also been reported to cause entrapment of the lateral plantar nerve,[27] possibly because of the heavy forces transmitted through the foot.

Morton's neuroma,[28] or Morton's metatarsalgia, is an entrapment neuropathy of an interdigital nerve between adjacent metatarsal heads. It usually affects the nerve lying between the third and fourth metatarsals. Histologically, a true neuroma is usually absent, and the condition develops, instead, secondary to fibrosis of the soft tissues surrounding the nerve, with subsequent neural compression. The main symptoms are aching or burning pain in the region of the metatarsal head, radiating into the two adjacent toes. The condition is typically exacerbated by walking and is alleviated by rest and removal of shoes. Symptoms may be constant or stabbing and shocklike and can be provoked by palpating or percussing the appropriate interdigital space close to the metatarsophalangeal joint or compressing the sides of the foot. Objective sensory loss is less commonly documented. Most sufferers are women between 30 and 60 years of age[29, 30]; one theory holds that the condition may be brought about by excessive stress on the forefoot perhaps from wearing high-heel shoes.[30] Neurectomy is often followed by good pain relief.[29] However, conservative medical treatment is also efficacious and consists of shoe orthoses and steroid or lidocaine injections into the area with avoidance of high-heel shoes.

Joplin's neuroma, the medial plantar proper digital nerve syndrome, results from damage to this nerve where it crosses the first metatarsophalangeal joint or the medial surface of the great toe. It is most often due to poorly fitting footwear. Pain and paresthesia are localized to the medial aspect of the great toe.

The role of NCS and EMG in these last three entrapment neuropathies is mainly to exclude other disorders that may mimic them. This is because NCSs of the affected nerves in these entrapments are not standardized and are technically difficult to perform.

Peroneal Nerve

The common peroneal nerve is most susceptible to compression as it winds around the head of the fibula where its branches, the deep and superficial peroneal nerve, may be compressed, usually subsequent to habitual leg crossing.[31] Along with weakness of foot eversion, lesions of the superficial peroneal nerve may present with sensory loss and paresthesia over the dorsum of the foot. The superficial peroneal nerve may also be entrapped after it has given off the motor branches to the peroneus longus and brevis muscles. The common site for this lesion is where the nerve emerges from the deep fascia, several centimeters above the lateral malleolus.[32] In these cases, the patient usually reports only the sensory symptoms mentioned previously.

Entrapment of the deep peroneal nerve usually produces only minimal sensory disturbances in the web space between the first and second toes. Weakness of foot and toe dorsiflexion are the predominant complaints. In both these conditions, NCS of the peroneal motor and sensory branches, along with EMG, are usually able to demonstrate and localize the abnormality.

In the "anterior tarsal tunnel syndrome," the deep peroneal nerve becomes entrapped anteriorly at the ankle under the extensor retinaculum[33, 34] or extensor digitorum brevis muscle.[35] Symptoms include pain and paresthesia in the ankle, dorsum of the foot, and great toe with sensory loss in the web space between the first and second toes. A positive Tinel's sign (reproduction of pain and paresthesia in the distribution in the nerve by percussion of the nerve) may be present over the inferior aspect of the extensor retinaculum. This condition may be diagnosed using NCS: stimulation of the deep peroneal nerve proximal to the extensor retinaculum and recording over the EDB muscle reveals a prolonged distal motor latency and sometimes also a reduced motor evoked response amplitude.[34] On needle EMG, abnormalities may be found in the EDB.[34] Surgical decompression may be required, but conservative measures are usually sufficient.

Sural Nerve

Compression of the sural nerve is uncommon but when it occurs it is usually at the ankle. Fractures and their related injuries (i.e., repeated ankle sprains) are the main causes. The primary symptoms are pain and paresthesia over the posterolateral lower leg and lateral portion of the dorsum of the foot. Because the sural nerve is commonly sampled for nerve biopsy, these symptoms can also occur after sural nerve biopsy. An absent sural sensory response or prolonged latency is diagnostic.

Peripheral Neuropathies

Peripheral neuropathies as a cause of foot pain are seen with many systemic diseases; diabetic neuropathy is the most common in the United States. Up to two thirds of all patients with diabetes (insulin and non–insulin-dependent diabetes) may have signs (clinical or electrodiagnostic) of polyneuropathy, whereas only about 20% overall have subjective symptoms. The two most frequently diagnosed forms of diabetic neuropathy that affect the foot and ankle are symmetric polyneuropathies and mononeuropathies; the former are more common.

Symmetric polyneuropathies affecting large fibers usually present with paresthesia in the feet and lower legs,[36] with loss of vibration and position sensation in a stocking distribution on neurologic examination. A certain degree of gait ataxia is common, and a positive Romberg's sign is variably present. Deep tendon reflexes will be attenuated if not absent, especially at the ankle. An acute painful neuropathy in diabetic patients, mediated by small nerve fibers, is also recognized.[37] This involves symptoms of severe burning, stabbing, or lancinating pain in the soles of the feet and intense hypersensitivity (allodynia). In addition to these predominantly sensory sequelae, a mild to moderate motor component may be present, with distally predominant weakness; patients, for example, may have difficulty walking on their heels.

Histologically, either large or small myelinated fibers may be involved by axonal loss, or both fiber types may be affected simultaneously. Patients with this latter type of histology are particularly prone to the development of diabetic foot ulcers. Some degree of segmental demyelination (and possibly evidence of remyelination) may also be present, but this is usually a less prominent phenomenon in diabetes.

Additionally, in the context of diabetes, lower leg and foot pain with paresthesia are occasionally seen after implementation of insulin or hypoglycemic drug therapy (insulin neuritis).[38] A 1994 study[39] suggests that hyperinsulinemia alone, induced in normoglycemic individuals, may cause sensory nerve dysfunction with decreased thermal sensation, but not pain per se. The sensations of pain and temperature are clearly related, and it is generally thought that they are conveyed by the same sensory fibers. Perhaps by altering the function of the small sensory fibers of the nervous system that transmit temperature information, insulin makes them more likely to signal pain or other noxious stimuli, but how this might occur is unknown. A clear biochemical pathogenesis for diabetic neuropathy has not yet been demonstrated, but a role has been posited for epidermally derived nerve growth factor, which is depleted in diabetic animal models.[40]

Electrophysiologic findings in diabetes are well described. When large-diameter nerve fibers are affected, NCSs reveal decreased evoked response amplitudes of both motor and sensory nerve fibers with some mild slowing of sensory and motor nerve conduction velocities. With pure axonal loss, such minimal decreases in nerve conduction velocity are generally thought to be due to loss of the largest diameter (and, therefore, most quickly conducting) nerve fibers and ought not to exceed 70% of the lower limit of normal. Larger decrements imply demyelinating disease, as found in other forms of polyneuropathy and to some extent in diabetes.

EMG in patients with diabetic polyneuropathy may reveal a variable degree of fibrillation potentials and positive sharp waves predominantly in the distal muscles of the lower limbs. In long-standing disease, more proximal lower extremity and distal upper extremity muscles may be involved as well.

Two caveats should be mentioned:

1. If small instead of large diameter fibers are primarily affected, as can occur in diabetes, NCSs will be normal because the potentials produced by these smaller fibers are not measured by current NCS techniques.

2. Electrophysiologic deficits, when present in the limbs, should be symmetric in the context of a polyneuropathy. If they are not, consideration should be given to the possibility of a different underlying process; one example might be mononeuritis multiplex, a usually asymmetric involvement of multiple individual nerves. Diabetes can cause this. However, diabetic nerves are more susceptible to compression, and any of the entrapment neuropathies discussed previously may also be manifest. A symmetric polyneuropathy with a superimposed, asymmetric entrapment neuropathy or mononeuropathy is thus a possibility.

Alcoholism, another very common cause of symmetric polyneuropathy, is characterized by weakness, pain, and paresthesia in the feet and lower legs.[41] This may develop acutely to subacutely or may follow a more insidious course. All sensory modalities are usually affected in a "stocking" distribution, with loss of deep tendon reflexes at the ankle; both small and large nerve fibers are histologically affected (axonal loss). NCSs usually show decreased motor and sensory amplitudes with normal distal latencies and conduction velocities, whereas EMG shows chronic changes in the form of decreased numbers of large polyphasic motor unit potentials without spontaneous activity.

Another increasingly encountered symmetric polyneuropathy is the distal polyneuropathy of human immunodeficiency virus (HIV); again, the major pathologic mechanism here is axonal loss. This often occurs during the early stages of the disease (acquired immunodeficiency syndrome–related complex), and patients may present with bilateral burning paresthesia of the soles, worsened by touch or standing. Accompanying this is a decrement to all sensory modalities, but vibration sense in particular. Attenuation of the ankle tendon reflexes is usual. A mild degree of weakness of the intrinsic foot muscles, with some wasting (especially the EDB) may be noted. Histologically, loss of both myelinated and unmyelinated nerve fibers is found with some secondary demyelination. Electrophysiologically, sensory responses in the lower extremities may be reduced (early on) or absent (with disease progression) but when present show only mildly decreased nerve conduction velocities. Motor nerve responses may be similarly affected. EMG of the intrinsic foot muscles and later the muscles of the leg may show abnormal spontaneous activity (positive sharp waves and fibrillations) together with decreased recruitment and motor unit remodeling typical of a neuropathic process (increases in motor unit potential duration, amplitude, and number of phases). The major significance of this form of polyneuropathy is that it may be the presenting feature of HIV-related disease, and should be considered when young, otherwise healthy people present with symptoms of polyneuropathy affecting the feet.

Although these are some of the most common entities to affect the foot, the differential diagnosis of foot pain associated with polyneuropathy is broad, and a complete review is beyond the scope of this chapter. It includes vasculitic neuropathies, such as polyarteritis nodosa, rheumatoid arthritis, and systemic lupus erythematosus as well as neuropathies associated with malignancies, paraproteinemias, and dysproteinemias. The latter are usually associated with demyelinating forms of polyneuropathy with prolonged distal latencies and pronounced slowing of motor and sensory nerve conduction velocities.

Reflex Sympathetic Dystrophy (Causalgia)

Nerve injury may infrequently result in a painful syndrome known as reflex sympathetic dystrophy or causalgia.[42–45] Symptoms are usually localized, at least initially, to the territory of the injured nerve and are described as a continuous burning pain that may be exacerbated by stress, movement, or even tactile stimuli as soft as a slight breeze. Sympathetic abnormalities such as vasodilation, hyperhidrosis, and edema are common. The pain may start a few hours to several days after injury, although it not uncommonly develops as late as 3 to 4 weeks after injury.[46] Reflex sympathetic dystrophy after calcaneal fracture results in severe burning pain in the heel associated with cold, shiny skin over and around the heel.[47] NCS and EMG abnormalities are those of the underlying nerve injury.

Differential Diagnosis of Neurogenic Foot Pain

In the evaluation of foot pain, it is essential to remember that proximal lesions involving the cauda equina, lumbosacral nerve roots, spinal nerves, and lumbosacral plexus may cause referred pain, paresthesias, and sensory disturbances in the foot. L4 root lesions may cause radiating pain from the knee down the medial aspect of the lower leg to the medial malleolus. An L5 lesion causes radiating pain and paresthesia over the lateral thigh, leg, and dorsum of the foot into the big toe, whereas an S1 root lesion radiates to the posterior thigh, leg, sole of the foot, and fifth toe. Sciatic mononeuropathy may also cause pain in the foot; the distribution is determined by the portion of the sciatic nerve affected. Each of these can be easily evaluated with NCSs and needle electromyography.

REFERENCES

1. Kimura J. Electrodiagnosis in diseases of nerve and muscle: principles and practice. Philadelphia: F. A. Davis, 1989.
2. DeLisa JA, Lee HJ, Baran EM, et al. Manual of Nerve Conduction Velocity and Clinical Neurophysiology, ed 3. New York: Raven Press, 1994.
3. Colachis SC III, Klejka JP, Shamir DY, et al. Amplitude of M responses: side to side comparability. Am J Phys Med Rehabil 72:19–22, 1993.
4. Dumitru D. Electrodiagnostic Medicine. Philadelphia: Hanley & Belfus, 1995.
5. Dellon AL, Mackinnon SE. Tibial nerve branching in the tarsal tunnel. Arch Neurol 41:645–646, 1984.
6. Mumenthaler M. Tarsal tunnel syndrome. Diagnosis and differential diagnosis. Wien Klin Wochenschr 105:459–461, 1993.
7. Matricali B. Tarsal tunnel syndrome caused by ganglion compression. J Neurol Sci 24:183–185, 1980.
8. Boyer MI, Hochban T, Bowen V. Tarsal tunnel syndrome: an unusual case resulting from an intraneural degenerative cyst. Can J Surg 38:371–373, 1995.
9. Sammarco GJ, Conti SF. Tarsal tunnel syndrome

caused by an anomalous muscle. J Bone Joint Surg Am 76:1308–1314, 1994.

10. Belding RH. Neurilemmoma of the lateral plantar nerve producing tarsal tunnel syndrome: a case report. Foot Ankle 14:289–291, 1993.

11. Smith W, Amis JA. Neurilemmoma of the tibial nerve. A case report. J Bone Joint Surg Am 74:443–444, 1992.

12. Myerson M, Soffer S. Lipoma as an etiology of tarsal tunnel syndrome: a report of two cases. Foot Ankle 10:176–179, 1989.

13. Jackson DL, Haglund BL. Tarsal tunnel syndrome in runners. Sports Med 13:146–149, 1992.

14. Grabois M, Puentes J, Lidsky M. Tarsal tunnel syndrome in rheumatoid arthritis. Arch Phys Med Rehabil 62:401–403, 1981.

15. Schwartz MS, Mackworth-Young CG, McKeran RO. The tarsal tunnel syndrome in hypothyroidism. J Neurol Neurosurg Psychiatry 46:440–442, 1983.

16. Oh SJ, Sarala PH, Kuba T, Elmore RS. Tarsal tunnel syndrome: electrophysiological study. Ann Neurol 5:327, 1979.

17. Galardi G, Amadio S, Maderna L, et al. Electrophysiological studies in tarsal tunnel syndrome. Diagnostic reliability of motor distal latency, mixed nerve and sensory nerve conduction studies. Am J Phys Med Rehabil 73:193–198, 1994.

18. Saeed MA, Gatens PF. Compound nerve action potentials of the medial and lateral plantar nerves through the tarsal tunnel. Arch Phys Med Rehabil 63:304–307, 1982.

19. Felsenthal G, Butler DH, Shear MS. Across-tarsal-tunnel motor-nerve conduction technique. Arch Phys Med Rehabil 73:64–69, 1992.

20. DeLisa JA, Saeed MA. AAEE case report #8: the tarsal tunnel syndrome. Muscle Nerve 6:664–670, 1983.

21. Gatens PF, Saeed MA. EMG findings in the intrinsic muscles of normal feet. Arch Phys Med Rehabil 1982;63:317–318, 1982.

22. Wiles CM, Whitehead S, Ward AB, Fletcher CDM. Not tarsal tunnel syndrome: malignant "triton" tumor of the tibial nerve. J Neurol Neurosurg Psychiatry 50:479–481, 1987.

23. Wolock BS, Baugher WH, McCarthy EJ. Neurilemmoma of the sciatic nerve mimicking tarsal tunnel syndrome. Report of a case. J Bone Joint Surg Am 71:932–934, 1989.

24. Wieman TJ, Patel VG. Treatment of hyperesthetic neuropathic pain in diabetics. Decompression of the tarsal tunnel. Ann Surg 221:660–664, 1995.

25. Baxter DE, Pfeffer GB, Thigpen M. Chronic heel pain, treatment rationale. Orthop Clin North Am 20:563–570, 1989.

26. Baxter DE, Thigpen M. Heel pain—operative results. Foot Ankle 5:16–25, 1984.

27. Johnson RE, Kudy K, Lieberman S. Lateral plantar nerve entrapment: foot pain in a power lifter. Am J Sports Med 20:19–20, 1992.

28. Morton TG. A peculiar and painful affection of the fourth metatarsophalangeal articulation. Am J Med Sci 71:37, 1876.

29. Jarde O, Trinquier JL, Pleyber A, et al. Treatment of Morton neuroma by neurectomy. Apropos of 43 cases. Rev Chir Orthop Reparatrice Appar Mot 81:142–146, 1995.

30. Wu KK. Morton's interdigital neuroma: a clinical review of its etiology, treatment and results. J Foot Ankle Surg 35:112–119, 1996.

31. Sidey JD. Weak ankles. A study of common peroneal entrapment neuropathy. BMJ 3:623–626, 1969.

32. Kernohan J, Levack B, Wilson JN. Entrapment of the superficial peroneal nerve. J Bone Joint Surg Br 67:60, 1985.

33. Marinacci AA. Neurological syndromes of the tarsal tunnels. Bull Los Angeles Neurol Soc 33:90–100, 1968.

34. Andresen BL, Wertsch JJ, Stewart WA. Anterior tarsal tunnel syndrome. Arch Phys Med Rehabil 73:1112–1117, 1992.

35. Reed SC, Wright CS. Compression of the deep branch of the peroneal nerve by the extensor hallucis brevis muscle: a variation of the anterior tarsal tunnel syndrome. Can J Surg 38:545–546, 1995.

36. Thomas PK, Brown MJ. Diabetic polyneuropathy. In Dyck PJ, Thomas PK, Asbury AK, et al., eds. Diabetic Polyneuropathy. Philadelphia: W. B. Saunders, 1987:57.

37. Ellenberg M. Diabetic neuropathic cachexia. Diabetes 23:418, 1974.

38. Llewelyn JG, Thomas PK, Fonseca V, et al. Acute painful diabetic neuropathy precipitated by strict glycemic control. Acta Neuropathol 72:157, 1986.

39. Delaney CA, Mouser JV, Westerman RA. Insulin sensitivity and sensory nerve function in non-diabetic human subjects. Neurosci Lett 180:277–280, 1994.

40. Anand P, Terenghi G, Warner G, et al. The role of endogenous nerve growth factor in human diabetic neuropathy. Nature Med 2:703–707, 1996.

41. Jackson J. On a peculiar disease resulting from the use of ardent spirits. N Engl J Med Surg 11:351, 1822.

42. Casten DF, Betcher AM. Reflex sympathetic dystrophy. Surg Gynecol Obstet 100:97–100, 1955.

43. Evans JA. Reflex sympathetic dystrophy. Report on 57 cases. Ann Intern Med 26:417–426, 1947.

44. Mitchell SW. Injuries of nerves and their consequences. Magnolia, MA: Peter Smith Publishers, 1972:363–368.

45. Sweet WH, Poletti CE. Causalgia and sympathetic dystrophy (Sudeck's atrophy). In Aronoff GM, ed. Evaluation and Treatment of Chronic Pain. Baltimore, MD: Yurban and Scharzenber, 1985:149–165.

46. Tracey DG, Cockett FB. Pain in the lower limb after sympathectomy. Lancet 1:12–14, 1957.

47. McLaughlin HL. Trauma. Philadelphia: W. B. Saunders, 1959.

6 The Foot and Ankle During Gait

Sherry I. Backus

The foot-ankle complex forms the link between the body and the ground. This is a dynamic mechanism, and the foot is not merely a static post to pivot over. Although frequently modeled in gait analysis as a rigid body, the foot is required to act as both a semirigid structure (as a spring and lever arm during roll-off) as well as a rigid structure that provides adequate stability to support body weight.[1]

The movements of the ankle, subtalar, tarsal, metatarsal, and phalangeal joints contribute to the smooth progression of the center of mass through space. There are constant adjustments in these joints, and by the muscles that cross them, to provide a smooth interaction between the body and the wide variety of supporting surfaces encountered when walking. The loss of normal motion or muscular function at these joints has a direct effect not only on the foot and ankle but on the remainder of the joints of the lower extremity as well.

The objective of this chapter is to provide information regarding the dynamic function of the normal foot-ankle complex during walking. A review of the gait cycle and phases of gait, kinematics, muscular control, and kinetics of the foot and ankle during normal gait is presented. After discussion of the entire gait cycle, the remainder of the chapter has been organized by functional joint segments. During observational and instrumented gait analysis, rather than attempting to visualize many segments at one instant or phase of time, it is often easier to follow one segment through the cycle. Therefore, this approach has been used here.

GAIT CYCLE AND THE PHASES OF GAIT

The basic objective of walking is to move the body forward so that the hands and the head can perform a task. During walking, the body must simultaneously move forward as well as maintain stance stability. Each lower limb, in turn, acts as a support and then advances to the next position. This sequence of support and advancement is referred to as a *gait cycle*. A gait cycle (or stride period) consists of two steps and is defined as the time from a specific event on one limb to the same event on the ipsilateral limb (Fig. 6–1). The distance covered during one gait cycle is termed *stride length*. In 60 normal adult males, Murray and associates[2] reported an average stride length of 156.5 cm. *Cadence* is defined as the number of steps taken per minute and averages 117 steps per minute in normal adult males.[2] *Walking velocity* (or the distance traveled over a unit of time) is dependent on both cadence and stride length.[3, 4] In normal adults, women walk at an average velocity of 77 m/min, which is 10% slower than that of men (86 m/min).[5]

Traditionally, initial contact serves as the start and the end of the gait cycle. During normal gait, initial contact is synonymous with heel strike. However, during pathologic gait, heel strike is not always present, so the generic term *initial contact* will be used. Equinus deformity, spasticity, and contracture are just a few examples of cases in which the heel may not even make contact with the ground.

The gait cycle can be broken down into two distinct phases: *stance* (when the foot is in contact with the ground) and *swing* (when the foot is not in contact with the ground) (see Fig. 6–1). Stance begins at initial contact and ends when the foot leaves the ground. In normal gait, the last segment of the foot to clear the ground is the hallux; thus, the final stance event is often referred to as "toe-off." Swing begins at toe-off and ends with the following initial contact.

In normal gait, stance is approximately 60% of the gait cycle, and swing is approximately 40% of the gait cycle (Fig. 6–2).[2] Walking velocity will influence the exact distribution of the gait cycle between stance and swing. Otis and Burstein[6] reported that at a free speed velocity of 80 m/min, stance and swing are 62% and 38% of the gait

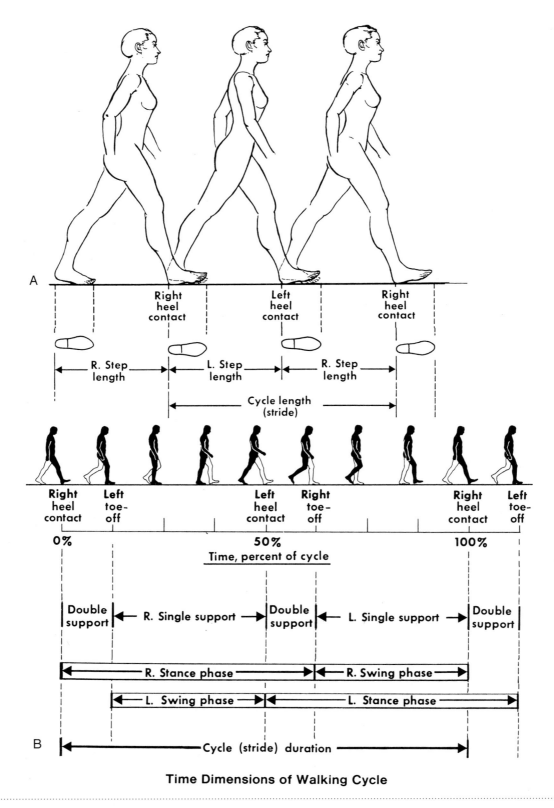

Time Dimensions of Walking Cycle

Figure 6–1. Distance and time parameters of walking. *A*, Distance: heel contact is equivalent to initial contact during normal walking. *B*, Time: gait cycle, stance (double and single support), and swing. (From Inman VT, Ralston HJ, Todd F. Human Walking. Baltimore: Williams & Wilkins, 1981.)

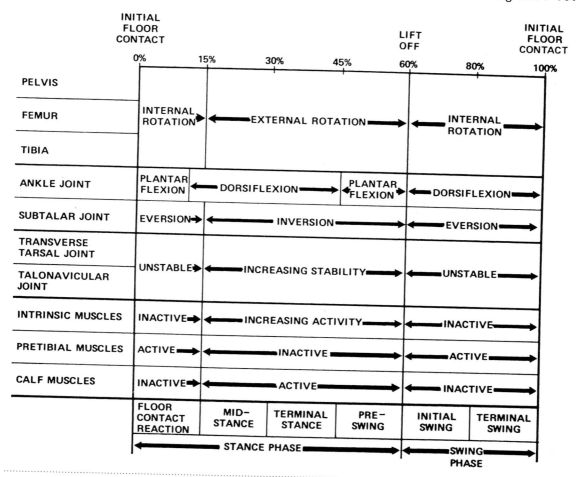

Figure 6–2. Complete walking cycle. Rotations of the lower extremity joints and activity in the leg muscles during the walking cycle. Floor contact reaction is equivalent to loading response. Also note swing in this figure is divided into only two phases. This chapter divides swing into three equal parts, which also includes a midswing phase. (From Mann RA, Mann JA. Biomechanics of the foot. In Goldberg B, Hsu JD, eds. Atlas of Orthoses and Assistive Devices, ed 3. St. Louis: Mosby–Year Book, 1997:149.)

cycle, respectively. At faster velocities, the relative percentage of swing is increased and stance is decreased.[7] In addition, increased walking velocity is associated with increases in both cadence and stride length and a decrease in the absolute time spent in swing and support.[3]

The gait cycle can be divided sequentially into events (e.g., initial contact and opposite toe-off) that occur at specific points and phases that occur over an extended percentage of the cycle (e.g., loading response and midswing). It is convenient to describe an entire gait cycle as lasting 100%, with initial contact occurring at 0% and 100%.

During the first 10 to 12% of the gait cycle after initial contact, the opposite limb remains in contact with the ground and double-limb stance occurs. As the opposite limb leaves the ground and swings forward, the stance limb is now in single-limb support. At the 50% point in the gait cycle, the opposite foot makes contact with the ground again (opposite initial contact), and a second period of double-limb stance begins. Again, lasting 10 to 12% of the gait cycle, both feet are in contact with the ground until swing begins on the ipsilateral side. To differentiate between the two double-limb stance phases, the one immediately after initial contact is referred to as initial double-limb stance, and the one immediately before swing is terminal double-limb stance. The presence of double-limb stance is one of the characteristics that differentiates walking from running, because there is no double-limb stance in running.[8]

Each gait cycle can be broken down into eight functional phases. Stance consists of the first five phases: initial contact, loading response, midstance, terminal stance, and preswing. Swing consists of the last three phases: initial swing, midswing, and terminal swing. During walking, the limb must accomplish three basic tasks: weight acceptance, single-limb support, and limb advancement. The first two tasks are the responsibility of the supporting or stance limb, and the final task is the responsibility of the swing limb.

During the first two phases (initial contact and loading response), the limb must meet the most demanding task in the gait cycle: weight acceptance. During weight acceptance, body weight is transferred onto a limb that has finished swinging and has an unstable alignment. Eccentric muscle activity during this phase of gait serves to control the rate of fall and to begin to stabilize the foot and limb.

The second task, single-limb support (midstance and terminal stance), begins once the opposite foot has left the ground. The stance limb is now solely responsible for supporting body weight while continuing the forward progression of the body.

Finally, the third task, limb advancement, begins during terminal double-limb stance (preswing) as the stance limb prepares for swing and continues throughout all of swing (initial swing, midswing, and terminal swing). During this phase, the swing limb is brought forward, and preparation for the next initial contact and the next phase of weight acceptance begins.

A more detailed description of each phase is presented here. The timing and specific objectives of each phase are adapted from Perry.[9]

Initial contact occurs at 0% of the gait cycle with contact of the foot to the floor. The objective of this phase is to position the foot so that stance can begin. The position of the foot and limb at initial contact determines the loading response pattern. During normal gait, the heel makes contact first.

Loading response occurs from 0% to approximately 10% of the gait cycle and is synonymous with initial double-limb stance. The objectives are shock absorption, load

acceptance, weight-bearing stability, and, finally, preservation of forward progression.

Midstance occurs from approximately 10 to 30% of the gait cycle and represents the first half of single-limb support. Midstance begins when the contralateral foot leaves the ground and ends as body weight (center of mass) is aligned over the stance limb forefoot. The objectives of midstance are progression over a stationary foot and maintenance of limb and trunk stability.

Terminal stance occurs from 30 to 50% of the gait cycle and is the last half of single-limb stance. It begins with heel rise and continues until opposite initial contact. The primary objective of this phase is the progression of the body past the supporting foot.

Preswing occurs from 50 to 60% of the gait cycle and is synonymous with terminal double-limb stance. This phase concludes stance and, with toe-off, marks the onset of swing. The objective of this phase is to position the limb for swing. During this phase, body weight is shifted to the opposite limb during loading response on the opposite leg.

Initial swing occurs from 60 to 73% of the gait cycle and consists of the first third of swing. Beginning at toe-off, initial swing ends when the swing limb is positioned directly opposite the stance foot. The objectives are foot clearance and advancement of the limb from its trailing position. *Midswing* occurs from 73 to 87% of the gait cycle and ends when the tibia is vertical. The objectives are foot clearance and further limb advancement. *Terminal swing* (87–100% of the gait cycle) is the last phase and ends with initial contact of the swing limb. The objectives are completion of limb advancement and preparation of the limb for stance.

During walking, forward fall of body weight serves as the primary propelling force. The center of mass of the human body is located just anterior to the second sacral vertebral body. During walking, the center of mass is highest during midstance and falls from this peak to the lowest point during loading response. Walking has sometimes been called a series of controlled falls. A critical factor in the ability to fall forward is mobility at the base of support: the foot. Throughout stance, the momentum of falling is preserved by a pivotal (rocker) system at the heel, ankle, and forefoot (Fig. 6–3).[10, 11] These rockers allow the body to

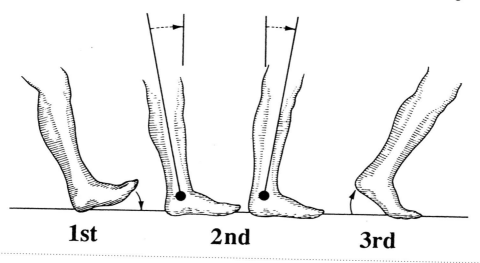

1st   **2nd**   **3rd**

Figure 6–3. The ankle in stance: three foot rockers. The first two are deceleration rockers, so their respective muscles are acting eccentrically (i.e., undergoing a lengthening contraction with energy absorption [negative work]). The third rocker is an acceleration rocker, so the plantar flexors must act concentrically (i.e., produce positive work). The point of application of the ground reaction force is forced to move forward with each successive rocker, thus allowing the center of mass to move forward with it. (From Gage JR. Normal gait. In Analysis in Cerebral Palsy. London: MacKeith Press, 1991:61.)

advance while the knee remains basically extended.

The first rocker, *heel rocker*, occurs from initial contact and continues through loading response. The heel rocker occurs as the rounded surfaces of the calcaneal tuberosities contact the ground and continues until the ankle plantar flexes into full ground contact (foot flat). The heel rocker behaves as an unstable lever system and the heel serves as a fulcrum. An eccentric (lengthening) contraction of the pretibial muscles (tibialis anterior, extensor digitorum longus, extensor hallucis longus, and peroneus tertius) restrains the rate of plantar flexion. With the foot fixed on the floor, the contraction of the pretibial muscles causes the tibia to become the moving segment to advance forward over the stationary foot.

The second rocker, *ankle rocker*, occurs during midstance. Once the forefoot has contacted the ground, the ankle becomes a fulcrum for continued forward progression of the body. Momentum causes the tibia to rotate forward over a stationary foot. The center of mass is rising to its highest level. The ankle rocker begins with foot flat and ends with the eccentric contraction of the plantar flexors to restrain further dorsiflexion.

The third rocker, *forefoot rocker*, occurs during terminal stance. The rounded contour of the metatarsal heads and the metatarsophalangeal joints serve as a fulcrum as heel rise occurs. During terminal stance, the center of mass of the body is accelerating downward past the base of support and is restrained by a concentric contraction of the gastrocnemius and soleus muscles. The forefoot rocker allows the acceleration of the limb needed in preswing.

KINEMATICS OF THE ANKLE JOINT

Kinematics refers to the description of joint motion without regard to the forces that act on the joint. Linear and angular displacements, location of the center of rotation for joints, and joint angles are all examples of kinematics.[12] There are 28 bones in each foot-ankle complex, including the tibia and fibula. The numerous joints between these bones can be functionally grouped into four major articulations that relate to the mechanics of walking. From proximal to distal, these are the ankle (tibiotalar), subtalar (talocalcaneal), midtarsal (talonavicular and calcaneocuboid), and forefoot (metatarsophalangeal) joints.

The ankle joint or tibiotalar joint is composed of the distal articulation of the tibia and the head of the talus. For the majority of the joints of the foot and ankle, different authors have proposed different locations for a given joint's axis; in fact, there is not always agreement on the number of axes for a given joint. The ankle joint is no exception. Barnett and Napier[13] and Hicks[14] described two different axes at the ankle joint: one for plantar flexion and one for dorsiflexion. Several other authors have demonstrated that the ankle axis of rotation is a variable axis that changes continuously as motion occurs.[15, 16]

However, three-dimensional video analysis of walking most commonly uses a single axis for ankle motion, and the results of

most gait studies use a definition that closely follows that of a single axis. Inman originally proposed a single axis of motion at the ankle joint that passes just distal to the medial and lateral malleoli.[17] For clinical purposes, this means that one can press one finger under the tip of each malleolus and determine with reasonable accuracy the inclination of the ankle axis.[18, 19]

The single ankle axis is inclined downward and laterally in the frontal plane and is rotated posterolaterally in the transverse plane (Fig. 6–4). In the frontal plane, the axis forms an angle of 83° (range, 74–94°) with the midline of the tibia. In the trans-

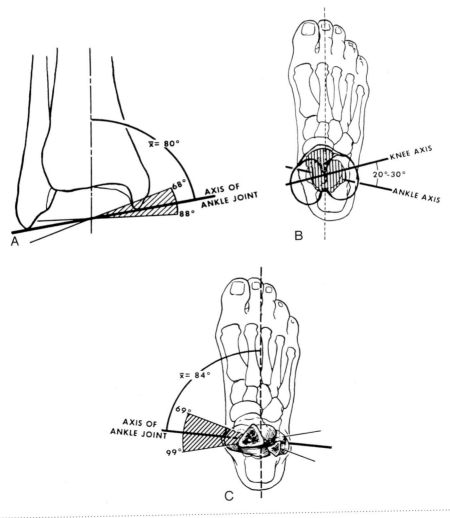

Figure 6–4. *A*, Angle between the axis of the ankle joint and the long axis of the tibia. *B*, Relationships of the knee, ankle, and foot axes. *C*, Relationship of the ankle axis to the longitudinal axis of the foot. (From Mann RA, Mann JA. Biomechanics of the foot. In Goldberg B, Hsu JD, eds. Atlas of Orthoses and Assistive Devices, ed 3. St. Louis: Mosby–Year Book, 1997:138.)

verse plane, the axis forms an angle of 20 to 30° with the transverse axis of the knee joint.[17] In adults, this can be seen as approximately 23° of "external tibial torsion."[20] As with all of the joints of the foot, this is a triplanar axis; it does not lie exclusively in one of the cardinal planes of the body. Therefore, as motion occurs about this axis, it does so in all three cardinal planes (Fig. 6–5). There is minimal or no transverse rotation within the ankle joint.

Like all of the other joints of the lower extremity, the arc of motion at the ankle joint required for gait is significantly less than the maximum passive motion available.[16] Although the arc of motion is not large, it is critical during stance to permit progression and shock absorption and in swing to allow limb advancement.[21] The range of motion used during walking averages 30°: from a maximum of 10° of dorsiflexion to 20° of plantar flexion. Figure 6–6 shows a schematic diagram of the complete walking cycle and the ankle motion seen during normal walking.

At the ankle, there are four arcs of motion in the gait cycle: plantar flexion followed by dorsiflexion, plantar flexion, and finally dorsiflexion. The first three arcs occur in stance, and the last arc of dorsiflexion occurs in swing.[22] Despite advances in three-dimensional motion-recording techniques,[23] the pattern of motion has changed little from the two-dimensional data recorded by Murray et al. in normal adults.[2] In combination with force platform recordings, however, the three-dimensional kinematic analysis provides improved calculation of the joint moments seen during walking.[24]

During normal gait, the initial contact by the heel on the ground occurs with the ankle at a nearly neutral position or in slight (3–5°) plantar flexion. During loading response, the first arc of plantar flexion motion begins and continues until the forefoot contacts the ground (heel rocker). This rapid plantar flexion reaches a maximum of approximately 7°. In addition, at the time of initial contact, the entire lower extremity undergoes internal (medial) rotation (see Fig. 6–2). While the foot is plantar flexing and not

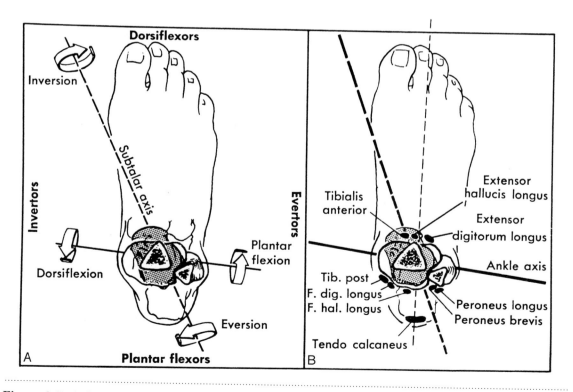

Figure 6–5. *A,* Rotation about the subtalar and ankle axes. *B,* Relationship of the various muscles about the subtalar and ankle axes. (From Mann RA, Mann JA. Biomechanics of the foot. In Goldberg B, Hsu JD, eds. Atlas of Orthoses and Assistive Devices, ed 3. St. Louis: Mosby–Year Book, 1997:145.)

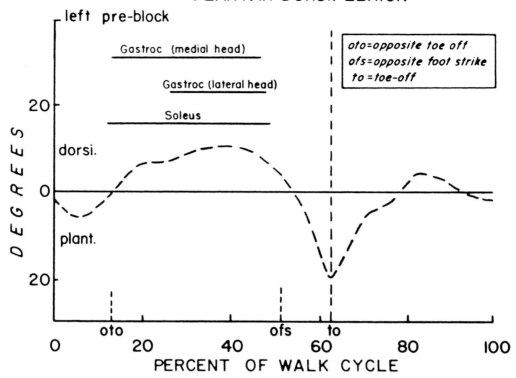

Figure 6–6. Ankle dorsiflexion and plantar flexion motion in normal subjects. (From Sutherland DH, Cooper L, Daniel D. The role of the ankle plantar flexors in normal walking. J Bone Joint Surg Am 62:354, 1980.)

in contact with the ground, it is free to move in space. There is a tendency for the foot to rotate medially (toe-in), which varies with the specific obliquity of the ankle joint.[20]

Once foot flat occurs and the forefoot is on the ground, ankle motion reverses its direction and dorsiflexion to 10° occurs. During this motion, the foot is stationary, and the tibia rotates anteriorly over the fixed foot (ankle rocker). The ankle passes through neutral at 20% of the gait cycle. By 48% of the gait cycle, just before opposite initial contact and the start of terminal double-limb stance, the ankle has reached its maximum dorsiflexion of 10°. With the foot fixed on the floor, there is medial rotation about the vertical axis of the leg with respect to the foot.[20]

As terminal double-limb stance begins, the ankle plantar flexes rapidly and reaches a maximum of 30° by the end of stance phase (forefoot rocker). As the toes stabilize the foot on the ground, the tibia advances forward proximally, resulting in rapid knee

flexion in preparation for swing.[21] With this plantar flexion during stance, because the forefoot is still in contact with the ground, the leg rotates laterally with respect to the foot.[20]

The last arc of motion, dorsiflexion, begins at toe-off and reaches neutral by midswing as the swing limb passes in front of the stance limb. The foot remains in neutral for the remainder of swing. During terminal swing, there is a minimal drop (3–5°) into plantar flexion. The foot is now ready for the next initial contact, and the cycle begins again.

MUSCLE CONTROL OF THE ANKLE JOINT

The relationship between the magnitude of electromyographic (EMG) signal, force generation, and ultimately torque production at a joint is complicated and not linear (except in limited isometric situations). This relationship is beyond the scope of this chapter, but it is important to note that one must not interpret larger EMG signals as stronger muscles. However, within a given muscle, greater electrical activity is usually associated with greater force generation.

The moment produced about a joint is dependent not only on the force generated by the muscle but also on the length of the lever arm on which the muscle acts. As the perpendicular distance between the axis and the muscle changes, so too does the moment generated about the joint. Therefore, in a simplistic sense, when interpreting EMG signals, although a larger signal indicates greater electrical activity and, in general, greater force generation, it does not follow that there must be greater torque about the joint. As a result, during gait analysis, it is the timing of the muscle firing (when muscle activation begins and ends) that is frequently used as the primary measure, and amplitude of the signal becomes a secondary consideration.

On the basis of EMG studies on the muscles that cross the ankle, the dorsiflexor muscles fire concentrically during swing to allow for foot clearance and eccentrically during loading response to control the foot (Fig. 6–7). The plantar flexors consistently fire eccentrically during stance to control the advancement of the tibia over the foot, stabilize the knee, and concentrically to assist roll-off or push-off.[22, 25, 26] To determine the role of a muscle at a joint, it is helpful to visualize the location of the muscle tendons in relationship to the axis on which they act (see Fig. 6–5). Muscle tendons that lie anterior to the ankle joint axis will result in ankle dorsiflexion. Muscle tendons that lie posterior to the ankle joint axis will cause the ankle joint to plantar flex.

The three major dorsiflexor muscles are the pretibial muscles: tibialis anterior, extensor digitorum longus, and extensor hallucis longus. The action of the peroneus tertius has been assumed to be that of the extensor digitorum longus, because these two muscle bellies blend into each other and share the lateral tendon. All of these dorsiflexors have lever arms across the ankle joint that are similar in length, but the size and cross-sectional area of these muscles vary considerably. The muscle with the largest cross-sectional area is the tibialis anterior, followed by the combined extensor digitorum longus and peroneus longus, and

the smallest is the extensor hallucis longus. The mass of the extensor digitorum longus is reported to be 40% of the tibialis anterior and the extensor hallucis longus just 20% of the tibialis anterior. Therefore, the dorsiflexion torques that the toe extensors are capable of producing are much smaller than that of the tibialis anterior.

The onset of muscle activity in the dorsiflexors begins just before foot-off during preswing. Winter and Yack[27] reported that these muscles remain active throughout swing and loading response; peak electrical activity is seen in the first 15% of the gait cycle during weight acceptance, when they must assist in controlling the fall of the center of mass (see Fig. 6–7). They are electrically silent during mid- and terminal stance.

The peak electrical activity corresponds to a high demand on the pretibial muscles as body weight is dropped onto the heel. These muscles fire eccentrically to decelerate the rate of ankle plantar flexion.[28] If there is insufficient control or strength in the pretibial muscles, a drop-foot or foot-slap gait pattern may be present.[29] In addition, restrained ankle plantar flexion provides some shock absorption during the loading response. During swing, the tibialis anterior and the toe extensors function to dorsiflex the foot for toe clearance. Loss of normal function in the pretibial muscle during swing frequently results in increased knee and hip flexion and a steppage-type gait.[8]

Seven muscle tendons lie posterior to the ankle joint and act as plantar flexors (see Fig. 6–5). Just as with the pretibial muscles, the size and cross-sectional area are widely divergent, as are the subsequent moments these muscles are able to create about the ankle joint. The two largest muscles are the gastrocnemius and soleus. Not only do these two muscles have the largest cross-sectional area, but they also have the longest lever arm distance from the ankle joint. It has been reported that these two muscles account for 93% of the theoretical plantar flexor torques.[30]

The soleus and the medial head of the gastrocnemius begin activation at approximately 10% of the gait cycle, as single-limb support begins (Fig. 6–8; see Fig. 6–7). They continue firing throughout the stance phase until preswing, when single-limb support ends and the opposite foot makes contact

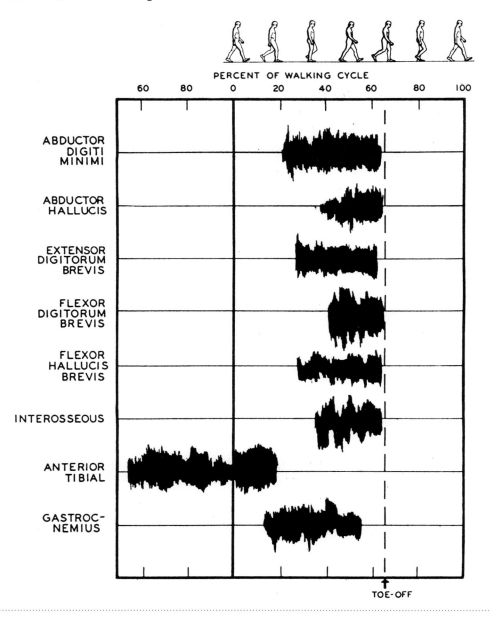

Figure 6–7. Electromyographic activity of selected calf and foot muscles during level walking. Also included are the phasic activity patterns of selected posterior calf muscles. (From Mann R, Inman VT. Phasic activity of the intrinsic muscles of the foot. J Bone Joint Surg Am 46:469, 1964.)

with the ground.[21, 22] The lateral head of the gastrocnemius may not begin activation until midstance.[22] During midstance, the plantar flexors eccentrically contract to restrain forward motion of the tibia.[31, 32] During terminal stance, as the heel begins to rise, the gastrocnemius continues to contract to begin active ankle plantar flexion.[11] During this phase, the soleus and gastrocnemius provide a stable tibia over which the femur may advance. Peak electrical activity is seen at 50% of the gait cycle.[27]

Although both the soleus and gastrocnemius muscles share a common insertion, the role of the soleus is somewhat different than that of the gastrocnemius because of the soleus' origin on the tibia. The soleus, as a one-joint muscle, provides a direct link between the tibia and the calcaneus and is thought to be the dominant decelerating

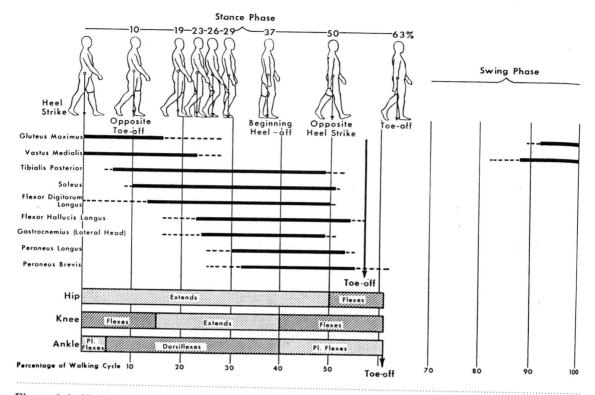

Figure 6–8. Walking cycle in normal adult males. Solid lines indicate the means; broken lines indicate the ranges of muscle activity. The dynamic changes in joint angles of the knee, ankle, and hip are indicated by the horizontal bars. (From Sutherland D. An electromyographic study of the plantar flexors of the ankle in normal walking on the level. J Bone Joint Surg Am 48:66, 1966.)

plantar flexion force. The gastrocnemius, as a two-joint muscle, plays a direct role in knee flexion during midstance.[21]

The remaining five posterior muscles— tibialis posterior, flexor hallucis longus, flexor digitorum longus, peroneus longus, and peroneus brevis—are smaller in size and, as perimalleolar muscles, lie closer to the ankle joint (see Fig. 6–5). These muscles play a greater role at the subtalar joint and the foot than at the ankle, but they still create a plantar flexion force at the ankle joint.

The tibialis posterior begins firing at initial contact and remains active through single-limb stance until opposite initial contact.[33] The flexor digitorum longus begins firing next at opposite toe-off and also continues until opposite initial contact. The flexor hallucis longus is active from 25% of the gait cycle into preswing. Peroneus brevis and longus activity begins early in stance and continues into preswing. Nota-

bly, the activity in these muscles is subject to considerable variation among individuals.[21, 33]

The posterior calf muscles function as a group and cease functioning by 50% of the gait cycle when opposite initial contact has occurred. The continuation of plantar flexion past this point probably serves only to balance the body, because the opposite foot has already accepted the body's weight. In a small group of healthy adults, Sutherland and associates[22] used a nerve block to the tibial nerve to further describe the role of the ankle plantar flexors, particularly the gastrocnemius and soleus during gait. They concluded that these muscles did not serve as a propulsion mechanism during preswing; rather, these muscles should be thought of as maintaining forward progression, step length, and gait symmetry. If the plantar flexors do not function normally, an increase in ankle dorsiflexion is seen with a shortened step by the swing limb.[22, 31] In addition, the swing limb strikes the ground prematurely because of the lack of restraint of tibial movement in the stance limb.[32]

In summary, during the first arc of plantar flexion after initial contact, the dorsiflexors fire eccentrically to decelerate the rate of plantar flexion and foot fall onto the ground. During the first arc of dorsiflexion, the plantar flexors fire eccentrically to control the rate of dorsiflexion and tibial progression over the stationary foot. During the second arc of plantar flexion, just before weight transfer onto the opposite limb, the plantar flexors fire to maintain walking velocity and step length. Finally, during the last arc of motion, dorsiflexion during swing, the dorsiflexors fire concentrically to allow foot clearance.

KINETICS OF THE ANKLE JOINT

Kinetics is the description of the forces and moments that cause movement at a joint. Both internal (muscular, ligamentous, frictional) and external (ground reaction) forces are examples of kinetics.[12] The joint reaction force of the ankle during walking has been calculated in two-dimensional analysis to be three times body weight during loading response.[34] The joint reaction force increases in magnitude to 4.5 to 5.5 times body weight during terminal stance as the heel rises and the gastrocnemius and soleus contract.[34] Using a three-dimensional analysis, Procter and Paul[35] reported peak compressive forces that were almost 4 times body weight.

For a joint to remain in equilibrium, the moment acting on the joint must be balanced by muscle activation in the opposite direction. Moments or torques at a given joint can be described by the motion that they tend to cause or by the muscle groups required to contract to maintain equilibrium. An ankle dorsiflexion moment (which tends to rotate the ankle joint into dorsiflexion) is balanced by an equal but opposite plantar flexor moment (which is produced by the activation of muscles that cause plantar flexion). All moments discussed here are in reference to the joint motion that would occur if unresisted. The magnitude of the moment (torque) about the joint is equal to the force times the perpendicular distance from the force to the joint axis.

At the ankle joint, during the first 5% of the gait cycle (initial contact), there is a brief, low-level plantar flexion moment (Fig. 6–9).[24, 36] The center of pressure during the stance phase starts at the posterior heel; therefore, the ground reaction force lies posterior to the ankle joint, and the resultant moment at the ankle is a plantar flexion moment.

As the center of pressure moves anterior along the foot during the remainder of stance, the ground reaction force acts anterior to the ankle joint, and the resultant moment at the ankle is a dorsiflexion moment.[22] This progressively increasing dorsiflexion moment reaches a maximum during terminal stance, just before opposite foot contact. Sutherland and associates[22] reported that this torque is nine times greater than the initial plantar flexion torque. The dorsiflexion moment rapidly decreases to zero by toe-off.

The actual movement that occurs at the ankle joint during walking is a result of the balance that exists between the external joint moments produced by the ground reaction force and the internal moments produced by the muscles that act across the joint. During midstance, the external joint moment (which is an increasing dorsiflexion moment) is larger than the torque produced by the plantar flexors, thus, the ankle dorsiflexes. As the plantar flexor muscle torque increases to the level of the external torques, the ankle stops dorsiflexing and begins to plantar flex (at approximately 41% of the gait cycle).[22]

Because there is no plantar flexion EMG activity during preswing as the ankle joint

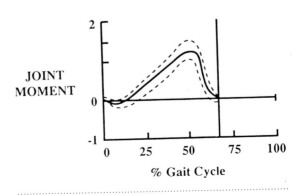

Figure 6–9. Normal ankle kinetics. The solid line represents the means; the dotted lines represent 1 standard deviation. Plantar flexion moments are negative, and dorsiflexion moments are positive. (Modified from Gage JR. Normal gait. In Gait Analysis in Cerebral Palsy. London: MacKeith Press, 1991:61.)

moves into more plantar flexion, both Perry[21] and Sutherland et al.[22] proposed that the plantar flexion occurring after opposite initial contact is a passive phenomenon. In contrast, Winter[37] reported that this phase of the gait cycle is a push-off and that retained mechanical energy from the plantar flexors is an important contribution to the propulsion of the body in the forward direction. According to Mann et al.,[38] only during the acceleration phase of running and sports do the posterior calf muscles provide a push-off.

KINEMATICS OF THE SUBTALAR JOINT

The subtalar joint is the junction between the talus and the calcaneus. The axis of the subtalar joint has been studied by Hicks,[14] Manter,[39] and Inman.[17] It is oblique, directed upward 42° from horizontal, anterior, and 23° medial to the axis of the foot passing through the second interdigital space (Fig. 6–10).[17] The subtalar axis has been reported as a single axis, a helical screw axis,[39] as well as a discrete bundle of axes.[40] In addition, there is substantial variability in the orientation of this axis in normal individuals; thus, the relative motions will also vary among normal individuals. Indi-

viduals with planovalgus feet have a subtalar joint that is more horizontal than those with neutral feet.[41]

Rotation about the subtalar axis allows the foot to tilt medially (*inversion* or varus) and laterally (*eversion* or valgus). The terms *pronation* and *supination* represent a combination of movement at the hindfoot and the forefoot. Hicks[14] described pronation of the foot as a combination of dorsiflexion of the ankle, eversion of the calcaneus, and abduction of the forefoot. He described supination of the foot as a combination of plantar flexion of the ankle, inversion of the calcaneus, and adduction of the forefoot. Therefore, the terms inversion and eversion are used to describe motion only about the subtalar axis.

The subtalar joint rotates in both stance and swing (Fig. 6–11), but it is the motion during stance that influences the weight-bearing alignment of the entire lower extremity. Like the ankle joint, the arc of motion at the subtalar joint is small compared with the knee and the hip, but it is the motion present at this joint that permits the foot to adapt to a variety of surfaces.[42] The subtalar joint functions as a mitered hinge during gait to transmit internal and external rotation from the tibia to rotations (eversion and inversion) about the foot.[41] In addition, the subtalar joint transmits inver-

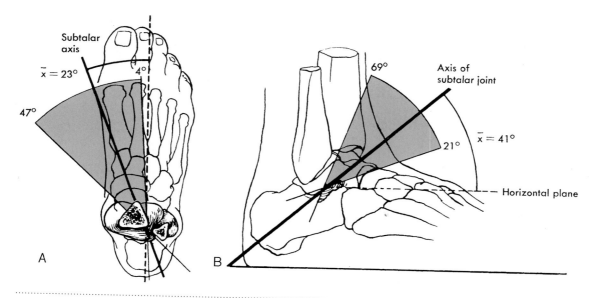

Figure 6–10. Subtalar axis in the transverse plane *(A)* and the horizontal plane *(B)*. (From Mann RA, Mann JA. Biomechanics of the foot. In Goldberg B, Hsu JD, eds. Atlas of Orthoses and Assistive Devices, ed 3. St. Louis: Mosby–Year Book, 1997:139.)

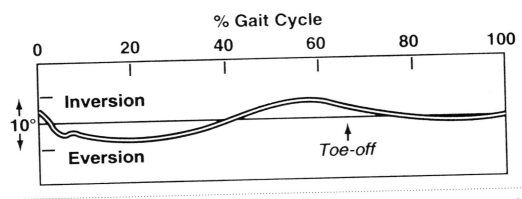

Figure 6–11. Normal subtalar joint motion during free walking. (Modified from Perry J. Ankle foot complex. In Gait Analysis: Normal and Pathological Function. Thorofare, NJ: Slack, 1992:51.)

sion and eversion from the foot to external and internal rotation about the tibia.

During loading response, the subtalar joint begins everting until peak eversion is reached by early midstance at 14% of the gait cycle (Fig. 6–11). Peak eversion averages 4° to 6°.[43] This rapid eversion is followed by gradual inversion; peak inversion is achieved by preswing. The foot drifts back to neutral during swing followed by minimal inversion during the last 20% of the gait cycle.

Subtalar eversion is one of the mechanisms for shock absorption as body weight drops onto the supporting foot during loading response and early midstance. Subtalar eversion is a normal passive response to initial contact with the heel. Because the body of the calcaneus is lateral to the longitudinal axis of the tibia at initial contact, as load is applied to the talus, eversion occurs at the subtalar joint.[44] Eversion of the subtalar joint unlocks the midtarsal joint to produce a relatively flexible forefoot.[8]

When the foot moves more laterally, the calcaneal support of the talus is decreased and the calcaneus falls into inversion. This is coupled with internal tibial rotation as a result of the shape of the ankle joint.[38] Subtalar inversion helps to bring about stability of the foot during single-limb stance.

There is an important inter-relationship between the motion at the ankle joint and the subtalar joint during gait, which permits compensation between the joints.[42] If this compensatory mechanism fails, there is increased stress in these joints and possibly an increased incidence of secondary degenerative arthritis.[44] For example, the degree of in-toeing (internal rotation at the ankle

joint) and out-toeing (external rotation at the ankle) affects the amount of motion required at the subtalar joint. In the case of an individual with excessive out-toeing, the range of motion required at the ankle joint is decreased, and at the subtalar joint the motion required is increased. This occurs because the greatest motion will always occur about the axis that is closest to perpendicular to the plane of progression. With out-toeing, the ankle joint axis is even less perpendicular to the plane of progression than normal. The subtalar joint axis becomes oriented more perpendicular to the plane of progression and subsequently undergoes a larger angular excursion.[42] The reverse occurs with increased in-toeing, the ankle joint axis becomes more perpendicular to the plane of progression, and the range of motion required at the ankle joint is increased; at the subtalar joint the motion required is then decreased. One compensation seen clinically for loss of ankle range of motion is increased out-toeing, so that the motion required for walking can occur at the subtalar joint.[8]

MUSCLE CONTROL OF THE SUBTALAR JOINT

Although no muscles directly originate on the talus and insert on the calcaneus, 10 muscles cross the hindfoot and act indirectly on the subtalar joint. These muscles not only control the subtalar joint but also frequently have actions at the forefoot and the toes.

Five muscles cross on the medial side of the subtalar joint and control inversion of the subtalar joint (see Fig. 6–5). Presented in order from greatest to least leverage, they are tibialis posterior, tibialis anterior, flexor digitorum longus, flexor hallucis longus, and soleus. With the exception of the tibialis anterior, these muscles lie posterior to the ankle joint. The sequence of activation of these muscles during stance occurs as muscular control progresses from the hindfoot to the toes. Activation occurs relative to the demands of the muscle at the more distal joints.

As the foot makes contact with the floor, subtalar eversion occurs as a shock-absorbing mechanism. The invertors fire to decelerate this eversion. The tibialis anterior acts to restrain the subtalar joint during loading response and the heel rocker. With its greatest activity seen during loading response, the tibialis anterior is quiet by midstance because dorsiflexion is no longer needed.

Although the activation patterns of the tibialis posterior have been reported with various patterns of activity by different investigators, there is agreement that it is a stance-phase muscle. It becomes active during loading response and remains active throughout stance until early preswing. Perry[21] proposed that the activation during loading response provides early subtalar control. In addition, the variability of activity in this muscle may be indicative of its function as a reserve force to supplement insufficient varus control by the ankle muscles.

Soleus activity is seen during midstance with progressively increasing activity in terminal stance. Despite its major function as an ankle plantar flexor, this muscle also has considerable inversion leverage, especially because of its large cross-sectional area. By preswing, there is a rapid decline in activity, and the muscle remains quiet during swing. The long toe flexors are the last invertors to be activated. The flexor digitorum longus and the flexor hallucis longus begin activation during midstance and cease firing during preswing.

The muscles that are responsible for eversion at the subtalar joint are the extensor digitorum longus, peroneus tertius, peroneus longus, and peroneus brevis. The first two lie anterior to the subtalar joint axis, whereas the last three lie posterior to the subtalar joint axis. Extensor digitorum longus is active during loading response and

quiet with the onset of midstance. There is little information about the firing of the peroneus tertius, but Perry[21] reported timing similar to that of the extensor digitorum longus.

The peroneus longus and brevis initiate activity during forefoot loading and demonstrate their peak activity at this time.[26, 33] Both timing and intensity of the EMG signals in the peroneus brevis and longus are very similar.[45] Activity in these muscles ceases during the middle of the preswing phase of the gait cycle. The peroneus longus has peak electrical activity at 50% of the gait cycle during push-off and an initial peak during loading response to control foot inversion.[27]

KINEMATICS OF THE MIDTARSAL JOINT

The midtarsal joint, also known as the transverse tarsal joint or Chopart's joint, is actually formed by two joints: the talonavicular and the calcaneocuboid joints. A functional unit is formed by the navicular and the cuboid, which move upon the talar head and the anterior calcaneal surface.[39]

Manter[39] determined two axes for the midtarsal joint: a longitudinal axis and a transverse axis. The longitudinal axis is the center of the pivotal movements of the cuboid on the calcaneus. This axis extends lengthwise through the foot and forms a 15° angle upward and anterior and a 9° angle medial to the second ray. Pronation of the subtalar joint causes abduction and dorsiflexion of the foot with respect to the talus and is accompanied by eversion of the midtarsal joint. The second, transverse axis is oblique and steeply oriented 52° from horizontal and 57° medially. Only minimal motion is allowed at this joint. The motion about this axis is combined abduction and minimal dorsiflexion, or adduction and minimal plantar flexion of the forefoot on a fixed talus and calcaneus.[8]

Motion about the transverse axis affects the longitudinal arch of the foot.[39] After forefoot contact, there is flattening of the longitudinal arch during single-limb support. The restoration of the arch occurs with heel rise.[21]

Midtarsal extension is another of the mechanisms for shock absorption as body weight falls onto the stance limb during loading response and early midstance. This motion, which accompanies forefoot contact at the onset of midstance, occurs after subtalar eversion.

Finally, the interaction between the subtalar joint and the midtarsal joint is such that if motion at the subtalar joint is limited, then motion at the midtarsal joint will be limited. Similarly, when motion at the talonavicular joint is prevented, almost no motion is permitted at the subtalar joint.[39]

MUSCLE CONTROL OF THE MIDTARSAL JOINT

The midtarsal joint is supported primarily by the tibialis posterior.[21] Because the activity of the long toe flexors and the lateral plantar intrinsic muscles begins before the toes flex, these muscles may well contribute to the support of the midtarsal joint.[21]

KINEMATICS OF THE FOREFOOT AND INTERPHALANGEAL JOINTS

The forefoot joint is the articulation between the metatarsals and the phalanges. Motion at this joint consists primarily of flexion and extension. The line drawn through the metatarsal heads is known as the metatarsal break. This axis is approximately 62° medial from the longitudinal axis of the foot. The interphalangeal joints of the toes have only flexion motion available with essentially no extension past neutral.

At initial contact, the toes are off the ground with the metatarsophalangeal joint in 25° of extension.[46] The toes then drop into neutral after forefoot contact at the end of loading response. A neutral position is maintained throughout midstance. During terminal stance, as the heel rises, the metatarsophalangeal joints extend to approximately 21°. During heel rise, the toes remain in contact with the ground as the hindfoot lifts up into the air. A maximum of 58° of toe extension is reached during preswing.[46] During swing, the toes drop slightly but remain in extension. Finally, there is a minimal increase in toe extension in preparation for initial contact.[21] There is little or no flexion at the metatarsophalangeal joint during walking, although some may be present during athletic activities.[8]

There is little or no motion at the interphalangeal joints during gait with the exception that, during foot-off, slight flexion is occasionally noted.[8]

MUSCLE CONTROL OF THE FOREFOOT AND INTERPHALANGEAL JOINTS

The flexor digitorum longus and the flexor hallucis longus begin activation during midstance and cease firing during preswing. These muscles stabilize the metatarsophalangeal joints and add toe support to supplement forefoot support.[11] The intrinsic muscles of the forefoot and interphalangeal joints include the abductor hallucis, adductor hallucis, flexor digitorum brevis, flexor hallucis brevis, and abductor digiti quinti. These muscles become active at approximately 30% of the walking cycle and cease when the foot leaves the ground.[47] These muscles aid in the stabilization of the longitudinal arch as well as the toes at the metatarsophalangeal joint.

Finally, although the motions and muscular control of the ankle, subtalar, midtarsal, and metatarsophalangeal joints have been presented as separate structures, these joints are functionally inter-related. Limitation or restriction of normal motion of any joint will have a subsequent effect on the other joints of the ankle-foot complex as well as on the other joints of the lower extremity. It is the complex integration of anatomy, biomechanics, and muscular control that permit normal walking.

REFERENCES

1. Mann RA, Mann JA. Biomechanics of the foot. In Goldberg B, Hsu JD, eds. Atlas of Orthoses and Assistive Devices, ed 3. St. Louis: Mosby–Year Book, 1997:135.
2. Murray MP, Drought AB, Kory RC. Walking patterns of normal men. J Bone Joint Surg Am 46:335, 1964.
3. Andriacchi TP, Ogle JA, Galante JO. Walking speed as a basis for normal and abnormal gait measurements. J Biomech 10:261, 1977.
4. Sutherland DH, Olshen RA, Cooper L, Woo SLY. The development of mature gait. J Bone Joint Surg Am 62:336, 1980.
5. Perry J. Stride analysis. In Gait Analysis: Normal and Pathological Function. Thorofare, NJ: SLACK Inc, 1992:431.
6. Otis JC, Burstein AH. Evaluation of the VA-Rancho gait analyzer, Mark I. Bull Prosthet Res 18:21, 1981.

7. Larsson LE, Odenrick P, Sandlund B, et al. The phases of the stride and their interaction in human gait. Scand J Rehabil Med 12:107, 1980.
8. Mann R. Overview of foot and ankle biomechanics. In Jahss MH, ed. Disorders of the Foot. Philadelphia: W. B. Saunders, 1991:385.
9. Perry J. Phases of gait. In Gait Analysis: Normal and Pathological Function. Thorofare, NJ: SLACK Inc, 1992:9.
10. Perry J. Kinesiology of lower extremity bracing. Clin Orthop Rel Res 102:20, 1974.
11. Gage JR. Normal gait. In Gait Analysis in Cerebral Palsy. London: MacKeith Press, 1991:61.
12. Rodgers MM, Cavanaugh PR. Glossary of biomechanical terms, concepts and units. Phys Ther 64:1886, 1984.
13. Barnett CH, Napier J. The axis of rotation at the ankle joint in man: its influence upon the form of the talus and the mobility of the fibula. J Anat 86:1, 1952.
14. Hicks JH. The mechanics of the foot. I. The joints. J Anat 187:345, 1953.
15. Lundberg A, Goldie I, Kaln B, Selvik G. Kinematics of the ankle/foot complex: plantar flexion and dorsiflexion. Foot Ankle 9:194, 1989.
16. Sammarco GJ, Burstein AH, Frankel VH. Biomechanics of the ankle: a kinematic study. Orthop Clin North Am 4:75, 1973.
17. Inman VT. The Joints of the Ankle. Baltimore, MD: Williams & Wilkins, 1976.
18. Johnson JE. Axis of rotation of the ankle. In Stiehl JB, ed. Inman's Joints of the Ankle, ed 2. Baltimore, MD: Williams & Wilkins, 1991:21.
19. Singh AK, Starkweather KD, Hollister AM, et al. Kinematics of the ankle: a hinge axis model. Foot Ankle 13:439, 1992.
20. Stiehl JB. Biomechanics of the ankle joint. In Stiehl JB, ed. Inman's Joints of the Ankle, ed 2. Baltimore, MD: Williams & Wilkins, 1991:39.
21. Perry J. Ankle foot complex. In Gait Analysis: Normal and Pathological Function. Thorofare, NJ: Slack Inc, 1992:51.
22. Sutherland DH, Cooper L, Daniel D. The role of the ankle plantar flexors in normal walking. J Bone Joint Surg Am 62:354, 1980.
23. Kadaba MP, Ramakaishnan HK, Wooten ME, et al. Repeatability of kinematic, kinetic and electromyographic data in normal adult gait. J Orthop Res 7:849, 1989.
24. Scott SH, Winter DA. Talocrural and talocalcaneal joint kinematics and kinetics during the stance phase of walking. J Biomech 24:743, 1991.
25. Brandell BR. Functional roles of the calf and vastus muscles in locomotion. Am J Phys Med 56:59, 1977.
26. Close JR, Todd FN. The phasic activity of the muscles of the lower extremity and the effect of tendon transfer. J Bone Joint Surg Am 41:189, 1959.
27. Winter DA, Yack HJ. EMG profiles during normal human walking: stride-to-stride and intersubject variability. Electroencephalogr Clin Neurophysiol 67:402, 1987.
28. Inman VT Ralston HJ, Todd F. Human Walking. Baltimore, MD: Williams & Wilkins, 1981.
29. Basmajian JV. Human locomotion. In Muscle Alive: Their Functions Revealed by Electromyography. Baltimore, MD: Waverly, 1978.
30. Haxon HA. Absolute muscle force in the ankle flexors of man. J Physiol 103:267, 1944.
31. Murray MP, Guten GN, Sepic SB, et al. Function of the triceps surae during gait: compensatory mechanisms for unilateral loss. J Bone Joint Surg Am 60:473, 1978.
32. Simon SR, Mann RA, Hagy JL, Larsen LJ. Role of the posterior calf muscles in normal gait. J Bone Joint Surg Am 60:465, 1978.
33. Sutherland D. An electromyographic study of the plantar flexors of the ankle in normal walking on the level. J Bone Joint Surg Am 48:66, 1966.
34. Stauffer R, Chao E, Brewster R. Force and motion analysis of the normal, diseased and prosthetic ankle joint. Clin Orthop Rel Res 127:189, 1977.
35. Procter P, Paul J. Ankle joint biomechanics. J Biomech 15:627, 1982.
36. Winter DA. Overall principle of lower limb support during stance phase of gait. J Biomech 13:923, 1980.
37. Winter DA. Energy generation and absorption at the ankle and knee during fast, natural and slow cadences. Clin Orthop 175:147, 1983.
38. Mann RA, Baxter DE, Lutter LD. Running symposium. Foot Ankle 1:190, 1981.
39. Manter JT. Movements of the subtalar and transverse tarsal joint. Anat Rec 80:397, 1941.
40. Van Langelaan EJ. A kinematical analysis of the tarsal joints. An x-ray photogrammetric study. Acta Orthop Scand Suppl 54:S204, 1983.
41. Sangeorzan BJ. Biomechanics of the subtalar joint. In Stiehl JB, ed. Inman's Joints of the Ankle. ed 2. Baltimore, MD: Williams & Wilkins, 1991.
42. Wright DG, Desai SM, Henderson WH. Action of the subtalar and ankle-joint complex during the stance phase of walking. J Bone Joint Surg Am 46:361, 1964.
43. Close JR, Inman VT, Poor PM, Todd FN. The function of the subtalar joint. Clin Orthop 50:159, 1967.
44. Perry J. Anatomy and biomechanics of the hindfoot. Clin Orthop 177:9, 1983.
45. Houtz SJ, Walsh FP. Electromyographic analysis of the function of the muscles acting on the ankle during weight bearing with special reference to the triceps surae. J Bone Joint Surg Am 41:1469, 1959.
46. Bojsen-Møller F, Lamoreux L. Significance of free dorsiflexion of the toes in walking. Acta Orthop Scand 50:471, 1979.
47. Mann R, Inman VT. Phasic activity of the intrinsic muscles of the foot. J Bone Joint Surg Am 46:469, 1964.

Edema and Foot Injuries: Pathophysiology and Differential Diagnosis

Jeffrey S. Borer
Brian Shaffer

Injuries of the foot commonly are associated with edema, a concomitant of local inflammation and mechanical obstruction to local venous blood flow. Edema also can result from a variety of systemic conditions, some of which are potentially life threatening. However, "swelling, like fever, is not a disease itself but a sign of an underlying disorder."[1] Therapy, both in its form and urgency, must be targeted to the causative process, not to the physical sign. The objective of this chapter is to review the pathophysiology of edema, differentiate the pathophysiologic characteristics associated with local injury from those associated with other diseases, and present the differential diagnosis of peripheral edema with particular reference to the clinical signs and symptoms by which the edema of localized injury might be differentiated from that resulting from other causes.

PATHOPHYSIOLOGY OF PERIPHERAL EDEMA

Ultimately, edema results from transudation of fluid across the capillary or proximal venular wall. Such fluid movement results from an imbalance between capillary permeability and the flow of fluid through the capillaries. Fluid flow is determined by capillary hydrostatic and oncotic pressures[2–4]; capillary permeability is a function of the performance of the endothelial cells (through which solute and fluid can move) and size of the spaces between these cells (which also serve as pathways for fluid and solute egress).[3, 5]

Interstitial and Capillary Hydrostatic Pressure

The usual cause of abnormal capillary hydrostatic pressure is increased total intra-vascular volume. Concomitant with the increased intraluminal pressure, the pressure gradient between the capillary lumen and the interstitium must rise, at least transiently, precipitating fluid transudation through interendothelial interstices. Most commonly, intravascular volume expansion results from abnormal sodium retention, as is found in the setting of congestive heart failure (CHF). In CHF, cardiac output is subnormal (low-output CHF) or relatively inadequate (high-output CHF). In either case, renal perfusion is compromised by a combination of neural and humoral responses triggered by signals emanating from a series of baroreceptors and chemoreceptors; these signals are influenced by cardiac output.[3, 4, 6–8] Subnormal renal perfusion (plasma volume deficiency) increases the release of renin through stimulation of the β-adrenoceptors in the juxtaglomerular cells of the renal cortex, which enhances the production of angiotensin I. In the blood stream, angiotensin I is rapidly converted to angiotensin II. Angiotensin II causes increased secretion of the salt-retaining hormone aldosterone from the adrenal cortex, renal vasoconstriction (specifically, constriction of efferent renal glomerular arterioles), and sodium reabsorption from the proximal convoluted tubule. Angiotensin-mediated vasoconstriction increases blood pressure and decreases renal perfusion, thus increasing filtration fraction and proximal tubular reabsorption of water and sodium in the kidney. Aldosterone acts on the distal convoluted tubule and collecting duct to reabsorb sodium. Thus, the result of activating the renin-angiotensin-aldosterone system is increased plasma volume potentiating the development of edema.[6–10]

Intravascular volume also can be expanded iatrogenically by intake of large fluid volumes at a rate that exceeds renal excretory potential.[11] Effective capillary volume can be increased even without an increase in total vascular volume by relaxation of precapillary arteriolar muscular sphincters, as occurs iatrogenically by administration of certain vasodilators, like nifedipine.[12] Similarly, capillary volume, and concomitant intracapillary hydrostatic pressure, can be increased by obstruction to venous flow, as by venous thrombosis. Such obstruction can prevent egress of fluid from the capillary lumen into the venular lumen while forward flow continues from the precapillary arterioles, resulting in abnormal filling of the capillary lumen. Similarly, in CHF, increased central venous pressure is reflected backward throughout the venous system, and the effects of relative obstruction to outflow potentiate those resulting from the increase in total vascular volume.[6, 11, 13]

Interstitial and Capillary Colloid Oncotic (Osmotic) Pressure

Capillary osmotic pressure primarily is a function of plasma protein concentration and, most specifically, the concentration of the relatively small protein albumin. Thus, capillary osmotic pressure is reasonably approximated as capillary oncotic pressure. Generally, plasma proteins do not pass through the capillary endothelial cells or the intercellular capillary pores. Therefore, the osmotic effects of the intraluminal plasma albumin counteract the effects of abnormal hydrostatic pressure and even tend to promote resorption of interstitial fluid. Plasma oncotic pressure is diminished by various systemic, renal, and hepatic diseases (e.g., nephrotic syndrome, malnutrition, cirrhosis, loss of protein in the gastrointestinal tract, severe catabolic state).[6, 11]

The effects of intravascular proteins are opposed by the interstitial colloid concentration. Tissue colloid osmotic pressure can be altered by extravascular protein accumulation as a result of abnormal capillary permeability or obstruction of flow within the lymphatic system.[3, 6, 13] Physiologically, the lymphatics remove the fluid, which is filtered by normal capillaries. Thus, normally, there is a slight flow gradient from the arterial to the venous side of the capillaries; the fluid and protein, which enter the capillaries from the arterioles, exceed the capacity of the capillaries, which filter the excess into the interstitial space. Some of this excess is resorbed into the capillary as this vessel communicates with the more compliant venule. However, the amount filtered generally exceeds the efficiency of the resorption process. The excess is removed directly by the lymphatic vessels, which drain the interstitial space, thus enabling tissue homeostasis to be maintained for water and solute.[3–6, 13] The lymph is returned to the venous system via anastomoses between lymphatic vessels and the larger central veins.

If the lymphatic system is obstructed (as may occur with certain malignancies and central venous obstruction), excess fluid and protein can accumulate in the extravascular space, increasing interstitial osmotic pressure and potentiating edema formation.[3, 5, 6, 13]

Capillary Permeability

Generally, only noncolloid solutes permeate the capillary wall freely. Injury to the capillary wall from chemical, bacterial, immunologic, thermal, or mechanical sources (as is characteristic of inflammation) can increase capillary transmural permeability to larger molecules, like albumin and other plasma proteins. Thus, for example, in extreme cases of capillary endothelial cell hypoxia (as might be seen with the ischemia of arteriolar or arterial obstruction or in the context of poison gas, burns, or allergic reactions), increases in permeability of capillaries and small venules can allow fluid, high in protein content, to enter the extravascular space within the injured tissue. Such abnormalities in microvascular permeability generally are not important factors in the pathophysiology of the common generalized edematous states but can be important in the genesis of localized edema.[3, 6, 11]

Several mechanisms may underlie pathologic alterations in capillary permeability. During acute and non-necrotizing injury to the skin, release of endogenous autacoids (e.g., histamine, serotonin), presumably most often from mast cells, can cause arterial constriction, possibly associated with capillary injury (itself potentially affecting capillary endothelial function and integrity). A period of constriction generally is followed by arterial dilation, which increases flow into the capillaries. Release of autacoids appears to be triggered by local release of calcium ions from injured cells. The effects of the autacoids are highly selective, resulting in separation of the lateral borders only of the endothelial cells lining the postcapillary venules of 10 to 30 μm in diameter and not, strictly speaking, of the capillaries themselves. Indeed, the effect can be quite marked: the width of the intercellular clefts can become greatly enlarged, sufficiently even to accommodate 7 to 10 μm of formed blood elements.[14] Although the microvascular basement membrane, which limits movement of colloidal particles (e.g., lipoproteins), is not affected by autacoid release, this barrier can be traversed by plasma proteins and smaller solutes, allowing edema formation to occur.[14]

Alteration in the function of the endothelial cells themselves also can be important in the pathophysiology of edema formation. Endothelium lining the microvasculature forms the critical barrier controlling the exchange of molecules between blood and interstitial fluid. Interaction of blood with the endothelial cell surface (the glycocalix) can restrict or increase transendothelial transport of specific ligands. Excessive movement of osmotically active molecules into the interstitium can promote edema formation, whereas their transport out of the interstitial space can have the opposite effect. Because these endothelial transport mechanisms depend on endothelial expression of cell surface glycoproteins, regional variations in endothelial transport can be expected and may be useful in developing tissue-directed drug therapies, which might limit edema formation in certain settings.[15]

The composition of the serum also can affect capillary permeability. This influence depends on the capacity of serum components to affect the configuration of the electrical charge of the glycocalix. Normally, the net negative charge configuration at the cell surface tends to restrict transcapillary transport of polyanionic molecules to a greater degree than neutral or polycationic molecules. Endothelial cell surface binding of certain plasma anionic macromolecules, such as albumin and orosomucoids, increases the charge negativity at the glycocalix, resulting in greater polyanion exclusion.[15] In addition to its effects via surface charge alteration, serum albumin acts as a steric molecular "filter" that can resist the transport of water, small solutes, and macromolecules across the microvascular wall.[15] Thus, reduction in serum proteins can promote edema formation both by reducing serum oncotic pressure and minimizing the electrostatic and physical effects that retard movement of osmotically active molecules into the extravascular space.

DIFFERENTIAL ETIOLOGIC DIAGNOSIS OF PERIPHERAL EDEMA

The pathophysiologic processes described previously can occur in various combinations among the many disease processes characterized by peripheral edema. Clues to the underlying cause can be inferred from associated clinical symptoms and physical signs. In approaching the differential diagnosis of edema, a useful framework for separating localized processes from systemic or diffuse diseases can be based on consideration of the following characteristics:

1. *History*
   a. Known potential causes or contributing factors (recent trauma, surgery, concurrent illness, drug therapy)
   b. Temporal factors
      (1) Rapidity of onset (gradual, more commonly associated with systemic diseases, vs. sudden, more commonly associated with localized processes)
      (2) Temporal pattern (short duration/first episode, chronic, recurrent, cyclic; note that variations in edema during 24-hour periods have limited diagnostic value because, irrespective of cause, peripheral edema is greatest in dependent regions and, therefore, typically is greater in feet and ankles during the daytime, when upright posture is most common)
   c. Symptoms (painless, more common in systemic diseases, vs. painful, very uncommon in most systemic diseases)[1, 2, 4, 6, 11]
2. *Physical signs*
   a. Laterality (unilateral, more common in localized processes, vs. bilateral, more common in systemic diseases)
   b. Condition of overlying skin (taut, thick, fibrotic skin generally is associ-

ated with a chronic process, more likely a result of systemic disease or venous insufficiency than musculoskeletal condition)

c. Density of edema (edema that is relatively low in protein commonly is soft and "pitting," typical of CHF or hypoproteinemia; edema that is relatively high in protein content or involves extensive subcutaneous fibrosis generally is nonpitting, as in pretibial myxedema)

d. Location (anasarca, edema plus ascites, simultaneous upper and lower extremity edema, and other generalized patterns suggest systemic diseases; localized edema, even if bilateral, may be more closely associated with a localized process)[1, 2, 4, 6, 11]

Laterality of edema is perhaps the most efficient initial discriminator of systemic versus localized processes. Therefore, the etiologic differential diagnosis of peripheral edema, presented next, is keyed to this characteristic, as modified from the classification schemes of Ruschhaupt and Graor[2] and Young.[1]

Bilateral Edema

Bilateral edema commonly begins simultaneously in both legs at feet and ankles and proceeds symmetrically up the legs.[2] Possible causes include the following:

CONGESTIVE HEART FAILURE.[1, 2] History of potential causes/contributing factors: hypertension, angina, or myocardial infarction; valvular diseases; cardiomyopathy; etc. Symptoms: dyspnea on exertion, orthopnea, paroxysmal nocturnal dyspnea; associated signs: tachypnea, rales, rhonchi, distended neck veins, tachycardia, hepatomegaly, ventricular gallop, heart murmur, etc.[1, 2, 11] Edema of CHF typically is soft and easily pitting, occurs predominantly in dependent parts of body and, therefore, diminishes in legs after a period of recumbency.[1, 2, 11] CHF edema can be distinguished from other forms of dependent edema by presence of engorged cervical veins, particularly if evidence of diffusely elevated systemic venous pressure (e.g., hepatomegaly) also is present.[6]

NEPHROTIC SYNDROME.[1, 2] History of causative/contributing factors: renal disease/uremia, proteinuria, hypoalbuminemia, hypercholesterolemia; symptoms: polyuria/polydipsia, nocturia. Renal biopsy can confirm the diagnosis.[1, 2, 6]

ACUTE GLOMERULONEPHRITIS.[2] History of causative/contributing factors: history consistent with recent group A beta-hemolytic streptococcal infection; proteinuria, hematuria, markedly subnormal creatinine clearance, recent-onset hypertension.[2]

HEPATIC CIRRHOSIS.[1, 2] History of causative/contributing factors: history of continuing jaundice or abdominal swelling, hepatosplenomegaly, gynecomastia, ascites, spider angiomas, palmar erythema[2]; abnormal fecal loss of albumin,[6] diagnostic liver biopsy or scan, abnormal serum liver enzymes, etc.[1]

HYPOPROTEINEMIA.[1, 2] History of causative/contributing factors: malnutrition, diarrhea, known malabsorption syndrome of any cause.[2]

IDIOPATHIC CYCLIC EDEMA.[1, 2] History of temporal factors: onset is quick and marked and disappearance is complete, with recurrences of a similar pattern; edema affects hands, face, legs, abdomen, and lower extremities. It often is related to the menstrual cycle and is limited almost entirely to obese women aged 20 to 40 years; may cause a 3- to 4- pound weight gain from morning to evening, reversed by bedrest; syndrome may be self-limited, sometimes disappearing after a few cycles (months). More commonly, it recurs during 1 to 20 years after initial episode. Associated symptoms: headache, irritability, anxiety, and depression.[1, 2, 16]

POSITION-RELATED EDEMA.[2] History of causative/contributing factors: any condition that severely limits ambulation (e.g., various arthritides[2]). History of temporal factors: temporal association with sitting and standing for long periods without use of calf and leg muscles (increasing capillary hydrostatic pressure by relative obstruction to capillary outflow because of gravity-mediated venous pressure elevation in lower extremities). Symptoms: generally painless, but if pain exists for other reasons (e.g., musculoskeletal injury), hanging affected foot over bed at night to relieve pain may result in unilateral edema[2]; sitting (to relieve ischemic pain) can result in bilateral edema[2]. Physical signs: skin generally increasingly compliant with age (causative factors also increase with age), resulting in diminishing interstitial fluid pressure and enabling considerable fluid accumulation[2]; edema can be unilateral if arterial insufficiency coexists with dependency or if dependency is systematically unilateral.

LIPIDEMA.[1, 2] History of causative/contributing factors: bilateral, symmetric distribution of fat confined to or predominantly present in the lower extremities, characteristically sparing the feet (and thus distinguishable from lymphedema[1, 2]), occurring only in women, often familial. Symptoms: generally painless,[1] although if complicated by exogenous obesity can be painful. Physical signs: this is not true edema and is not associated with pitting unless a comorbid condition causes water retention.[1] Support hose, often useful in other forms of edema, do not provide benefit and can potentiate pain; avoidance of abnormal weight gain may be useful, but intensive weight loss generally is not effective therapy because site of abnormal fat accumulation (buttocks and legs) generally does not respond to dietary alteration.[1]

DRUG EFFECTS.[1, 2] History of causative/contributing factors: temporally related use of nonsteroidal anti-inflammatory medications (e.g., phenylbutazone, oxyphenbutazone, ibuprofen[2]), certain vasodilating and antihypertensive drugs (e.g., nifedipine, alpha-methyldopa, guanethidine sulfate, hydrazaline, diazoxide, rauwolfia alkaloids),[1] hormone therapy (e.g., progesterone, estrogen, testosterone, corticosteroids, adrenocorticotropins), monoamine oxidase inhibitor antidepressant drugs, etc. Physical signs: edema is soft and pitting, similar to that observed with cyclic edema or hypoproteinemia.[1]

PRIMARY LYMPHEDEMA.[1, 2] History of temporal factors: onset gradual, over days, weeks, or months[2] (and thus distinguishable from idiopathic cyclic edema) and is chronic. Symptoms: generally painless unless a concurrent painful process is extant. Physical signs: often accompanied by abnormal epi-

dermal proliferation and dermal subcutaneous fibrosis[17] but rarely by skin ulceration; often not bilateral and, in any event, generally less uniformly distributed and extensive than edema caused by lymphatic or venous obstruction.[1]

EXTREME HIGH-TEMPERATURE EXPOSURE.[2] History of causative/contributing factors: temporally related exposure to high temperatures (which cause peripheral vasodilatation, increasing flow through, and hydrostatic pressure in, affected capillary beds), typically occurring in healthy individuals. History of temporal factors: moderately rapid onset (many minutes to hours depending on temperatures, dependency of limbs, etc.), moderately rapid resolution (again depending on temperature change, as well as intercurrent ambulation).

Unilateral Edema

The causes of unilateral edema are more numerous than bilateral edema and, most commonly, are due to local rather than systemic conditions.[2]

CHRONIC VENOUS INSUFFICIENCY.[1, 2] This is the most common cause of unilateral edema,[1, 2] occasionally resulting from congenitally absent or abnormal valves of the deep veins but more commonly caused by acquired deep venous valvular dysfunction; in either case, valvular insufficiency results in abnormal venous pressure when affected body parts are dependent, with associated relative obstruction to capillary outflow. History of causative/contributing factors: remote deep venous thrombosis (veins subjected to engorgement distal to thrombi often are permanently dilated because of damage and remodeling of vascular wall, commonly rendering valves incompetent; additionally, venous valves often are damaged or destroyed during the healing process[1]). Deep venous thrombophlebitis can be symptomatic, but often is asymptomatic and must be detected by objective testing. A specific "subacute" form of this syndrome regularly is observed after coronary artery bypass grafting in which a venous bypass conduit is used; removal of the saphenous vein leads to transient volume overload of the remaining veins in the ipsilateral leg, with resulting soft, pitting edema that resolves over several months as the deep veins remodel to handle their new load. Chronic stasis changes (see later) seldom occur unless additional, pre-existing venous disease is present. Physical signs: in early stages, edema typically is soft and pitting, consisting mainly of fluid transudation resulting from excessive microvascular hydrostatic pressure[1, 2]; with time, inefficient capillary inflow and abnormal interstitial pressure lead to chronic skin changes, including pigmentation (iron deposition can occur as a result of extravasation of red blood cells), dermatitis, and fibrosis, occasionally accompanied by indurated cellulitis and ulceration.[1] The result is so-called brawny edema, which can be contrasted with the soft, easily pitting edema of hypoproteinemia. These changes commonly are associated with venous stasis. Prominent superficial veins may appear shortly after an attack of phlebitis and may become varicose in the chronic stage of venous insufficiency. In the very late stages, chronic venous insufficiency can result in secondary hemodynamic stresses in the superficial veins, which are sufficient to cause soft, pitting edema in addition to the chronic, brawny edema.[1]

SUPERFICIAL THROMBOPHLEBITIS. History of causative/contributing factors: temporally related development of tender, indurated, superficial "cord" extending a variable distance along path of superficial vein, associated with erythema, warmth, and tenderness during the acute stage; thrombus usually remains palpable for days or weeks after diminution of the acute inflammation. Although systemic symptoms usually are absent, a low-grade fever may be present.[1, 18] Physical signs: although pitting, edema is not soft, because inflammatory process can be expected to alter microvascular permeability; importantly, edema usually is uniform in consistency in the area drained by the obstructed vein.[18]

DEEP VEIN THROMBOSIS AND/OR THROMBOPHLEBITIS.[1, 2] History of causative/contributing factors: temporally related conditions associated with enforced bedrest or physical inactivity, particularly if extremities are immobilized (e.g., orthopedic or abdominal surgery, prolonged airplane flight, childbirth, traumatic injury, or any particularly debilitating illness). Diagnosis generally requires support from objective testing (e.g., contrast venography, Doppler ultrasonography, radionuclide-based thrombus imaging), and leads to chronic venous hypertension of the affected lower extremity when the leg is dependent.[2] History of temporal factors: edema may develop gradually, over a few days, or more rapidly, over hours, depending on the location and extent of the underlying process.[1, 2, 18] When thrombosis is unusually extensive, edema can occur relatively abruptly, with massive sudden swelling and intense cyanosis of extremity. The latter presumably results from particularly complete oxygen extraction from blood flowing very slowly through the capillaries, combined with compromise of arterial and arteriolar flow resulting from the external mechanical pressure of the rapidly accumulating edema and engorged veins. Indeed, in this setting, pulses in the limb are subnormal or absent, and gangrene can result if obstruction to arterial flow is particularly severe,[1] as in the condition known as phlegmasia cerulea dolens, which can cause shock by trapping a large quantity of blood in the swollen extremity. Phlegmasia cerulea dolens primarily is associated with advanced or metastatic malignancies.[1] Even in somewhat less severe deep venous obstruction, fluid can accumulate beneath the deep fascia. Symptoms: deep venous thrombosis or thrombophlebitis can cause localized dull, aching pain, which can be quite severe, particularly when limb is dependent,[4] but lack of pain does not rule out this cause. Low-grade fever may be common, but rigors are uncommon and lymphadenopathy and lymphangitic streaking are absent.[1] Physical signs: soft, pitting edema often develops within 24 to 48 hours of the thrombosis and can be extensive. Associated inflammation can cause local warmth, tenderness, erythema, and even cyanosis; it can occur as in chronic venous insufficiency.[1, 2] Superficial veins can be prominent[1] (a single "sentinel" vein may be observed), and tenderness on deep palpation can be present.[1, 2]

LYMPHEDEMA.[2] History of causative/contributing factors: any condition associated with obstruction of lymphatics or incompetence of lymphatic valves, resulting in lymph stasis, increased intralymphatic pressure, and inefficient drainage of the interstitium (e.g., femoral artery bypass surgery, which appears to damage and interfere with surrounding lymphatics, local infection).[1] Lymphedema can be subclassified according to cause: (1) primary lymphedema (idiopathic) can be congenital or acquired, commonly affects drainage of cutaneous or subcutaneous lymphatics in the legs[1, 2]; primary lymphedema can be further subclassified into (a) lymphedema tarda, which becomes apparent only after age 40, raising concern of other common causes (e.g., malignancy)[1]; (b) primary congenital lymphedema (either nonfamilial ["simple"] or familial [Milroy's disease]), present at birth, and usually involving only one lower extremity that manifests aplasia, hypoplasia, or varicose dilation of the lymphatic vessels[1, 2]; (c) primary acquired lymphedema (lymphedema praecox), idiopathic but apparently involving a subnormally developed lymphatic system, not seen before adolescence but usually presenting before age 30 and predominantly affecting women.[2] Characteristically, this form is associated with a "hump" on the dorsum of the foot, although upper extremities can be involved, and edema development is slow, typically involving an entire limb over the course of months to years; although commonly unilateral, both limbs may be affected. In early stages, edema is soft and painless and disappears overnight. Lymphangitis and/or cellulitis occur within weeks to months of edema in a minority of cases[1, 2]; (2) secondary (obstructive) lymphedema may be inflammatory or noninflammatory[1] and most commonly is secondary to malignancy. The noninflammatory form almost always is unilateral and typically results from metastatic carcinoma involving regional lymph nodes or after irradiation or surgical lymph node resection,[2] but can occur with retroperitoneal fibrosis and other conditions[1]; the inflammatory form results from lymphangitis (sometimes recurrent) or cellulitis, commonly caused by infection, local traumatic injury, filariasis, etc.,[1] and often associated with fever. History of temporal factors: all forms usually develop slowly, over months or years. Symptoms: usually painless.[1] Physical signs: soon after onset, edema is soft and pitting; in chronic stages, as subcutaneous fibrosis develops, the skin thickens, and edema may resist pitting and is firmer than that associated with chronic venous obstruction; superficial veins are not dilated, another point of differentiation from chronic venous obstruction.[1] Clinically, differentiation from deep venous thrombosis may be difficult unless pain is present (generally not present with lymphatic obstruction); venograms can rule out venous obstruction, but lymphangiograms then may be necessary to confirm lymphangitic abnormality.[1]

LYMPHANGITIS. Like lymphedema, lymphangitis features lymphatic obstruction, in this case by thrombosis and fibrosis, which occurs secondary to local parasitic (dermatophytoses) and bacterial infections, typically introduced in the foot and ankle. The lymph stasis that is produced predisposes to recurrent cellulitis, in turn causing recurrent lymphangitis. Physical signs: although typically restricted to the foot and ankle, inflammation and edema may spread up the leg.[1, 2]

INFECTION.[1, 2] Although infection can cause lymphangitis and lymphedema, occasionally a particularly virulent infection presents acutely with characteristics that justify a separate classification. History of causative/contributing factors: trauma breaking the skin (wound, cut, abrasion, ulcer, contusion, scratch, hangnail, pinprick, or vesicle) allows for invasion; the area between the toes is the most common site, because it is often softened from chronic tinea pedis infection.[1, 2] History of temporal factors: dramatic development of edema, with subsequent complete disappearance, occasionally featuring similarly characterized recurrences.[2] Infections that commonly cause sudden, unilateral edema include filariasis, particularly in tropical climates, clostridia infections causing gas gangrene, and agents associated with chronic osteomyelitis.[1] Symptoms and physical signs: pronounced fever, rigors, malaise, other nonspecific systemic symptoms, and localized pain[2] associated with rapid and even explosive development of local warmth, tenderness, erythema, "lymphangitic" streaks following the course of affected lymphatics from the infection site, and regional lymphadenopathy. Dermatophytosis of the toes may enable recurrent attacks, probably caused by secondary bacterial invaders; inflammation and edema are restricted to the foot and ankle but can spread up the leg.[2]

TRAUMA.[1, 2] Mechanical injury can affect characteristics of microvasculature directly, resulting in edema. In addition, traumatic injury to veins can result in venous thrombosis and provide a skin portal for entry of infectious agents.

POSITION-RELATED EDEMA.[2] See Bilateral Edema.

VASCULAR ANOMALIES.[1, 2] Arteriovenous fistulas must be considered in the differential diagnosis of edema because they can cause edema (e.g., by mechanical pressure on microvasculature) and can result in limb enlargement, which can mimic edema. History of causative/contributing factors: traumatic penetrating injury. Physical signs: thrill and bruit overlying the lesion, abnormal limb circumference; hemangiomas or other vascular anomalies and severe, unilateral, varicose or dilated veins in unusual places may indicate a congenital fistula.[1] Angiography and venous oxygen saturation determinations can confirm the diagnosis.[2]

KLIPPEL-TRÉNAUNAY-WEBER SYNDROME. Presentation of muscular, bony, and soft tissue hypertrophy, persistent nevus flammeus, and varicose veins usually involving a single lower limb, which may be associated with arteriovenous fistulas.[1]

TUMORS.[1, 2] Lipomas, hemangiomas, hemangiolymphangiomas, sarcomas, neuroepitheliomas, and osteosarcomas can cause unilateral limb edema, usually relatively localized to the proximity of the tumor,[1] unlike the more extensive and diffuse edema of several other common processes. Tumors also can cause more extensive edema by extrinsic mechanical compression of vascular structures.

FACTITIOUS EDEMA.[2] Edema caused by self-inflicted constriction of veins, as with a tourniquet. When reported, such edema generally follows no pattern suggestive of a known cause; on examination, there may be a sharply defined region of edema consistent with the application of the constricting apparatus.[2]

GASTROCNEMIUS RUPTURE.[2] Typically the result of athletic effort, gastrocnemius rupture is sudden, acutely painful (usually mid-calf), commonly associated with a large ecchymosis in dependent areas (foot, ankle) from internal hemorrhage. The increased limb circumference must be differentiated from edema and also causes edema as vascular structures are compressed by the internal hemorrhage and hematoma.[1, 2]

POPLITEAL CYST, POPLITEAL SYNDROME.[2] Mechanical compression of venous structures by cyst or aneurysm can cause edema like that of venous thrombosis; differential clue is the palpation of the cystic structure on examination.[2]

COMPARTMENT SYNDROME.[2] Increased tissue pressure in the region of the anterior tibial artery as a result of trauma, thrombosis, or embolism can cause severe ischemia, edema, and pain over the anterior tibial compartment.[2] Edema within the confined space may compress arterial structures sufficiently to compromise viability of muscle and nerve structures within the compartment, requiring fasciotomy to prevent gangrene.[1]

RETROPERITONEAL FIBROSIS.[2] As noted previously, this entity can cause secondary lymphedema. In addition, retroperitoneal fibrosis can compromise arterial flow to the affected limb.[1, 2]

ANGIONEUROTIC EDEMA (HEREDITARY ANGIOEDEMA).[2] This is a noninflammatory and hereditary disease characterized by localized swelling of the skin, internal organs, and mucous membranes and caused by lack of $C'1$ esterase inhibitor of the first component of complement $C'1$ esterase, resulting in increased capillary permeability and precapillary arteriolar dilatation. History of temporal factors: attacks are episodic, usually begin in adolescence, and are often preceded by anxiety and triggered by trauma or infection, although an identifiable trigger may not exist. Initial site of edema may be one of minor trauma (e.g., athletic contact).[19] Frequency of attacks varies, from weekly to yearly or longer. Symptoms: abdominal pain, tightness, or tingling of skin, followed by a nonpruritic and painless rash. Symptoms are usually short lived.[20] Attacks commonly are preceded by bloating, anorexia, vomiting, constipation, and nausea.[19] Signs: stridor (resulting from potentially lethal edematous airway obstruction), edema in upper extremities and oropharynx (upper face, trunk, extremities; lower trunk and lower extremities are rarely swollen); lesions are nonpitting and erythematous.[19]

PRETIBIAL MYXEDEMA.[1, 2] Unlike the myxedema associated with hypothyroidism, which may result from alterations in capillary permeability and in the synthesis and degradation rates of plasma proteins, pretibial myxedema is an unusual manifestation of hyperthyroidism.[22] The pathogenesis may be related to an increase in osmotically active mucopolysaccharide production in the interstitium, producing a brawny, nonpitting edema, often with plaque formation of the overlying skin, affecting the pretibial region and dorsum of the foot. The basis for the rarity of this finding in the hyperthyroid population is unclear. Pretibial myxedema is seen in combination with exophthalmos and may not resolve with treatment of the underlying disease.[21]

THERMAL INJURY AND EXPOSURE TO EXTREME HIGH TEMPERATURES.[2] See Bilateral Edema.

BAKER'S CYST. This synovial structure can rupture behind the knee into the calf muscle, producing severe pain,[2] swelling, and tenderness, which can mimic the presentation of thrombophlebitis.[1] Baker's cysts have been associated with rheumatoid arthritis, osteoarthritis, and internal knee malfunction[1]; may be bilateral; and can be confirmed by arthrography.[2]

CONCLUSION

Peripheral edema results from well-defined pathophysiologic processes that can be variously combined in many disease entities. The clinical presentation, specifically, the character and distribution of edema, depend on the pathophysiologic mechanisms involved in each case. The operative pathophysiology is at least partially inferable from the clinical evaluation. Although beyond the scope of this chapter, such recognition is important in selection among therapeutic modalities for the conditions of which edema is a feature.

REFERENCES

1. Young JR. The swollen leg. Am Fam Physician 15:163–173, 1977.
2. Ruschhaupt WF, Graor RA. Evaluation of the patient with leg edema. Postgrad Med 78:132–139, 1985.
3. Tobian L. The influence of hydrostatic pressure and colloid osmotic pressure and fluid transfer across the capillary membrane. In Moyer JH, Fuchs M, eds. Edema: Mechanisms and Management: A Hahnemann Symposium on Salt and Water Retention. Philadelphia: W. B. Saunders, 1960, pp. 3–6.
4. Johnson HD, Pflug J. The Swollen Leg: Causes and Treatment. Philadelphia: J. B. Lippincott, 1975, pp. 70–86, 134–46.
5. Witte CL, Witte MH, Dumont AE. Pathophysiology of chronic edema, lymphedema, and fibrosis. In Staub NC, Taylor AE, eds. Edema. New York: Raven Press, 1984, pp. 521–542.
6. Friedberg CK. Edema and pulmonary edema: pathologic physiology and differential diagnosis. Prog Cardiovasc Dis 3:546–579, 1971.
7. Harris P. Role of arterial pressure in the oedema of heart disease. Lancet 1:1036–1038, 1988.
8. Braunwald E. Pathophysiology of heart failure. In Heart Disease: A textbook of Cardiovascular Medicine, ed 4. Philadelphia: W. B. Saunders, 1992, pp. 411–412.
9. Firth JD, Raine AEG, Ledingham JGG. Raised venous pressure: a direct cause of renal sodium retention in oedema? Lancet 1:1033–1036, 1988.
10. Pastan SO, Braunwald E. Renal disorders and heart disease. In Braunwald E, ed. Heart Disease: A Textbook of Cardiovascular Medicine, ed 4. Philadelphia: W. B. Saunders, 1992, pp. 1856–1858.
11. Braunwald E. Edema and heart failure. In Wilson JD, Braunwald E, Isselbacher KJ, et al, eds. Harrison's Principles of Internal Medicine, ed 12. New York: McGraw-Hill, 1991, pp. 228–232, 890–900.
12. Rutherford JD, Braunwald E. Chronic ischemic heart disease. In Braunwald E, ed. Heart Disease: A Textbook of Cardiovascular Medicine, ed 4. Philadelphia: W. B. Saunders, 1992, pp. 1311–1313.
13. Streeten DHP. Othostatic Disorders of the Circulation: Mechanisms, Manifestations, and Treatment. New York: Plenum Medical, 1987, pp. 13–57.
14. Wissig SL, Charonis AS. Capillary ultrastructure. In Staub NC, Taylor AE, eds. Edema. New York: Raven Press, 1984, pp. 117–142.
15. Schnitzer JE. Update on the cellular an molecular basis of capillary permeability. Trends Cardiovasc Med 3:124–130, 1993.
16. Streeten DHP. Idiopathic edema: pathogenesis, clinical features, and treatment. Metabolism 27:353–383, 1978.
17. Gniadecka M. Localization of dermal edema in lipodermatosclerosis, lymphedema, and cardiac insufficiency. J Am Acad Dermatol 35:37–41, 1996.
18. Young JR. Evaluation of the patient with spontaneous thrombophlebitis. Postgrad Med 78:149–156, 1985.
19. Elnicki ME, Mansmann PT. Hereditary angioedema. In Conn RB, Borer WZ, Snyder JW, eds. Current Diagnosis. Philadelphia: W. B. Saunders, 1997, pp. 1172–1180.
20. Granger DN, Barrowman JA. Gastrointestinal and liver edema. In Staub NC, Taylor AE, eds. Edema. New York: Raven Press, 1984, p. 645.
21. Smith TJ. Localized myxedema. In Braverman LE, Uitger RD, eds. Werner and Ingbar's The Thyroid: A Fundamental and Clinical Text. Philadelphia: J. B. Lippincott, 1991, pp. 676–681.
22. Kleeman CR, Mackovic-Basic M. The kidneys and electrolyte metabolism in hypothyroidism. In Braverman LE, Uitger RD, eds. Werner and Ingbar's The Thyroid: A Fundamental and Clinical Text. Philadelphia: J. B. Lippincott, 1991, pp. 1009–1016.

8 Tarsal Tunnel Syndrome

David M. Wallach
Stuart D. Katchis

Tarsal tunnel syndrome (TTS) is a compressive neuropathy of the tibial nerve or one of its branches (medial plantar, lateral plantar, or calcaneal nerve). Like carpal tunnel syndrome (CTS), TTS can be extremely disabling, but it is far less common.

Compression of the tibial nerve within the tarsal canal was first described by Pollack and Davis in 1932.[1] In 1960 Clark[2] and Kopell and Thompson[3] reported on tibial nerve compression, but it was not until 1962 that Keck[4] and Lam[5] described this compressive neuropathy in detail. Keck is credited with coining the term *tarsal tunnel syndrome.*

In his report, Keck described a male army recruit who, during basic training, experienced bilateral paresthesias of his toes and plantar feet. The patient failed to respond to conservative management and was ultimately treated with surgical release of the laciniate ligament, resulting in complete resolution of symptoms.

In 1965, Goodgold and associates[6] were the first to correlate clinical examination with electrophysiologic studies. Using motor evoked potentials, they documented normative values for the tibial nerve to the abductor hallucis and abductor digiti quinti and then used this information to confirm a TTS diagnosis.

In 1967, Lam[7] described the surgical release that is used today. Of the 10 patients (14 feet) on which he operated, complete relief of symptoms was achieved in 12 feet and partial relief in 2 feet. Lam proposed several possible causes of TTS, including anatomic, vascular, regional, and occupational factors.

ANATOMY

Srinivasan and coworkers[8] documented the normal anatomy of the tarsal tunnel after dissecting 40 cadaveric feet in 1980. The authors divided the flexor retinaculum, a "fan-shaped band," into three regions, each of which (superior, middle, and inferior) demonstrated increased thickening in a caudal direction. The tarsal tunnel's most superior aspect begins at the superior border of the flexor retinaculum. Beneath the retinaculum are the tendons, nerves, and vessels from the posterior compartment of the leg that descend into the ankle. From anterior to posterior are the tibialis posterior tendon, flexor digitorum longus tendon, the neurovascular bundle, and the flexor hallucis longus tendon. The fibers of the flexor retinaculum travel obliquely in a superolateral direction from the medial malleolus, joining with the transverse fascial septum to become one unit. Septa pass from the undersurface of the retinaculum to encase the tendons and neurovascular bundles in separate synovial sheaths. The neurovascular bundle normally has abundant room.

The middle portion of the retinaculum originates from the inferior margin of the medial malleolus and spreads radially to the distal Achilles insertion and medial calcaneus. On division of the tibial nerve into medial and lateral plantar branches, the fibrous septa divide to travel with the respective branches. The medial calcaneal nerve and vessels exit through the retinaculum.

The most inferior aspect of the reticulum joins the fascia of the deltoid ligament, abductor hallucis, and plantar aponeurosis. The flexor retinaculum extends proximally 100 mm from the inferoposterior aspect of the medial malleolus to the sustentaculum tali.

As mentioned, the tendons within the tarsal tunnel are the posterior tibial, flexor digitorum longus, and flexor hallucis longus. The posterior tibial tendon is the most anterior of the three and lies in a separate fibro-osseous tunnel and synovial sheath. The flexor digitorum longus is just posterior to the posterior tibial tendon and anterior to the neurovascular bundle. The flexor digitorum longus enters the plantar aspect of the foot by passing deep to a fibrous arch that connects the abductor hallucis muscle to the navicular bone. The flexor hallucis longus is the most posterior structure of the tarsal tunnel, which passes beneath the sustentaculum tali and penetrates the sole of the foot.

The posterior tibial artery lies medial to the tibial nerve. It is typically joined by two venae comitantes, which encompass the artery. The vascular bundle is wrapped in a thick sheath. The artery then assumes a posterior position to the vein. On passing inferior to the medial malleolus, it supplies the ankle with an articular branch. The main arterial trunk then passes superficial to the medial and lateral plantar nerves to form an arterial arch and tarsal branch 18 mm distal to the bifurcation of the tibial nerve. In 95% (38/40) of Srinivasan and colleagues'[8] specimens, the bifurcation occurred at the upper border of the abductor hallucis.

In another cadaveric study, Dellon and Mackinnon[9] determined the branching pattern of the tibial nerve. They defined a "calcaneal axis" as a line from the center of the medial malleolus to the calcaneus. In 90% of feet examined, the nerve divided within 1 cm proximal or distal to the calcaneal axis and in 95% within 2 cm. Dellon and Mackinnon, therefore, concluded that 95% of specimens had division of the nerve within the tarsal tunnel.

The medial plantar nerve is the largest of the three branches of the tibial nerve. It lies anterior to the lateral plantar nerve as it enters an opening in the fascial origin of the abductor hallucis. It then passes inferolateral to the spring (calcaneonavicular) ligament. The medial plantar nerve is analogous to the median nerve in the hand, having both motor and sensory function. It supplies the abductor hallucis brevis, flexor digitorum brevis, flexor hallucis brevis, and first lumbrical muscle. Its sensory distribution is to the medial sole, the medial three and one-half toes, and the articular surfaces of the respective tarsal, metatarsal, and phalangeal joints.

The lateral plantar nerve travels distally and posterior to the medial branch. It too enters a fascial opening in the abductor hallucis muscle. The nerve passes lateral to the quadratus plantae on entering the fascial opening. The nerve enters deep within the foot beneath the abductor hallucis and the flexor digitorum. It remains plantar to the quadratus plantae, moving to a more super-ficial position between the abductor digiti minimi and the flexor digitorum brevis. The lateral plantar nerve is analogous to the ulnar nerve in the hand. The nerve supplies motor innervation to the quadratus plantae, interossei, flexor digiti minimi, adductor hallucis, abductor digiti minimi, and lateral three lumbricals. Sensation is supplied to the lateral sole and lateral one and one-half toes. The tarsal, metatarsal, and phalangeal joints of these regions are also supplied by the branches from the lateral plantar nerve.

The calcaneal (medial) nerve supplies sensation to the heel. It has a highly variable branching pattern. In 25% (8/31) of Dellon and Mackinnon's cases, the nerve arose from the tibial nerve proximal to the tarsal tunnel and entered the heel superficial to the retinaculum. In 16% (5/31), one calcaneal nerve originated proximal to the tunnel, and the other originated from the tibial nerve within the tunnel. In 23% (7/31), the nerve arose from the tibial nerve within the tunnel (16% before bifurcation and 6% from the lateral plantar nerve). The calcaneal branch has no motor function. It supplies sensation to the medial and plantar heel and the calcaneus.

Havel and associates,[10] in a similar cadaveric study, determined the bifurcation of the tibial nerve within the tarsal tunnel. They found that the tibial nerve divided within the tunnel 93% (63/68 feet) of the time. The other 7% (5/68) of cases divided proximal to the tarsal tunnel. Havel et al. described nine branching patterns of the calcaneal nerve. The calcaneal nerve arose from the posterior aspect of the tibial nerve in 75% (51/68) of cases and from the lateral plantar nerve in the remaining 25% (17/68). The nerve formed multiple branches in 21% of cases and remained a single branch in 79%. Like Dellon and Mackinnon, Havel and associates found that, in almost 40% of cases, the calcaneal nerve originated proximal to the tibial tunnel. Again, like Dellon and Mackinnon, Havel and associates proposed that the early branching of the calcaneal nerve before entering the tunnel may account for the relative infrequency of calcaneal sensory complaints. In addition, both proposed that early branching of the tibial nerve may predispose an ankle to TTS. According to Dellon and Mackinnon, this occurs when multiple nerves present "a larger cross-sectional area at the narrowed entrance to the tarsal tunnel."

Nerve compression leading to TTS is most frequently found in three anatomic areas: the first beneath a tight flexor retinaculum; the second and third at the individual fascial openings of the abductor hallucis through which the medial or lateral plantar nerve passes.

DEMOGRAPHICS AND ETIOLOGY OF TARSAL TUNNEL SYNDROME

In 1990, Cimino[11] reviewed 25 TTS reports and found that the syndrome was slightly more common in females (56% female, 44% male). His study included patients ranging in age from 14 to 80 years.

Much has been written in the literature regarding the causes and conditions associated with TTS. Lam[7] in 1967 wrote of the adherence of fibrous septa to calcaneus periosteum, causing reduced mobility of the neurovascular bundle, increased susceptibility of the nerve to traction injuries, and minimal room for edema. One cause of TTS is a space-occupying lesion, such as a ganglion, neuroma, or tumor. TTS may also be caused by trauma or may develop iatrogenically. However, in many cases, TTS has no apparent cause.

Mann and Coughlin[12] found that the cause of TTS was identifiable in 60% of their cases, whereas Cimino reported an 65% rate. Of the 186 cases that Cimino reviewed, 122 had a proposed cause. Twenty-five cases were idiopathic in origin, followed by trauma-related cases (21), varicosities (16), heel varus (14), fibrosis (11), and heel valgus (10). The remaining factors (each of which caused three or fewer reported cases) included ganglia, diabetes, obesity, accessory or hypertrophic muscles, and systemic disease.

TTS has been associated with several conditions, including diabetes, rheumatoid arthritis, scleroderma, hypothyroidism, and hyperlipidemia. Oloff and coworkers[13] reviewed 73 cases (49 patients) with TTS over a 3-year period. All patients had verification of disease by prolonged motor latency. Systemic disease was present in 34.6% of the cases (diabetes, 20.4%; inflammatory arthritis, 12.2%; and hypothyroidism, <2%. There were three cases of rheumatoid arthritis, two cases of systemic lupus erythematosis, and one case of mixed connective tissue disease.

Several studies report on TTS in rheumatoid patients.[14–19] The tenosynovitis found in rheumatoid arthritis causes TTS in some patients. Grabois and coworkers[18] conducted electrodiagnostic tests (motor nerve latency) in 39 patients with rheumatoid arthritis, and found a 15% (6/39) incidence of peripheral neuropathy and a 5% (2/39) incidence of TTS. In 1981, Baylan and associates[19] measured motor nerve latency in 44 patients with rheumatoid arthritis, after excluding 4 patients with peripheral neuropathy in regions outside the tarsal tunnel. Nerve conduction studies demonstrated abnormal conduction velocity in 25% (11/44) of the patients. Only 2 of the patients with abnormal studies had pain in the distribution of the medial plantar nerve; however, 18% (8/44) with normal conduction velocities had foot pain. In 1983, McGuigan and associates[20] evaluated 30 patients with rheumatoid arthritis and foot pain. All patients underwent compound muscle action potential and sensory conduction testing. Four patients (13.3%) demonstrated diagnostic evidence of TTS. Unlike Baylan et al., McGuigan and associates corrected for skin temperature, and their lower value was likely more accurate.

Mondelli et al.[21] based their study on prior evidence that other systemic diseases predispose to entrapment syndromes.[22] In their study, 17 asymptomatic patients (no clinical evidence of peripheral nervous system involvement) with progressive systemic sclerosis were subjected to electrodiagnostic study. All 17 patients experienced a delay in conduction velocity, and 1 demonstrated abnormalities within the tibial nerve consistent with TTS. TTS has also been seen in patients with ankylosing spondylitis. Kucukdeveci et al.[23] evaluated sensory nerve conduction and motor distal latencies in 30 patients with ankylosing spondylitis. Ten percent (3/30) of the patients had abnormal results consistent with TTS.

Dellon[24] in 1988 proposed that diabetics were susceptible to compression neuropathies secondary to "endoneural edema" as well as diminished transport via the axon. In a rat model, Dellon et al.[25] induced diabetes with injections of streptozotocin. He recorded hindfoot gait by observing footprints on white paper after painting the hindfeet of the rats. After tarsal tunnel release, gait was reanalyzed, and all of the normal gait returned in all diabetic rats after surgery.

Dellon et al. concluded that decompression of the tarsal tunnel would prevent development of the abnormal walking pattern of the diabetic rat. Weiman and Patel[26] in 1995 applied this rationale to 26 diabetic patients with painful neuropathic feet by performing tarsal tunnel releases. Neuropathic pain "subsided" in 92% (24/26) within 1 month. Furthermore, at 1 to 6 months follow-up, in 73% (19/26) of patients, two-point discrimination improved an average of 4 mm. In addition, there was an improvement between preoperative and postoperative electrodiagnostic studies. Complications included four wound infections (all of which resolved) and fifth toe numbness in one patient.

Hypothyroidism may also lead to peripheral neuropathies, myopathies, and compression neuropathies such as CTS and TTS. In 1983, Schwartz and associates[27] reported on nine patients with hypothyroidism who had been referred for evaluation of CTS. Three of the nine patients had symptoms consistent with TTS. All three, plus one asymptomatic patient, had increased distal motor latencies in the tibial nerve. Torres and Moxley[28] described a patient with hypothyroidism who, with thyroid hormone replacement, experienced almost complete relief of TTS. Elevated serum lipid is found with many peripheral neuropathies. Ruderman et al.[29] described a case of TTS in a male patient with type V hyperlipidemia (cholesterol, 1565 mg/dL; triglycerides, 9370 mg/dL) and multiple xanthomas on his arms and legs. The patient had prolonged distal latency of the medial and lateral plantar nerves of his right foot. After several rounds of plasmaphoresis, a low-fat diet, and treatment with insulin, the patient's pain resolved fully, although he complained of sporadic paresthesias in his plantar foot.

As discussed, heel valgus and varus are associated with TTS. In 1991 El-Shahaly and El-Sherif[30] reported 95 female and 19 male patients with ligamentous laxity without an identifiable connective tissue disorder. Their patients suffered from multiple musculoskeletal disorders, including TTS (n = 16). The patients with TTS were predominantly female, with disease onset later in life. Radin[31] described 14 patients with TTS, which he attributed to heel varus and a pronated forefoot. According to Kopell and Thompson,[3] placing the foot in an "overpro-nated" position leads to compression of the tibial nerve.

TARSAL TUNNEL SYNDROME IN ATHLETES AND LABORERS

There have been several reports of TTS resulting from athletic participation.[32–36] TTS has been found in skiers (attributed to the use of tight ski boots) and in runners (from heel valgus). Schon[33] stated that the foot that is more frequently in a position of hyperpronation, whether from being on the inside when racing on a track or on the "high side" when running on a banked road, will be the foot more frequently affected by TTS. TTS has also been found to be prevalent in several occupations. Lam[7] discussed TTS in jockeys, and Sammarco and Miller[37] documented TTS in dancers.

PRESSURES WITHIN THE TARSAL TUNNEL

Kumar and coworkers,[38] using Whiteside and coworkers'[39] compartment pressure technique, measured pressures within the tarsal tunnel in eight normal subjects. Pressure measurements were made with the ankle in three positions: plantigrade, plantar flexion, and dorsiflexion. The recorded pressures ranged between 4 and 6 mm Hg, 10 and 15 mm Hg, and 10 and 20 mm Hg in plantigrade, plantar flexion, and dorsiflexion of the ankle, respectively.

CLINICAL PRESENTATION

The patient with TTS complains of pain in the heel, sole, or toes, or a combination. The pain may be characterized as burning. TTS symptoms usually develop gradually, except in children. In severe cases, paresthesias or anesthesias may develop.

TTS pain may also radiate proximally. However, the radiating pain typically lacks the intensity experienced along the sole of the foot. Romansky and associates[40] reviewed 44 patients with TTS and sciatica or low back pain. All patients underwent treatment directed at relieving the TTS. Electrodiagnostic studies were positive in 65% (29/44) of the patients (8 patients tested negative). Twenty-six patients were radiographically (computed tomography or myelography) confirmed to be without spinal disease. Thirty-three patients had tarsal tunnel releases, 11 had local injections, and 5 had physical therapy or traction. All 44 patients reported that their sciatic symptoms were relieved by these varied treatment modalities.

As in CTS, TTS pain may worsen at night, causing sleep disturbance. Many activities, including walking, may aggravate the condition. Thus, patients may complain that they are bothered by TTS both day and night. Massage may provide temporary relief.

Physician inquiries regarding trauma and systemic disease are essential in forming the differential diagnosis for TTS.

PHYSICAL EXAMINATION

Physical examination begins with a careful inspection of foot alignment. Both varus and valgus malalignment have been implicated in TTS and should be sought. Tenderness over the nerve within the flexor retinaculum or a positive percussion sign suggests nerve injury. In thin patients with a localized region of compression, a fusiform swelling of the nerve may be palpable.

A thorough neurologic examination is essential. Diminished sensation can be demonstrated by reduced two-point discrimination or by monofilament pressure testing. Sensory disturbances may be present along the distribution of some or all of the branches of the posterior tibial nerve. The calcaneal branches are least often involved.

Muscle weakness and wasting in the distribution of the medial and lateral plantar nerves may occur. Early in the disease, the abductor hallucis may be enlarged, and it may be the offending structure that compresses the medial or lateral plantar nerve. Over time, however, its innervation may be affected, and the abductor hallucis muscle will atrophy.

There are several provocative tests in addition to the compression test. Thirty percent of patients experience the Valleix phenomenon, exhibiting tenderness to palpation of the nerves proximal and distal to the area of compression. Placing the foot in a position of inversion (decreasing the tunnel volume; Lam[7]) or eversion (stretching the nerve; Distefano and associates[41]) may reproduce the symptoms. Elevation of a pressure cuff may elicit symptoms more rapidly in the affected than the nonaffected extremity. Venous engorgement and ischemia have been proposed as causes of this effect.

DIFFERENTIAL DIAGNOSIS

TTS is an uncommon disease. Other conditions must be given careful consideration and ruled out before making a TTS diagnosis. The differential diagnoses may be divided into mechanical abnormalities, peripheral neuropathies from systemic disease, and nerve abnormalities that are not secondary to compression. Plantar callosities, metatarsalgia, and plantar fasciitis cause foot pain far more frequently than TTS. Other systemic diseases, such as diabetes, may lead to a peripheral neuropathy. Patients with peripheral vascular disease may also present with foot pain. Last, other nerve abnormalities such as Morton's neuroma, peripheral neuritis, and sciatica can lead to confusion in making a diagnosis.

IMAGING

Plain radiographs are helpful in cases of trauma in which a suspected fracture may be the cause of TTS. However, before magnetic resonance imaging (MRI), there was no good method of visualizing the tarsal tunnel. In 1988, Kneeland and coworkers[42] used MRI to image the normal ankle, and they described the anatomy in detail. Two years later, Erickson and coworkers[43] studied tarsal tunnel disease using MRI. In addition to describing the anatomy, they also imaged six patients with a clinical history of TTS. Four of the six patients had confirmatory electrical diagnostic testing. The MRI detected neurilemomas in two patients, two cases of "probable posttraumatic fibrosis," one case of tenosynovitis, and a ganglion cyst in one patient. Three patients had lesions within the tarsal tunnel, and the rest were found above the flexor retinaculum. The patient with tenosynovitis was treated conservatively; therefore, there were no confirmatory surgical findings. The other patients had demonstrable lesions detected at surgery that corroborated the MRI findings. In another report, Ho and associates[44] detected an extra muscle, the accessorius flexor digitorum longus, by MRI. This muscle originated from the peroneus brevis superior to the tarsal tunnel and then traveled posterior to the posterior tibial nerve and flexor hallucis longus, entering deep to the plantar branches of the nerve and inserting on the quadratus plantae. The muscle demonstrated increased signal on T2-weighted imaging, a finding consistent with the edema found in an injured muscle. The authors believed that the finding was pathognomonic for a muscle strain. The patient responded to conservative treatment.

A larger series of ankles were evaluated by Kerr and Frey.[45] In 1991, they evaluated 33 feet (27 patients) using MRI. All 17 patients who ultimately underwent surgery had confirmatory electrodiagnostic testing. Findings included five masses, eight dilated veins, five fractures or soft tissue injuries, two fibrous scarrings, six cases of flexor hallucis longus tenosynovitis, one case of abductor hallucis hypertrophy, and six normal feet. The surgical findings of 89% (17/19) of the feet were consistent with preoperative MRI diagnosis. One ganglion and one venous varicosity were found, which had not been detected by MRI.

MRI is helpful not only with preoperative planning but also in evaluating failed surgical releases. Zeiss and associates[46] described a 47-year-old man with TTS after a calcaneal fracture. The patient had recurrent symptoms despite two tarsal tunnel releases. An MRI after the second recurrence demonstrated that the flexor retinaculum was still intact, distal to the region released at the two prior surgeries. This finding was confirmed and corrected at surgery, and the patient was asymptomatic at 6-month follow-up.

ELECTRODIAGNOSTIC STUDIES

Goodgold and associates[6] were the first to use electrodiagnostic studies to document TTS objectively. They defined normal conduction velocity value as 49.9 ± 5.1 ms and normal latency as 4.4 ± 0.9 ms and 4.7 ± 1.0 ms for the abductor hallucis and the abductor digiti quinti, respectively.

Kaplan and Kernahan[47] refined Goodgold's technique and applied it to 21 patients with a clinical diagnosis of TTS.

There was no difference in conduction velocity between controls and TTS patients in the tibial nerve proximal to the flexor retinaculum. There was, however, a significant difference in regard to amplitude and duration of evoked potentials in the abductor hallucis and the abductor digiti quinti. The values for distal latency were 6.4 ± 0.8 ms and 7.5 ± 0.6 ms for abductor hallucis and abductor digiti quinti, respectively. Fu et al.,[48] in an effort to standardize the measuring of motor nerve conduction, obtained a range of normative values of healthy volunteers, and controlled for skin temperature as well as distance from reproducible points on the lower extremity.

In an effort to compare the sensitivity of sensory nerve conduction versus motor nerve conduction, Oh and associates[49] in 1979 tested 21 feet with clinically diagnosed TTS. Motor nerve conduction detected abnormal terminal latency in 52% (11/21) of the feet. Sensory nerve conduction detected an abnormality in 90% (19/21) of the feet. Oh and associates concluded that sensory testing was superior to motor testing. This result was supported by Takakura and coworkers,[50] who evaluated 31 TTS patients with sensory nerve conduction studies. Eighty-four percent (26/31 feet) of patients with clinical symptoms of TTS had reduced or absent sensory conduction velocities. Increased distal motor latency was present in only 25% (8/31 feet). In 1985, Oh et al.[51] analyzed their results with a refinement of their sensory nerve conduction technique (near-nerve sensory conduction) in the foot. Ninety-six percent (24/25) of feet had abnormal sensory nerve conduction whereas motor nerve conduction was abnormal in only 16% (4/25) of feet.

Dumitru and coworkers[52] developed a technique of using somatosensory evoked potentials (SEPs) to assess the medial plantar, lateral plantar, and calcaneal nerves. Forty-six healthy volunteers were tested. The values for latency were as follows: tibial, 37.5 ± 2.1 ms; medial plantar, 42.3 ± 3.0 ms; lateral plantar, 43.5 ± 3.0 ms; and calcaneal, 46.9 ± 3.2 ms. The values for amplitude were as follows: tibial, 4.7 ± 2.7 µV; medial plantar, 3.3 ± 1.9 ms; lateral plantar, 2.9 ± 1.7 µV; and calcaneal, 1.4 ± 0.9 µV. In two cases, mixed nerve action potentials failed to reveal an abnormality; however, SEPs demonstrated findings of compressive neuropathy. The first patient responded to conservative therapy (orthotics and injection); the second patient had confirmation of a tarsal tunnel lesion at surgery. Both patients had normalization of SEPs and resolution of symptoms after treatment.

Pressure-specified sensory device (PSSD) is another technique that has shown promise. Tassler and Dellon[53] applied PSSD to 34 normal controls and 28 feet with TTS. There were four different types of stimuli: one-point and two-point discrimination, each of which was paired with both static and dynamic probes. Patients had to determine which type of stimuli they were receiving at varying degrees of applied pressure and in different regions of the foot. Of 26 patients previously examined with electrodiagnostic testing, 65% (17/26) had electrodiagnostic confirmation of TTS. All the patients in the study with clinical evidence of TTS were PSSD positive (with two-point static) for TTS. This raises the question of whether or not PSSD is more sensitive than conventional electrodiagnostic testing. In another study of PSSD performed 1 year earlier, Tassler and Dellon[54] found that, when compared with the "gold standard" of electrodiagnostic testing, PSSD was 100% sensitive and 0% specific for TTS. They attributed the very low specificity to PSSD demonstrating abnormalities in patients when electrodiagnostic testing was found to be normal despite positive clinical findings.

In summary, electrodiagnostic testing is of value for detecting abnormalities in the tibial and plantar nerves. The standard tests (motor and sensory nerve conduction) are less able to detect abnormalities in the calcaneal branch. However, for the tibial and plantar nerves, there is high specificity and low sensitivity. This is especially true when ruling out peripheral neuropathies or spinal lesions. When using motor evoked potentials, values higher than 6.2 ms and 7 ms for the medial and plantar nerves, respectively, are considered abnormal. Some of these deficiencies may be corrected with PSSD; however, further testing is warranted. Mann and Coughlin[12] proposed that a definitive diagnosis of TTS be made only when history, physical examination, and electrodiagnostic tests corroborate. If all three are not in agreement, a search for another diagnosis should be strongly considered.

TREATMENT

Few controlled studies analyze the merits of conservative treatment. Mann[55] wrote in 1974 that conservative treatment is of temporary benefit and "the treatment is surgical release of the flexor retinaculum and neurolysis of the medial and plantar nerve." Conservative treatment includes orthotics, anti-inflammatory medication, tricyclic medication for chronic pain, and steroid injections. The success of conservative treatment is directly related to the underlying cause of the TTS. A patient with synovitis may respond to a steroid injection. However, no controlled studies exist to support this observation. Schon[33] recommended that athletes with hyperpronation of the foot try strengthening the tibialis posterior muscle in addition to placing a medial heel and sole wedge in their shoes.

SURGICAL RELEASE

Lam[5] was the first to describe the surgical release of the tarsal tunnel in detail. This is accomplished through a curved medial incision. The nerve is traced from proximal to distal, extending beyond the flexor retinaculum and entering deep to the abductor hallucis. All branches should be explored and freed. The surgical release must be complete, including the entire flexor retinaculum, according to Srinivasan and associates[8] which extends proximally 10 cm above the calcaneus. Preoperative identification of the region of maximum tenderness is one of the most effective means of localizing the abnormal lesion.

At surgery, the nerve is examined for a fusiform swelling consistent with compression. If this is not present, the tourniquet can be momentarily deflated to look for a delayed vascular blush over the tibial nerve. The absence of both of these conditions may indicate a poor prognosis secondary to an improper diagnosis (CS Ranawat, personal observation, 1997).

As in carpal tunnel release, endoscopic decompressions have been performed. Day and Naples[56] reported their experience with 16 TTS patients with a 4- to 28-month follow-up. The operations were performed using a 4-mm, 30° endoscope and a retrograde knife through a slotted cannula. After release of the flexor retinaculum, the authors could visualize "both branches of the tibial nerve." No mention was made of the calcaneal branch. Dexamethasone was then injected into the tunnel before closure. Fourteen of the 16 patients who had this procedure were available for follow-up. Ninety percent were found to have an excellent result. The authors cautioned against incomplete release as well as failure to recognize when the fascia is continuous with the deep fascia of the foot. More troubling is when scarring and adhesions within the tunnel lead to injury of neurovascular structures, a complication that occurred in 10% of their patients. We have no experience with this technique at our institution, and we await further reports to judge more accurately its place in the treatment armamentarium.

POSTOPERATIVE CARE

Recommendations in the literature concerning postoperative regimen vary. We believe that the most reasonable approach is to wait 2 weeks for the wound to heal before weight bearing. However, range-of-motion exercise can be started as soon as the patient is comfortable. After removing the sutures, weight bearing is advanced as tolerated.

RESULTS OF DECOMPRESSION

Lam,[7] in 1967, presented one of the first reported series of tarsal tunnel releases. He reviewed 13 TTS patients who were treated with surgical release. Eighty-five percent (11/13) experienced complete relief of symptoms; the remaining 2 patients had partial relief. Unfortunately, the study lacked long-term follow-up.

In 1985, Takakura and coworkers[50] evaluated 50 feet in TTS patients who underwent surgical release. The patients with coalitions and ganglia had the best results, and those who were posttraumatic or idiopathic had the worst results. A delay in treatment of greater than 10 months was associated with poor recovery. Stern and Joyce[57] reviewed their experience with 13 patients (15 feet) after surgical release. They reported eight excellent, three good, three moderate, and one poor result (1 patient was lost to follow-up). All 8 of the patients with posttraumatic causes reported

excellent results. The poor result in 1 patient (who was lost to follow-up) was attributable to a peripheral neuropathy.

An objective measure of the success of a tarsal tunnel release can be made by performing postoperative nerve conduction studies. Oh and associates[58] evaluated three patients with 14 months to 3.5 years follow-up. Despite improved sensory symptoms, all three patients had a continued percussion sign. Motor nerve conduction improved in two and was normal in one. Sensory nerve conduction improved in all patients.

Pfeiffer and Cracchiolo[59] reviewed 32 feet after surgical release for TTS with an average 31-month follow-up. There was a 44% (14/32 feet) good to excellent result and a 38% (12/32 feet) poor result. Half of the patients with a poor result reported decreased pain but retained some functional disability. The complications included three wound infections and one delayed wound healing.

In a review of 25 reports, Cimino[11] documented a 91% (111/122 patients) good or improved result after surgery. Seven percent (8/122) of patients had a poor result, and an additional 2% (3/122) of patients suffered a recurrence. The review also included patients who were treated conservatively. Of the patients treated with orthotics, 45% (10/22 patients) had a good result; however, 55% (12/22 patients) either refused treatment or were awaiting treatment. Only seven patients had a corticosteroid injection, and symptoms resolved in three.

There are three possible explanations for a failed release of a TTS: the diagnosis was incorrect, the compression occurred in a region other than the tarsal tunnel, or the surgical release was inadequate.

RESULTS AFTER REVISION TARSAL TUNNEL RELEASE

Zahari and Ly[60] presented their study of two patients with recurrent TTS after surgical release. In both cases "abundant scar tissue" was found at reoperation. With release, full relief from pain was obtained for both patients over a 1- to 2-year follow-up period.

In 1992 Mann and Coughlin[12] cautioned against re-exploration of an ankle for recurrent or failed tarsal tunnel release when an adequate release had been performed previously. They stated that the results of neurolysis of postoperative scar tissue are poor. These observations were supported in 1994 by Skalley and associates,[61] who reviewed the results of 13 cases of recurrent TTS treated with reoperation. The indication for surgery was persistent pain and paresthesias in the affected feet. Electrodiagnostic studies had been performed preoperatively and were found to be abnormal in 75% (9/12) of feet. The patients were divided into three groups on the basis of operative findings. In group A, scar tissue was found about the nerves, and the surgical release was judged to have been adequate. Group B also had abundant scar tissue; however, the prior release was believed to be inadequate. Group C had both inadequate release and minimal scar tissue. There was 7%, 64%, and 81% pain relief in groups A, B, and C, respectively. Improvement in symptoms was reported in 10 of 12 patients. Persistent paresthesias plagued 8 patients, and 7 patients continued to have an antalgic gait. There were two wound infections, one of which resulted in a below-knee amputation.

TARSAL TUNNEL SYNDROME IN CHILDREN

TTS primarily affects adults, although there have been scattered reports in the literature concerning TTS in children.[55, 62–64] One of the largest series was that of Albrektsson et al.,[64] who in 1982 described 10 female patients, ranging in age from 9 to 15 years, with unilateral TTS. The diagnosis was established by clinical examination only. No electrodiagnostic studies were performed. In contrast to adults, the children presented with pain, which was "sharp" in three and would lead to total "disability" in four. At surgery, the findings were as follows: two local nerve swellings, three narrow tarsal canals, three fibrous adhesions, two constricting bands, one "kinking" of the medial plantar nerve over an edematous abductor hallucis, and two normal findings. At follow-up (13 months to 10 years), nine of the patients were asymptomatic. Two patients experienced recurrences, one of whom improved with reoperation.

ANTERIOR TARSAL TUNNEL SYNDROME

Anterior tarsal tunnel syndrome (ATTS) is a distinct entity. First described by Kopell and Thompson[65] in 1963, this is a compression neuropathy of the deep peroneal nerve as it courses under the inferior extensor retinaculum. Marinacci[66] is credited with naming this condition ATTS.

The boundaries of the anterior tarsal tunnel include superficially the inferior extensor retinaculum and deeply the fascia overlying the navicular and talus. Zongzhao et al.[67] described the course of the deep peroneal nerve based on 25 anatomic specimens. The tunnel length was 15.7 mm laterally and 55.3 mm medially. The width of the tunnel was 46 mm and 64 mm for the superior and inferior margins, respectively. The confluence of the Y-ligament (the lateral region where the superior and inferior limbs coalesce) was 20 mm long × 18 mm wide. The peroneus tertius and extensor digitorum longus muscles were enclosed within this compartment. The upper limb of the extensor retinaculum encased the extensor hallucis longus. The dimensions of this limb were 11 mm long × 9 mm wide. The deep peroneal nerve split into medial and lateral branches at a distance of 15.5 mm (± 5.3 SD) from the head of the talus in 92% (23/25) of the specimens. Before division, the deep peroneal nerve was 2 to 3.5 mm wide × 1 mm thick. The medial branch was larger than the lateral branch, measuring 2.0 mm × 0.7 mm.

Cangialosi and Schnall[68] stated that the predisposing cause of ATTS was tethering of the peroneal nerve at the "fibular neck and distally by its subcutaneous attachment." In the setting of edema or scar tissue, traction from plantar flexion or inversion may lead to ATTS. They further proposed that a foot with a "rigid-type forefoot valgus" commonly had supination at the hindfoot. The resultant excessive motion was likened to a lateral ankle instability, with even greater nerve irritation. They supported these statements with a study of eight ATTS patients with hindfoot valgus. Six of the eight patients responded to orthotic and steroid injection without surgery.

There is a slight female preponderance (1.7:1) in ATTS. The patient ages reported have ranged from 18 to 66 years. Within the foot, the deep peroneal nerve supplies sensation to the first web space and innervates the muscle of the extensor digitorum brevis. Although the nerve also innervates the muscles of the anterior compartment of the leg, these muscles are superior to the extensor retinaculum and are not affected.

ATTS is characterized by ankle and dorsal foot pain. The pain is burning in nature, and paresthesias along the course of the deep peroneal nerve may be present. The pain may awaken the patient at night and typically radiates to the first and second toes. High-heeled shoes or tightly laced boots may precipitate the condition.

The cause of the compression may be injury (fracture or soft tissue), ankle instability, navicular or talonavicular osteophytes, ganglia, pes cavus, or tight-fitting footwear. Walking may relieve the pain temporarily, but it returns at rest. Because of normal anatomic variation, the nerve may supply regions normally in the distribution of the sural or superficial peroneal nerve. Motor abnormalities are subtle, because the extensor hallucis longus and extensor digitorum longus are able to compensate for the weakened brevis muscle. One can test for a weakened extensor digitorum brevis by palpating the muscle while having the patient dorsiflex the toes against resistance. A percussion sign can be elicited by tapping the nerve just lateral to the extensor hallucis longus. Two-point discrimination may be reduced. Extreme plantar flexion of the ankle may also elicit symptoms.

As in TTS, electrodiagnostic studies are valuable in making a diagnosis. An increase of distal latency to more than 5 ms in the deep peroneal nerve is considered a positive finding. In Zongzhao and associates'[67] series, the range of motor latency was 5.4 to 8.3 ms (mean, 6.3 ms). In addition, a denervation of the extensor digitorum brevis is consistent with a compression neuropathy. However, 16 to 87%[69, 70] of "normal" individuals have abnormal electromyographic (EMG) findings of their extensor digitorum brevis. Andersen et al.[71] reported their experience with two ATTS patients. Normal EMG findings were found, despite strong clinical evidence of ATTS. In one patient, surgical exploration revealed the presence of an accessory peroneal nerve. Because the accessory peroneal nerve innervates the extensor digitorum brevis, they speculated that it was possible to have a false-negative result by EMG for ATTS. They further cautioned against failing to warm the dorsum of the foot, because a reduced skin temperature may lead to a misleading electrodiagnostic test result.

Similar to TTS, treatment results are best when directed at an identifiable cause of nerve compression. When constrictive shoes are the culprit, modification of footwear has been helpful. The literature lacks significantly large series to make recommendations about treatment. However, one can make suggestions on the basis of the few reports in the literature. Gessini and associates[72] reported four patients—two men and two women ranging in age from 35 to 66 years—who had pain and paresthesias in the distribution of the deep peroneal nerve. Three of the patients were treated with steroid injections and one with shoe modification. One of the patient's symptoms resolved completely; however, the other three had decreased pain, and residual sensory disturbances were present in two. No subsequent follow-up was reported.

Surgical release is performed with a longitudinal incision along the lateral border of the extensor hallucis longus. The superficial peroneal nerve is identified and mobilized medially. The extensor retinaculum is incised. The deep peroneal nerve and the dorsalis pedis are exposed and isolated. Any masses or other identifiable lesions are then addressed at this juncture. It is prudent to close subcutaneous tissue and skin without first repairing the extensor retinaculum.

Zongzhoa and associates[67] reported on 10 cases of ATTS. Unlike Gessini et al.,[72] 8 of the 10 patients went on to surgery. One of the conservatively treated patients had no improvement, and a second had only "slight relief of aching paresthesias." Six of the eight patients who had surgical release experienced total recovery. The remaining two patients had minor residual weakness. Sensory recovery was complete or reduced in all eight patients. No bowstringing of the tendons was noted in any of the patients treated operatively.

REFERENCES

1. Pollack LJ, Davis L. Peripheral nerve injuries. Am J Surg 18:361–401, 1932.
2. Clark K. Peripheral nerve injuries associated with fractures. Postgrad Med 27:476–479, 1960.
3. Kopell HP, Thompson WAL. Peripheral entrapment neuropathies of the lower extremity. N Engl J Med 262:56–60, 1960.
4. Keck C. The tarsal tunnel syndrome. J Bone Joint Surg Am 44:180–182, 1962.
5. Lam SJS. A tarsal-tunnel syndrome. Lancet 2:1354, 1962.

6. Goodgold J, Kopell HP, Spielholz NI. The tarsal-tunnel syndrome: objective diagnostic criteria. N Engl J Med 273:742–745, 1965.
7. Lam SJS. Tarsal tunnel syndrome. J Bone Joint Surg Br 49:87, 1967.
8. Srinivasan R, Rhodes J, Seidel MR. The tarsal tunnel. Mt Sinai J Med 47:17–23, 1980.
9. Dellon AL, Mackinnon SE. Tibial nerve branching in the tarsal tunnel. Arch Neurol 41:645–646, 1984.
10. Havel PE, Ebraheim NA, Clark SE, et al. Tibial nerve branching in the tarsal tunnel. Foot Ankle 9:117–119, 1988.
11. Cimino WR. Tarsal tunnel syndrome: review of the literature. Foot Ankle 11:47–52, 1990.
12. Mann RA, Coughlin MJ. Surgery of the Foot and Ankle, ed. 6. St. Louis, MO: C. V. Mosby, 1992.
13. Oloff LM, Jacobs AM, Jaffe S. Tarsal tunnel syndrome: a manifestation of systemic disease. J Foot Surg 22:302–307, 1983.
14. Chater EH, Wilson AL. Tarsal tunnel syndrome. J Irish Med Assoc 61:326–328, 1968.
15. Lam SJ. Tarsal tunnel syndrome. Ann R Coll Surg Engl 50:325–327, 1972.
16. Lloyd K, Agarwal A. Tarsal-tunnel syndrome, presenting feature of rheumatoid arthritis. BMJ 3:32, 1970.
17. Marmor L. Surgery in Rheumatoid Arthritis. Philadelphia: Lea & Febiger, 1967:213–214.
18. Grabois M, Puentes J, Lidsky M. Tarsal tunnel syndrome in rheumatoid arthritis. Arch Phys Med Rehabil 62:401–403, 1981.
19. Baylan SP, Paik SW, Barnert AL, et al. Prevalence of the tarsal tunnel syndrome in rheumatoid arthritis. Rheum Rehabil 20:148–150, 1981.
20. McGuigan ML, Burke D, Fleming A. Tarsal tunnel syndrome and peripheral neuropathy in rheumatoid disease. Ann Rheum Dis 42:128–131, 1983.
21. Mondelli M, Romano C, Porta PD, Rossi A. Electrophysiologic evidence of "nerve entrapment syndromes" and subclinical peripheral neuropathy in progressive systemic sclerosis (scleroderma). J Neurol 242:185–194, 1995.
22. Potts F, Shamani BT, Young RR. A study of the coincidence of carpal tunnel syndrome and generalized peripheral neuropathy. Muscle Nerve 3:440A, 1990.
23. Kucukdeveci AA, Kutlay S, Seckin B, Arasil T. Tarsal tunnel syndrome in ankylosing spondylitis. Br J Rheum 34:488–489, 1995.
24. Dellon AL. Optimism in diabetic neuropathy. Ann Plast Surg 20:103–105, 1988.
25. Dellon AL, Dellon ES, Seiler WA. Effect of tarsal tunnel decompression in the streptozotocin-induced diabetic rat. Microsurgery 15:265–268, 1994.
26. Wieman TJ, Patel VG. Treatment of hyperesthetic neuropathic pain in diabetes: decompression of the tarsal tunnel 221:660–665, 1995.
27. Schwartz MS, Mackworth-Young CG, McKeran R. The tarsal tunnel syndrome in hypothyroidism. J Neurol Neurosurg Psychiatry 46:440–442, 1983.
28. Torres CF, Moxley RT. Hypothyroid neuropathy and myopathy: clinical and electrodiagnostic longitudinal findings. J Neurol 4:271–274, 1990.
29. Ruderman MI, Palmer RH, Olarte MR, et al. Tarsal tunnel syndrome caused by hyperlipidemia: reversal after plasmapheresis. Arch Neurol 40:124–125, 1983.
30. El Shahaly HA, El-Sherif AK. Is the benign joint hypermobility syndrome benign? J Rheumatol 10:302–307, 1991.
31. Radin EL. Tarsal tunnel syndrome. Clin Orthop 181:167–170, 1983.
32. Jackson DL, Haglund B. Tarsal tunnel syndrome in athletes: case reports and literature review. Am J Sports Med 19:61–65, 1991.
33. Schon LC. Nerve entrapment, neuropathy, and nerve dysfunction in athletes. Orthop Clin North Am 25:47–59, 1994.
34. Lorei MP, Hershman EB. Peripheral nerve injuries in athletes. Treatment and prevention. Sports Med 16:130–147, 1993.
35. Antonini G, Gragnani F, Vicihi R. Tarsal tunnel syndrome in skiers. Case report. Ital J Neurol Sci 14:391–392, 1993.
36. Yamamoto S, Tominaga Y, Yura S, Tada H. Tarsal tunnel syndrome with double causes (ganglion, tarsal coalition) evoked by ski boots. J Sports Med Phys Fitness 35:143–145, 1995.
37. Sammarco J, Miller EH. Forefoot conditions in dancers: part II. Foot Ankle 4:93–98, 1982.
38. Kumar K, Deshpande S, Jain M, Nayak MG. Evaluation of various fibro-osseous tunnel pressures (carpal, cubital and tarsal) in normal human subjects. Ind J Physiol Pharmacol 32:139–145, 1987.
39. Whiteside TE, Haney TC, Harda H, et al. A simple method of tissue pressure determination. Arch Surg 110:1311–1314, 1975.
40. Romansky NM, Fried LC, Frugh A. Relief of low back pain from treatment of tarsal tunnel syndrome. J Foot Surg 25:327–329, 1986.
41. Distefano V, Sack JT, Whittaker R, Nixon JE. Tarsal tunnel syndrome: review of the literature and two case reports. Clin Orthop 88:76–79, 1972.
42. Kneeland JB, Macrander SJ, Middleton WD, et al. MR imaging of the normal ankle: correlation with anatomic sections. AJR Am J Roentgenol 151:117–123, 1988.
43. Erickson SJ, Quinn SF, Kneeland JB, et al. MR imaging of the tarsal tunnel and related spaces: normal and abnormal findings with anatomic correlation. AJR Am J Roentgenol 155:323–328, 1990.
44. Ho VW, Peterfy C, Helms CA. Tarsal tunnel syndrome caused by strain of an anomalous muscle: an MRI-specific diagnosis. J Comput Assist Tomogr 17:822–823, 1993.
45. Kerr R, Frey C. MR imaging in tarsal tunnel syndrome. J Comput Assist Tomogr 15:280–286, 1991.
46. Zeiss J, Fenton P, Ebraheim N, Coombs RJ. Magnetic resonance imaging for ineffectual tarsal tunnel surgical treatment. Clin Orthop 264:264–266, 1990.
47. Kaplan PE, Kernahan WT. Tarsal tunnel syndrome: an electrodiagnostic and surgical correlation. J Bone Joint Surg Am 61:96–99, 1981.
48. Fu R, DeLisa JA, Kraft GH. Motor nerve latencies through the tarsal tunnel in normal adult subjects: standard determinants corrected for temperature and distance. Arch Phys Med Rehabil 61:243–248, 1980.
49. Oh SJ, Sarala PK, Kuba T, Elmore RS. Tarsal tunnel syndrome: electrophysiologic study. Ann Neurol 5:327–330, 1979.
50. Takakura Y, Kitada C, Sugimoto K, et al. Tarsal tunnel syndrome. J Bone Joint Surg Br 73:125–128, 1985.
51. Oh SJ, Kim HS, Ahmad BK. The near-nerve sensory nerve conduction in tarsal tunnel syndrome. J Neurol Neurosurg Psychiatry 48:999–1003, 1985.

52. Dumitru D, Kalantri A, Dierschke B. Somatosensory evoked potentials of the medial and lateral plantar and calcaneal nerve. Muscle Nerve 14:665–671, 1991.

53. Tassler PL, Dellon AL. Pressure perception in the normal lower extremity and in the tarsal tunnel syndrome. Muscle Nerve 19:285–289, 1996.

54. Tassler PL, Dellon AL. Correlation of measurements of pressure perception using the pressure-specified sensory device with electrodiagnostic testing. J Occup Environ Med 37:862–866, 1995.

55. Mann RA. Tarsal tunnel syndrome. Orthop Clin North Am 5:109–115, 1974.

56. Day FN, Naples JJ. Tarsal tunnel syndrome: an endoscopic approach with 4- to 28-month follow-up. J Foot Ankle Surg 33:244–248, 1994.

57. Stern DS, Joyce MT. Tarsal tunnel syndrome: a review of 15 surgical procedures. J Foot Surg 28:290–294, 1989.

58. Oh SJ, Arnold TW, Park KH, Kim DE. Electrophysiological improvement following decompression surgery in tarsal tunnel syndrome. Muscle Nerve 14:407–410, 1991.

59. Pfeiffer WH, Cracchiolo A III. Clinical results after tarsal tunnel decompression. J Bone Joint Surg Am 76:1222–1230, 1994.

60. Zahari DT, Ly P. Recurrent tarsal tunnel syndrome. J Foot Surg 31:385–387, 1992.

61. Skalley TC, Schon LC, Hinton RY, Myerson MS. Clinical results following revision tibial nerve release. Foot Ankle Int 15:360–367, 1994.

62. Mumenthaler M, Probost CH, Mumenthaler A, et al. Das Tarsaltunnelsyndrom. Schweiz Med Wochenschr 94:373–382, 1964.

63. Edwards WG, Lincoln CR, Basset FH III, Goldner JL. The tarsal tunnel syndrome. JAMA 207:716–720, 1969.

64. Albrektsson B, Rydholm A, Rydholm U. The tarsal tunnel syndrome in children. J Bone Joint Surg Br 64:215–217, 1982.

65. Kopell HP, Thompson WAL. Peripheral Entrapment Neuropathies. Baltimore, MD: Williams & Wilkins, 1963.

66. Marinacci AA. Neurological syndromes of the tarsal tunnels. Bull Los Angeles Neurol Soc 33:90–100, 1968.

67. Zongzhao L, Jiansheng Z, Li Z: Anterior tarsal tunnel syndrome. J Bone Joint Surg Br 73:470–473, 1991.

68. Cangialosi CP, Schnall SJ. The biomechanical aspects of anterior tarsal tunnel syndrome. J Am Podiatr Med Assoc 70:291–292, 1980.

69. Gatens PF, Saeed MA. Electromyographic findings in the intrinsic muscles of normal feet. Arch Phys Med Rehabil 63:317–318, 1982.

70. Weichers D, Guyton JD, Johnson EW. Electromyographic findings in the extensor digitorum brevis in a normal population. Arch Phys Med Rehabil 57:84–85, 1976.

71. Andersen BL, Wertsch JJ, Stewart WA. Anterior tarsal tunnel syndrome. Arch Phys Med Rehabil 73:1112–1117, 1992.

72. Gessini L, Jandolo B, Peitrangeli A. The anterior tarsal tunnel syndrome. J Bone Joint Surg Am 66:786–787, 1984.

9 Biomechanics of the Heel Pad and Plantar Aponeurosis

Finn Bojsen-Møller

Critical shock absorption depends on a proper combination of springs and dampers, and this is what the plantar aponeurosis and the heel pad have in common. The necessary shock absorption at each of the innumerable foot touch-downs in walking and running is brought about by two high-hysteresis and one low-hysteresis mechanisms. The former are the deformation of the heel pad at impact and the eccentric activity of the tibialis anterior muscle group in the rest of the heel phase. Their function is to protect the suprastructure, reduce the transmission of vibrations, and reduce any tendency for the heel to bounce off. After full foot contact, the foot is converted into a spring with a low-hysteresis deformation mainly located in the plantar aponeurosis, adding to other energy-conserving measures in the leg.

HEEL PAD

Fat is nature's choice of material for insulation and is, therefore, the main constituent of the soles of the feet, which are especially exposed to cold. Contained in chambers, fat provides the soles with the necessary compliance to allow the feet to adapt to rough and uneven surfaces, thereby securing a proper grip. Furthermore, fat acts as a mechanical buffer between a hard ground and the impacting parts of the skeleton, which are the tuber of the calcaneus and the heads of the five metatarsal bones.

Fat tissue is built up of fat cells 100 to 200 μm in diameter surrounded by a reticulum of supporting fibers. Fat has a melting point below body temperature and is, therefore, a fluid, which means that, among other properties, it is incompressible. The temperature of the sole is often well below 37°C, which in cold surroundings can fall to 20°C and even lower. It is, therefore, noteworthy that the fat of the soles contains a higher proportion of unsaturated fatty acids, which depresses the melting point and reduces the viscosity at these temperatures.[1]

The ball of the heel consists of a 17- to 18-mm thick padding (range, 13–21 mm) that covers the tuber of the calcaneus.[2, 3] The padding is built up of superficial micro- and deep macrochambers filled with fat and separated by tough septa of collagenous and some elastin fibers. The deep chambers measure 5 to 8 mm in transection, whereas the superficial chambers, which are arranged in a single layer just beneath the dermis, only measure 1 to 2 mm.[4, 5] The two sets of chambers are separated by a layer of collagenous tissue, shaped like the ball of the heel and called the internal cup (Fig. 9–1B). The macrochambers are especially well developed in the posterior part of the heel, where the impacts from walking and running are received.[6] The same arrangement is found in the ball of the foot, but is more complicated because of the longitudinal passage of a series of structures for the toes.[7, 8]

The chambers are sealed off by the septa, so that there is no outflow of fat when the heel is loaded. The fluid-containing chambers act as small pressure units that support the calcaneus and allow it to sink into the tissue when loaded, thereby spreading the collision forces in time as well as in space.[5, 9] The construction endows the heel with a high Poisson ratio (i.e., the heel has a relatively large lateral expansion when loaded), a fact that can be used in prescribing external support cups for increased shock absorption.[10]

The heel pad has a rich supply of nerves and blood vessels. The density of Pacini's corpuscles is high inside the fat chambers, whereas Meissner's corpuscles and other end organs are seen more superficially.[5, 8] The former are known to sense high-frequency shocks and tissue displacements, whereas the latter probably register low-frequency shocks. Together the two modalities allow the organism to perceive the

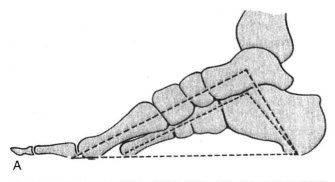

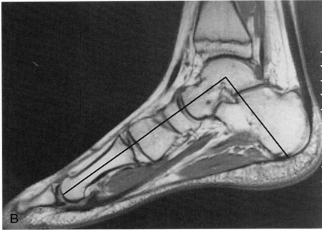

Figure 9-1. The load frame consists of a tibial and a fibular triangle. The compression members of the triangles are straight and can, therefore, be loaded in pure or almost pure compression. The plantar aponeurosis forms the tension member in both triangles. *A,* Drawing showing the two triangles. *B,* Magnetic resonance imaging scan through the tibial triangle. The deep macrochambers and the small superficial chambers separated by the internal cup of the heel pad are visible.

character of the ground and the foot's movements against it, and enable it to react properly in case of sudden skidding. Pacini's corpuscles are large (> 1 mm in diameter), and it was actually here and in the palm of the hand that Pacini discovered them.[11] With their long nerve supply, the end organs of the foot sole are especially endangered in their function, and loss of vibration sensation is an early sign in diabetic neuropathy.[12]

Blood reaches the heel through medial and lateral branches. On the venous side, small and large plexuses are located in the dermis, in the fat chambers, and further forward in the plantar muscle compartments.[13] The blood is drained into the deep veins of the leg and through perforating branches from deep to superficial to continue around the medial and lateral margins of the foot and on to the saphenous veins. The perforating veins are either devoid of valves or have valves that direct the flow outward, which is opposite to what is found in other regions of the leg.[14, 15]

The veins in the heel pad mainly course

transversely.[16] Blood is, therefore, squeezed into the margins of the foot and is not propelled forward when the foot rolls over the heel. The small and larger venous plexuses of the planta are compressed by the body weight at each step, and thus act as the chamber of a hydraulic pump, which returns the blood from the foot. Stroke volume has been estimated at 20 to 30 ml,[13] and the blood pressure in the deep as well as in the superficial veins of the leg is known to rise abruptly with each step or compression of the sole.[17–19]

This pumping explains part of the high hysteresis found during deformations of the heel. Load-deformation studies of human heels have been carried out both in vivo and in vitro, and large differences in the degree of energy loss have been reported.[20] However, only in vivo experiments can show the importance of a full vascular bed with a hydrostatic pressure laid upon it. Cavanagh and associates used a pendulum to hit the heel of a test person standing with the experimental shank horizontal and the knee in contact with the wall of the laboratory.[21]

They found that 85% of an input energy of 3 to 4 J was absorbed by the total heel-foot-leg system. To lift the just-mentioned 20 to 30 mL to heart level takes approximately 0.5 J, an amount that can be raised if there are constrictions at the outlet from the heel and lowered if the deep veins can contain the stroke volume.

Bojsen-Møller and Jørgensen performed drop tests on a vertical shank of three test persons with and without normal hydro-static pressure in the foot.[22] The persons first sat upright with the heel on a force platform and the knee receiving the impact. Subsequently, they laid prone with the knee resting on the platform, the foot immobi-lized, and the heel exposed to the impacts. A mass of 1.6 kg instrumented with a uniaxial piezoelectric accelerometer was dropped with a velocity of 1 m/s. Coefficients of en-ergy return estimated from the flight time of the mass at rebound were 30% for the prone position and only 18% for the persons sitting upright, indicating that an im-portant part of the energy is taken out for antigravity propelling of the venous blood. Further energy is dissipated by the defor-mation of the heel pad and the internal flow of fat inside the chambers. The heel restores itself in the swing phase from the arterial supply and probably by some reflux from the valveless part of the veins.

TIBIALIS ANTERIOR MUSCLE GROUP

In the stand phase, heel contact is followed by the forefoot touch-down. In barefoot walking on hard ground as in the labora-tory, the touch-down phase lasts 80 to 100 ms and 150 ms when the feet are protected by running shoes. The tibialis anterior mus-cle group acts eccentrically as a brake dissi-pating mechanical energy. The result is a high-hysteresis shock absorption added to that of the heel.

PLANTAR APONEUROSIS

The plantar aponeurosis connects like a tie beam the two ends of what conventionally is called the longitudinal arch of the foot. The foot has, however, also been compared to a triangle with two rigid linkages con-nected by the viscoelastic plantar aponeuro-sis acting as a Kelvin element. Kim and Voloshin used this model and added a tor-sional spring and a torsional damper in par-allel between the two linkages.[23] They were thereby able to calculate the spring con-stants and the two damping coefficients.

The triangle model can be elaborated fur-ther by taking the talocalcaneal movements into consideration. Thus, in the skeleton of the foot, there is a cleavage plane that sepa-rates a fibular and a tibial set of bones (Fig. 9–2). Each set forms its own triangle joined by the posterior talocalcaneal facet and with the calcaneus as a common member (see Fig. 9–1). Almost all named ligaments in the foot span this cleavage from posterior-fibular to anterior-tibial, namely the plantar aponeurosis, the long plantar ligament, the calcaneonavicular and calcaneofibular, the interosseous talocalcaneal, part of the bifur-catum, and the transverse metatarsal liga-ments (Fig. 9–3A). The cleavage is also bridged by the short muscles for the great toe (Fig. 9–3B).

The plantar aponeurosis is strong and has the best leverage of the foot ligaments. It extends from the tuber calcanei to the ball of the foot, where it inserts with super-ficial fibers into the skin and with deep fi-bers onto the base of the proximal phalan-ges of the toes. The plantar aponeurosis is

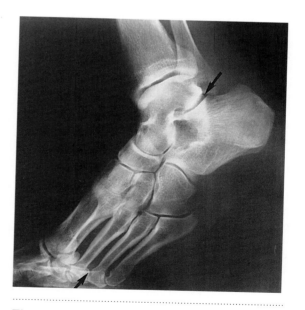

Figure 9–2. X-ray film of supinated foot. A cleavage plane extending proximally from the spatium between the third and fourth toes separates the foot into a tibial and a fibular part.

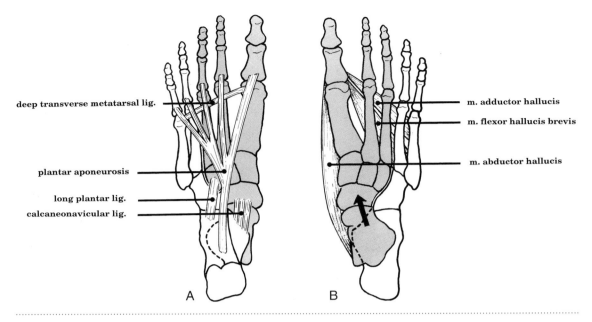

deep transverse metatarsal lig.

plantar aponeurosis

long plantar lig.

calcaneonavicular lig.

m. adductor hallucis

m. flexor hallucis brevis

m. abductor hallucis

A   B

Figure 9–3. Plantar aspect of the right foot with plantar ligaments *(A)* and dorsal aspect of the right foot with the short muscles for the hallux *(B)*. The cleavage plane is shown and the tibial set of bones is dotted. The ligaments as well as the muscles cross the cleavage and are located so that they can catch and regulate the forward movement of the tibial part.

thus hooked to a set of levers that tense the aponeurosis at each dorsiflexion in the so-called windlass mechanism.[24] The deep fibers are also connected to the fascia covering the interossei through a set of sagittal septa arranged to allow the longitudinal passage of muscles, tendons, nerves, and vessels for the toes.[7, 25] In the distal part of the sole, the ligament is divided into five longitudinal strands. Kitaoka and associates divided the distal part into medial, central, and lateral zones and found an overall average stiffness of 209 ± 52 N/mm for all zones.[26]

With the posterior talocalcaneal facet tilting anteriorly, the talus, when loaded, will swing medially and slide forward, pushing the navicular, the three cuneiform, and the three tibial metatarsals ahead, thereby engaging more and more of the fibers of the above named ligaments (Fig. 9–4).[27] By adding the short muscles for the hallux, the stiffness of the foot will be increased in a regular and regulated manner and eventually set a limit to its deformation (Figs. 9–4 and 9–5). With the foot exposed to loads from a few kilograms up to 8 to 10 times body weight, a mechanism such as that just described seems necessary for having a com-

pliant foot at low loadings while avoiding a bottoming out under heavy loads.

It is noteworthy that the triceps surae and the peroneus longus muscles are the only long muscles to have an effect on the load frame stiffness. The Achilles tendon is connected by reinforcements in the crural fascia to the talus and the distal end of the tibia and the fibula. Through tension in the muscle, it can thereby check the anterior sliding of the talus (see Fig. 9–4B, C). The peroneus longus tendon crosses the cleavage plane from the fibular to the tibial side and thus supports the short muscles of the foot.

The flexor hallucis longus reaches under the sustentaculum tali of the calcaneus on its way to the great toe. It does not cross the cleavage plane, but has an effect on the pronation of the foot, which is also a part of the foot yielding.

In bone-ligament specimens, we found a tangent modulus at 3-mm vertical compression of the load frame varying from 480 N for a small female foot to 915 N for a large male foot. The stiffness decreased 30 to 40% when the plantar aponeurosis was cut and an additional 15 to 20% when the deep ligaments were severed.[28] In other specimens, the subtalar joint was blocked by two

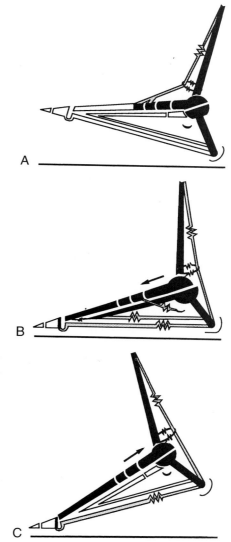

Figure 9–4. Diagram of the foot in its three working phases. The larger tibial and the smaller fibular triangle, the subtalar joint, and the tibia with the tibialis anterior and the soleus muscles are shown. Compression members are black and tension members dotted. *A,* Heel phase. The foot pivots around the tuber of the calcaneus, and the tibialis anterior muscle group acts eccentrically. *B,* The foot in full contact. The tibial and fibular triangles are both loaded, and the tibial triangle has slid forward (*arrow*) relative to the fibular. The displacement is caught by the tensed soleus muscle, the calcaneonavicular ligament, the plantar aponeurosis, and the transverse metatarsal ligament. *C,* During push-off. The tibial triangle is retracted (*arrow*) by tension in the Achilles tendon and by the plantar aponeurosis, which is tensed through the dorsiflexion of the toes in the so-called windlass mechanism. Elastic energy in the other ligaments also contributes. The fibular triangle is unloaded.

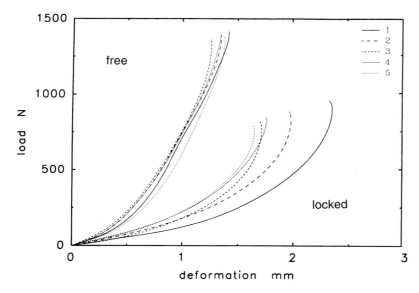

Figure 9–5. Load-deformation curves for five foot specimens with the subtalar joint free to move and with the joint locked by arthrodesis screws. Deformation is vertical through the tibia. Overall stiffness is determined by subtalar slide while the stiffness of the triangles themselves is unmasked by the arthrodesis.

arthrodesis screws to prevent the talar sliding. The stiffness of the load frame itself (i.e., the two foot triangles) was thereby unmasked (see Fig. 9–5).[29]

CONCLUSION

The foot can be pictured as a hydraulic damper combined with a muscular brake and a spring working in sequence. The damper is the circulating and the stationary fluids of the heel, whereas the brake is the eccentric action of the tibialis anterior muscle group. The spring is a double-triangle load frame joined by the posterior talocalcanean facet and with the plantar aponeurosis as a (visco)elastic tie beam. Of the two triangles, the larger tibial one acts as a forward sliding outrigger with strain-dependent, exponentially increasing stiffness. The elements and their concerted action for the foot need to be quantified under different functional conditions, including different shoes and playing surfaces.

REFERENCES

1. Winter WG, Reiss OK. The plantar fat pads. Anatomy and physiology of the heel pad. In Jahss MH, ed. Disorders of the Foot and Ankle, ed 2. Philadelphia: W. B. Saunders, 1991, pp. 2745–2752.
2. Gooding GAW, Stress RM, Graf PM, Grunfeld C. Heel pad thickness: determination by high-resolution ultrasonography. J Ultrasound Med 4:173–174, 1985.
3. Steinbach HL, Russel W. Measurement of the heel pad as an aid to diagnosis of acromegaly. Radiology 82:418–423, 1964.
4. Blechschmidt E. Die Architectur des Fersenpolsters. Morphologisches Jahrbuch 73:20–68, 1934.
5. Jahss MH, Michelson JD, Desai P, et al. Investigations into the fat pads of the sole and the foot: anatomy and histology. Foot Ankle 13:233–242, 1992.
6. Tietze A. Concerning the architectural structure of the connective tissue in the human sole. Foot Ankle 2:252–259, 1982.
7. Bojsen-Møller F. Anatomy of the forefoot, normal and pathologic. Clin Orthop 142:10–18, 1979.
8. Bojsen-Møller F, Jørgensen U. The plantar soft tissue: functional anatomy and clinical application. In Jahss MH, ed. Disorders of the Foot and Ankle, ed 2. Philadelphia: W. B. Saunders, 1991, pp. 532–540.
9. Bojsen-Møller F. Biomechanical effects of shock absorbing heels in walking. In Nigg BM, Kerr BA, eds. Biomechanical Aspects of Sport Shoes and Playing Surfaces. Calgary: University of Calgary, 1983, pp. 73–76.
10. Jørgensen U, Ekstrand J. The significance of heel pad confinement for the shock absorption at heel strike. Int J Sports Med 9:468–473, 1989.
11. Pacini F. Nuovi organi scoperti nel corpo umano. Pistoja: Tipografia Cino, 1840, pp 1–60.
12. Steiness IB. Vibratory perception in diabetes. Acta Med Scand 158:327–335, 1957.
13. Gardner AMN, Fox RH. The venous footpump: influence on tissue perfusion and prevention of venous thrombosis. Ann Rheum Dis 51:1173–1178, 1992.
14. Gottlob R, May R. Venous Valves. New York: Springer-Verlag, 1986, p 19.
15. Pegum JM, Fegan WG. Anatomy of venous return from the foot. Cardiovasc Res 1:241–248, 1967.
16. Spalteholz W. Die Vertheilung der Blutgefässe in der Haut. Arch Anat Entwgesh 1–54, 1893.
17. Arnoldi CC, Greitz T, Linderholm H. Variations in cross sectional area and pressure in the veins of the normal human leg during rhythmic muscular exercise. Acta Chir Scand 132:507–522, 1966.

18. Killewich LA, Sandager GP, Nguyen AH, et al. Venous hemodynamics during impulse foot pumping. J Vasc Surg 22:598–605, 1995.
19. Pegum JM, Fegan WG. Physiology of venous return from the foot. Cardiovasc Res 1:249–254, 1967.
20. Aerts P, Ker RF, Clercq DD, et al. The mechanical properties of the human heel pad: a paradox resolved. J Biomech 28:1299–1308, 1995.
21. Cavanagh PR, Valiant GA, Misevich KW. Biological aspects of modeling shoe/foot interaction during running. In Frederick EC, ed. Sport Shoes and Playing Surfaces. Champaign: Human Kinetics Publishers Inc., 1984, pp. 47–75.
22. Bojsen-Møller F, Jørgensen U. Heel pad critical damping. Abstract presented at the 5th meeting of the European Society of Biomechanics, Berlin, 1986.
23. Kim W, Voloshin AS. Role of plantar fascia in the load bearing capacity of the human foot. J Biomech 28:1025–1033, 1995.
24. Hicks JH. The mechanics of the foot: II. The plantar aponeurosis and the arch. J Anat 88:25–30, 1954.
25. Hedrick MR. The plantar aponeurosis. Foot Ankle Int 17:646–649, 1996.
26. Kitaoka HB, Lou ZP, Growney ES, et al. Material properties of the plantar aponeurosis. Foot Ankle 15:557–560, 1994.
27. Ebraheim NA, Mekheil AO, Yeasting RA. Components of the posterior calcaneal facet: anatomic and radiologic evaluation. Foot Ankle 17:751–757, 1996.
28. Bojsen-Møller F, Misevich KW, Simonsen EB, Voigt M. The human foot: a composite spring with strain dependent exponentially increasing stiffness. Abstract presented at the 12th meeting of the International Society of Biomechanics, Los Angeles, 1989.
29. Bojsen-Møller F, Misevich KW, Voigt M. The foot load frame. Manuscript in preparation.

Plantar Fascia:
Mechanical and Clinical Perspectives

Chris J. Snijders

ARCH OF THE FOOT BIOMECHANICS

The architecture of the foot resembles a Roman arch. We put confidence on mechanics when we walk below the piled-up heavy stones that form an arch on historic ground without cement (Fig. 10–1). The arch mechanism relies on the protection against lateral movement of both ends. In the foot, this function is ascribed to the plantar aponeurosis.

The functional interpretation of the skeleton of the foot as an arch is an old concept.[1] Snijders and colleagues[2] supplemented descriptions of foot arch mechanics with a theory on form and function of joint surfaces. This led to a comparison between the pelvic arch and the arch of the foot (Fig. 10–2).

Similarity exists in the shape of the tarsal joints and the sacroiliac joints, because of the predominantly flat joint surfaces. Therefore, a similar physiologic loading mode is required that is ensured by the bony configuration of an arch by which shear load of flat joints is avoided. In the pelvic arch, protection against lateral movement of the hip bones comes from the sacroiliac and sacrotuberous ligaments, the coccygeus and piriformis muscles, the transverse and oblique abdominal muscles, and other structures. Failure of these structures in lower back, pelvis, and legs is assumed to be related to nonspecific low-back and pelvic pain.

Form and function of joint surfaces can be explained as follows. The loading mode of joints can be transverse, tensile, compres-

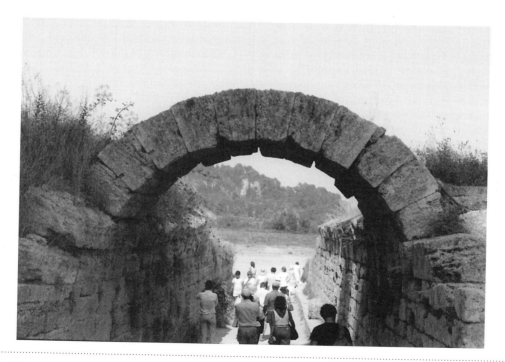

Figure 10–1. Loose stones form a stable arch when both ends cannot move laterally. This arch is the entrance to the field of play where the original Olympic games were held in ancient Olympia, Greece.

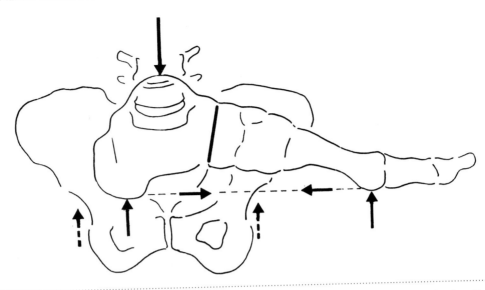

Figure 10–2. Analogy between the load on a tarsal joint and a sacroiliac joint. Both have predominantly flat joint surfaces and belong to an arch. The (horizontal) line of action of forces in the plantar fascia and foot muscles preserves the arch. The pelvic arch is supported by sacrospinal and sacrotuberous ligaments, coccygeus and piriformis muscles, and other structures. (From Snijders CJ, Vleeming A, Stoeckart R. Transfer of lumbosacral load to iliac bones and legs. Part I: biomechanics of self-bracing of the sacroiliac joints and its significance for treatment and exercise. Clin Biomech 8:285, 1993.)

sive, bending, or torsional. Spherical and flat joint surfaces have different capabilities in transferring these respective loading modes. In tension and torsion, the form of the joint surfaces has no influence as long as they are purely spherical or purely flat. In compression, the best conformity of adjacent surfaces gives the best capability of load transfer. The type of joint surface becomes of interest when comparing transverse forces and bending (Fig. 10–3).

Application of a transverse force near the joint in Figure 10–3A leads to a shift of the

upper bone with respect to its adjacent bone until this shear is stopped by ligaments or muscles. The bones do not remain in line, which points to the risk of subluxation. This significant disadvantage does not exist in spherical joints (Fig. 10–3B). In Figure 10–3C, the flat joint is loaded with a pure bending moment. The joint cavity tends to a wedge shape, and the bone contact point shifts to the edge. The bone contact force (F_n) is perpendicular to the joint surface and equal to the ligament force (F_l). In Figure 10–3D, the bone contact force, which must

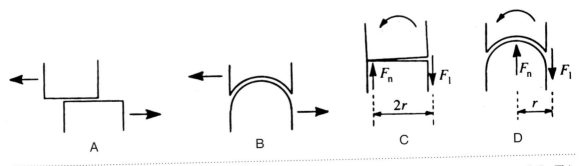

Figure 10–3. *A*, Flat joint surfaces are vulnerable to shear load; the bones do not "stay in line." *B*, This disadvantage does not occur with a ball and socket joint. *C, D*, Because of a greater lever arm, a flat joint is more appropriate than a ball-and-socket joint to transfer a bending moment. (From Snijders CJ, Nordin M, Frankel VH. Biomechanica van Het Spier-Skeletstelsel; Grondslagen en Toe Passingen. Utrecht, The Netherlands: Lemma, 1995. Used with permission.)

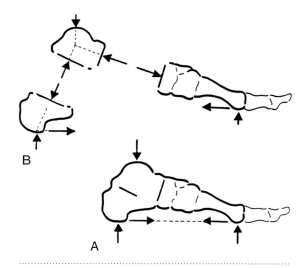

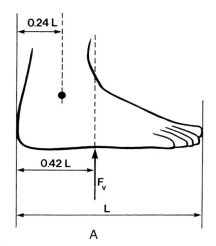

Figure 10–4. *A,* Simplified model of load transfer by the arch of the foot. *B,* Plantar tensile forces provide for compression of the tarsal joints. This principle, resembling a Roman arch, helps to avoid shear in the direction of the flat joint surfaces. (From Snijders CJ, Vleeming A, Stoeckart R. Transfer of lumbosacral load to iliac bones and legs. Part I: biomechanics of self-bracing of the sacroiliac joints and its significance for treatment and exercise. Clin Biomech 8:285, 1993. Used with permission.)

be parallel to the force from ligaments or muscles (F_l), cannot shift to the edge and remains on top of the sphere. Thus, the lever arm of the couple formed by F_n and F_l

in the joint with the flat surface (Fig. 10–3*C*) is about twice as large as that in the ball-and-socket joint (Fig. 10–3*D*). We can conclude that a joint with predominantly flat surfaces is well suited to transfer great moments of force but is vulnerable to shear load. Therefore, flat joint surfaces go with restricted joint excursions.[3] The foregoing principles may well be applied to the predominantly flat joint surfaces of the hindfoot.

Figure 10–4 shows that shear load of flat joint surfaces is avoided in the architecture of the arch of the foot. This also holds when the weight force of the body is located a few centimeters before the ankle axis in unconstrained standing (Fig. 10–5) and when the heel is lifted from the floor at push-off (Fig. 10–6). This raises the forces in the arch considerably. The often repeated drawing of D'Árcy Thompson (1917) (Fig. 10–7), which originated with Meijer (1867), shows how bones in the foot are selectively and anisotropically deposited to resist the patterns of forces to which they are subjected. The orientation of the hydroxyapatite crystals is highly correlated with the directions in which trabeculae point and also correlates with predominant forces acting on cortical bone.[4] The stress lines in Figure 10–7 correspond well with the forces derived from the free body diagrams in Figure 10–4*B*. From the foregoing, we conclude that in stance

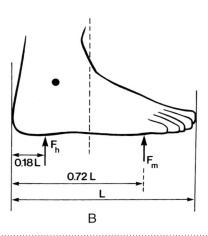

Figure 10–5. *A,* In unconstrained standing, the resultant force under the foot (F_v) is located below the mass center of gravity of the body, which is always located in front of the ankle joint. *B,* Division of total ground reaction force (F_v) on rearfoot (F_h) and forefoot (F_m). Average values for a group of healthy subjects. (From Strüben HWA, Snijders CJ. De Velatie Tussen Hekverhogging en Voor Voet Belasting Bij Het Ongewongen Staan. Eindhoven: Eindhoven University of Technology, 1977.)

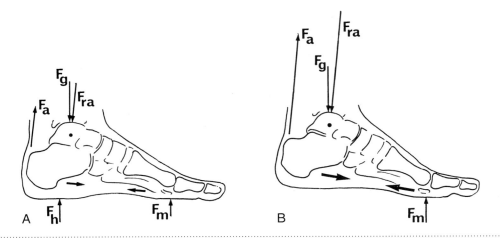

Figure 10–6. *A,* Addition of Achilles tendon force (F_a) to Figure 10–4 requires more tension in the plantar fascia for equilibrium of the calcaneus and other bony structures. This loading mode equals that in Figure 10–5. *B,* The arch mechanism is also valid at heel-off. The ground reaction force is shifted to the forefoot. The required Achilles tendon force is much larger because of the larger lever arm of F_v (here = F_m) with respect to the ankle joint. Because of higher stresses, the plantar fascia will elongate, which can be compensated by dorsiflexion of the toes.

and gait the main loading mode of the joints in the hindfoot remains the same—compressive forces and bending moments are transferred while shearing of flat joint surfaces is avoided in the healthy foot.

Addition of Achilles tendon force is always connected to larger stresses in the whole arch (see Fig. 10–6). In unconstrained standing, body weight is almost equally distributed over hindfoot and forefoot. In Figure 10–5, the resultant ground reaction force (F_v) is located at almost half the foot length (0.42 L from dorsal) with 56% of body weight (F_h) at the posterior part and 44% of body weight (F_m) at the anterior part of the foot sole.[5] Thus, the vertical through the mass center of gravity of the body always falls anterior to the ankle axis, and calf

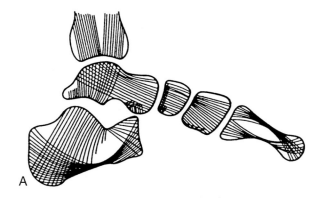

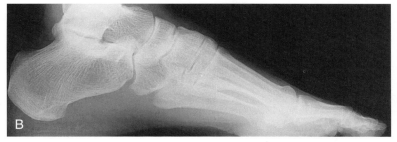

Figure 10–7. *A,* Stress lines in the human foot, originally drawn by D'Árcy Thompson (derived from Bacon and colleagues[4]). The compressive load of the flat joint surfaces in Figure 10–4B meets with the direction of these stress lines. *B,* Stress lines are also visible on x-ray photographs.

muscle activity must be present continuously for equilibrium (see Fig. 10–6A). With no support below the heel (see Fig. 10–6B), Achilles tendon force must be considerably larger.

STRESSES IN ARCH STRUCTURES

Manter[6] measured the pressures that occur in the different intratarsal joints and concluded that an arrangement of internal stresses opposed the action of external forces, in which the whole foot structure was involved in weight bearing, the raised portion of the longitudinal arch being of major import. Hicks[1] showed that the plantar aponeurosis was under tension during weight bearing and, therefore, was necessary for the fixation of the metatarsal heads.

Scott and Winter[7] measured the ground reaction force for subjects running at 5.1 m/s (18.36 km/h) and calculated the magnitude of the loads at common injury sites of the lower extremity during running. The range of peak loads, normalized to subject body weight (BW), estimated from five running trials were as follows: Achilles tendon force, 6.1 to 8.2 BW; ankle bone-on-bone compressive force, 10.3 to 14.1 BW; and plantar fascia force, 1.3 to 2.9 BW. All peak loads were associated with midstance and push-off when muscle activity was maximal. The impact force at heel contact was estimated to have no effect on the peak force seen at the chronic injury sites. The peak force calculated in the plantar fascia estimated load required for tissue failure. This points that greater support of the arch must occur from other tissues, including the ligaments, the intrinsic muscles, and the tendons from the leg muscles, in particular the plantar flexors that are active during push-off.

Thordarson and colleagues[8] studied the dynamic support provided to the human longitudinal arch by the leg muscles in the stance phase of gait and by the plantar aponeurosis. The tendons of the posterior tibialis, flexor digitorum longus, flexor hallucis longus, peroneus longus, peroneus brevis, and Achilles were attached to force transducers. Plantar loads of up to 700 newtons (N) were applied. The tendons were tensioned individually, the Achilles tendon with an amount equal to the plantar load, and the other tendons to a fractional amount proportional to their cross-sectional area relative to the gastrocnemius-soleus complex. The plantar aponeurosis, via dorsiflexion of the toes, contributed to most significant arch support in the sagittal plane with a 3.6° increase between the first metatarsal and talus at 350 N and a 2.3° increase at 700 N (approximate BW). The posterior tibialis tendon consistently provided arch support, and the peroneus longus consistently abducted the forefoot in the transverse plane. From in vivo studies on the arch support by muscles,[9] it is concluded that in the standing-at-ease posture muscle activity is not required and the muscles are inactive, whereas muscles do react at the take-off phase of gait.

The stiffness of the longitudinal arch (i.e., the degree of displacement with load along the long axis of the tibia) was studied in vitro by Huang and colleagues.[10] The degree of arch vertical displacement was greatest after sectioning of the plantar fascia, followed by the long and short plantar ligaments and finally the plantar calcaneonavicular or spring ligament. After all three of these structures were sectioned, the longitudinal arch retained 63% of its stiffness; thus, other static factors also contribute to maintaining arch stability. This study agrees with the statement of Sarrafian[11] that "when under tension, the plantar aponeurosis relieves the tensile forces from the plantar surface of the foot skeleton, which is subjected then to compressive forces only" (see Fig. 10–4B). Plantar fasciotomy would result in increased bending load of the tarsal joints, which is an appropriate loading mode for flat joint surfaces as well (see Fig. 10–3C) but is attended with shear load. Huang and colleagues[10] measured radiologically significant change in arch alignment toward flatfoot deformity in patients who had undergone plantar fasciotomy an average of 8 years previously (talometatarsal −1 angle, arch height).

MATERIAL PROPERTIES

Plantar aponeurosis loading tests by Kitaoka and colleagues[12] showed that the plantar aponeurosis in most of the specimens failed at the proximal level (i.e., near the calcaneal attachment). Specimens from men failed at a significantly higher level

(1540 ± 250 N) than those from women (1000 ± 100 N). Average stiffness of the intact fascia was 204 ± 50 N/mm. There was no significant difference in stiffness at loading rates of 11, 110, and 1100 N/s. Here stiffness is defined as the slope of the load-deformation curve, omitting the initial portion of 0.6 mm of the curve, which shows little deformation with increasing load. Deformation of elastic structures means storage of elastic strain energy. Ker and colleagues[13] showed that the arch of the foot stores enough strain energy to make running more energy efficient. Their data indicated that 17 joules (J) or slightly more is stored as strain energy in the compliant elements of the arch of the foot and 35 J in the Achilles tendon, whereas the total energy turnover in each stance phase of a 70-kg man running at 4.5 m/s is approximately 100 J.

PATHOLOGY OF PLANTAR FASCIA

Plantar fasciitis is an injury to the medial border of the tissue at the origin to the calcaneus. It is considered one of the more serious injuries because of the long recovery period. Repetitive tensile overloads of the plantar fascia can result in this clinical representation, although it is important to realize that plantar fasciitis is multifactorial in cause.[14] Anatomic factors such as pronation, cavus foot, or heel valgus, and environmental effects such as an increase in running intensity or frequency or changes in shoes will increase the likelihood of tensile loading. However, at the muscular level, it appears that plantar fasciitis is caused by gradual overload of the posterior tissues of the calf and foot. Kibler and colleagues[14] found deficiencies in muscle strength and flexibility in a large majority of patients with plantar fasciitis. For treatment, observations on relaxation of the plantar fascia are significant. Bojsen-Møller[15] showed that in vitro inversion of the foot with the hindfoot abducted and flexed in relation to the forefoot slackened the plantar aponeurosis because the distance from the tuber calcanei to the metatarsophalangeal joints became shorter. The opposite occurred in pronation. Campbell and Inman[16] described how this phenomenon can be readily demonstrated on oneself or on the patient by rotating the

leg. External rotation of the leg causes the heel to invert and the forefoot to supinate, whereas the longitudinal arch rises simultaneously. Palpation will reveal that with this maneuver tension is reduced in the plantar fascia. The theory of their UC-BL shoe insert is to hold the foot in a position that relieves tension on the plantar fascia; this is accomplished by holding the heel in inversion and applying forces against the navicular and the outer side of the forefoot, without direct pressure on the soft tissues under the longitudinal arch. When treating plantar fasciitis, the primary objective is to relieve any tenderness along the medial plantar surface, usually just distal to the attachment of the plantar fascia to the calcaneus, to reduce any excessive pressure in that area and to reduce any tendency toward pronation.[17] Abnormal stretching of the plantar fascia can be the result of excessive pronation, which can be related to a tight Achilles tendon, which limits ankle dorsiflexion. Abnormal plantar fascial tension created by biomechanical factors may be subclinical unless other stressors such as running, sudden increase in activity, obesity, inadequate shoes, or prolonged standing or walking occur.[18] Furthermore, a correlation exists between decreased range of motion at the first metatarsophalangeal joint and the onset of plantar fasciitis. Kibler and colleagues[14] studied groups of athletes who underwent physical examination, including checking ankle range of motion and peak torque ankle dorsiflexion and plantar flexion. They found deficiency in muscle strength and flexibility in a large majority of patients with plantar fasciitis. These deficiencies are thought to produce a functional biomechanical defect of excessive pronation, which may cause the clinical overload syndrome if combined with other factors of overload, such as training errors or anatomic hyperpronation. Perry[19] reported that absence of triceps pull on the calcaneus leads to plantar fascial contracture and a proportionally high arch. Conversely, failure to oppose this force, through lack of plantar musculature, allows the arch to sag.

Contracture of plantar structures as well as overactivity of intrinsic foot muscles can contribute to varus, cavus, and adduction deformity of the fore part of the foot in clubfoot.[20] In a study of records and radiographs of children with clubfeet reoperated for residual deformity after operative repair, the investigators[20] found that not releasing the plantar fascia and short plantar muscles correlated with a high level of statistical significance to residual cavus deformity and to residual adduction deformity.

It is a common clinical dictum that the higher the arch (pes cavus), the higher is the predisposition for overuse injuries.[21] Cavanagh and colleagues[22] studied peak plantar pressure in symptom-free feet during walking and made radiographic measurements. In their study, the widely held belief that the cavus foot type is associated with high plantar pressure has been confirmed; a greater inclination of the first metatarsal bone, which occurs in a cavus foot type, is predicted to lead to elevated pressure under the rearfoot and the forefoot. The respective increases per degree are predicted to be 17.5 and 47.3 kilopascals (kPa) under the heel and the first metatarsal head, respectively. Navicular height correlated with the inclination of the first metatarsal bone. This study also confirms that when the second metatarsal head protrudes more distally than the first, a lower pressure results under the first metatarsal head than when the heads are aligned or when the first is more distally placed.

REFERENCES

1. Hicks JH. The mechanics of the foot: II. The plantar aponeurosis and the arch. J Anat 88:25, 1954.
2. Snijders CJ, Vleeming A, Stoeckart R. Transfer of lumbosacral load to iliac bones and legs: part I. Biomechanics of self-bracing of the sacroiliac joints and its significance for treatment and exercise. Clin Biomech 8:285, 1993.
3. Snijders CJ, Nordin M, Frankel VH. Biomechanica Van Het Spier-Skeletstelsel; Grondslagen en Toepassingen. Utrecht, The Netherlands: Lemma, 1995.
4. Bacon GE, Bacon PJ, Griffiths RK. A neutron diffraction study of the bones of the foot. J Anat 139:265, 1984.
5. Strüben HWA, Snijders CJ. De Relatie Tussen Hakverhoging en Voorvoetbelasting Bij Het Ongedwongen Staan. Eindhoven: Eindhoven University of Technology, 1977.
6. Manter JT. Distribution of compression forces in the joints of the human foot. Anat Rec 96:313, 1946.
7. Scott SH, Winter DA. Internal forces at chronic running injury sites. Med Sci Sports Exerc 22:357, 1990.
8. Thordarson DB, Schmotzer H, Chon J, Peters J. Dynamic support of the human longitudinal arch. Clin Orthop Rel Res 316:165, 1995.
9. Basmajian JV, Stecko G. The role of muscles in arch support of the foot. J Bone Joint Surg Am 45:1184, 1963.
10. Huang CK, Kitaoka HB, An KN, Chao EYS. Biomechanical evaluation of longitudinal arch stability. Foot Ankle 14:353, 1993.
11. Sarrafian SK. Functional characteristics of the foot and plantar aponeurosis under tibiotalar loading. Foot Ankle 8:4, 1987.
12. Kitaoka HB, Luo ZP, Growney ES, et al. Material properties of the plantar aponeurosis. Foot Ankle 15:557, 1994.
13. Ker RF, Bennett MB, Bibby SR, et al. The spring in the arch of the human foot. Nature 325:147, 1987.
14. Kibler WB, Goldberg C, Chandler TJ. Functional biomechanical deficits in running athletes with plantar fasciitis. Am J Sports Med 19:66, 1991.
15. Bojsen-Møller F. Calcaneocuboid joint and stability of the longitudinal arch of the foot at high and low gear push-off. J Anat 129:165, 1979.
16. Campbell JW, Inman VT. Treatment of plantar fasciitis and calcaneal spurs with the UC-BL shoe insert. Clin Orthop Rel Res 103:57, 1974.
17. Janisse DJ. Indications and prescriptions for orthoses in sports. Foot Ankle Inj Sports 25:95, 1994.
18. Karr SD. Subcalcaneal heel pain. Foot Ankle Inj Sports 25:161, 1994.
19. Perry J. Anatomy and biomechanics of the hindfoot. Clin Orthop Rel Res 177:9, 1983.
20. Tarraf YN, Carroll NC. Analysis of the components of residual deformity in clubfeet presenting for reoperation. J Pediatr Orthop 12:207, 1992.
21. Simkin A, Leichter I, Giladi M, et al. Combined effect of foot arch structure and an orthotic device on stress fractures. Foot Ankle 10:25, 1989.
22. Cavanagh PR, Morag E, Boulton AJM, et al. The relationship of static foot structure to dynamic foot function. J Biomech 30:243, 1997.

11 Heel Pain Syndrome: Etiology, Diagnosis, and Conservative Treatment

Rock G. Positano
Michael J. Brunetti

David M. Dines
John J. Doolan

Plantar heel pain is a common foot complaint encountered in foot and ankle clinics.[1-5] Approximately 15% of adult foot complaints are attributed to heel pain.[4, 6, 7] Heel pain is referred to by many different names, including heel spur, heel spur syndrome, plantar fasciitis, heel pain syndrome, painful heel syndrome, calcaneodynia, subcalcaneal bursitis, and stone bruise.[1, 2, 4, 5, 8, 9] Although some authors make a distinction between heel pain syndrome and plantar fasciitis, the two terms are used interchangeably throughout this presentation.[10] These two foot pathologies are clinically difficult to differentiate because often each presents with identical symptomatology. Although causes of heel pain are multifactorial and must be included in the differential diagnosis, these two causes are most commonly encountered in the clinical setting.

ANATOMY AND FUNCTION OF THE PLANTAR FASCIA

The plantar fascia is a fibrous band of connective tissue, originating from the plantar medial tubercle of the calcaneus. It is composed of three major bands: medial, central, and lateral. The central segment is the strongest and thickest of the three. The central segment courses distally and, at the level of the metatarsal bases, separates into five slips that attach to the plantar plates of each of the metatarsophalangeal joints.[1, 11] The thinner medial and lateral segments run distally and coalesce with fibers of the central segment to form the origins of the intermuscular septa.

The plantar fascia is an integral component of the foot, because it provides support and rigidity throughout the gait cycle. During heel strike, the plantar fascia permits the midfoot to become flexible, facilitating this structure's ability to conform to the ground and provide adequate shock absorption. At toe-off, when the metatarsophalangeal joints are extended, the plantar fascia becomes taut, causing the height of the arch to increase, the rearfoot to resupinate, and the foot to become a rigid lever, thereby facilitating propulsion. This is known as the "windlass mechanism." This further defines the important role of the plantar fascia in maintaining the integrity of the longitudinal arch of the foot.[8, 9, 12]

In addition, many of the intrinsic muscles of the foot find their origins on the medial tuberosity of the calcaneus, mainly the abductor hallucis, abductor digiti minimi, flexor digitorum brevis, and quadratus plantae muscles.

The posterior tibial and sural nerves innervate the areas of the medial and lateral heel, respectively. The posterior tibial nerve gives rise to the medial calcaneal nerve branches at the site of the medial malleolus, most commonly piercing the flexor retinaculum innervating the medial aspect of the heel.[1, 11] The sural nerve gives rise to the lateral calcaneal nerve and branches at the level of the lateral malleolus, providing innervation to the lateral heel and continuing distally to supply the lateral aspect of the foot. The posterior tibial nerve continues distally, giving rise to the medial and lateral plantar nerves, passing deep to the abductor hallucis muscle, and providing motor and sensory innervation to the plantar aspect of the foot.[11]

CLINICAL PRESENTATION

The symptoms of heel pain syndrome—plantar fasciitis present as gradual onset of pain, often described as a "burning" sensation in the heel. There is concomitant maximum tenderness just anterior to the plantar medial calcaneal tubercle.[1] This also is the origin site of the plantar fascia. Often the patient may not recall any history of trauma. The tenderness is described as most intense in the morning, after the "first steps out of bed." The pain often follows a period of non-weight bearing and rest, such as sleeping and sitting. The pain usually subsides with ambulation, but recurs with prolonged weight-bearing activity and may continue during non–weight-bearing episodes.[4, 8, 12] In mild cases of plantar fasciitis, pain may only be present after exercise or repetitive stress trauma. This is frequently seen in athletes and obese people.[8, 10, 13, 14]

The occurrence of pain during early ambulation after a period of nonweight bearing and rest is pathognomonic for heel pain syndrome.[6] Patients also report a decrease in pain when wearing shoe gear with an elevated heel (i.e. high-heel shoes). Occasionally, one might observe patients with heel pain walking with a limp or referred pain to the calf, knee, or hip.[4] These symptoms usually present unilaterally, although bilateral pain associated with plantar fasciitis has been reported in 4 to 30% of patients.[8]

Bilateral presentation of plantar heel pain–plantar fasciitis as well as concomitant skin and integument changes warrants further investigation by the physician to rule out systemic disorders such systemic lupus erythematosus, diffuse idiopathic skeletal hyperostosis, rheumatoid arthritis, gout, and the seronegative arthropathies (i.e., psoriatic arthritis, inflammatory bowel disease, ankylosing spondylitis, and Reiter's syndrome).[8, 15, 16] In support of this observation, Amor and colleagues reported that 86.5% of a patient population involved in a clinical trial (148 of 171 patients) with spondyloarthropathy had suffered from inferior heel pain.[17]

ETIOLOGY AND PATHOPHYSIOLOGY

Plantar heel pain may present secondary to local and systemic disorders. Local causes of heel pain include anatomic variations, pathologic gait patterns, trauma, obesity, shoe gear, nerve entrapments, bony spurs, tendinitis, plantar fasciitis, calcaneal bursitis, and fat pad atrophy.[1, 2, 4, 7, 8, 12, 13, 18, 19] Systemic causes of plantar heel pain include rheumatoid arthritis, seronegative arthritides, Paget's disease, and collagen vascular disorders.[1, 2, 4, 7, 8, 12, 13, 18, 19]

The tenderness associated with plantar fasciitis–heel pain syndrome may be attributed to maximal strain on the plantar fascia, which results in fascial and perifascial inflammation, microtears, and fibrosis of the plantar fascia at the site of origin.[1, 7, 8, 14] Biopsies of the plantar fascia have revealed collagen degeneration and necrosis, mucinoid degeneration, angioplastic hyperplasia, chondroid metaplasia, and matrix calcification. These findings are most consistent with inadequate and incomplete healing and repair, chronic inflammation, and fatigue failure of the plantar fascia.[8, 10, 14, 19]

Major factors responsible for fatigue failure of the plantar fascia include anatomic, biomechanical, and environmental. Situations that increase the tension of the plantar fascia include structural abnormalities such as excessive subtalar pronation, pes valgus, pes cavus, increased body weight, tight Achilles tendon, and limb-length inequality.[7–9, 12, 20] It is of interest that two totally different structural and pathologic foot types, pes valgus and pes cavus, may cause plantar heel pain and present with identical symptoms. Snook and Chrisman stated that "it is reasonably certain that a condition which has so many different theories of etiology and treatment does not have valid proof of any one cause."[8]

There is much controversy as to whether plantar heel pain can be attributed to the presence of plantar calcaneal heel spurs. An anatomic study conducted by Schepsis and coworkers found that the plantar spur is located at the origin of the short flexor tendon, not at the origin of the plantar fascia as originally thought.[1] This study supports the theory that it is not the spur that is solely responsible for causing pain but rather an inflammatory process or nerve entrapment. According to a study by Rubin and Witten, 125 of 461 patients who were asymptomatic for heel pain had plantar calcaneal heel spurs, and of those with heel spurs 10% subsequently experienced plantar heel pain.[1, 19, 21] Tanz's study included 100 patients with no heel pain and found that 16 had plantar calcaneal spurs. Tanz also found that 50% of his patients with plantar heel pain had a plantar calcaneal spur.[1, 22] Another study revealed that 11% of the adult U.S. population had a calcaneal hyperostosis. The same study also found that 73% of people with heel pain had radiographic evidence of a calcaneal hyperostosis.[6] These data illustrate that heel pain can be a result of a plantar spur or other related causes. Figure 11–1A shows a prominent calcaneal heel spur, yet this patient was asymptomatic for plantar heel pain. Although Figure 11–1B shows no evidence for a calcaneal spur, this patient presented with typical plantar heel pain.

There are numerous neurologic causes associated with plantar heel pain, such as nerve entrapments, neuropathies, tarsal tunnel syndrome, and radiculopathies.[2, 7, 8, 12, 18, 19, 23] A number of nerves have been identified as being responsible for nerve entrapment associated with plantar heel pain. Branches of the medial calcaneal and lateral plantar nerves are most often responsible for plantar heel pain.[10, 23] Rask reported the presence of heel pain secondary to entrapment of the medial plantar nerve.[7] Kenzora reported entrapment of the deep calcaneal nerve, the nerve to the abductor digiti quinti muscle, as contributing to heel pain.[7] Baxter identified the nerve to the abductor digiti quinti muscle as a cause of heel pain.[24] Heel pain is also attributed to entrapment of the tibial nerve at the level of the laciniate ligament, a structure often associated with tarsal tunnel syndrome.[7]

CLINICAL AND DIAGNOSTIC EVALUATION

Physical examination and palpation will elicit tenderness on the medial plantar tubercle of the calcaneus. In addition, atrophy of the plantar heel pad may be noted. The tenderness may radiate to the center of the heel, including the lateral tubercle of the calcaneus, and to the plantar fascia more proximally.[1] Pain may also be elicited with passive stretching of the plantar fascia. This pain is reproduced by taking the foot and dorsiflexing the metatarsal heads with one hand while holding the heel firmly and posteriorly with the other hand, as seen in Figure 11–2, which illustrates the "windlass mechanism."

Gait analysis and range-of-motion measurements of the foot, ankle, and knee can be of great clinical value in establishing the cause and diagnosis of heel pain syndrome–plantar fasciitis. It is important to examine the flexibility, length, and func-

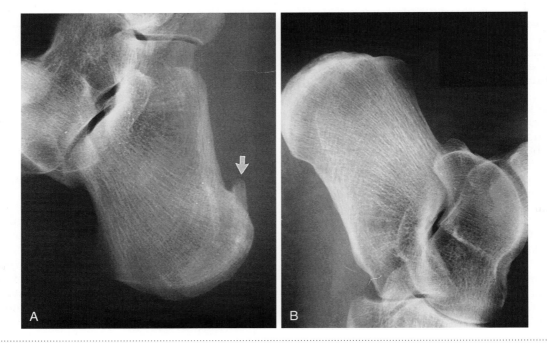

Figure 11–1. *A,* A typical plantar calcaneal heel spur *(arrow).* It was noticed as an incidental finding on routine foot x-ray films (this patient was asymptomatic for heel pain). *B,* This is an x-ray film from a patient who had severe plantar heel pain. Notice the absence of a calcaneal spur compared with Figure 11–1A.

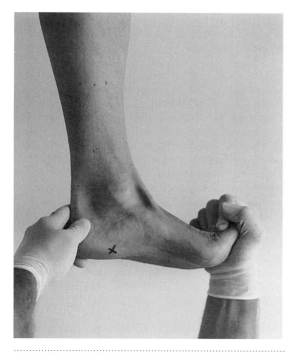

Figure 11–2. "The windlass mechanism" is demonstrated by firmly grasping the heel posteriorly and dorsiflexing the forefoot. This may elicit pain at the insertion of the plantar fascia. "X" marks the location of the medial aspect of the plantar fascia insertion.

tional integrity of the Achilles tendon when evaluating a patient with plantar heel pain, because a tight heel cord and a short Achilles tendon may contribute to pain in this location.[7]

A neurologic examination is also essential when evaluating heel pain because the differential diagnosis includes nerve entrapment and neuropathy.

Several different diagnostic modalities can be used to confirm the diagnosis of heel pain syndrome or plantar fasciitis. These diagnostic tests may also be very useful in ruling out other causes of plantar heel pain such as seropositive and seronegative arthritides, neuropathies, and other systemic disorders. Diagnostic modalities that can be of use when determining the cause of plantar heel pain are discussed next.

ROENTGENOGRAM (PLAIN FILM X-RAY). Lateral, anteroposterior, medial oblique, and calcaneal axial views of the foot are recommended for all patients who present with plantar heel pain. This not only confirms the presence or absence of a spur, but also assists in ruling out less frequent causes of heel pain, such as a calcaneal cyst, foreign body, bony tumor, osteomyelitis, or stress fracture.[7] If a spur is present, it is most often horizontal in orientation and projects from the calcaneal tuberosity. Occasionally, the spurring may be more diffuse along the plantar aspect of the foot and may correspond to the attachment of the plantar fascia or intrinsic musculature of the foot.[1, 6] Calcaneal spurs that project downward or plantarly have been associated with rheumatoid arthritis.

COMPUTED TOMOGRAPHY. Computed tomographic (CT) imaging has been found to offer no significant advantage when evaluating heel pain syndrome and plantar fasciitis.

MAGNETIC RESONANCE IMAGING. The clinical presentation of plantar fasciitis may be mimicked by a number of painful heel conditions. Magnetic resonance imaging (MRI) offers superior imaging of soft tissue and bone, thereby making this procedure the diagnostic modality of choice when evaluating plantar fascia or heel pain. The plantar fascia of an asymptomatic patient by MRI (sagittal T1-weighted, T2-weighted, sagittal short τ inversion recovery [STIR], and coronal dual-echo pulse sequences) appears to have a low signal intensity and a thickness of 3 to 4 mm. The plantar fascia in patients with symptomatic plantar fasciitis was found to have a mean thickness of 7 to 8 mm and an observed increase in signal intensity near the origin of the plantar fascia.[10] Berkowitz and colleagues[14] studied eight symptomatic patients and nine asymptomatic patients. The plantar fascia of the asymptomatic control group was of uniform low signal intensity with uniform thickness (range, 3.00–3.44 mm) and minimal tapering along its course. In the symptomatic patients, the plantar fascia thickness was found to be significantly increased, ranging from 7.40 to 7.56 mm. The plantar fascia of the symptomatic patients was also found to have increased signal intensity along the thickened portion of the plantar fascia.[14] The measurements of plantar fascia thickness found in this study, however, were view dependent (i.e., the same plantar fascia had different thickness measurements depending on the view [e.g., T1, T2, STIR]).

In this same study, the thickness of the

plantar fascia of both feet of an asymptomatic 58-year-old obese woman was measured. The results showed a bilateral thickening of the plantar fascia and some signal abnormalities that were similar to those seen in the symptomatic patient group. This observation was explained by the likelihood of more frequent chronic repetitive trauma secondary to obesity or age, resulting in changes similar to those seen in plantar fasciitis. It may be inferred by this finding that morphologic changes are not specific to plantar fasciitis alone.[14]

DIAGNOSTIC ULTRASONOGRAPHY. Ultrasound has been used to confirm the diagnosis of plantar fasciitis by more objective means. In a study by Wall and associates,[25] the thickness of the plantar fascia of patients with heel pain (clinical plantar fasciitis) was compared with that of the plantar fascia of a patient cohort who were asymptomatic for heel pain. The study concluded that the plantar fascia of patients with heel pain (clinical plantar fasciitis) had a significantly thicker plantar fascia than that of the asymptomatic group.[25] The study also concluded that plantar fascia of a symptomatic foot was thicker than in the contralateral foot in patients with unilateral heel pain (clinical plantar fasciitis). Ultrasonic studies of the Achilles tendon by Fornage demonstrated the appearance of inflammatory changes. These changes were consistent with the ultrasonic appearance of the plantar fascia of patients with clinical plantar fasciitis.[25] Ultrasound studies also indicate no difference in plantar fascia thickness between the male and female populations or left and right feet in asymptomatic people.[25]

The objective standard measurement for the diagnosis of plantar fasciitis by plantar fascia thickness is 4.00 mm or greater.[25] This value can be useful to diagnose plantar fasciitis as well as determine the effectiveness of treatment with serial measurements over the period of rehabilitation time. One potential limitation when performing ultrasound studies is that studies are operator dependent; therefore, one should try to avoid using different ultrasound technicians.

ELECTRODIAGNOSTIC TESTING. When nerve involvement is suspect as to the cause of heel pain, electromyography and nerve conduction velocity testing should be considered. If a positive Tinel's or Valleix's sign is elicited or if heel pain is burning or shooting in nature, then electrodiagnostic testing is indicated. Schon and colleagues demonstrated that 23 of 38 patients with neuritic heel pain had abnormal electrodiagnostic test signals in the medial or lateral plantar nerves, or both.[23] Electrodiagnostic testing is essential when evaluating neuritic heel pain to identify correctly the nerve or nerves that are entrapped, compressed, or damaged. Lumbosacral radiculopathy must always be in the differential diagnosis of heel pain.

BLOOD WORK/LAB RESULTS. In clinical situations in which heel pain is refractory to conservative therapy or bilateral in nature, a rheumatologic lab work-up should be considered.

NUCLEAR MEDICINE. The use of bone scintigraphy when evaluating painful heel syndrome can be of great diagnostic value. Although it is not practical to perform nuclear medicine studies on all cases of painful heel syndromes, specific situations exist in which such studies are necessary. Bone scans provide valuable information when ruling out a stress fracture of the calcaneus, which is not always evident on plain x-ray films.[26] Studies have shown an increased frequency for the diagnosis of calcaneal stress fracture based on radionucleotide uptake.[1, 8, 27, 28] Bone scintigraphy has been useful in diagnosing plantar fasciitis–heel pain syndrome in the absence of plain x-ray film changes.

Another use of bone scans with regard to heel pain has been provided by Dasgupta and Bowles.[29] Technetium-labeled bone scans were used to localize the site of maximum inflammation and provide guidance to the most appropriate site of injection in patients with heel pain. These patients were initially unresponsive to an initial injection. Using this method, the authors reported that injecting into the site of maximum inflammation resulted in a reduction of tenderness in all 12 patients.[29] Anatomically, this study also suggested that the most common location of heel pain encountered in this group was medial and posterior to the point of maximal tenderness.[29]

Plantar fasciitis has been associated with an increased soft tissue uptake of Tc-99m-HMDP during the early blood pool imaging phase of scintigraphic studies, whereas delayed images were normal.[16, 26] In a study by Williams and associates, 52 painful heels were evaluated, 11 (21%) of which showed immediate uptake, whereas 31 (59.6%) showed an increased uptake of Tc-99 isotope on delayed scan. The area of increased uptake varied from the site of insertion of the plantar fascia to areas more diffuse over the calcaneus.[27] Using bone scintigraphy, Graham[28] showed that 97.7% of patients with painful heel syndrome had positive uptake in the symptomatic heel. Although bone will often show an increased uptake or focal uptake in the area of the medial calcaneal tubercle, it is often consistent with soft tissue or periosteal inflammation secondary to the pull of the plantar fascia or to the existence of enthesopathy.[10]

TREATMENT

There are numerous proposed causes associated with plantar heel pain. Because of the nature of this condition, there is a variety of treatments, both nonsurgical and surgical. Most clinicians will agree that conservative therapy is most effective when treating plantar heel pain and is preferred to surgery.[24] Failure of all forms of conservative therapy should be the only indication for surgical intervention. There is no definitive rule of thumb that dictates the duration or type of conservative therapies that should be implemented.[18] The literature reports a wide range of efficacy percentages concerning conservative therapy, ranging from 46 to 100%.[18] This wide range is most likely attributable to the patient population selected for the study. Although the numbers varied from 46 to 100%, these investigators often found successful results in the range of 80 to 95%.[1, 3, 4, 12, 18]

In a study by Davis and others, 89.5% of patients with plantar heel pain had successful outcomes with conservative treatment, with an average follow-up of 29 months, whereas 5.7% had continued pain.[2] The remaining 4.8% elected to have surgical intervention.[2] The patients with successful results had either complete resolution of symptoms or occasional symptoms that were not disabling.[2] According to Wolgin and coworkers,[18] conservative therapy had a success rate of 82%. Baxter[13] found that 95% of the study population with plantar

heel pain recovered with a conservative therapy regimen.

Although it is often difficult to ascertain the cause of plantar heel pain, conservative therapy programs should be designed to address the suspected cause. For example, if the suspected cause is a tight heel cord, therapy should initially be focused at the Achilles tendon insertion. If the suspected etiology is inflammation at the plantar fascial insertion, therapy should be directed at eliminating the inflammation at this site. Treatment of a tight heel cord might include stretching of the Achilles tendon, heel lift, or night splints. Treatment for inflammation at the insertion of the plantar fascia might include steroid injections (not recommended initially), nonsteroidal anti-inflammatory drugs (NSAIDS), physical therapy, or immobilization. Once the cause is identified, one can pursue the many conservative therapy modalities that are available.

Surgical treatment for heel pain syndrome–plantar fasciitis is indicated only after an extensive course of conservative therapy has proven to be unsuccessful.

Conservative Modalities

MODIFICATION OF DAILY ACTIVITIES. Reducing weight-bearing activities (walking, running, standing) is a preliminary strategy used to eliminate the tenderness associated with the mechanical stresses causing heel pain. For patients who are involved in athletic programs, a modification of training is often necessary. For example, long-distance runners should supplement some of their running with biking or swimming.[8] This will maintain their overall cardiovascular fitness, reduce the duration of weight-bearing activity, and decrease the repetitive trauma of running. When training modification does not alleviate heel pain, total non-weight bearing may be necessary. Short leg casts have been used as a method of treatment with great success.[30, 31] This conservative method, however, should be used only as a last resort.

Changes in lifestyle, including weight reduction and stretching exercises, can greatly reduce the factors contributing to plantar heel pain.[8] Weight reduction decreases the load absorbed by the calcaneus and reduces the tension in the plantar fas-

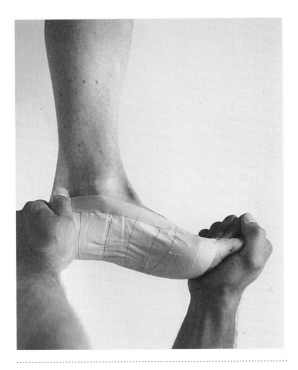

Figure 11–3. Modified Campbell's–low-dye strapping. A medial arch support may be incorporated into this strapping. This strapping may remain on for 1 week.

cia on ambulation.[8] Stretching of the posterior muscle groups of the thigh and leg (biceps femoris, gastrocnemius, and soleus) as well as the plantar fascia can be helpful in reducing contractures and tension that contribute to heel pain.

STRAPPING, SHOE MODIFICATION, AND OR-THOSES. Strapping, shoe modification, and orthoses have proven to be effective modalities in the relief of heel pain caused by plantar fasciitis and heel spurs. The main goal of foot strappings and orthotic devices is to minimize the pathologic forces of the gait cycle and try to restore the desired biomechanical function of the foot as well as support the medial and lateral longitudinal arch.

There are many different methods of strapping a foot to provide relief for plantar fasciitis. Some popular strappings that provide relief are the low-dye strap, Campbell's rest strap, and plantar figure-of-eight strap.[32] In our practice, a combination of these strappings is used. They are effective because they support the medial arch and limit the pronatory forces applied during

gait. When a patient reports a significant reduction of symptoms after being strapped, it is a strong indication that an orthotic device will be useful in treatment and maintaining a therapeutic correction. Figure 11–3 demonstrates a modified Campbell's–low-dye strapping.

Many orthotics are designed to reduce pathologic pronation or the amount of time the foot participates in the pronatory phase of the gait cycle. Increased heel height as well as medial longitudinal arch support are common features incorporated into an orthotic device used to treat heel pain syndrome and plantar fasciitis. A deep heel cup in a slightly varus attitude may also be useful to maintain the rearfoot in the desired position. Figure 11–4 displays many of the different types of orthoses used in the treatment of heel pain.

Orthoses and shoe gear are also designed to increase the shock absorption capability of the foot. Many orthotics have padding as well as weight-dispersion qualities added to the device and assist in reducing pressure resulting from excessive weight bearing.

Shoe gear is also an important component when treating heel pain syndrome–plantar fasciitis. The shoe should possess a firm counter and rigid shank as well as a

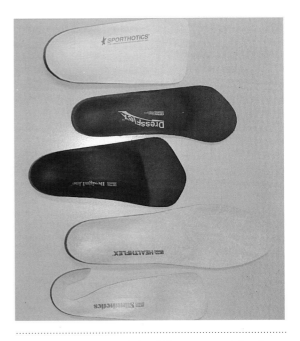

Figure 11–4. Some of the different types of orthoses used in the management of plantar heel pain. Note the variation in size, shape, and depth.

heel cup that will grasp the rearfoot. The sole of the shoe must also have a flexible area under the metatarsal heads. This permits proper propulsion as well as proper orthotic function.[8]

Night splints and ankle-foot orthoses have proven useful in the treatment of refractory plantar heel pain. In a study conducted by Wapner and Sharkey, ankle-foot orthoses that maintained the foot in 5° of dorsiflexion were used at night to treat recalcitrant plantar fasciitis. The patients in the study had experienced subcalcaneal heel pain for more than 1 year and had pain on the first steps of ambulation in the morning. Contracture of the plantar fascia and Achilles tendon occurs at night as a result of the plantar flexed attitude of the foot during sleep. The theory behind the splinting is to stretch the Achilles tendon and plantar fascia during the night, thereby reducing the pain associated with the first steps on waking.[33]

PHYSICAL THERAPY. Many physical therapy modalities can be used to treat heel pain syndrome–plantar fasciitis, as either a primary therapeutic measure or an adjunct to other types of therapy. Physical therapeutic modalities used in the treatment of heel spur–plantar fasciitis include the following: ultrasound, electric muscle stimulation (EMS), transcutaneous electrical nerve stimulation (TENS), iontophoresis, high-voltage pulsed galvanic stimulation (HVPGS), massage therapy, cryotherapy (ice/cold packs), thermotherapy (heating pads), and hydrotherapy (whirlpool, either hot or cold). These modalities may be used solely or in conjunction with each other depending on the nature of the disease.[8, 34]

Ultrasound is effective in the treatment of heel spur syndrome–plantar fasciitis for various reasons. It can be used either as continuous waves or pulsed modes. Continuous ultrasound mechanisms of action are found in Table 11–1.[8, 34]

Table 11–2. Therapeutic Effects of Electrical Stimulation and Galvanic Currents

1. Reduction of muscle atrophy
2. Reduction of pain
3. Muscle re-education at a controlled rate
4. Reduction of inflammation
5. Mild thermal effect
6. Increases local circulation

Pulsed ultrasound has a similar mode of action with the exception of heat delivery. Therefore, pulsed ultrasound can be used when direct heat is contraindicated. For example, pulsed ultrasound is recommended in an acute situation or if the patient has any hardware in the area of treatment (screws, plates, pins). Pulsed ultrasound is also advantageous when pinpointing an area of treatment, because it is not necessary to move the ultrasound head continuously.

Ultrasound can also be used to drive medication through the skin into the inflamed soft tissue by an alternative method called phonophoresis. This is accomplished by applying the desired medication (e.g., topical steroid) mixed with ultrasound gel to the inflamed area and then applying the ultrasound head to the area. The ultrasound "drives" the medication through the skin. In addition, medications can also be delivered through the skin into soft tissue by two other modalities: electrophoresis and iontophoresis.[8, 34]

The electrical devices used to treat heel spur syndrome–plantar fasciitis (EMS TENS, HVPGS) are effective for the various reasons listed in Table 11–2.[8, 34]

Heat and cold are effective adjunctive treatment for heel spur syndrome–plantar fasciitis. Heat via whirlpool, hot packs, and heat compresses, for example, can be used to treat chronic heel pain (Table 11–3).[8, 34]

Cold therapy via ice packs, whirlpool,

Table 11–1. Therapeutic Effects of Ultrasound

1. Heat penetrates to 5 cm subcutaneously
2. Reduction of muscle spasm
3. Reduction of pain
4. Increases local blood circulation
5. Increases peripheral blood flow

Table 11–3. Therapeutic Effects of Heat

1. Vasodilation of local vessels
2. Loosens tight muscles, ligaments, and tendons before activity
3. Expedites soft tissue healing
4. Reduction of muscle spasm
5. Reduction of pain

Table 11–4. Therapeutic Effects of Cold

1. Produces anesthetic effect
2. Reduces acute inflammation
3. Decreases muscle spasm

cold compresses, and so on can be used to treat acute heel pain as well as chronic inflammation related to heel pain. Cold therapies action is summed up in Table 11–4.[8, 34] Hydrotherapy is summarized in Table 11–5.[8, 34]

MEDICAL THERAPEUTICS. Two of the most common conservative medical therapeutics used to treat heel pain syndrome–plantar fasciitis are NSAIDs and injectable steroids.

NSAIDs are useful when treating heel spur syndrome–plantar fasciitis for two main reasons: They are effective in reducing inflammation, and they provide analgesia. This class of drugs inhibits the enzyme cyclooxygenase, which in turn blocks the synthesis of prostaglandins, which mediate pain and inflammation.[35] It is noteworthy to mention that NSAIDs must be administered at therapeutic doses for an anti-inflammation effect when treating heel pain syndrome–plantar fasciitis, because the dosage for analgesia is often lower than the dose for anti-inflammation.[35] NSAIDs should be discontinued after eliminating or controlling the patient's pain and inflammation. If pain and inflammation are not controlled after 2 to 4 weeks of NSAID therapy, alternative modes of therapy should be considered. One should also be wary of the side effects of NSAID therapy, which include gastrointestinal irritation, bleeding, and cross-reactions with other medications.

Some clinicians advocate the use of an injection of a steroid-containing mixture for the treatment of heel pain syndrome–plantar fasciitis.[2, 3, 8, 18] In a 1991 study, 95%

of the patients experienced significant relief of symptoms associated with plantar heel pain within a short period of time after receiving a single injection containing a corticosteroid and local anesthetic.[5] There are many considerations when choosing a steroid injection for treatment of heel spur syndrome. First, one must choose the appropriate steroid to be used and decide whether a local anesthetic will be added to the solution. Corticosteroids vary in solubility, potency, and duration of action. The addition of local anesthetic provides rapid analgesia at the injected region and decreases the pain from the injection. Pain on injection can also be minimized with the use of a high-gauge needle (22–25 gauge) and topical skin anesthetics such as ethyl chloride spray.[36] Speed of injection can influence the level of discomfort during injection. Injections should be administered slowly to avoid rapid volume increases in a small area. In addition, using a large volume of injectables is discouraged.[2] An absolute contraindica-

Table 11–5. Therapeutic Effects
of Hydrotherapy

Warm	Cold
1. Sedative	1. Reduces acute inflammation
2. Relief from painful sensory conditions and spasm	
3. Increases local circulation	2. Increases muscle tone
4. Increases range of motion	

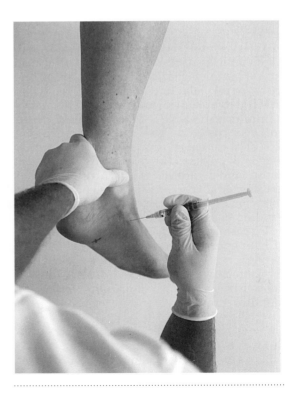

Figure 11–5. Technique for an injection at the insertion of the plantar fascia. The needle should enter medially, not plantarly, and should be aimed transversely. "X" marks the location of the insertion of plantar fascia.

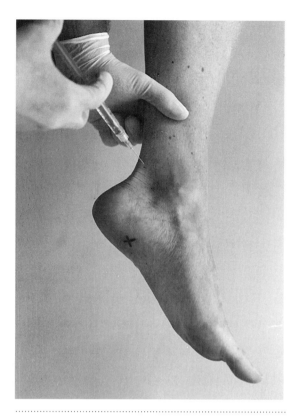

Figure 11–6. A posterior tibial nerve injection. One should palpate the posterior tibial artery at this location. Always aspirate to avoid intravascular injection. This nerve block will "knock out" the sympathetic nerve supply to the foot and cause a hyperemic effect.

tion to steroid injection is local infection as well as acute trauma in the area, surrounding osteoporosis, and any violation of skin integrity around the site of injection.

Some clinicians recommend an injection of ½ mL of betamethasone sodium phosphate, 3 mg/mL, and betamethasone acetate, 3 mg/mL (Celestone Soluspan), and 1 mL of 1% plain lidocaine (Xylocaine). This injection should be directed medially, aiming at the insertion of the plantar fascia into the medial tubercle of the calcaneus using a 25-gauge needle 1½ inches long. Figure 11–5 demonstrates an injection aimed at the medial tubercle of the calcaneus from a transverse medial injection site.

Side effects of local corticosteroid injection are both local and systemic in nature. Local effects include tendon (fascia) rupture, infection, local skin and soft tissue atrophy, and other dermatologic changes. Systemic side effects include anaphylaxis,

vasovagal reaction, hyperglycemia in diabetics, and emotional disturbances.[36] The incidence of plantar fascia rupture is significantly increased with repeated corticosteroid injections.[37–40] This practice discourages the use of corticosteroid injection when treating heel pain for this very legitimate reason.

Table 11–6. Positano Algorithm for Plantar Heel Pain

Initial visit—Detailed History and Physical, X-ray Films
If
Neoplasm: surgery/oncology consult
Stress fracture: immobilization, non-weight bearing
Osteomyelitis: infectious disease consult
Rupture/tear of plantar fascia: immobilization, consider surgery
Nerve entrapment: neurology consult, NCV/EMG
Plantar fasciitis/heel pain syndrome
Seronegative, seropositive arthritis: rheumatology consult
↓
Weeks 1–3
- Diagnostic ultrasound for baseline value (measurement of plantar fascia thickness)
- Start 3-week course of physical therapy, 3 days a week
    1. Ultrasound
    2. Electric stimulation plus galvanic currents
    3. Massage
    4. Whirlpool
    5. Hot/cold compresses
    6. Plantar rest strap
- Recommendation of weight loss if applicable; begin posterior leg and posterior thigh stretching if no improvement
↓
Weeks 4–5
- Iontophoresis with steroid solution added to regimen
- NSAIDs
- Cast patient for orthoses if no improvement
- MRI
↓
Weeks 6–9
- Posterior tibial nerve block (4–6 total injections over 4 weeks) if no improvement
- Repeat diagnostic ultrasound and compare with original measurement
↓
Weeks 10–11
- Cast for night splints if no improvement
↓
Week 12
- Short leg cast or Cam walker (4–6 weeks if no improvement)
↓
6 months–1 year
- Consider surgical intervention

MRI = magnetic resonance imaging; NCV = nerve conduction velocity; EMG = electromyography; NSAIDs = nonsteroidal anti-inflammatory drugs.

An alternative method of injection therapy includes administration of local anesthetic aimed at the neurovascular bundle surrounding the posterior tibial nerve at the level of the medial malleolus. This technique has two modes of action. First, it provides a temporary analgesic effect by blocking the innervation to the heel for pain sensation. Second, it provides a nonspecific vasodilation by blocking the sympathetic innervation of the heel provided by the posterior tibial nerve.[11] Figure 11–6 illustrates the technique used for a posterior tibial nerve block.

CONCLUSION

Heel pain should never be addressed as a simple musculoskeletal complaint. It is obvious from the previous discussion that the cause of heel pain is multifactorial.

To evaluate this very common complaint better, we have devised an algorithm (Table 11–6) that one can follow when evaluating and treating a patient with heel pain.

Conservative therapeutic regimens should always be the first course of action. In addition, the appropriate diagnostic protocols should be fully used by the clinician to design and implement the most effective clinical regimen. Only when heel pain becomes more severe and unresponsive to a conservative therapy regimen should more aggressive and invasive measures be considered.

REFERENCES

1. Schepsis AA, Leach RE, Gorzyca J. Plantar fasciitis. Clin Orthop Rel Res 266:185, 1991.
2. Davis P, Severud E, Baxter D. Painful heel syndrome: results of nonoperative treatment. Foot Ankle Int 15:531, 1994.
3. Miller R, Torres J, McGuire M. Efficacy of first-time steroid injection for painful heel syndrome. Foot Ankle Int 16:610, 1995.
4. Dailey JM. Differential diagnosis and treatment of heel pain. Clin Podiatr Med Surg 8:153, 1991.
5. Barrett SL, Day SV. Endoscopic plantar fasciotomy for chronic plantar fasciitis/heel spur syndrome: surgical technique—early clinical results. J Foot Surg 30:568, 1991.
6. McGlammary ED, Banks AS, Downey MS. Comprehensive Textbook of Foot Surgery, ed 2. Baltimore, MD: Williams & Wilkins, 1992.
7. Black JR, Bernard JM, Williams LA. Heel pain in the older patient. Clin Podiatr Med Surg 10:113, 1993.
8. Demaio M, Paine R, Mangine RE, Drez D. Plantar fasciitis. Sports Med Rehabil 16:1153, 1993.
9. Windsor RE, Dreyer SJ, Lester JP. Overuse injuries of the leg, ankle, and foot. Phys Med Rehabil Clin North Am 5:195, 1994.
10. Deutsch AL, Mink JH, Kerr R. MRI of the Foot And Ankle. New York: Raven Press, 1992.
11. Draves DJ. Anatomy of the Lower Extremity. Baltimore, MD: Williams & Wilkins, 1986.
12. LeMelle DP, Kisilewicz P, Janis LR. Chronic plantar fascial inflammation and fibrosis. Clin Podiatr Med Surg 7:385, 1990.
13. Baxter DE. The heel in sport. Clin Sports Med 13:683, 1994.
14. Berkowitz JF, Kier R, Rudicel S. Plantar fasciitis: MR imaging. Radiology 179:665, 1991.
15. Shumacher HR, Klippel JH, Koopman WJ. Primer on Rheumatic Disease. Atlanta: Arthritis Foundation, 1993.
16. Vasavada PJ, DeVries DF, Nishiyama H. Plantar fasciitis—early blood pool images in diagnosis of inflammatory process. Foot Ankle 5:74, 1984.
17. Amor B, Dougados M, Khan MA. Management of refractory ankylosing spondylitis and related spondyloarthropathies. Rheum Dis Clin North Am 21:117, 1995.
18. Wolgin M, Cook C, Graham C, Mauldin D. Conservative treatment of plantar heel pain: long-term follow-up. Foot Ankle 15:97, 1994.
19. Sammarco GJ, Helfrey RB. Surgical treatment of recalcitrant plantar fasciitis. Foot Ankle Int 17:520, 1996.
20. Warren BL. Plantar fasciitis in runners. Treatment and prevention. Sports Med 10:338, 1990.
21. Rubin G, Witten M. Plantar calcaneal spurs. Am J Orthop 5:38, 1963.
22. Tanz SS. Heel pain. Clin Orthop 28:169, 1969.
23. Schon LC, Glennon TP, Baxter DE. Heel pain syndrome: electrodiagnostic support for nerve entrapment. Foot Ankle 14:129, 1993.
24. Baxter DE, Thigpen CM. Heel pain—operative results. Foot Ankle 5:16, 1984.
25. Wall JR, Harkness MA, Crawford A. Ultrasound diagnosis of plantar fasciitis. Foot Ankle 14:465, 1993.
26. Intenzo CM, Wapner KL, Park CH, Kim SM. Evaluation of plantar fasciitis by three-phase bone scintigraphy. Clin Nucl Med 16:325, 1991.
27. Williams PL, Smibert JG, Cox R, et al. Imaging study of the painful heel syndrome. Foot Ankle 7:345, 1987.
28. Graham CE. Painful heel syndrome: rationale of diagnosis and treatment. Foot Ankle 3:26, 1983.
29. Dasgupta B, Bowles J. Scintigraphic localization of steroid injection site in plantar fasciitis. Lancet 346:1400, 1995.
30. Gill LH, Kiebzak GM. Outcome of nonsurgical treatment for plantar fasciitis. Foot Ankle Int 17:527, 1996.
31. Dreeben SM, Mann RA. Heel pain: sorting through the differential diagnosis. J Musculoskel Med 9:21, 1992.
32. Kaplan C, Natale PD, Spilken TL. Paddings and Strappings of the Foot. Mount Kisco, NY: Futura, 1982.
33. Wapner KL, Sharkey PF. The use of night splints for treatment of recalcitrant plantar fasciitis. Foot Ankle 12:135, 1991.

34. Poole RM. Physical therapy in the treatment of sports injuries. In Birrer RB, ed. Sports Medicine for the Primary Care Physician, ed 2. Boca Raton, FL: CRC Press, 1994:267.

35. Cirlincione A, Doolan J, Larsen J. NSAIDs: a review and administration in special populations. Podiatr Med Rev 1:24, 1995.

36. Fick DS, Kelly MW. Use of injectable corticosteroids for chronic musculoskeletal inflammation. Fam Pract 18:37, 1996.

37. Pai VS. Rupture of the plantar fascia. J Foot Ankle Surg 35:39, 1996.

38. Sellman JR. Plantar fascia rupture associated with corticosteroid injection. Foot Ankle Int 15:376, 1994.

39. Ahstrom JP. Spontaneous rupture of the plantar fascia. Am J Sports Med 16:306, 1988.

40. Leach R, Jones R, Silva T. Rupture of the plantar fascia in athletes. J Bone Joint Surg Am 60A:537, 1978.

12

Surgical Correction of Heel Spur and Plantar Fascia Tears

Thomas M. DeLauro
Rock G. Positano

Surgical therapies for painful heel spur are historically diverse and still evolving. This has undoubtedly resulted from changes in our beliefs regarding pathogenesis. The earliest operative procedures focused on the calcaneal spur as the cause of a patient's discomfort. Present-day surgeries, however, discard this notion in favor of approaches designed to alter the plantar fascial origin from the calcaneus. The latter reflects the current belief that the spur is more of an effect from, rather than a cause of, heel spur pain, with a disorder of the plantar fascia playing the pivotal etiologic role.

This new direction has strong empirical and research support: namely, the all-too-often existence of heel spur pain without radiographic evidence of an inferior calcaneal spur (heel spur syndrome), the discovery of the fascia's nonattachment to the spur, and the resolution of symptoms in patients with a visible spur who elect plantar fascial surgery alone. Operations aimed at removing a radiographically evident spur invariably involve sectioning or otherwise lengthening the plantar fascia, which may explain their success. As patients continue to insist that a visible spur be excised, the critical facet of heel spur surgery (fascial vs. osseous) will remain obscure.

ANATOMY

The anatomy of the plantar fascia origin and the inferior calcaneal spur have been fairly well established.[1] The plantar fascia is believed to consist of three bands: medial, central, and lateral. The central band comprises the most significant portion of the plantar fascia. This central band has its thick, broad origins from the medioplantar calcaneal tubercle, and sends out septa into the transverse and sagittal planes to anchor the subcutaneous fascia and the plantar heel pad.

The medial band originates from the medial aspect of the medioplantar calcaneal tubercle, but it is thin and serves only as the superficial fascial covering of the abductor hallucis muscle belly. It fans distally into a medial and lateral crux; the gap between the medial and central bands is referred to as the medial sulcus.

The lateral band begins from the lateral aspect of the medial plantar calcaneal tubercle, also fans distally into a medial and lateral crux, and forms what is known as the lateral sulcus between its origin and that of the central band. The lateral band is unique, however, in that its development may be anomalous: (1) complete, (2) complete but thinned and atrophic, or (3) incomplete in that its fibers end at the midfoot (Fig. 12–1).

Although the plantar fascia appears to be a passive structure, it is capable of serving a number of functions during the gait cycle. Its elastic and collagen fibers allow a small degree of stretch when stress is first applied but render the fascia stiffer as force continues; therefore, the foot can accommodate to the weight-bearing surface at initial contact and yet fully support the body as full weight bearing is reached. In static stance, this interpretation of function was further confirmed when electromyographic studies revealed little extrinsic or intrinsic muscle activity: the passive structures of the foot entirely supported the skeleton above.[2] Sequential sectioning of the plantar fascia, the long and short plantar ligaments, and the spring ligament demonstrated that the plantar fascia was responsible for the greatest degree of arch stability.[3] Hick's windlass effect leads to arch elevation, heel inversion, and external leg rotation, all from tightening of the plantar fascia when the toes dorsiflex at heel-off (presumably, the fascia's origin from the medial calcaneus also contributes to this action).[2]

The inferior calcaneal spur consists of

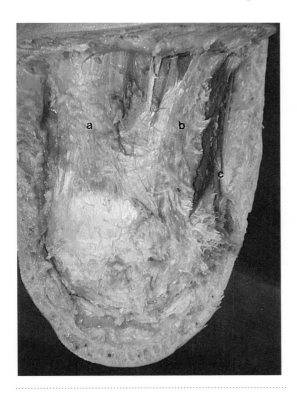

Figure 12–1. Plantar view of cadaveric heel. Note prominent central band (a), lesser lateral band (b), and abductor digiti quinti muscle belly (c).

bone that is arranged in both cortical and trabecular layers. Although lateral radiographs of the heel depict the spur as an osseous projection without width, surgeons and anatomists recognize that the inferior spur is, in fact, a shelf of bone that extends across most of the medial calcaneal tubercle. When viewed from the plantar aspect, the spur extends most distally in its central portion (Fig. 12–2).

Another controversial issue is the anatomic relationship of the inferior calcaneal spur to the plantar fascia. Until recently, the belief that the fascia attached directly into the spur was widely accepted and popularized the traction theory of spur formation. Subsequent dissections found that a significant number of spurs were located superior to the fascial origin, resulting in surgical procedures that advocated fasciotomy without spur resection. The most recent dissections, however, placed the incidence of each finding at approximately 50%.[4] In other words, patients with radiographically demonstrable inferior calcaneal spurs had

an equal chance of the spur either connecting to or existing separate from the fascia.

SURGICAL INCISION PLACEMENT

The cutaneous blood supply to the human heel comes from tributaries of the posterior tibial and lateral plantar arteries medially, the peroneal and lateral malleolar arteries laterally, and communicating branches posteriorly.[5] Knowledge of this network is usually necessary only in radical surgeries of the region; it is rarely compromised in current-day approaches. Complications such as hematoma, infarction, dehiscence, and infection (which are discussed in later sections) in today's procedures are probably more often the result of improper tissue handling than incision placement and technique.

The incisions that have been described in approaching heel spur excision and plantar fasciotomy include, chronologically, a transverse U-shaped plantar flap (Griffith), goblet for access to inferior and superior calca-

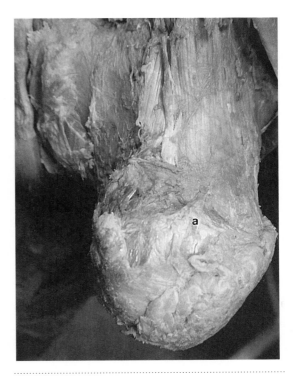

Figure 12–2. Plantar view of cadaveric heel. Note that the inferior calcaneal spur projects most distally in its midportion (a).

neal spurs (Chang and Miltner), linear on the plantar heel (Kenzora),[6, 7] transverse on the plantar heel (Kahn), medial linear (separately by DuVries and Steindler), medial oblique (Duggar), medial and lateral portals (Barrett and Day), single percutaneous plantar stab (White,[8] Licopantis[9]), and multiple plantar stabs (unpublished).

Although the skin flap and island created by the Griffith and Chang/Miltner approaches remain viable, to our knowledge these incisions are rarely used today because of their extensive nature. Each of the plantar approaches provides excellent access to and visualization of the fascia and spur, but requires longer incisions or greater undermining because of the extensive attachment of the plantar heel pad to the calcaneus. Large, broad retractors are needed to keep the plantar fat pad out of the surgeon's way. A second relative disadvantage is the care required of plantar incisions in general (i.e., 3 weeks of non-weight bearing to avoid painful cicatrix formation).

A departure from this need occurs in the case of multiple plantar stab incisions for percutaneous plantar fasciotomy alone. A total of eight incisions are normally used, consisting of two tranverse rows of four incisions each. The two rows are placed directly inferior to the plantar fascial origin from the calcaneus, and are staggered so the distal row interdigitates with the proximal one (Figs. 12–3 and 12–4). As in the case of other percutaneous plantar stab incision techniques, the minute size of the incision obviates the need for suturing, and patients bear weight immediately after the surgery as comfort allows.

The medial approaches, as well as the medial and lateral endoscopic portals, probably represent the most popular incisions used today. Although the literature warns of possible trauma to the lateral plantar nerve branch that supplies the abductor digiti quinti muscle,[6] this branch is superior to the spur and runs transversely across the heel. Again, in our opinion, medial incisions place the plane of dissection (when performing the fascial release) either below or within the nerve's direction, thereby avoiding its accidental injury or severance.

Two variations of the medial incision exist: one that is approximately 4 cm long and running from proximal superior to distal inferior, and the other being only 1 to 2 cm long and coursing from proximal inferior to

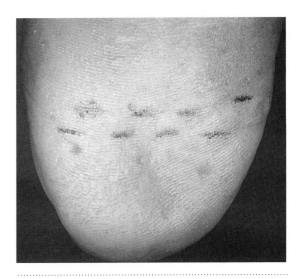

Figure 12–3. Plantar view of heel illustrating placement of plantar stab incisions approximately at the site of plantar fascial origin from the calcaneus.

distal superior. Advocates of the former incision cite that it runs parallel to the first branch of the lateral plantar nerve, thereby decreasing the incidence of nerve transection or injury. Surgeons who use the latter approach believe that (1) the incision is distal to the nerve's course, and (2) by paralleling the inferior calcaneal surface, dissection is minimized. In our opinion, the second incision is preferred.

Arthroscopic procedures using medial and lateral portals transect the fascia under direct supervision and do not excise the spur. The lateral plantar nerve branch should, as a result, not be in the surgical field.

OSSEOUS PROCEDURES

Early efforts to reduce an inferior calcaneal spur were quite dramatic, no doubt a result of the prevailing belief that the spur itself was the primary cause of a patient's pain. After performing a tendo-Achilles lengthening and removing a section of bone from the inferior calcaneal surface, Steindler advocated the use of a rotating calcaneal osteotomy. This procedure would bury the spur within the defect created on the inferior calcaneal surface. Equally remarkable was the countersinking osteotomy of Michele and Krueger, designed to reduce the "high point"

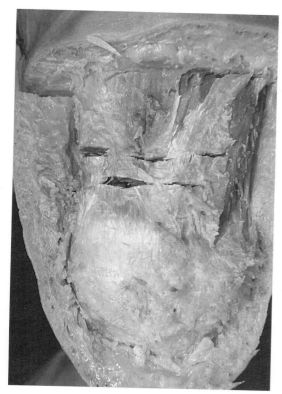

Figure 12–4. Result of multiple plantar stab incisions on cadaveric heel (plantar view). If tendon slides are not created, the multiple incisions allow at least a meshing of the fascia so it can elongate. In either case, overall fascial integrity is maintained. The instrument used, a no. 67 miniblade, is incapable of penetrating more deeply than the most superficial fibers of the most plantar layer, thereby avoiding transection of the named blood vessels and nerves.

created by the spur. These procedures have been abandoned; their use in any circumstance is contraindicated.

Hassab and El-Sherif[10] popularized drilling of the os calcis as a means of "decompressing" the bone and left the spur intact. They based their technique on the anatomic finding of nerve endings adjacent to microvascular channels within bony lacunae. Inflammatory congestion would, therefore, compress these nerve endings, giving rise to discomfort. Drilling five to seven holes from lateral to medial through the calcaneal walls was clinically successful in a small number of patients. Widespread application of this concept, however, has demonstrated that it can sometimes be effective when used adjunctively but not as the primary procedure. In addition, the multiple drill

holes can serve as stress risers resulting in calcaneal fracture.

Osteotripsy (i.e., reduction of the spur via a rotating bur) can work well in experienced hands. The high speed of the bur and lack of visualization (which is an aspect of the procedure) leaves little room for error, potentially resulting in overzealous removal of the spur and erosion of the inferior cortical wall. The latter can lead to fracture on weight bearing.

Remaining procedures use various surgical instruments to excise the spur: rongeur, osteotome and mallet, or a number of different rasps. Some are performed in an open fashion and others percutaneously. Obviously, percutaneous procedures do not lend themselves to rongeurs and osteotomes with mallets because the small incision size does not allow successful manipulation of the instrument and the fragment. This limitation also applies to procedures performed under fluoroscopy. In our experience, hand rasp techniques offer the safest approach to spur excision. Coarse, transverse rasps such as the Cottle rasp are most effective; because of their relatively less abrasive tooth pattern, fine rasps add an undesirable amount of procedural effort and time.

Once the spur has been freed of its fascial attachments, the rasp should be placed directly on the summit of the spur and moved in a back-and-forth fashion. After several strokes, the rasp should be used as a probe to palpate the concave inferior calcaneal surface. If the spur's prominence is still palpable, further rasping is required. Rasping should not be continued once the inferior calcaneal surface has been restored to its smooth, arciform shape.

PLANTAR FASCIAL PROCEDURES

In clinical practice, closed plantar fascial tears are rarely, if ever, repaired. The literature is noticeably lacking in this regard; in fact, trauma surgeons generally consider fascia to be expendable.

In contrast, the procedures discussed in this section center on plantar fasciotomy and partial plantar fasciectomy (at the calcaneal origin). Although fasciectomy is advocated by some foot and ankle surgeons, an overwhelming majority favor fasciotomy because the stress of postoperative weight bearing allows the fascia to heal in a lengthened position. An early and radical form of fascial release included the first layer of plantar musculature (the Steindler stripping) and is uncommonly performed. A definitive answer regarding the extent of less aggressive fasciotomy and the potential for adverse effect is under considerable debate.

Present-day disagreement revolves around the need to transect the fascia completely versus transecting only its medial portion. Advocates of the first school cite a calcaneal spur's shelflike expansion from medial to lateral and the increased stress that would be placed on an unsectioned portion of fascia. Disciples of the second school focus on the need to protect the long and short plantar ligaments from undue tension, at the same time avoiding a total disruption of the plantar fascia's windlass function. Interestingly, Sammarco and Helfrey[11] advocated resecting a 1-cm² section of the medial fascial border near its calcaneal origin for two reasons: preserving fascial integrity and decompressing the nerve branch to the abductor digiti quinti. They cited nerve compression as a possible cause for heel spur pain, hence the rationale for their procedure.[11]

Over the course of time, comparatively equal success rates have been achieved with either technique. Some degree of temporary lateral discomfort is often encountered with either procedure, although the structure or structures giving rise to that complaint remain enigmatic. Empirically, adhesive felt padding beneath the cuboid, functional foot orthoses, or the passage of time have resulted in a gradual disappearance of symptoms. Preoperatively, patients must be warned of this possibility as well as the protracted recovery period for heel spur surgery in general (4–6 months before preoperative symptomatology resolves).

Regardless of the procedure used, immediate postoperative weight bearing is usually recommended unless the surgical outcome has become complicated by excessive spur resection or drilling. In prior years, plaster immobilization with softening of the heel region of the cast was used to place tension stress on the transected fascia when weight bearing. Surgeons believed that this would prevent a recurrence of symptoms secondary to fascial healing in a contracted position. This technique is rarely, if ever, used today.

ENDOSCOPIC PLANTAR FASCIOTOMY

Although just another form of fascial release, the endoscopic plantar fasciotomy (EPF) is the newest and, therefore, most controversial technique in heel spur surgery. As a result, we believe it deserves special consideration. Even the title of the procedure has been patented.

When originally described by Barrett and Day in 1991,[12] a single portal approach was advocated. This was revised by a two-portal approach in 1993,[13] which continues to be the favored present-day methodology. Although percutaneous techniques were not new, endoscopy removed their "blindness." An additional departure from current practice was the concept of partial plantar fasciotomy (i.e., only its medial third). Investigators argued that the lesser degree of fascial separation prevented or lessened the complications witnessed with total fascial release. Those complications are discussed later. A final distinction of the EPF was its partial fascial release without the excision of a radiographically visible spur. Historically, this is inaccurate, because Spitzy advocated a similar procedure as early as 1937.[14] Like investigators of today, he believed that fascial strain was more the cause of a patient's pain than the spur itself.

The instrumentation and steps in performing the EPF have already been well described[12, 13, 15] and, therefore, are not reiterated in this chapter. Instead, we hope to present a compilation of data obtained in the most recently published large series.

In 1995, Tomczak and Haverstock presented a retrospective comparison of EPF versus open fasciotomy with heel spur resection.[16] Their series consisted of 68 patients, 34 undergoing EPF and 34 undergoing open fasciotomy. Although both procedures were found to be equally effective in relieving pain, the time required to return to work or full activity averaged 29 days for the EPF group and 84 days for the open fasciotomy cohort. Although seemingly significant, we question the validity of studying a soft tissue procedure with one involving bone and expecting the healing rates to be comparable. An investigation of EPF against open fasciotomy alone seems more sound.

Later in the same year, Barrett and colleagues published a multisurgeon prospective analysis of 652 patients undergoing

EPF.[15] They cited at least five prior studies documenting the effectiveness of plantar fasciotomy without spur resection. Twenty-five surgeons participated in the Barrett study; 633 patients were relieved of heel pain. Seventy-seven percent of the patients returned to wearing regular shoes by the 7th day, and 87% had less pain than preoperatively by the 21st postoperative day.

In 1996, Stone and Davies reported their own experiences retrospectively with 40 patients who underwent the EPF between 1992 and 1994.[17] On the basis of return-mail questionnaires, they concluded that approximately 3 months were required postoperatively before heel pain resolved. Seventy percent of patients stated they would recommend the procedure to other patients; 30% claimed they would not.

On the basis of these reports, as well as our own experiences, it is fairly safe to conclude that plantar fasciotomy without heel spur resection can be markedly effective. In clinical practice, however, we have noticed that most patients will demand resection of a radiographically visible spur. In addition, a number of surgical facilities are reluctant to invest in the required endoscopy equipment if it is not already available. Because alternate percutaneous techniques for plantar fasciotomy already exist that do not require special equipment, more data on the outcome of EPF procedures are needed before it can be considered the procedure of choice among foot and ankle surgeons.

The data on all heel spur surgeries, however, do reveal a number of complications that are discussed in the following section.

COMPLICATIONS

Overly aggressive tissue handling and poor surgical hemostasis have resulted in complications of hematoma and wound dehiscence.[16] Of course, these outcomes can potentially occur in any wound and are not endemic to heel spur surgery. Patients will typically complain of excessive pain postoperatively, and the removal of one or more sutures will release a hemorrhagic discharge. Unless monitored closely to allow early detection and treatment, tissue necrosis develops rapidly as a result of the abundant adipose tissue in the heel pad.

The fatty layer of the heel will also allow microorganisms to colonize quickly and spread to the calcaneus, which consists of predominantly trabecular bone. Osteomyelitis results, leading to reoperation and weeks of parenteral antibiotic therapy for what was supposed to have been, in the eyes of both patient and surgeon, a fairly routine procedure. Some centers now advocate either oral or parenteral antibiotic prophylaxis,[17] although we believe this is unnecessary and does not replace good surgical technique.

Severance of or trauma to the sensory branches of the medial calcaneal nerve or first branch of the lateral plantar nerve to the abductor digiti quinti muscle has been mentioned. Although medial surgical approaches have been implicated as the potential cause of this complication, experience has shown that permanent numbness or hypesthesia postoperatively is more the result of improper wound management during the procedure (Figs. 12–5 and 12–6). As in

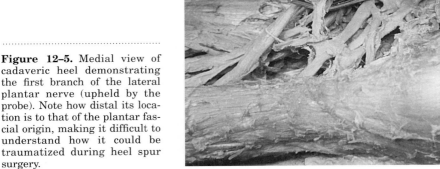

Figure 12–5. Medial view of cadaveric heel demonstrating the first branch of the lateral plantar nerve (upheld by the probe). Note how distal its location is to that of the plantar fascial origin, making it difficult to understand how it could be traumatized during heel spur surgery.

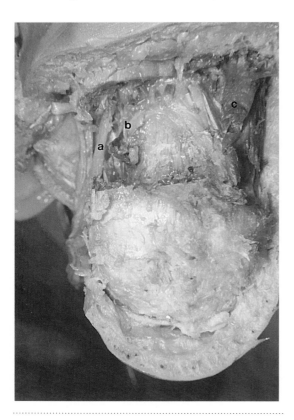

Figure 12–6. Plantar view of cadaveric heel with plantar fascia removed. Note location of lateral plantar nerve (a) and artery (b) in relation to site of heel spur. Abductor digiti quinti muscle is labeled (c).

all incisions, temporary alteration of sensation along the incision line is to be expected but resolves spontaneously within several weeks or months. In two separate cadaver studies, endoscopic plantar fasciotomy failed to pose any danger to adjacent neurovascular structures (i.e., the lateral plantar nerve or its first branch to the abductor digiti quinti muscle).[18, 19] Partial transection of the flexor digitorum brevis muscle occurred in 46% of the specimens in one study, but the degree of transection was considered insignificant (an average of 0.8 mm).[19]

As a complication, hypertrophic scar formation usually follows an untoward event such as hematoma, wound dehiscence, or infection. Unless a patient demonstrates hypertrophic and keloid scars elsewhere, present-day heel spur surgery should not result in painful scarring. Its development signals excessive intraoperative tissue trauma and can lead to painful nerve compression requiring surgical release. In our experience,

this has typically been the case in surgeries involving release of the foot's intrinsic musculature (i.e., Steindler stripping). Here, the plantar nerves becomes entrapped in the porta pedis (the fibrous hiatus through which these nerves pass deep to the abductor hallucis muscle belly). In such cases, patients experience the signs and symptoms of tarsal tunnel syndrome, that is, plantar paresthesia and intrinsic muscle atrophy. Tinel's sign is present at the porta pedis rather than at the entrance of the tarsal tunnel.

As mentioned earlier, calcaneal fracture can develop secondary to overdrilling or aggressive heel spur removal. The cortical wall of the calcaneus is relatively thin, so breaks in its continuity lead to stress risers that often fail. The patterns of presentation include sudden overt fractures or subacute stress fractures. Procedures that do not involve bone have not, to our knowledge, ever resulted in calcaneal fracture unless complicated by infection with resultant osteomyelitis.

In comparison to the aforementioned, plantar fascia release (and not heel spur excision per se) more frequently results in lateral column complaints secondary to increased stress placed on the long and short plantar ligaments and the cuboid postoperatively. This was reported in 36% of all postoperative patients in one series[17] and in another 52% of those patients experiencing complications of any kind.[15] We have had the same experiences regardless of whether partial or complete transection of the plantar fascia was performed. Laboratory data have confirmed that plantar fascia interruption can lead to a lowering of the longitudinal arch and lateral weight transfer.[20] One case study implicated this phenomenon as the cause of subsequent pronation and unilateral hammertoe formation.[21]

Particularly in patients undergoing endoscopic plantar fasciotomy, this has led to experimentation in terms of just how much of the fascia can and should be incised. Champions of the partial plantar fasciotomy (the EPF group) seem to favor sectioning the medial one half of the fascia, because it appears that transecting less than one half of the fascia leads to continued heel pain and incising more than one half results in tearing of the remaining fibers. Despite the introduction of internal markings on the endoscope cannula to aid the surgeon in determining the precise extent of fasciotomy, the cadaver studies mentioned earlier discovered that true precision was elusive because of the variable width of the fascia.[18, 19] Interestingly, in an effort to diminish the tearing of the lateral fibers that have been left intact, below-knee walking cast immobilization for 4 to 6 weeks has been advocated.[17] Because the same investigators reported that most of these problems resolve with "therapy, orthoses, and time," it appears that patience and patient education would be more beneficial than an arduous postoperative course. The reader is asked to keep in mind that, as stated earlier, the recovery from heel spur surgery in general is prolonged and in the range of 4 to 6 months. During that period, patients are still able to walk, work, and engage in an active lifestyle; for unknown reasons, heel spur symptoms persist postoperatively until this "golden period" passes. On the basis of the available results, none of the present-day surgical techniques have been able to shorten that interval significantly.

CONCLUSIONS

Heel spur surgery continues to be considered a procedure of last resort and only after a prolonged course of conservative therapy. Despite the presence of a radiographically evident inferior calcaneal spur, the surgical pendulum appears to be swinging in the direction of partial plantar fasciotomy or fasciectomy alone. Although a variety of other surgical approaches work equally well, this evolving shift in rationale may be the result of recent discoveries concerning the role of the plantar fascia as well as a trend toward decreasing invasiveness.

REFERENCES

1. Sarrafian, SK, Anatomy of the Foot and Ankle. Philadelphia: J. B. Lippincott, 1983.
2. Hedrick MR. The plantar aponeurosis. Foot Ankle Int 17:646–649, 1996.
3. Huang C, Kitaoka HB, An K, et al. Biomechanical evaluation of longitudinal arch stability. Foot Ankle 14:353–357, 1993.
4. Barrett SL, Day SV, Pignotti TT, et al. Endoscopic heel anatomy: analysis of 200 fresh frozen specimens. J Foot Ankle Surg 34: 51–56, 1995.
5. Malay DS, Duggar GE. Heel surgery. In McGlamry ED, Banks AS, Downey MS, eds. Comprehensive Textbook of Foot Surgery, 2nd ed. Baltimore, MD: Williams & Wilkins, 1992.
6. Pfeffer GB, Baxter DE. Surgery of the adult heel. In Jahss MH, ed. Disorders of the Foot and Ankle, ed 2. Philadelphia: W. B. Saunders, 1991.
7. Sundberg SB, Johnson KA. Painful conditions of the heel. In Jahss MH, ed. Disorders of the Foot and Ankle, ed 2. Philadelphia: W. B. Saunders, 1991.
8. White DL. Plantar fascial release. J Am Podiatr Med Assoc 84: 607–613, 1994.
9. Licopantis DP. Heel spur surgery: another new approach. J Am Podiatr Med Assoc 85:100–103, 1995.
10. Hassab HK, El-Sherif AS. Drilling of the os calcis for painful heel with calcanean spur. Acta Orthop Scand 45:152–157, 1974.
11. Sammarco GJ, Helfrey RB. Surgical treatment for recalcitrant plantar fasciitis. Foot Ankle Int 17:520–526, 1996.
12. Barrett SL, Day SV. Endoscopic plantar fasciotomy for chronic plantar fasciitis. J Foot Surg 30:568, 1991.
13. Barrett SL, Day SV. Endoscopic plantar fasciotomy: two portal endoscopic surgical techniques. Clinical results of 65 procedures. J Foot Ankle Surg 32:248, 1993.
14. Spitzy H. Surgical treatment of painful calcaneal spur. Munch Med Wochenschr 84:807–808, 1937.
15. Barrett SL, Day SV, Pignetti TT, et al. Endoscopic plantar fasciotomy: a multi-surgeon prospective analysis of 652 cases. J Foot Ankle Surg 34:400–406, 1995.
16. Tomczak RL, Haverstock BD. A retrospective comparison of endoscopic plantar fasciotomy to open plantar fasciotomy with heel spur resection for chronic plantar fasciitis/heel spur syndrome. J Foot Ankle Surg 34:305–311, 1995.
17. Stone PA, Davies JL. Retrospective review of endoscopic plantar fasciotomy—1992 through 1994. J Am Podiatr Med Assoc 86:414–420, 1996.
18. Hawkins BJ, Langermen RJ, Gibbons T, et al. An anatomic analysis of endoscopic plantar fascia release. Foot Ankle Int 16: 552–558, 1995.
19. Hofmeister EP, Elliott MJ, Juliano PJ. Endoscopic plantar fascia release: an anatomical study. Foot Ankle Int 16: 719–723, 1995.
20. Daly PJ, Kitaoka HB, Chao EY. Plantar fasciotomy for intractable plantar fasciitis: clinical results and biomechanical evaluation. Foot Ankle 13:188, 1992.
21. Pontious J, Flanigan KP, Hillstrom HJ. Role of the plantar fascia in digital stabilization: a case report. J Am Podiatr Med Assoc 86:43–47, 1996.

13

Heel Pain in the Setting of Metabolic, Infiltrative, and Bone Disorders

Stephen A. Paget   L. Ricardo Zuniga-Montes
Joseph A. Markenson   Helen Bateman

Heel pain, also termed calcaneodynia or talalgia, is among the most common complaint of patients presenting with foot and ankle disorders. Sources of heel pain include all tissue components of the region, including disorders of skin, tendon, fascia, bone, and nerve.[1] It is generally accepted that the vast majority of these heel complaints are mechanical in cause.[2] However, heel pain may be secondary to a variety of conditions not directly mechanical in nature and may be the presenting feature of a previously undiagnosed medical condition.

Talalgia is defined as heel pain located either posteriorly (along the Achilles tendon and its insertion to the calcaneus) or at the attachment of the superficial aponeurosis on the plantar surface of the calcaneus. Talalgia of varying intensity may be observed during the course of most rheumatologic conditions (e.g., Reiter's syndrome and rheumatoid arthritis), but also in patients with metabolic and systemic diseases.

Metabolic and endocrine diseases that may contribute to heel pain include conditions such as crystalline arthropathies: gout and pseudogout or chondrocalcinosis, hyperlipidemias, hypothyroidism, diabetes, and hypo- and hyperparathyroidism. Systemic disorders include infiltrative diseases such as sarcoidosis and amyloidosis. Primary bone disorders such as Paget's disease may also lead to heel pain.

METABOLIC DISORDERS

Although the following disorders differ in their pathogenesis and basic metabolic defect, they have in common the capability of causing musculoskeletal dysfunction or inflammation.

Crystalline Arthropathy

Gout

An elevated serum uric acid level may be due to either a renal excretory abnormality (the cause in 90% of cases) or hyperproduction of uric acid. Deposition of urate crystals in connective tissue, including tendons, synovial fluid, and tissue, is thought to occur in areas of high connective tissue metabolism in association with supersaturation of these tissues with monosodium urate.[3] The most common site for an attack of acute gout is the first metatarsophalangeal joint, commonly presenting as a painful, hot and red tender toe.[4] Other joints and tissues can be involved, including the subtalar joint and tendons. Gouty deposits may occur in the Achilles tendon, causing tendinitis pain and can even lead to tendon rupture.[5] Plantar fasciitis may be due to urate deposition. The term is often used to designate a clinical condition in which the patient has pain in the plantar aspect of the heel, characteristically worse when arising in the morning and after periods of sitting. The only physical finding is severe localized tenderness at the heel.[6] Evidence of plantar fasciitis can be detected by magnetic resonance imaging (MRI), but the diagnosis is usually made clinically, and MRI is reserved only for those cases that are not clear-cut or do not respond to therapy. Treatment is usually conservative, starting with rest and avoidance of trauma, nonsteroidal anti-inflammatory drugs (NSAIDs) such as indomethacin (25 mg three times per day with meals), and a heel pad. In the elderly patient, especially those with other medical problems or a history of NSAID-related side effects, one should avoid these medications and consider a short course of oral prednisone (e.g., 5 mg twice a day with a taper by 2.5 mg each day for 4 days). Occasionally, local steroid injections may be helpful when the pain is acute, severe, and unresponsive to a conservative approach, but in general should be avoided because of the risk of tendon rupture.

Pseudogout/Chondrocalcinosis

Calcium pyrophosphate deposition with chondrocalcinosis in the Achilles tendon may lead to an acute tendinitis.[7, 8] The development of Achilles tendinitis in an elderly patient can be an inflammatory reaction to calcium pyrophosphate dihydrate (CPPD). This is illustrated by a study in which such crystals were found in the biopsy of the tendon. Characteristic linear calcifications in patients with chondrocalcinosis may be seen on radiograph near the insertion of the Achilles to the calcaneum, but the patients may be asymptomatic.[4, 9–11, 13] Treatment is similar to that recommended for gout. Hypercalcemia resulting from hyperparathyroidism may, at times, lead to inflammatory joint or tendon disease.

Hyperlipidemia

In a review of 88 patients with hyperlipidemia, musculoskeletal complaints that were significantly increased compared with controls were tendon xanthomas associated with Achilles tendinitis. This finding was present in patients with adult familial hypercholesterolemia and mixed hyperlipidemia. Oligoarthritis was significantly increased in patients with mixed hyperlipidemia but not adult familial hyperlipidemia. Migratory polyarthritis and transient Achilles tendon pain were rare. Musculoskeletal system manifestations antedated the diagnosis of hyperlipidemia in 62% (24 of 39), and in 63% (19 of 30) manifestations improved or completely resolved with lipid-lowering treatment. Interestingly, there was no difference in musculoskeletal symptoms between patients with juvenile familial hypercholesterolemia and controls.[14] However, in one report, symptoms of Achilles tendinitis were the presenting feature of familial type II hyperlipoproteinemia in 14 patients ranging from ages 20 to 63.[15] In another study of children aged 6 to 18 who presented with tendinitis lasting approximately 72 hours, all were found to have type II hyperlipidemia.[16] In the latter two studies, non-specific arthritis often preceded the Achilles symptoms. Tendinitis in patients with hyperlipidemia needs to be carefully evaluated because diagnostic confusion may arise. This is illustrated in the case in which a patient with Achilles tendon pain, in the setting of hypercholesterolemia and premature coronary artery disease, was found on aspiration of the retrocalcaneal bursa and tendon nodule to have positively birefringent lipid crystals that could be confused with CPPD crystals. However, in contrast to calcium pyrophosphate crystals, these lipid crystals were large, not rhomboid, and had bright birefringence and a negative reaction to calcium stain, alizarin red S.[17] Distinguishing the two is important therapeutically because NSAIDs would be used to treat the patients with CPPD, whereas lipid lowering therapy would be used for those with lipid crystals.

Achilles tendon thickness can, in fact, be used to discriminate between familial hypercholesterolemia and secondary hypercholesterolemia; the thicker tendon is associated with the former.[18] Primary hyperlipidemias (hyperlipoproteinemias) are due to an abnormal metabolism of lipoproteins, resulting in an increase in their blood levels. Tendon xanthomas comprise lipid infiltrates, which result in irregular thickening of the involved tendon.[19] When one is considering treatment of tendinitis or prophylaxis against tendon rupture, ultrasound can be helpful in supporting or excluding Achilles tendon abnormalities in patients with familial hypercholesterolemia. Patients with secondary hypercholesterolemia do not differ significantly from those of normal controls.[20] The xanthomas can decrease in size with appropriate therapy as described in the study of 13 patients with heterozygotic familial hypercholesterolemia with tendinous xanthomatosis, in which 11 had regression of the size of the xanthomas with appropriate diet and bezafibrate therapy over 2 years. This correlated with a favorable change in lipid profile.[21] Surgical treatment is reserved for cosmetic and, more importantly, symptomatic xanthomas, but there is a tendency for recurrence in Achilles lesions.[22]

Diabetes Mellitus

The morbidity, cost, and mortality associated with lower extremity complications among patients with diabetes mellitus are well known, with increased risk of foot ulcerations, infections, neuropathic fractures, and amputation.[23, 24] The involvement of the forefoot is most common, but 8% of the ulcers in patients with neuropathic foot ulceration are localized to the heel with an additional 4% in the midfoot.[25] The most common articular involvement in the diabetic, neuropathic foot is the tarsal and tarsometatarsal or Lisfranc's joint (60%), followed by metatarsophalangeal joints (30%) and the tibiotalar joints (10%).[26, 27]

The diabetic foot is common and affects approximately 15% of diabetic individuals during their lifetime.[28] It has been estimated that 20% of all diabetic patient admissions to the hospital are for the treatment of foot lesions, with a 15-fold higher risk of major amputation in diabetic than nondiabetic patients.[29] These amputations are preceded by diabetic foot ulcers in 84 to 85% of cases.[30] Callus predicts subsequent ulceration[31]; therefore, the foot should be examined closely to determine whether there are sites of excessive pressure resulting from footwear. Foot lesions occur in both insulin and non–insulin-dependent patients, with an annual incidence of foot ulcers of 2.4% in younger diabetic patients (diagnosed before age 30 and taking insulin) and 2.6% in older diabetics (diagnosed after age 30).[32]

A complete physical examination, including a close inspection of the shoes, is the most important step to detect diabetic-related lesions of the foot early and to prevent further damage. Because of sensory loss resulting from neuropathy, it is not uncommon that patients are completely unaware of any foot problems, and the problems are found "by accident" on a complete physical examination.[33] However, the absence of symptoms in the feet in some neuropathic patients sometimes cause physicians to miss examining the foot, as was highlighted in a study in which physicians were unlikely to examine their patients' feet unless the patients removed their socks and shoes before the consultation began.[34]

A significant number of diabetic patients present with hyperostotic changes noted in various bony locations. There is an especially high incidence of bony exostoses, reactive bone proliferation, debris and periarticular calcifications in the feet, with osteophytosis of the calcaneus in 80% of diabetic patients. Also, in diabetic patients with a history of neuropathy, episodes of spontaneous fractures of the calcaneus and avulsion fractures of the posterior tubercle of the calcaneus have been documented.[35, 36]

Diabetic foot ulcers are traditionally considered to be the consequence of peripheral vascular disease and peripheral neuropathy, frequently complicated by infection. However, in recent years, our understanding of the pathogenesis of the diabetic foot has greatly increased, and several contributory risk factors leading to diabetic foot lesions have been reported. This includes both somatic and autonomic neuropathy, peripheral vascular disease, foot deformity, blindness, diabetic nephropathy (especially with chronic renal failure), high alcohol intake, aging, and confusion.[37]

Sensorimotor neuropathy produces a combination of insensitivity to pain, abnormal proprioception, and abnormalities of thermal and vibration perception, all contributing to abnormal loading during standing and walking[38, 39] and thus ulceration at pressure points.[40] Autonomic dysfunction, which frequently coexists with somatic neuropathy, is characterized by reduced or absent perspiration[41] and increased blood flow in the absence of large-vessel arterial disease (autosympathectomy).[37] Dry, warm skin with swollen veins during standing suggests diabetic autonomic neuropathy of the foot, and this dry skin predisposes to callus formation and fissuring. Abnormalities of microvascular hemodynamics have been demonstrated in patients with foot ulceration, as well as a higher incidence of macrovascular disease in diabetic patients.[42]

Initially described by Charcot in 1868 in three patients with syphilitic tabes dorsalis,[43] Charcot's joint or neuroarthropathy is defined as a relatively painless progressive arthropathy of single or multiple joints caused by an underlying neurologic deficit. The term, however, is now used to describe the bone and joint changes associated with all neuropathic arthropathies.[27] Although 17.8% of diabetic patients have neuropathy, the prevalence of the neuropathic joint in diabetes is 0.4%. However, early signs of neuroarthropathy are present in up to 16% of diabetic patients with neuropathy.[44] Usually patients with neuropathy are in the fifth to seventh decade of life, with history of diabetes for at least 15 years.[26] The patient may present either with an acute or chronic unilateral problem, but the problem may be bilateral in 9.1%.[27] In the acute case, the onset is similar to a septic arthritis with an acutely swollen, painful foot, frequently with a history of minor trauma. It is usually related to arch collapse after a Charcot fracture of the foot, with rapidly progressive destruction, sometimes with disintegration of one or more tarsal bones within a period of only a few weeks.[26] Patients with acute Charcot's arthropathy and concomitant neuropathy have larger wounds that heal faster than in patients without Charcot's arthropathy,[25] and patients frequently seek medical care because of generalized pain in the feet. The chronic Charcot foot develops insidiously with a painless, deformed, and unstable foot.

The pathophysiology of Charcot's foot is not well understood. Two mechanisms have been described that might be responsible for the bony resorption in the early phase: increased blood flow, possibly associated with autonomic neuropathy, and increased osteoclastic activity, which is aggravated by loss of pain and loss of proprioceptive sensation. In the presence of repetitive micro- or macrotrauma, the changes are initiated.[27] The final results are fatigue fractures of cartilage and bone and soft tissue injury (ulcers). It must not be forgotten that deep infection may act synergistically with other factors, such as neuropathy, trauma, or small blood vessel disease, to promote the osteoarticular alterations. In general, two forms of neuroarthropathy have been described in the diabetic foot: the atrophic neuroarthropathy, most frequently occurring in the forefoot, which is characterized by osteoporosis, bone resorption, and dislocation. The second form is the hypertrophic neuroarthropathy, most frequently seen in the midfoot or hindfoot, characterized by osteophyte formation, bone sclerosis, eburnation, fragmentation, and dislocation.[26] As described by Gold,[26] the radiographic features of hypertrophic neuroarthropathy are the five D's: joint *d*istention, *d*islocation, bony *d*ebris, *d*isorganization, and increased bone *d*ensity.

Most serious foot problems are preventable if a few basic rules in patient education are followed. Therefore, patient education and the provision of adequate footwear for "at-risk" feet are the most important physician responsibilities to avoid greater dam-age. Shoes may present dangers as well as protection for insensitive feet. The most important basic rules to advise "at-risk" patients are (1) inspect feet daily, (2) wash both feet every day in warm water, (3) apply lotion or oil to feet after drying, (4) change shoes often, (5) inspect feet at each clinic visit, and (6) avoid extremes of temperature.[37]

In the early stages of diabetic feet, once infection has been eliminated, an intensive program of wound care, including debridement, dressing, education, and adequate mechanical unloading, must be started. The application of a total-contact plaster cast allows the patient to walk, helps to reduce swelling, and preserves the shape of the foot.[45] Infection must always be treated aggressively. Surgery has a definite role to play in the management of these deformed feet. Simple trimming of the bony exostosis is invaluable and is usually followed by healing of the ulcer. Also, stabilization of the hind- or midfoot by arthrodesis can be effective. Arthrodesis of any of the involved joints, including the ankle, subtalar, midtarsal, and tarsometatarsal joints, can be performed.[27, 46]

Parathyroid Disease

Hyperparathyroidism is an endocrine disorder resulting in an increased secretion of parathyroid hormone caused by glandular hyperplasia or adenoma, which leads to hypercalcemia and hyperphosphatemia. There is, however, a great variation in the clinical presentation, varying from asymptomatic hypercalcemia to renal stones, pancreatitis, and osteoporosis. It can be a primary parathyroid gland disorder or secondary to another underlying disease such as chronic renal failure. A patient with hyperparathyroidism is at risk for crystal-induced synovitis from either urate or CPPD or both, and the relationship between hyperparathyroidism and a high incidence of chondrocalcinosis has been well established.[47] Articular calcification in primary hyperparathyroidism takes the form of CPPD and has been found in the knee, triangular cartilage of the wrist joint, and Achilles tendon.[48]

CPPD-induced acute or subacute inflammatory arthritis is very common and involves the tibiotalar, subtalar, talonavicular, and midtarsal joints. However, very little is known concerning local factors that determine the specific site of crystal deposition in hyperparathyroidism.

Spontaneous tendinous laxity and rupture are not uncommon in patients with hyperparathyroidism secondary to chronic renal failure.[49] This type of secondary hyperparathyroidism has been considered an additional factor contributing to the development of Jaccoud's syndrome (i.e., finger soft tissue reversible deformities) and tendinous laxity and rupture in patients with systemic lupus erythematosus (SLE).[50, 51] In this setting, the patella, Achilles, and quadriceps tendons, in this order, are the tendons most frequently affected.[52] In these patients, tendon damage might be due to direct action of the parathyroid hormone on the highly polymerized glycoprotein matrix, and dystrophic calcium deposits may further weaken the tendons.[53] Additionally, in a study of 14 patients with SLE and ligamentous derangement demonstrated by Jaccoud's syndrome or patellar tendon elongation (or both), 4 patients had Achilles tendinitis simultaneously.[54]

Shortening of the metacarpals occurs in 70% of pseudohypoparathyroidism cases, and shortening of the metatarsals occurs in 40%. This is a disorder in which the end organ is unresponsive to parathyroid hormone. In contrast, brachydactyly has not been reported to occur in patients with hypoparathyroidism.[55] No forefoot bony growth abnormalities have been reported to date in either of these disorders.

Hypothyroidism

Hypothyroidism is caused by metabolic effects of a decreased production of thyroxine. Common causes include glandular damage from an autoimmune process such as Hashimoto's thyroiditis, acute infectious (subacute, de Quervain's) thyroiditis, and goiter. The clinical manifestations vary from mild fatigue and weight gain with carpal tunnel syndrome to myxedema with myopathy, cardiac disease, bone collapse, and coma.

The tarsal tunnel is located behind and below the medial malleolus, and compression of the posterior tibial nerve and its branches (medial plantar nerve, lateral plantar nerve, or medial calcaneal nerve) may occur as they pass between the medial surface of the ankle and the overlying flexor retinaculum.[56] Any decrease in the size of the subretinacular space resulting from myxomatous tissue infiltration related to the hypothyroid state may cause pressure on the nerve. Multiple published reports about its causes have appeared, and the differential diagnosis includes many disparate disorders such as hypothyroidism–myxedema, posttraumatic, inflammatory diseases such as rheumatoid arthritis, and benign tumors (lipomas).[57–59] Tarsal tunnel syndrome (TTS) has become a frequently recognized cause of heel pain that may be accompanied by a tingling, burning, or numb feeling around the heel and foot and sometimes complaints of pain radiating upward on the medial side of the calf. The diagnosis is based on the clinical history, physical findings (tenderness over the tarsal tunnel, positive Tinel's sign), and a prolonged nerve conduction time in 70 to 80% of patients studied.[60]

TTS is often mistaken for other heel or foot disorders, and clinicians should include this entrapment neuropathy in the broad differential diagnosis of heel pain, especially if there are associated neurologic symptoms. If related to an underlying disease such as hypothyroidism or diabetes, the treatment is directed against the primary disorder. Conservative treatment of TTS includes local corticosteroid injection, NSAIDs, and orthotics; however, if persistent, a surgical decompression is indicated.

SYSTEMIC, INFILTRATIVE DISORDERS

Sarcoidosis

The most common type of arthropathy seen in sarcoidosis is acute polyarthritis in the setting of erythema nodosum and bilateral hilar adenopathy. This is usually symmetric and additive, starting in the ankles but also affecting the knees, hands, wrists, elbows, and feet. Heel pain, however, may be a major characteristic of the disease, as illustrated by Shaw and colleagues.[61] The seven patients they reviewed presented with heel pain as the initial disease feature. The pain may be bilateral and can precede or accompany the other manifestations. Treatment consists of NSAIDs initially, followed by corticosteroids (e.g., 10–20 mg prednisone/day with a taper over 5–7 days) in resistant patients. The course may be variable with relapses and remissions.

Amyloidosis

Amyloidosis is defined as the extracellular local or systemic deposition of an insoluble proteinaceous material. There are multiple, biochemically different forms of amyloid that are differentiated into AA and AL types, according to the unique fibrous structure that they all possess.[62]

Amyloid can directly involve articular structures by its presence in the synovial membrane, synovial fluid, or articular cartilage. AA amyloidosis is a complication of chronic inflammatory diseases, and renal involvement (nephrotic syndrome and renal insufficiency) is its primary clinical manifestation. AL amyloidosis can occur in association with multiple myeloma, in which the para-articular deposition of amyloid is found in 1 to 4% of cases, mainly in the shoulders, wrists, knees, and metacarpophalangeal and interphalangeal joints.[63]

Skin lesions localized to the lower legs, heels, and feet have been reported in patients with familial amyloidosis with polyneuropathy. In many respects, these lesions are similar to those of long-standing diabetes mellitus. In both entities, which involve the microvasculature, necrotic and traumatic skin lesions might be due not only to the impaired sensitivity but also to an altered reaction to trauma.[64] Sural nerve biopsy may be useful to help diagnose amyloid-related polyneuropathy.[65] In patients with polyneuropathy related to diabetes or amyloidosis, skeletal destruction in the feet has been described without previous skin lesions.[66] These skeletal lesions in patients with familial amyloidosis and polyneuropathy are apparently different from amyloid joint disease in connection with, for example, myeloma, in which bone amyloid deposits have been demonstrated by histopathologic investigation.[67] Any of these mechanisms may lead to heel pain, and treatment should be directed at the underlying cause; many of the previously described simple measures are used for the diabetic foot.

BONE DISORDERS

Paget's Disease

Paget's disease of bone may be the source of heel pain in the elderly and is demonstrable on all forms of bone imaging.[68] The underlying pathogenesis of this disease is unknown, but it involves localized remodeling of bone; some areas may be osteoporotic and others sclerotic. It can affect any bone in the body. The pain is thought to be caused by increased vascular activity within the bone and may occur both at rest and on weight bearing. The diagnosis is made by imaging and the finding of increased bone turnover, biochemically indicated by elevated serum alkaline phosphatase and increased hydroxyproline and N-telopeptide in the urine. Therapy is directed at suppressing the bone formation and may include calcitonin and bisphosphonates.[69] Some indications for therapy include involvement of long bones and joints to try to prevent fractures and deformity, skull involvement to prevent deafness and nerve entrapment, and vertebral disease to prevent cord compression. Bisphosphonates in particular can keep the disease well controlled.[70]

CONCLUSION

As can be seen from this review, many conditions can lead to heel pain, and the evaluating physician needs to keep these in mind for accurate diagnosis and treatment. This demands that a complete history and physical be taken to define whether or not there are extra-articular abnormalities. In fact, the presentation of heel pain may be the only clue to previously unrecognized, underlying medical conditions such as diabetes, myeloma, and endocrinopathies. Hyperlipidemia is also very prevalent and is often undertreated unless suspected. Less common diseases such as hyperparathyroidism or Paget's disease can be treated early in the course of the disease if the presentation of heel pain is adequately investigated. Early treatment of the underlying disorder could prevent more extensive disease.

REFERENCES

1. Kier R. Magnetic resonance imaging of plantar fasciitis and other causes of heel pain. Ankle Foot Int 2:97, 1994.
2. Lichniak JE. The heel in systemic disease. Clin Podiatr Med Surg 7:225, 1990.
3. Katz WA. Deposition of urate crystals in gout. Arthritis Rheum 18:751, 1975.
4. Raymakers R. The painful foot. Practitioner 215:61, 1975.

5. Mahoney PG, James PD, Howell CJ, Swannell AJ. Spontaneous rupture of the Achilles tendon in a patient with gout. Ann Rheum Dis 40:416, 1981.
6. Furey JG. Plantar fasciitis. J Bone Joint Surg Am 57:672, 1975.
7. Gerster JC, Hauser H, Fallet GH. Xeroradiographic techniques applied to assessment of Achilles tendon in inflammatory or metabolic diseases. Ann Rheum Dis 34:479, 1975.
8. Gerster JC, Saudan, Fallet GH. Talalgia: a review of 30 severe cases. J Rheumatol 5:210, 1978.
9. Gerster JC, Lagier R, Boivin G. Achilles tendinitis associated with chondrocalcinosis. J Rheumatol 7:82, 1980.
10. Gibson T. Is there a place for corticosteroid injection in the management of Achilles tendon lesions? Br J Rheumatol 30:436, 1991.
11. Gomes DR. Acute gout of subtalar joint in a 56-year-old white female. J Am Podiatr Med Assoc 67:568, 1977.
12. Raymakers R. The painful foot. Practitioner 215:61, 1975.
13. Kier R. Magnetic resonance imaging of plantar fasciitis and other causes of heel pain. Magn Reson Imaging Clin N Am 2:97, 1994.
14. Klemp P, Halland AM, Majoos FL, Steyn K. Musculoskeletal manifestations in hyperlipidemia, a controlled study. Ann Rheum Dis 52:44, 1993.
15. Glueck C, Levy R, Fredrickson DS. Acute tendinitis and arthritis: a presenting symptom of familial type 2 hyperlipidemia. JAMA 206:2895, 1968.
16. Shapiro JR, Fallat RW, Tsang RC, et al. Achilles tendinitis and tenosynovitis. Am J Dis Child 128:486, 1978.
17. Schumacher HR, Michaels R. Recurrent tendinitis and Achilles tendon nodule with positively birefringent crystals in a patient with hyperlipidemia. J Rheumatol 16:1387, 1989.
18. Mabuchi H, Ito S, Haba T, et al. Discrimination of familial hypercholesterolemia and secondary hypercholesterolemia by Achilles tendon thickness. Atherosclerosis 28:61, 1977.
19. Bardin T, Kuntz D. Primary hyperlipidemias and xanthomatosis. In Klippel JH, Dieppe PA, eds. Rheumatology, ed 1. St. Louis, MO: C. V. Mosby, 1994: 7.27.1.
20. Kainberger F, Seidl G, Traindl S, et al. Ultrasonography of the achilles tendon in hypercholesterolemia. Acta Radiol 34:408, 1993.
21. Rouffy J, Chanu B, Bakir R, et al. Changes in lipid and Achilles tendon diameters in familial hypercholesterolemic patients with tendinous xanthomatosis treated by diet and bezafibrate for 2 years. Curr Med Res Opin 11:123, 1988.
22. Fahey JJ, Stark H, Donavan WF, Drennan DB. Xanthoma of the Achilles tendon. J Bone Joint Surg Am 55:1197, 1973.
23. Lavery LA, Ashry HR, Van Houtom WH, et al. Variation in the incidence and proportion of diabetes-related amputations in minorities. Diabetes Care 19:48, 1996.
24. Van Houtom WH, Lavery LA, Harkless LB. The costs of diabetes-related lower extremity amputations in the Netherlands. Diabet Med 12:777, 1996.
25. Lavery LA, Armstrong DG, Walker SC. Healing rates of diabetic foot ulcers associated with midfoot fracture due to Charcot's arthropathy. Diabet Med 14:46, 1997.
26. Gold RH, Tong DJF, Crim JR, Seeger LL. Imaging in the diabetic foot. Skeletal Radiol 24:563, 1995.
27. Klenerman L. The Charcot joint in diabetes. Diabet Med 13:S52, 1996.
28. Palumbo PJ, Melton LJ. Peripheral vascular disease and diabetes. In Harris MI, Hamman RF, eds. Diabetes in America (NIH Pub. No 85-1468). Washington, DC: U.S. Government printing Office, 1985:1.
29. Most RS, Sinnock P. The epidemiology of lower extremity amputation in diabetic individuals. Diabetes Care 6:87, 1993.
30. Pecoraro RE, Reiber GE, Burgess EM. Pathways to diabetic limb amputation: basis of prevention. Diabetes Care 13:513, 1990.
31. Boulton AJM. The pathogenesis of diabetic foot problems. An overview. Diabet Med 13:S12, 1996.
32. Moss SE, Klein R, Klein B. The prevalence and incidence of lower extremity amputation in a diabetic population. Arch Intern Med 152:610, 1992.
33. De Heus-van Putten MA, Schaper NC, Bakker K. The clinical examination of the diabetic foot in daily practice. Diabet Med 13:S55, 1996.
34. Cohen SJ. Potential barriers to diabetes care. Diabetes Care 6:499, 1983.
35. Coventry MB, Rothacker GW Jr. Bilateral calcaneal fracture in a diabetic patient. J Bone Joint Surg Am 61:677, 1970.
36. El-Khowy G, Kathol M. Neuropathic fractures in patients with diabetes mellitus. Radiology 134:313, 1980.
37. Boulton AJM. The diabetic foot. Med Clin North Am 72:1513, 1988.
38. Lippmann HI, Perotto A, Farrar R. The neuropathic foot of the diabetic. Bull N Y Acad Med 52:1159, 1976.
39. Boulton AJM, Kubrusly DB, Bowker JH, et al. Impaired vibratory perception and diabetic foot ulceration. Diabet Med 3:335, 1986.
40. Boulton AJM. The importance of abnormal foot pressures and gait in the causation of foot ulcers. In Connor H, Boulton AJM, Ward JD, eds. The Foot in Diabetes. Chichester, England: Wiley, 1987:11.
41. Ahmed ME, Delbridge L, Le Quesne LP. The role of autonomic neuropathy in diabetic foot ulceration. J Neurol Neurosurg Psychiatry 49:1002, 1986.
42. Janku HU, Standl E, Mehnert H. Peripheral vascular disease in diabetes mellitus and its relationship to cardiovascular risk factors: screening with Doppler's ultrasound technique. Diabetes Care 3:207, 1980.
43. Charcot JM. Sur quelques arthropathies qui paraissant depende d'une lesion du cerveau ou de la maelle epiriere. Arch Physiol Norm Pathol 1:161, 1868.
44. Bavanagh PR, Vickers KL, Young MJ, et al. Radiographic abnormalities in the feet of patients with diabetic neuropathy. Diabetes Care 17:201, 1994.
45. Laining PW, Cogley DI, Klenerman L. Neuropathic foot ulceration treated by total contact casts. J Bone Joint Surg Am 74:261, 1992.
46. Myerson MS, Henderson MR, Saxby T, Short KW. Management of midfoot diabetic neuroarthropathy. Foot Ankle Int 15:233, 1994.
47. Grahame R, June Sutor D, Mitchener MB. Crystal deposition in hyperparathyroidism. Ann Rheum Dis 30:597, 1971.
48. Mintz DH, Canary JJ, Carreaon G, Kyle LH. Hyperuricemia in hyperparathyroidism. N Engl J Med 265:112, 1961.

49. Babini SM, Arturi A, Marcos JC, et al. Laxity and rupture of the patellar tendon in systemic lupus erythematosus: association with secondary hyperparathyroidism. J Rheumatol 15:1162, 1988.

50. Liote F, Fitzcharles MA, Osterland CK. Jaccoud's arthropathy and hypermobility syndrome in systemic lupus erythematosus. Clin Exp Rheumatol 5:186, 1987.

51. Morgan J, McCarty DJ. Tendon ruptures in patients with systemic lupus erythematosus treated with corticosteroids. Arthritis Rheum 17:1033, 1974.

52. Khan MA, Ballou SP. Tendon rupture in systemic lupus erythematosus. J Rheumatol 8:308, 1981.

53. Preston FS, Adicoff A. Hyperparathyroidism with avulsion of three major tendons. N Engl J Med 266:968, 1962.

54. Babini SM, Cocco JA, De La Sota M, et al. Tendinous laxity and Jaccoud's syndrome in patients with systemic lupus erythematosus: possible role of secondary hyperparathyroidism. J Rheumatol 16:494, 1989.

55. Moses AM, Rao J, Coulson R, Miller M. Parathyroid hormone deficiency with Albright's hereditary osteodystrophy. J Clin Endocrinol Metab 39:496, 1974.

56. Srinivasan R, Rhodes J, Seidel MR. The tarsal tunnel. Mt Sinai J Med 47:17, 1980.

57. Linscheid RL, Burton RC, Frederiks EJ. Tarsal tunnel syndrome. South Med J 63:1313, 1970.

58. Nakano KK. The entrapment neuropathies of rheumatoid arthritis. Orthop Clin North Am 6:837, 1975.

59. Mann R. Tarsal tunnel syndrome. Orthop Clin North Am 5:109, 1974.

60. Johnson EW, Ortiz PR. Electrodiagnosis of tarsal tunnel syndrome. Arch Phys Med 47:776, 1966.

61. Shaw RA, Holt PA, Stevens MB. Heel pain in sarcoidosis. Ann Intern Med 109:675–677, 1988.

62. Cohen AS. Amyloidosis. In Isselbacher K, Braunwald E, Wilson JD, et al, eds. Harrison's Principles of Internal Medicine, ed 13. New York: McGraw-Hill, 1994:1625.

63. Van Rijswijk MH. Amyloidosis. In Klippel JH, Dieppe PA, eds. Rheumatology, ed 1. St. Louis, MO: C. V. Mosby, 1994:7.24.1.

64. Lithner F. Skin lesions of the legs and feet and skeletal lesions of the feet in familial amyloidosis with polyneuropathy. Acta Med Scand 199:197, 1976.

65. Dyck PJ, Lofgren EP. Nerve biopsy: choice of nerve, method, symptoms, and usefulness. Med Clin North Am 52:885, 1968.

66. Lithner F. Cutaneous erythema, with or without necrosis, localized to the legs and feet: a lesion in elderly diabetics. Acta Med Scand 198:319, 1975.

67. Wiernik PH. Amyloid joint disease. Medicine 51:465, 1972.

68. Gibbon WW, Cassar-Pullicino VN. Heel pain. Ann Rheum Dis 53:344, 1994.

69. Milgram JW. Metabolic disorders and Paget's disease of bone. In Jahss MH, ed. Disorders of the Foot and Ankle: Medical and Surgical Management, ed 2. Philadelphia: W. B. Saunders, 1991:1761.

70. Nagant de Deuxchaisnes C. Paget's disease of bone. In Klippel JH, Dieppe PA, eds. Rheumatology. St. Louis, MO: C. V. Mosby, 1994:7.39.1.

14

Heel Pain and Achilles Pain Associated with Rheumatoid Arthritis and Seronegative Spondyloarthropathies

Stephen A. Paget   Helen Bateman
Joseph A. Markenson   L. Ricardo Zuniga-Montes

Although rheumatoid arthritis (RA) and the seronegative spondyloarthropathies, (SNSs) such as psoriatic arthritis (PsA), Reiter's syndrome (RS), the colitic arthropathies and ankylosing spondylitis (AS) are all inflammatory types of arthritis, they have distinct clinical characteristics. The area of the hindfoot affected in the two categories of diseases is quite different.

SERONEGATIVE SPONDYLOARTHROPATHIES

Seronegative spondyloarthropathies include several heterogeneous diseases, characterized by inflammatory disease of the spine and sacroiliac joints and a largely asymmetric, peripheral joint synovitis, and any one of the following: positive family history, psoriasis, inflammatory bowel disease, buttock pain, and enthesopathy, defined as pain or inflammation at the site of tendon or ligament insertion.[1] The sera of these patients usually do not contain rheumatoid factor, and thus have been called seronegative. In patients with some of these disorders, there is a strong association with the class I histocompatibility antigen HLA-B27.

The diseases included within the spondyloarthropathies are (1) RS, characterized by episodes of mainly large joint, lower extremity, asymmetric arthritis of more than 1 month duration occurring in association with conjunctivitis, urethritis, or cervicitis[2]; (2) AS, an inflammatory disease that primarily involves the spine, sacroiliac joints, hips, and shoulders[3]; (3) PsA; and (4) the arthritis associated with inflammatory bowel disease, including Crohn's disease and ulcerative colitis. Insertional tendinitis and enthesopathic pain are hallmarks of the HLA-B27 spondyloarthropathies and are usually the dominant clinical factors that lead to functional limitation.[4] It is not known why AS and other SNSs localize to the entheses, but this pathologic localization differs from the peripheral synovitis characteristic of RA.[3]

Clinical Features

Talalgia, defined as heel pain located either posteriorly (along the Achilles tendon and its insertion into the calcaneus) or at the attachment of the superficial aponeurosis on the plantar surface of the calcaneus, is a common manifestation and usually the first symptom of the SNSs, primarily PsA and RS. In a study by Gerster and others[5] of 30 patients with severe heel pain, 24 were found to have one of the SNSs. Most of the patients were carriers of the antigen HLA-B27.[5] In one series of 36 Northern Indian patients with RS, approximately 44% had heel pain as one of their clinical manifestations.[6] Severe heel enthesopathy may also occur in more than 25% of patients with juvenile-onset SNS; involvement of the plantar fascia is more common than the Achilles tendon. The incidence is similar to that in adults.[7] In another study of 39 children with SNS, 20 patients had tenderness at the calcaneal insertion of the Achilles tendon and 26 at the calcaneal insertion of the plantar aponeurosis.[8] One case of isolated HLA-B27–associated Achilles tendinitis suggests that heel enthesopathy may be the sole clinical manifestation of HLA-B27 disease.[9] Another case highlights the fact that peripheral enthesitis may occur at several sites, such as the ischial tuberosities, greater trochanter, tendinous and ligamentous insertions on the head of the fibula, as well as the calcaneal insertion of the plantar aponeurosis and Achilles insertion.[10]

The differential diagnosis of heel pain includes tendon chondrocalcinosis, local infection resulting from *Mycobacterium tuberculosis* or other organisms, and nodular tendinitis related to a partial rupture of the Achilles tendon. Severe tarsalgia is rarely found in RA, and in the series by Gerster and colleagues[7] no case was associated with gout-related tophi or a hypercholesterolemia-related xanthoma of the Achilles tendon.[5] Heel pain has been reported in sarcoidosis[11] and secondary to enthesopathy in a patient with Behçet's syndrome, a disorder that some believe is part of the spectrum of the SNSs.[12] It is important to emphasize that, although heel pain may be prominent in patients with one of the SNSs, mechanically induced heel pain is a more common cause. The former can be distinguished from more common forms of heel pain by recognizing certain clinical features such as inflammatory changes posteriorly at the paratenon of the Achilles tendon and bursa between the anterior surface of the tendon and posterior surface of the calcaneus (retrocalcaneal recess). Alternative sites of involvement may include the ankle and interphalangeal joints of the digits, the latter producing a "sausage-shaped" toe (dactylitis) characteristic of PsA. Clinical clues that should alert the physician to the possibility of SNS include inflammatory peripheral joint disease that tends to involve four or less joints (i.e., oligoarticular) in an asymmetric pattern, inflammatory axial disease and sacroiliitis with morning stiffness in the low back, eye inflammation (e.g., iritis or conjunctivitis), and psoriasiform skin disorders.[13]

In assessing heel pain, the examiner must also exclude pain referred from a more proximal source such as the back. X-ray film–defined heel spurs are common in patients with and without heel pain; their presence, however, does not always explain the problem, and simple excision may not relieve the pain.[14] Although posterior involvement is common in the enthesopathy of SNS, it is rarely seen in the heel spur syndrome.[13] It is important to try to distinguish between enthesopathy and heel spur syndrome to prevent misdiagnosis and delayed or incorrect treatment.[15]

Investigations

The evolution of radiologic findings in enthesopathy begins with heel erosions and is followed by the development of heel spurs. These occur at sites of prior inflammation at entheses where the Achilles tendon and plantar fascia attach to the calcaneus.[16] Fluffy periostitis at entheses can also be seen.[4] Radiologic bony lesions of the calcaneus are usually present only after several months of heel pain.[5] In a series of 42 patients with RS, arthritis of the heels was seen by roentgenogram in 23. Scintigraphy of the heel of one patient with symptoms for approximately 3 months showed an abnormality at the left calcaneus in the absence of roentgenographic findings.[17]

Pathology

Enthesopathy histologically is characterized by multiple, focal microscopic inflammatory lesions localized to the ligamentous and tendinous attachments, which produce the erosion or defect in the cortical bone. The number of inflammatory cells in the tissue block are very variable but suggests an inflammatory reaction. Lymphocytes and plasma cells predominate, with a few polymorphonuclear leukocytes.[18] The inflammatory process begins in the soft tissues (Achilles peritendinitis, plantar fasciitis) and later may involve the calcaneus bone, with the development of spurs, erosions, and periosteal new bone formation.[19]

Treatment

Nonsteroidal anti-inflammatory drugs (NSAIDs) are often used as the first-line treatment modality in patients with SNS. In a 6-week, double-blind, randomized, prospective study of 32 patients with AS, naproxen, indomethacin, and fenoprofen calcium were the most effective of the six NSAIDs studied. In contrast, patients with RA showed no preference.[20] Olivieri and colleagues reported a patient with juvenile-onset SNS with disabling bilateral heel pain from Achilles enthesopathy who had complete resolution of symptoms with naproxen, 500 mg daily, after failure of adequate trials of diclofenac, local corticosteroid injections, and laser therapy.[21] Olivieri also used naproxen successfully in another patient with isolated peripheral enthesitis.[22] Other adjunctive therapies include a trial of heel cord–stretching exercises, shoes with soft impact–absorbing heels, and cushions within the shoes. Orthotics can be helpful, especially if the patient pronates excessively.[14] Second-line drugs, such as sulfasalazine and methotrexate, are used when the inflammatory process is unremitting or leads to joint or soft tissue damage. Corticosteroid injections into the site of local tissue inflammation are fraught with the possibility of subsequent tendon rupture. Local radiotherapy has also been used with some success in resistant cases of Achilles enthesopathy, with lower risk of leukemia than spinal irradiation because of the smaller area of bone marrow exposed. The risk of long-term tumor and osteonecrosis, however, is unknown.[4, 23, 24]

RHEUMATOID ARTHRITIS

RA is the most common inflammatory disease, affecting about 1% of the general population worldwide.[25] Small joints tend to be affected earlier than large joints, and the lower extremity joints generally are affected earlier in the disease process than upper extremity joints. Although RA may affect any diarthrodial joint, foot and ankle involvement is frequent and many times heralds the onset of the disease process.[26] It has been estimated that 89% of patients with RA have problems with the feet.[27] A prospective study of foot and ankle involvement in 99 outpatients with RA found that 94% of patients had significant foot and ankle complaints.[28] Rheumatoid foot disorders may have a variable clinical course from patient to patient. In general, however, forefoot involvement has been reported to occur more frequently[29] and earlier in the disease course than hindfoot involvement.[30] However, in contrast to previous studies,[31] the hindfoot is also identified as an area of fairly frequent involvement, particularly at the subtalar joint.[32] In a study of 99 rheumatoid patients, when specifically asked about distal lower extremity complaints, 94% reported having symptoms of the ankle and forefoot and 56% identified the ankle region as a primary problem. The longer patients have active RA, the more likely they are to experience foot disease. In one study, 50% of patients had significant foot and ankle symptoms if they had RA for less than 10 years, but the percentage increased to 75% in those patients who had RA for

more than 20 years.[28] Forefoot, subtalar, and ankle disease not only leads to significant functional limitation as a result of local symptoms but can alter the patient's gait pattern and lead to proximal joint stress and progressive damage.

Pathogenesis

The nature and frequency of hindfoot disease are not universally agreed on. Because hindfoot changes occur later in the disease course, it has been suggested that the mechanical stresses of weight bearing are primarily responsible for the development of progressive hindfoot deformity. The more common hindfoot abnormalities include valgus deformity, varus deformity, and planovalgus deformity (consisting of increased heel valgus angulation and tendency toward flattening of the sustentaculum tali and medial and downward slippage of the talar head). Valgus deformity of the hindfoot is the most common disabling defect in patients who have RA and has been reported to be 25 times more common than a varus deformity.[26] Little is known about the pathogenesis of valgus deformity of the hindfoot in patients who have RA or about the implications of this deformity for function of the foot. Several hypotheses as to the cause of this valgus deformity in patients with RA have been advanced. These include cartilaginous and osseous changes in the subtalar and midtarsal joints, laxity of the joint capsules and ligaments secondary to repeated episodes of inflammation and swelling, and rupture and tenosynovitis of the tibialis posterior resulting in decreased function during gait because of pain and weakness.[26, 33, 34]

Although hindfoot disease in RA is a significant cause of disability for patients, the cause of the planovalgus deformity is controversial in terms of whether it is secondary to subtalar joint instability, rupture of the spring ligament, or posterior tibial tendon dysfunction. Although there have been reports of specific instances of posterior tibial tendon rupture in rheumatoid patients, the prevalence of this association is unknown.[35] Some believe that all of the hindfoot deformity seen in RA is a consequence of rheumatoid-related joint laxity without a significant element of posterior tibial tendon dysfunction.[36] Downey and associates[37] have reported on two patients in whom rupture of the posterior tibial tendon coexisted with RA. RA was believed to be the primary deforming factor and showed that RA-related tenosynovitis is the most frequent tendinous lesion and corresponds to a first stage of tendon deterioration in its potential progression toward rupture. However, according to a study of 50 patients with RA[38] and another study based on surgical exploration,[39] the progressive longitudinal arch collapse and hindfoot valgus deformity are a consequence of hindfoot joint destruction rather than posterior tibial tendon insufficiency, which may be relatively unaffected by the rheumatoid process. Fortunately, because treatment of either condition (i.e., primary hindfoot instability or primary posterior tibial tendon rupture) is similar, the distinction is not important clinically.

Clinical Features

Physical examination of the rheumatoid hindfoot should include an observation of the patient's gait and shoes, which provide important information about deformity and areas of increased pressure. When the patient stands on tiptoes, inversion of the hindfoot is noted. With a competent posterior tibial tendon and normal hindfoot motion, the heel should normally shift from a valgus to a varus position during single-leg toe rise. It is important to evaluate the alignment of the heel, because when bony changes and ligamentous laxity affect the hindfoot and midfoot, they lead to a variety of alignment abnormalities, including heel valgus, pes planovalgus, and hindfoot subluxation.[40] Such hindfoot involvement may lead to pain and impaired gait.

In patients who have RA, the alignment of the hindfoot is rarely markedly abnormal during the early stages of the disease. However, changes in the talonavicular and subtalar joints appear to play a dominant role in the development of subsequent deformities. As the duration of disease increases, deformities of the hindfoot begin to determine function and disability.[41]

Because the subtalar articulation is probably the most important joint of the foot,[42] any derangement of this joint has major implications. The range of motion of the ankle and subtalar joints should be evaluated. Restriction of motion, instability, pain or crepitus may be noted. It has been em-phasized clinically that a lack of motion in a joint may not represent a significant problem if it is not associated with disabling pain. This is particularly true in the foot and ankle, where lack of motion can be easily accommodated without greatly altering gait mechanics.[43]

Posterior tibial tendon tenosynovitis sometimes appears obvious when there is typical swelling on the tendinous tract that is localized behind and beneath the medial malleolus up to the tuberosity of the navicular; localized pressure and active inversion against resistance are painful. The tendon is palpated during this last test. The diagnosis of dysfunction of the posterior tibial tendon is difficult to make on clinical grounds, and because relatively few patients ultimately undergo surgery, it has been difficult to correlate these clinical findings with pathologic results. Moreover, there is extreme variability among widely used diagnostic criteria for posterior tibial tendon dysfunction.

Using the presence of all three of the most stringent criteria for diagnosis (loss of the longitudinal arch, inability to perform a heel rise, and lack of a palpable posterior tibial tendon), a study of 99 patients with RA for approximately 13.5 years demonstrated that 11% had posterior tibial tendon dysfunction.[44] Otherwise, based on single diagnostic criteria alone, anywhere from 13 to 64% of patients could be diagnosed as having posterior tibial tendon dysfunction.[45] However, objective evidence of posterior tibial muscle-tendon unit dysfunction was lacking in this study.

Investigations

Plain film radiographic imaging is an important part of the evaluation of patients with rheumatoid foot and ankle problems. In most patients, involvement will be symmetric with joint space narrowing, periarticular bony erosions, juxta-articular osteoporosis, and soft tissue swelling. Sometimes joint space widening from exuberant synovitis, capsular laxity, and joint effusion may also be noted. Lateral radiographic films are useful in patients with planovalgus deformity to determine the exact level of the deformity and the relative contributions of each joint to the deformity. This may be secondary to rheumatoid ankle involvement or secondary to the hindfoot deformity itself.[26]

Computed tomography (CT) scans of the rheumatoid foot reported talonavicular involvement in 39%, calcaneocuboid involvement in 25%, and subtalar involvement in 20%. The benefits of CT include its ability to depict the foot's bone and soft tissue anatomy in the coronal plane and to provide quantitative information about bony relationships and alignment abnormalities in patients who have RA. The ability to make objective, reproducible measurements could facilitate monitoring the course of arthritis and, if more data could be acquired, identify patients who would benefit from surgery.[46] On CT scans, patients with RA would show a characteristic constellation of abnormalities, including soft tissue swelling, cartilage space narrowing, bony erosions, and a pes planovalgus alignment abnormality.

When tendon involvement is suspected, the magnetic resonance imaging (MRI) scan, because of its excellent soft tissue contrast and ability to image sagittal planes, proves to be very effective for highlighting partial ruptures, and especially longitudinal tears, not visualized by the CT. Moreover, using an MRI-enhanced with gadolinium, it is possible to distinguish an inflammatory tenosynovitis (synovial pannus enhancing after gadolinium) from a mechanical tenosynovitis (no enhancement).[47] The CT and the MRI with gadolinium show that the tendinous lesions of the rheumatoid hindfoot are much more frequent, diffuse and important than could have been imagined from the clinical examination and plain roentgenograms.

In addition to CT and MRI, ultrasonography (US) is another procedure that is cheaper and easier to perform,[48] although technician experience must be taken into consideration. US has been helpful in evaluating abnormalities of soft tissues around the ankle joint.[49] High-resolution, real-time US of the heel provides good spatial resolution and selects lesions appropriate for injection, such as bursitis and tenosynovitis. It is inexpensive, readily performed, well tolerated, does not use ionizing radiation, and it is an accurate means for diagnosing tendon and other soft tissue lesions.[50] Although it has been reported that other ankle tendons, besides the Achilles tendon, are difficult to visualize with US,[51] in one study, successful US-guided local steroid injection between the sheath and tendon in patients with posterior tibialis tenosynovitis was performed.[52]

Treatment

In patients with RA, the high prevalence of foot and ankle symptoms stands in contrast to the low frequency of therapeutic interventions.[28] Given the patient-identified severity of ankle and hindfoot problems, more aggressive medical or surgical intervention is warranted. It is also consistent with the observations that symptoms and abnormal mechanics of the forefoot can be the result of hindfoot disease.[34]

Nonoperative foot care is very important in the management of patients with RA, but conservative management of the rheumatoid foot requires a working knowledge of foot mechanics, orthotic devices, and footwear. A pedorthist should be involved in the management of any rheumatoid patient to coordinate the proper footwear with the fabrication of an orthotic device. Simple shoe modifications can improve mobility in patients with limited ankle motion, such as the addition of a long rocker-bottom sole to the shoe; this helps patients to accommodate to the lack of motion in the ankle.[53] The shoe should be supportive and comfortable, allowing for accommodation of a deformity if present, and keep the patient as functional as possible. Improved gait patterns and decreased pain will also decrease the stress on more proximal joints. For patients with hindfoot or midfoot pain from instability or deformity, an ankle-foot orthosis can be used to help to regain their ambulatory capacity. The device extends from the leg across the ankle and incorporates the foot, which provides stability to the foot, absorbing and transmitting a portion of the stresses across the foot and permitting more comfortable ambulation.[26]

Local injection of steroid can be useful in patients with tendinitis and is usually given using palpation to guide needle placement. Ultrasound (US) can be used to confirm precise needle tip placement, which is especially important in the treatment of tenosynovitis, because steroid injection into the tendon substance may cause tendon necrosis, predisposing to rupture.[54] US guidance may be the injection technique of choice but is particularly indicated for patients with lesions unresponsive to injections guided by palpation.[55]

In the absence of deformity, surgery is rarely indicated. However, occasionally synovectomy may be considered if nonsurgical measures fail to control pain and inflammation. If hindfoot disease becomes particularly painful, deforming, or disabling, surgical intervention should be strongly considered, usually including at least a subtalar arthrodesis for stabilization and correction of the deformity. Once the medial longitudinal arch of the foot begins to collapse because of involvement of the subtalar joint, talonavicular joint, or both, one should consider early surgical intervention. The foot should not be allowed to collapse completely before surgical intervention is offered to the patient.[26] Unfortunately, in the foot and ankle, total joint replacements have been less than satisfactory, and at this time ankle fusion still provides the best long-term results.[56]

The primary question regarding arthrodesis is related to which and how many joints to involve in the procedure. Some studies recommend a triple odesis (fusion of the subtalar, talonavicular, and calcaneocuboid joints) for the patient in whom soft tissue repairs seem inadequate.[57] In contrast, others believe that only the transverse tarsal joints need to be fused but that arthrodesis of both is necessary for long-term stability.[58] Finally, some authors have reported that a single arthrodesis is effective. Some prefer to stabilize the subtalar joint alone,[59] which produces the least amount of functional loss for the patient, whereas others have reported performing reduction and arthrodesis on only the talonavicular joint.[60] Increased hindfoot valgus may benefit from posterior tibial tendon and spring ligament reconstruction. This frequently involves triple arthrodesis to correct severe fixed hindfoot valgus and first metatarsophalangeal fusion with less metatarsal head resections. However, although a triple arthrodesis results in a stable, well-aligned foot, after 5 or more years the ankle joint undergoes some degenerative changes in about 30% of cases; for this reason, the triple arthrodesis is reserved for patients with a significant deformity that does not respond to conservative management.[61]

If the posterior tibial tendon has ruptured or shows longitudinal tears, a surgical tendinous transfer does not seem to be the best solution in RA because, even if the other tendons are healthy at the time, they will probably be involved and weakened in this progressive disease. An immediate arthrodesis appears more judicious and will probably help to avoid a later operation. In a 1996 study,[60] 27 patients with posterior tibial tendon insufficiency, but not RA, were treated with talonavicular arthrodesis as the primary stabilizing procedure. All of the patients had a history of a progressive painful flatfoot deformity and exhibited an asymmetric planovalgus deformity of the affected foot, with excessive hindfoot valgus and forefoot abduction. After an average follow-up of 27 months, results were rated as excellent or good in 89%.[60] An isolated talonavicular arthrodesis seems to offer patients with this disorder both reliable pain improvement and lasting stability and perhaps could be tried in patients with similar deformities in RA.

CONCLUSION

Both RA and SNSs have prominent manifestations of heel and Achilles pain, which are often overlooked when other joints may also be involved. It is essential to keep in mind that tendon as well as joint abnormalities are common and may, in fact, be presenting features of these diseases, highlighting the importance of performing a complete physical examination, not merely focusing on the area of complaint. Relatively simple, conservative measures such as orthoses and the right footwear can make the difference between a functional, ambulating patient and one who is disabled.

REFERENCES

1. Khan MA, Van Der Linden SM. Ankylosing spondylitis and other spondyloarthropathies. Rheum Dis Clin North Am 16:551, 1990.
2. Wilkens RF, Arnett FC, Bitter T, et al. Reiter's syndrome: evaluation of preliminary criteria for definite disease. Arthritis Rheum 24:844, 1981.
3. Wollheim FA. Ankylosing spondylitis. In Kelley WN, Harris ED, Ruddy S, Sledge CB, eds. Textbook of Rheumatology, ed 4. Philadelphia: W. B. Saunders, 1993:943.
4. Zvaifler NL, Seagran SL. Local radiotherapy for the painful heels of patients with spondyloarthropathy. In Klippel JH, Dieppe PA, eds. Rheumatology. St. Louis, MO: Mosby-Year Book Europe Limited, 1994:3.30.7.

5. Gerster JC, Saudan Y, Fallet GH. Talalgia: a review of 30 severe cases. J Rheumatol 5:210, 1978.

6. Prakash S, Mehra NK, Bhargava S, Malaviya AN. Reiter's disease in northern India: a clinical and immunogenetic study. Rheumatol Int 3:101, 1983.

7. Gerster JC, Piccinin P. Enthesopathy of the heels in juvenile onset seronegative B27 positive spondyloarthropathy. J Rheumatol 12:310, 1985.

8. Rosenberg AM, Petty RE. A syndrome of seronegative enthesopathy and arthropathy in children. Arthritis Rheum 25:1041, 1982.

9. Olivieri I, Gemignani G, Gherardi S, et al. Isolated HLA B27 associated Achilles tendonitis. Ann Rheum Dis 46:626, 1987.

10. Olivieri I, Gemiganani G, Giovanni B, et al. Isolated HLA B27 associated peripheral enthesitis. J Rheumatol 16:1519, 1989.

11. Shaw RA, Holt PA, Stevens MB. Heel pain in sarcoidosis. Ann Intern Med 109:675, 1988.

12. Olivieri G, Gemignani G, Braccini G, Pasero G. Bechet's syndrome and spondyloarthritis. Br J Rheumatol 29:409, 1990.

13. Turlick MA. Seronegative arthritis as a cause of heel pain. Clin Podiatr Med Surg 7:369, 1990.

14. Deland JT, Wood B. Foot pain. In Kelley WN, Harris ED, Ruddy S, Sledge CB, eds. Textbook of Rheumatology, ed 4. Philadelphia: W. B. Saunders, 1993:459.

15. Scherer PR, Gordon D, Kashanian A, Belvill A. Misdiagnosed recalcitrant heel pain associated with HLA-B27 antigen. J Am Podiatr Assoc 85:538, 1995.

16. Jacobs JC. Spondyloarthritis and enthesopathy. Arch Intern Med 143:103, 1983.

17. Sholkoff SD, Glickman MG, Steinbach HL. The radiographic pattern of polyarthritis in Reiter's syndrome. Arthritis Rheum 14:551, 1971.

18. Ball J. Enthesopathy of rheumatoid and ankylosing spondylitis. Ann Rheum Dis 30:213, 1970.

19. Gerster JC, Hauser H, Fallet GH. Xeroradiographic techniques applied to assessment of Achilles tendon in inflammatory or metabolic disease. Ann Rheum Dis 34:479, 1975.

20. Wasner C, Britton MC, Kraines G, et al. Nonsteroidal anti-inflammatory agents in rheumatoid arthritis and ankylosing spondylitis. JAMA 246:2168, 1981.

21. Olivieri I, Gemignani G, Grassi L, Pasero G. Diffuse Achilles tendon thickening in juvenile onset seronegative HLA B27 positive spondyloarthropathy. J Rheumatol 15:381, 1988.

22. Olivieri I, Pasero G. Longstanding isolated juvenile onset HLA B27-associated peripheral enthesitis. J Rheumatol 19:164, 1992.

23. Mantell BS. Radiotherapy for painful heel syndrome. BMJ 90:1, 1978.

24. Grill BV, Smith M, Ahern M, Littlejohn G. Local radiotherapy for pedal manifestations of HLA-B-27-related arthropathy. Br J Rheumatol 27:390, 1988.

25. Firestein GS. Etiology and pathogenesis of rheumatoid arthritis. In Kelley WN, Harris ED, Ruddy S, Sledge CB, eds. Textbook of Rheumatology, ed 5. Philadelphia: W. B. Saunders, 1997:851.

26. Mann RA, Horton GA. Management of the foot and ankle in rheumatoid arthritis. Rheum Dis Clin North Am 22:457, 1996.

27. Vainio K. The rheumatoid foot: a clinical study with pathological and roentgenological comments. Ann Chir Gynaecol 45:1, 1956.

28. Michelson J, Easley M, Wigley FM, Hellman D. Foot and ankle problems in rheumatoid arthritis. Foot Ankle Int 15:608, 1994.

29. Solomon G. Inflammatory arthritis. In Jahss MH, ed. Disorders of the Foot and Ankle: Medical and Surgical Management, ed 2. Philadelphia: W. B. Saunders, 1991:1681.

30. Vidigal E, Jacoby RK, Dixon AS. The foot in chronic rheumatoid arthritis. Ann Rheum Dis 34:292, 1975.

31. Van Der Heijde DM, Van Leeuwen MA, Van Riel PL. Biannual radiographic assessments of hands and feet in a three-year prospective follow-up of patients with early rheumatoid arthritis. Arthritis Rheum 35:26, 1992.

32. Anderson EG. The rheumatoid foot: a sidewalk look. Ann Rheum Dis 49(Suppl):S851, 1990.

33. Cracchiolo A. Surgery for rheumatoid disease: instructional course lectures. Am Acad Orthop Surg 33:386, 1984.

34. Platto MJ, O'Connell PG, Hicks JE, Gerber LH. The relationship of pain and deformity of the rheumatoid foot to gait and an index of functional ambulation. J Rheumatol 18:38, 1991.

35. Simkin PA, Downey DJ, Richardson ML. More on the posterior tibial tendon in rheumatoid arthritis (letter). Arthritis Rheum 32:1050, 1989.

36. Keenan MA, Peabody TD, Gronley JK, Perry J. Valgus deformities of the feet and characteristics of gait in patients who have rheumatoid arthritis. J Bone Joint Surg Am 73:237, 1991.

37. Downey DJ, Simpkin PA, Mack LA. Tibialis posterior tendon rupture: a cause of rheumatoid flatfoot. Arthritis Rheum 31:441, 1988.

38. Kirkman BW, Gibson T. Comment on the article by Downey et al (letter). Arthritis Rheum 32:359, 1989.

39. Jahss MH. Tendon disorders of the foot and ankle. In Jahss MH, ed. Disorders of the Foot and Ankle: Medical and Surgical Management, ed 2. Philadelphia: W. B. Saunders, 1991:1461.

40. Pastershank SP. Mid-foot dissociation in rheumatoid arthritis. J Can Assoc Radiol 32:166, 1981.

41. Spiegel TM, Spiegel JS. Rheumatoid arthritis in the foot and ankle: diagnosis, pathology and treatment. The relationship between foot and ankle deformity and disease duration in 50 patients. Foot Ankle Int 2:318, 1982.

42. Jahss MH. The subtalar complex. In Jahss MH, ed. Disorders of the Foot. Philadelphia: W. B. Saunders, 1982:727.

43. Buck P, Morrey BS, Chao EYS. The optimal position of arthrodesis of the ankle: a gait study of the knee and ankle. J Bone Joint Surg Am 69:1052, 1987.

44. Funk DA, Cass JR, Johnson KA. Acquired adult flat foot secondary to posterior tibial tendon pathology. J Bone Joint Surg Am 68:95, 1986.

45. Michelson J, Easley M, Wigley FM, Hellman D. Posterior tibial tendon dysfunction in rheumatoid arthritis. Foot Ankle Int 16:156, 1995.

46. Seltzer SE, Weissman BN, Braunstein EM, et al. Computed tomography of the hindfoot with rheumatoid arthritis. Arthritis Rheum 28:1234, 1985.

47. Bouysset M, Tavernier T, Tebib J, et al. CT and MRI evaluation of tenosynovitis of the rheumatoid foot. Clin Rheum 14:303, 1995.

48. Van Holsbeeck M, Katcherian D, Wu KK, Introcaso JH. Patterns of posterior tibial tendon abnormality (abstract). Radiology 185:143, 1992.

49. Kalebo P, Allenmark C, Peterson L. Diagnostic value of ultrasonography in partial ruptures of the Achilles tendon. Am J Sports Med 20:378, 1992.

50. Gibbon WW, Cassar-Pullicino VN. Heel pain. Ann Rheum Dis 53:344, 1994.

51. Cheung Y, Rosenburg ZS, Magee T. Normal anatomy and pathological conditions of ankle tendons: current imaging techniques. Radiographics 12:429, 1992.

52. Cunnane G, Brophy DP, Gibney RG, Fitzgerald O. Diagnosis and treatment of heel pain in chronic inflammatory arthritis using ultrasound. Semin Arthritis Rheum 25:383, 1996.

53. Ouzonian TJ, Kleiger B. Arthrodesis in the foot and ankle. In Jahss MH, ed. Disorders of the Foot and Ankle: Medical and Surgical Management, ed 2. Philadelphia: W. B. Saunders, 1991:2614.

54. Balasubramaniam P, Prathap K. The effect of injection of hydrocortisone into rabbit calcaneal tendons. J Bone Joint Surg Br 54:729, 1972.

55. Brophy DP, Cunnane G, Fitzgerald O, Gibney G. Technical report: ultrasound guidance for injection of soft tissue lesions around the heel in chronic inflammatory arthritis. Clin Radiol 50:120, 1995.

56. Clayton ML. Management of the rheumatoid ankle. In Clayton ML, Smyth CJ, eds. Surgery for Rheumatoid Arthritis. New York: Churchill Livingstone, 1992:295.

57. Jahss MH. Miscellaneous soft tissue lesions. In Jahss MH, ed. Disorders of the Foot and Ankle: Medical and Surgical Management, ed 2. Philadelphia: W. B. Saunders, 1991:828.

58. Clain MR, Baxter DE. Simultaneous calcaneocuboid and talonavicular fusion: long term follow-up study. J Bone Joint Surg Am 76:133, 1994.

59. Johnson JE, Johnson KA, Unni KK. Persistent pain after excision of interdigital neuroma: results of reoperation. J Bone Joint Surg Am 70:651, 1988.

60. Harper MC, Tisdel CL. Talonavicular arthrodesis for the painful adult acquired flatfoot. Foot Ankle Int 17:658, 1996.

61. Graves SC, Mann RA, Graves KO. Results of triple arthrodesis in older adults following long-term follow-up. J Bone Joint Surg Am 75:355, 1995.

15

Heel and Hindfoot Pain in the Pediatric and Adolescent Patient

Cathleen L. Raggio

The pediatric and adolescent populations generally do not suffer from pain as do adults. When children complain of pain, a logical differential diagnosis should be entertained (Tables 15–1, 15–2, 15–3). On the basis of a careful history and thorough physical examination, the practitioner can narrow the list of possible diagnoses to a few. This chapter attempts to give the reader an overview of the unique pediatric causes of pain in the heel and hindfoot. It does not attempt to address all congenital abnormalities of the foot but only those associated with pain as a presentation.

TARSAL COALITION

Tarsal coalition is defined as the fusion of two or more tarsal bones. The coalition may be fibrous, cartilaginous, or bony. Fibrous coalitions or syndesmoses of the tarsal bones are generally asymptomatic. Cartilaginous, synchrondroses, and bony synostosis fusions may be symptomatic. The coalition may be an isolated anomaly or may be part of a syndrome (e.g., Apert's and Nievergelt Pearlman syndromes). They may also be as-

Table 15–1. Differential Diagnosis of Tendo-Achilles Tightness

1. Functional: secondary to normal growth, especially in adolescents
2. Congenital (familial): short Achilles
3. Neurologic disorders
   Cerebral palsy
   Myelomeningocele
   Muscular dystrophies
4. Spinal disorders
   Tethered spinal cord
   Intraspinal anomalies (e.g., lipoma)
   Syrinx
5. Residual clubfoot deformity
6. Pes planus "valgus ex equinus" (see Table 15-2 for differential diagnosis)
7. Congenital vertical talus associated with syndromes
8. Sever's disease (see text)

Table 15–2. Differential Diagnosis of Pes Planus

Flexible
  Idiopathic: no treatment
Inflexible/painful
  Idiopathic: associated with tight tendo-Achilles; normal subtalar motion; treatment consists of physical therapy
  Tarsal coalition (see text)
  Accessory navicular (see text)
  Ruptured posterior tibialis tendon (rare in children)
  Inflammatory conditions (see text)
  Tumors (see text)

sociated with other synostoses of the carpus and finally may be part of major limb anomalies such as fibular hemimelia, proximal focal femoral deficiency, and absence of rays.[1]

Tarsal coalitions were first described by Buffon[2] in the late 1700s, but it was not until the late 1800s that the clinical significance of the coalitions became apparent.

Etiology

The majority of tarsal coalitions are secondary to the failure of differentiation or segmentation of the fetal primitive mesenchymal tissue. The genetic inheritance is commonly autosomal dominant with variable penetrance. Secondary tarsal coalitions may occur and result from a variety of conditions, including (1) intra-articular fractures, (2) juvenile rheumatoid arthritis, (3) infection, and (4) tumors.

Table 15–3. Differential Diagnosis of Decreased Subtalar Arc of Motion

1. Tarsal coalition
2. Inflammatory conditions
3. Infection
4. Tumors

Incidence

Although an exact incidence in the entire population is impossible to calculate, most studies of large population segments reveal no more than 1% of the population with a coalition. Coalitions are bilateral in approximately 50% of cases. The most common sites for a coalition are the calcaneonavicular and the medial talocalcaneal joints. These two sites account for 90% of all coalitions. Other sites such as talonavicular, calcaneocuboid, and naviculocuneiforms are generally rare and variably symptomatic.

Presentation

In infancy and early childhood, the coalition is generally asymptomatic. As a child's tarsals mature and ossify, symptoms may appear. The common age of presentation for a calcaneonavicular bar is 8 to 12 years, although cases in children as young as 2 have been reported.[3]

Talocalcaneal coalitions become symptomatic later in early adolescence at ages 12 to 16. The age-related symptoms are a factor of (1) normal bony ossification of the tarsals, (2) increased weight of the individual with maturity, and (3) increased activity, especially sports.

Symptoms and Signs

The patient comes to the physician with one of two presentations: (1) an asymptomatic flatfoot, the cosmetic appearance of which bothers the parent or the child; (2) a symptomatic painful foot with an associated flatfoot deformity. The symptoms are an achy pain in either the foot or ankle region. The pain increases with activities and may preclude participation in sports. There is often a history of repeated ankle sprains. On close questioning, a history of difficulty walking on uneven or rough terrain may be elicited. A family history may reveal others with flatfeet and difficulty with pain in their advancing years.

Physical examination consists of a full pediatric orthopedic evaluation to rule out associated anomalies. In the typical coalition, the patient will be between 8 and 16 years of age. Any child younger than 8 should be carefully examined for one of the conditions to which reference has been made (see Etiology).

The most common presentation is that of a rigid planovalgus foot. There is decreased motion of the subtalar complex, and the tendo-Achilles will be tight when heel valgus correction is attempted. The heel valgus does not correct with toe walking, which may, in itself, be difficult. The most extreme presentation is the "peroneal spastic foot." The deformity is secondary to the pain reflex in which the heel is in extreme valgus. The irritation of weight-bearing activities in heel valgus and restricted subtalar arc of motion leads to tightness of the peroneal tendons over time. The persistent contracture leads to forefoot abduction and valgus, leading to peroneal irritation, the so-called "spasm."

Roentgenographic Evaluation

As with most conditions, a thorough history and physical examination will narrow the differential diagnosis. X-ray films, computed tomography (CT), and magnetic resonance imaging (MRI) scans, however, are necessary to make a firm diagnosis. The recommended x-ray films are standing anteroposterior (AP), lateral, and obliques of the feet. Diagnosis of a calcaneonavicular bar is made on the oblique x-ray film (Fig. 15–1).

Associated findings include subtalar process blunting, elongation of the anterior calcaneal process, talar beaking, and narrowing of the posterior subtalar joint. The CT scan is the next step to evaluate the middle facet subtalar coalitions often not apparent on plane films (Fig. 15–2). The facet may be obviously fused, but angulation of the facet of more than 20% from horizontal is consistent with coalition. The MRI is also sensitive for coalitions, especially the fibrous or cartilagenous bars. In the younger child, an MRI may be the first choice because the coalitions will be less ossified.[4]

Previous imaging included 45° axial x-ray views of the heel, tomography, and bone scans; however, these have been supplanted by both MRI and CT scans as the second imaging study to obtain in coalition definition.

Treatment

Once the definitive diagnosis has been made, treatment is begun. An asympto-

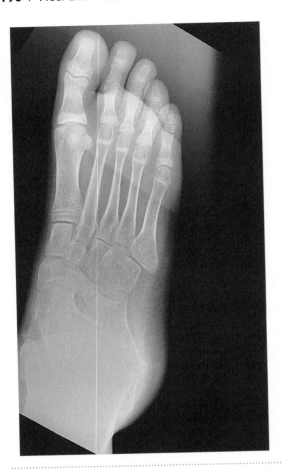

Figure 15–1. Oblique x-ray film of calcaneonavicular coalition.

Calcaneonavicular coalitions are best treated by a wide excision of the coalition and interposition of the extensor digitorum brevis muscle in the interval. Postoperative care should include a brief period of immobilization followed by an extensive physical therapy program to regain motion. Weight bearing should be withheld until full range of motion is achieved. Orthotic use may help in the initial weight-bearing period to maintain alignment. The success of the surgery is generally close to 80% with excellent or good results and only 7% with poor results.[5] The best results were achieved in those patients younger than 16 and in the synchondrotic bars.

The surgical treatment of middle-facet coalitions is more difficult and controversial. Some authors advocate resection and interposition grafting regardless of the percentage of the facet joint involvement.[6] Others[7] recommend resection only if less than 50% of the middle facet is affected. In patients with additional significant posterior-facet degenerative changes, an isolated subtalar fusion may offer the best pain relief.[8] Finally, if there are degenerative changes in both the midfoot and hindfoot, a triple arthrodesis is indicated. A hindfoot osteotomy may be needed for severe deformity.[8]

matic foot should probably not be treated because no long-term studies of adults who had asymptomatic coalitions as adolescents and who experience painful feet have been reported.

Symptomatic patients should be placed in a short leg walking cast for several weeks if the foot is extremely tender or if tightness of the peroneal exists. Once the foot is relaxed after casting, a well-molded orthotic can be made. A UCBL is a good orthotic device that supports the hindfoot and can maintain a painless foot for sports activities. I recommend a program of physical therapy consisting of stretching the tendo-Achilles and peroneals and strengthening the posterior tibialis. Heel and toe walking are also good exercises to maintain muscle balance. If compliant, nonoperative treatment fails to relieve the patient's symptoms, then surgical intervention is indicated.

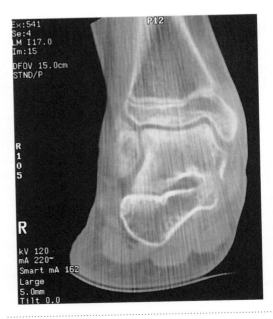

Figure 15–2. Computed tomographic scan of talocalcaneal coalition.

ACCESSORY NAVICULAR

Accessory bones of the foot in children are seen in 4 to 21% of the populations studied. The accessory navicular is often an incidental finding on x-ray examination, but it may be the source of pain in the hindfoot because of associated symptoms and so is discussed in this chapter. The accessory navicular can be described as one of three types. Type I is the os tibiale externum, in which there is a sesamoid bone in the posterior tibialis tendon. There is a small distance (<3 mm) between the sesamoid and the navicular. Type II consists of an accessory bone, up to 1.2 cm in diameter, in which a synchondrosis exists between it and the navicular (Fig. 15–3A, B). Type III is the fused accessory navicular to the navicular, resulting in a large cornuate navicular (Fig. 15–4A, B). Generally, types I and III are asymptomatic; type II can be symptomatic and accounts for 50 to 70% of all accessory naviculars reported.

Signs and Symptoms

The typical patient is a young female (10–20 years) who complains of chronic midfoot and arch pain. There is pain over the prominence, and the patient will report difficulty with footwear. There may be pain over the posterior tibialis tendon from a tendinitis and tightness of the tendo-Achilles. There is often a pes planovalgus (flatfoot) deformity. Physical examination reveals an exquisite tenderness over the accessory navicular, which often has an inflamed bursa over it.

Roentgenographic Data

Routine AP/lateral and oblique x-ray films are taken to assess the feet. The x-ray find-

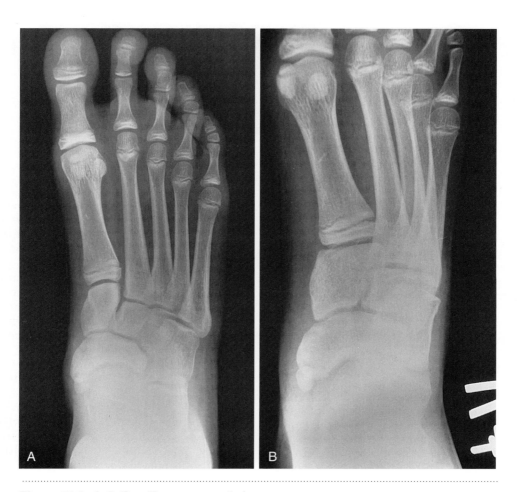

Figure 15–3. *A, B,* Type II accessory navicular.

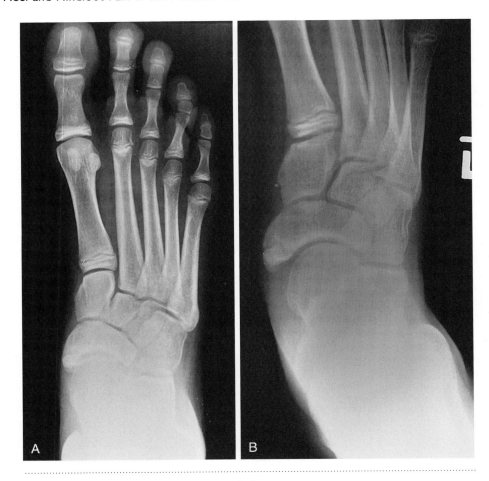

Figure 15–4. *A, B,* Type III accessory navicular.

ings are straightforward (see Figs. 15–3 and 15–4). However, it is important not to assume that the painful foot is secondary to the accessory navicular. Other conditions such as stress fractures, tight heel cords, tumors, tendinitis, and tarsal coalitions may be the true cause of the pain.

Treatment

In light of the incidental nature, the secondary muscle imbalances, and the tendinitis associated with an accessory navicular, nonoperative treatment should be maintained for at least 6 months before any surgical intervention. Depending on the severity of the posterior tibialis tendinitis, a short leg walking cast should be applied for 3 weeks. After this, a well-padded shoe orthotic should be worn. A physical therapy program

of Achilles and peroneal stretching and posterior tibialis strengthening should be instituted. The patient may then resume normal activities and maintain good foot balance through the exercise regimen. If the symptoms recur, the casting can be reinstituted. Surgical intervention is indicated for relentless, symptomatic feet in spite of all modalities of treatment. The surgical procedure of choice is a simple resection of the accessory navicular. The medial prominence is removed flush to the medial border of the midtarsal area. The posterior tibialis tendon is longitudinally split for exposure and is not advanced, as described by Kidner.[14]

The flatfoot deformity associated with the accessory navicular is not corrected by the surgery. This should be discussed with the patient and parents before surgery to avoid any misconceptions. Postoperatively, the foot is maintained in a short leg walking cast for several weeks. A physical therapy program is begun after cast removal, and the shoe is padded to avoid pressure over the wound. The operation is successful in 90% of the patients as long as expectations and criteria are clear.[9]

SEVER'S DISEASE

Sever's disease is a traction apophysitis at the Achilles tendon insertion in a skeletally immature patient. Like most cases of traction apophysitis in children and adolescents, there is a localized muscle tightness, which comes first; the "itis" or inflammation or the contracture of the Achilles tendon has not been established. The patient is generally a male involved in running-related sports, especially over hard surfaces. The age of onset is between prepubertal to adolescent (9–14 years) and correlates with growth spurts.[10]

The patient complains of heel pain with running and, if untreated, pain with walking. The physical examination is specific for tenderness to palpation and transverse compression of the calcaneal apophysis. Dorsiflexion of the ankle is limited and may reproduce the symptoms. X-ray films are nondiagnostic but may rule out other conditions. The x-ray finding of sclerosis and fragmentation of the apophyses is nonspecific and is a normal variant. The treatment consists of rest, a heel lift, if there is limited dorsiflexion, and ice. The use of antisteroids is an individual preference. In severe cases, a plantar flexed cast (25°) may be worn for several weeks to rest the area completely. The key is a physical therapy program of stretching and strengthening of the tendo-Achilles and dorsiflexors. The patient must be instructed on the recurrent nature of the disease and the importance of stretching and application of ice before and after athletic endeavors.[11]

Sever's disease is a condition that children outgrow, but the quality of their athletic endeavors can be enhanced with appropriate care and prophylactic stretching programs.

RETROCALCANEAL BURSITIS

The retrocalcaneal bursa can be inflamed secondary to improperly fitted shoes. Compared with Sever's disease the complaints include pain and swelling in the posterior and lateral aspects of the heel. Treatment consists of a heel pad in well-fitting shoes. Ice and open-heel shoes offer some immediate relief. Radiographs are negative, although a report by Heneghan and Wallace[12] noted loss of the lucent retrocalcaneal recess in an otherwise normal x-ray film.

KÖHLER'S DISEASE

Köhler's disease is a self-limited osteochondrosis of the immature navicular (Fig. 15–5). It was first described by Köhler in 1908[13] on radiograph evaluation. The cause is postulated to be mechanical. Repetitive compression forces to the navicular lead to irregular ossification. Biopsies, performed before current knowledge, reveal areas of necrosis, resorption, and new bone formation.[14] The average age at presentation is 4 years (range, 2–9 years). Köhler's disease is more common in boys and is bilateral in 30% of cases. The patient presents with an antalgic limp and tends to bear most of the weight on the lateral border of the foot. In the very young child, there may be a refusal to weight bear, and this young group (ages 2–3) present a dilemma in making the ini-

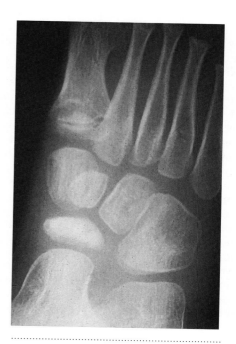

Figure 15–5. Köhler's disease.

tial diagnosis. A careful pediatric orthopedic exam can generally rule out spine, hip, and knee disorders and localize the pain to the foot. There is tenderness on palpation of the navicular. Swelling may or not be present. The remainder of the exam is normal, especially subtalar and ankle range of motions.

Treatment depends on the severity of symptoms. In cases of intense pain, refusal to bear weight, or limited weight bearing, a short leg cast should be placed for several weeks. The cast can be placed with the foot in 10 to 15° of varus and equinus, as suggested by Tachijian.[8] However, this author places the foot in as near neutral a heel position as possible to allow weight bearing. In milder cases, a soft longitudinal arch support is all that is needed. The outcome is excellent. Studies of long-term outcome[15] show that the navicular reconstitutes within 1 to 3 years from onset. There is no residual deformity in adulthood.

INFECTIONS

Cellulitis, osteomyelitis, soft tissue abscesses, and septic arthritis are causes of heel pain. Patients often present without constitutional symptoms or signs of infection. Puncture wounds, commonly caused by stepping on a nail, may lead to cellulitis, osteomyelitis, osteochrondritis, and septic arthritis in children. Patients have tenderness and swelling around the puncture site. They rarely have leukocytosis, but the erythrocyte sedimentation rate may be moderately elevated. Most children who sustain this injury have no sequelae. They should be treated with irrigation of the puncture tract, tetanus prophylaxis, and, if there is evidence of cellulitis, oral gram-positive antibiotics. *Staphylococcus aureus* is the most common cause of cellulitis.

Osteomyelitis develops in 0.6 to 1.8% of patients with plantar puncture wounds. *Pseudomonas aeruginosa* accounts for as many as 93% of all cases of puncture wound osteomyelitis.[16] Sneakers, work boots, and other forms of warm moist footwear are known to harbor *P. aeruginosa* species. When a nail penetrates through the sole, it drives bacteria from the shoe into the skin and the wound.[17] Because *P. aeruginosa* has an affinity for cartilage, it invades the physis and articular surfaces of joints in the foot. In addition to osteomyelitis, osteo-

chondritis, septic arthritis, or an intraosseous abscess may develop.[18] Irrigation, surgical debridement, and administration of intravenous antibiotics must be performed immediately in all of these entities.

Other causes of infectious heel pain can come from bites and sexually transmitted diseases. Underlying conditions may also predispose patients to infections in the hindfoot. Cellulitis after a dog or cat bite is caused by *Pasteurella multocida*. Cellulitis or septic arthritis may develop secondary to Lyme disease. Lyme disease, caused by the infectious spirochete *Borrelia burgdorferi* is transmitted by the Ixodes tick.[19] Patients with chlamydial reactive arthritis or sickle cell anemia may experience osteomyelitis in the hindfoot. Hematogenous calcaneal osteomyelitis has been reported in schoolchildren.[20] There is a case report of an 8-year-old boy with chronic granulomatous disease who experienced a soft tissue infection of the heel after riding a motor scooter. The infection was insidious with minor heel pain. His hindfoot infection was caused by *Paecilomyces varioti*.[21] Although infections of the hindfoot are uncommon, a careful history is essential for establishing the appropriate diagnosis.

INFLAMMATORY DISEASES

Juvenile rheumatoid arthritis and seronegative spondyloarthropathies are causes of hindfoot pain in children and adolescents. Also known as talalgia, heel pain is frequently the first symptom of the seronegative spondyloarthritides[22]: Reiter's syndrome, anklyosing spondylitis, and psoriatic arthritis. Most of these patients are carriers of the antigen HLA-B27.

Patients with juvenile rheumatoid arthritis frequently have foot and ankle pain that can most often be managed nonoperatively with special shoes and orthotics. Whereas the subtalar joint or ankle is affected in pauciarticular disease, both of these joints as well as the midfoot and forefoot are involved in polyarticular disease. The ankle often contracts in equinus, whereas the subtalar joint may develop a varus or valgus deformity. Osteotomies or arthrodesis should be considered only if these deformities cannot be corrected by conservative measures (i.e., footwear, orthotics, or casting). The goal is to maintain a plantigrade, mobile, and pain-free foot.[23]

Seronegative spondyloarthropathies include those types of arthritis associated with sacroiliitis, spinal arthritis, and enthesitis.[24] Patients have an absence of rheumatoid factor in their blood. Boys are affected four times as often as girls. These patients experience heel pain secondary to Achilles tendinitis and plantar fasciitis. The pain is exacerbated by weight bearing and is relieved with rest. Patients may also have associated "sausage" digits and bony lesions on the calcaneus. When the pain is located in the calcaneus itself, other diagnoses should be considered, notably stress fractures or bone tumors.[25] Surgery is contraindicated during the inflammation phase, because it may cause local aggravation and risk ankylosis of the talocalcaneal articulation. Most patients respond well to medical therapy.

TRAUMA

Fractures of the talus and calcaneus as well as osteochondral fractures of the talus are traumatic causes of heel pain in children and adolescents. A thorough history will disclose the mechanism of injury so that the appropriate management is administered. A nondisplaced fracture of the hindfoot may be missed with plain films; therefore, a bone scan may be helpful in establishing the diagnosis.

Talus fractures and subtalar dislocations in children are rare. Because the talus is largely cartilaginous, it is more resilient to compression injury than bone. Also children are lighter than adults, so less force is generated across the bone during a fall from a height. The usual mechanism of injury is forced ankle dorsiflexion. If the fracture is displaced more than 2 mm, open reduction and internal fixation should be performed.[26] Subtalar dislocation occurs with high-energy trauma. The foot is usually medially displaced. Unless the dislocation is more than 3 weeks old, closed reduction and casting in a neutral position is appropriate treatment.[27]

Like the talus, the calcaneus is largely cartilaginous; it too is more resilient to compressive forces. The mechanism of injury is high-energy trauma, a fall from a height, or a motor vehicle accident. Contrary to adults, in whom 60% of calcaneal fractures are intra-articular and 40% are extra-articular, children sustain intra-articular calcaneal fractures 40% of the time and extra-articular fractures 60% of the time.[28] In addition, associated injuries, such as lumbar spine fractures, are much less frequent in children. Because the majority of calcaneal fractures are extra-articular and the calcaneus undergoes remodeling in children with further growth, the long-term sequelae (i.e., posttraumatic arthrosis, difficulty with footwear, and lateral impingement) seen in adults after calcaneal fractures are less frequent in children. Open reduction and internal fixation technique is reserved for large-fragment avulsions or joint disruption.

Osteochondral fractures of the talus may cause heel pain. They usually occur after an ankle sprain. The posterior medial aspect of the talus is the most common location for this lesion. The lesion is a microscopic fracture of subchondral bone, often missed on plain films. The staging system for the lesions is as follows: stage 1, subchondral fracture without collapse; stage 2, incomplete separation of the fragment; stage 3, unattached, undisplaced fragment; stage 4, unattached, displaced fragment (Fig. 15–6). If symptoms persist after an ankle sprain but the roentgenograms are normal, a bone scan or MRI will highlight the injury. Treatment depends on the stage of the injury: stage 1 and 2 injuries, cast immobilization for 6 weeks; stage 3 and 4 injuries, arthroscopic curettage and drilling or excision.

TUMORS

Tumors in the hindfoot are uncommon but must be considered when evaluating a child

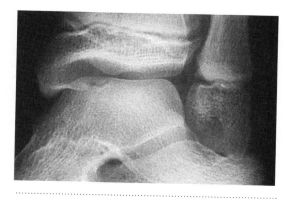

Figure 15–6. Osteochondral fracture.

or adolescent with heel pain. Persistent pain in a child with an otherwise normal examination, normal lab results, and negative x-ray films should be evaluated by a bone scan. This will localize a lesion, if present. If normal, then expectant watching of the patient is indicated. The types of tumors vary with the site of origin. Soft tissue tumors that may occur in the hindfoot region are epithelioid sarcoma and plantar fibromatosis. Osteoid osteoma and osteosarcoma originate from bone; osteochondroma and chondroblastoma stem from cartilage. Nonossifying fibroma, unicameral bone cyst, and intraosseous lipoma are all fibrous tumors. Aneurysmal bone cyst, Ewing's sarcoma, and leukemia are entities derived from marrow.

Although epithelioid sarcoma is the most common soft tissue sarcoma of the hand, it may also occur in the subcutaneous and deep tissues of the foot. More common in males in their second or third decade of life, epithelioid sarcoma is rarely painful because it is slow growing.[29] Plantar fibromatosis also occurs more frequently in males in their second or third decade. It is a locally aggressive tumor found in the plantar fascia and should be treated nonoperatively.[30] A case of infantile digital fibromatosis in a 3-year-old girl has been reported. Two tumors were present on the fourth toe and over the lateral aspect of the heel. The tumors showed spontaneous regression without therapy.[31]

Osteoid osteoma usually occurs in the second decade in males and is characterized by night pain, relieved with aspirin. Physical exam reveals a tender mass or joint effusion, and the patient may walk with a limp.[32] Radiographs demonstrate dense reactive bone surrounding a radiolucent nidus that is smaller than 1 cm in diameter. A CT scan may be used to better localize the nidus in areas where the bony architecture is complex, such as the hindfoot. Although the lesion is benign and self-limiting, complete or en bloc excision is the treatment of choice.[33]

Isolated osteochondromas are rare in the foot, but may be seen in patients with the inherited autosomal dominant disease multiple familial osteochondromatosis. Like osteoid osteomas, these lesions occur in the second decade; however, they are usually not painful. Heel pain occurs when the os-

teochondroma fractures, compresses a nerve, or interferes with footwear.

Chondroblastoma is a benign tumor seen more often in males during their second and third decades. When it exists in the foot, this entity is most commonly located in the calcaneus. Symptoms are heel pain and effusion associated with a traumatic event. Curettage with bone graft is the treatment of choice. Malignant transformation is not reported in the foot.[33]

Nonossifying fibroma is one of the most common primary lesions of bone, with a peak incidence in the second decade. It is rarely symptomatic; in certain cases, however, a pathologic fracture or a nonossifying fibroma in another location may lead to heel pain. In one study, an adolescent girl complaining of chronic heel pain was found to have acquired hypophosphatemic rickets and a nonossifying fibroma of the femur. The hypophosphatemic rickets was completely corrected by surgical excision of the bone lesion.[34]

Unicameral bone cysts also occur in the second decade. They are usually painless and are commonly found in the proximal humerus and proximal femur. The calcaneus is an uncommon site for a unicameral bone cyst. However, because of the concentration of forces through the heel, such calcaneal cysts are usually symptomatic and require treatment. For the asymptomatic patient, observation or aspiration and steroid injection is the appropriate treatment. For the symptomatic patient or the high-impact athlete, the treatment of choice is curettage with bone graft.[35]

Aneurysmal bone cyst, Ewing's sarcoma, and leukemia are all tumors of marrow origin that create heel pain. They are radiolucent on roentgenograms. Although the aneurysmal bone cyst is benign and leukemia is malignant, both are extremely rare in the hindfoot. Ewing's sarcoma presents in the second decade and in only 2% of patients with foot and ankle lesions. The disease has a better prognosis if it exists in the appendicular skeleton. Patients complain of pain, especially at night; swelling; fever; night sweats; and weight loss. Treatment includes chemotherapy, radiation therapy, and wide local resection.[30]

REFERENCES

1. Grogan DP, Halt GR, Ogden JA. Talocalcaneal coalition in patients who have fibular hemimelia or

proximal femoral focal deficiency: a comparison of the radiographic and pathological findings. J Bone Joint Surg Am 76:1363–1370, 1994.

2. Buffon GL. Historic Naturelle, Generale et Particuliere, Tome 3. Paris: Panekaucke, 1769:47.

3. Cowell HR. Diagnoses and management of peroneal spastic flatfoot. AAOS Instr Course Lect 24:94, 1975.

4. Munk PL, Vellet AD, Livin MF. Current status of magnetic resonance imaging of the ankle and hindfoot. Can Assoc Radiol J 43:19–30, 1992.

5. Gonzalez P, Kumar SJ. Calcaneonavicular coalition treated by resection and interposition of the extensor digitorium brevis muscle. J Bone Joint Surg Am 72:71–77, 1990.

6. Kumar SJ, Guille JT, Lee MS, Cuoto JC. Osseous and non-osseous coalition of the middle facet of the talocalcaneal joint. J Bone Joint Surg Am 74:529–535, 1992.

7. Swiontkowski MF, Scranton PE, Hansen S. Tarsal coalitions: long term results of surgical treatment. J Pediatr Orthop 3:287–292, 1983.

8. Tachijian MD. Textbook of Pediatric Orthopaedics, ed2. Philadelphia: W. B. Saunders, 1990:2600.

9. Bennett GL, Weiner DS, Leighley B. Surgical treatment of symptomatic accessory tarsal navicular. J Pediatr Orthop 10:445–449, 1990.

10. Madden CC, Mellion MB. Sever's disease and other causes of heel pain in adolescents. Am Fam Physician 54:1995–2000, 1996.

11. McKenzie DC, Taunton JE, Clement DB, et al. Calcaneal epiphyses in adolescent athletes. Can J Sport Sci 6:123–125, 1981.

12. Heneghan MA, Wallace T. Heel pain due to retrocalcaneal bursitis—radiographic diagnosis. Pediatr Radiol 15:119–122, 1985.

13. Köhler A. Übereine Haufige besher ansheinend unbekannte Erkiankung, eingelner Kenderlicker Knohen Muncher Mi. Wachenschr 55:1923, 1908.

14. Kidner FC, Muro F. Köhler's disease of the tarsal scaphoid or os navicular, pedis retardatum. JAMA 83:650, 1924.

15. Ippolito E, Pallini PTR, Falez F. Köhler's disease of the tarsal navicular: longterm followup of 12 cases. J Pediatr Orthop 4:416, 1984.

16. Jacobs RF, McCarthy RE, Eiser JM. *Pseudomonas* osteomyelitis complicating puncture wounds of the foot in children: a 10 year evaluation. J Infect Dis 160:657–661, 1989.

17. Fisher MC, Goldsmith JF, Gilligan PH. Sneakers as a source of *Pseudomonas aeruginosa* in children with osteomyelitis following puncture wounds. Pediatrics 106:607, 1985.

18. Jarvis JG, Skipper J. *Pseudomonas* osteochondritis complicating puncture wounds of the foot in children. J Pediatr Orthop 14:755–759, 1994.

19. Steere AC, Malowista SE, Snydman DR. Lyme arthritis: an epidemic of oligoarticular arthritis in children and adults in three Connecticut communities. Arthritis Rheum 20:7, 1977.

20. Winker H, Scharli AF. Hematogenous calcaneal osteomyelitis in children. Euro J Pediatr Surg 1:216–220, 1991.

21. Williamson PR, Kwan-Chung, KJ, Gallin JI. Successful treatment of *Paecilomyces varioti* infection in a patient with chronic granulomatous disease and a review of *Paecilomyces* species infections. Clin Infect Dis 14:1023–1026, 1992.

22. Gerster JC, Saudan Y, Fallet GH. Talalgia: a review of 30 severe cases. J Rheumatol 5:210–216, 1978.

23. Morrissy RT, Weinstein SL. Lovell and Winter's Pediatric Orthopaedics. Philadelphia: Lippincott-Raven, 1996.

24. Schaller JG. The seronegative spondyloarthropathies of childhood. Clin Orthop 143:76, 1979.

25. Winfield AD, Dennis JM. Stress fractures of the calcaneus. Radiology 72:415–418, 1959.

26. Kasser JR. Orthopaedic Knowledge Update. Rosemont, IL: American Academy of Orthopaedic Surgeons, 1996.

27. Richards BS. Orthopaedic Knowledge Updates: Pediatric Orthopaedics. Rosemont, IL: American Academy of Orthopaedic Surgeons, 1997.

28. Rockwood CA, Wilkins KE, Beaty JH. Fractures. Philadelphia: Lippincott-Raven, 1996.

29. Chase DR, Enzinger FM. Epithelioid sarcoma: diagnosis, prognostic indications, and treatment. Am J Surg Pathol 9:242–263, 1985.

30. Lewis MM. Musculoskeletal Oncology: A Multidisciplinary Approach. Philadelphia: W. B. Saunders, 1992.

31. Shi N, Matsui K, Takahashi Y, Nakajima H. A case of infantile digital fibromatosis showing spontaneous regression. Br J Dermatol 121:129–133, 1978.

32. Jackson RP, Reckling FW, Mants FA. Osteoid osteoma and osteoblastoma: similar histologic lesions with different natural histories. Clin Orthop 128:303–313, 1977.

33. Lutter LD, Mizel MS, Pfeffer GB. Orthopaedic Knowledge Update Foot and Ankle. Rosemont, IL: American Academy of Orthopaedic Surgeons, 1994.

34. Asnes RS, Berdon WE, Bassett CA. Hypophosphatemic rickets in an adolescent cured by excision of a nonossifying fibroma. Clin Pediatr 20:646–648, 1981.

35. Moreau G, Letts M. Unicameral bone cyst of the calcaneus in children. J Pediatr Orthop 14:101–104, 1994.

16

Thrombophlebitis as a Cause of Heel and Rearfoot Pain

Geoffrey H. Westrich

Although pain in the lower extremity may arise from many causes such as trauma and surgery, thrombophlebitis is common after injury to the lower extremity and may also elicit pain. Deep venous thrombosis (DVT) alone may or may not be symptomatic; however, subsequent pulmonary embolism is potentially life threatening. Therefore, common knowledge about the prevention, diagnosis, and treatment of thromboembolic disease is essential to any physician who treats patients with disorders of the lower extremity. Furthermore, DVT should always be included in the differential diagnosis of pain and swelling in the lower limb.

Patients who have undergone orthopedic operations such as total joint replacement and fracture fixation are at greatest risk for the development of thromboembolism; however, such a complication may also occur, although less commonly, after foot and ankle surgery and foot and ankle trauma. Although the literature is replete with articles about thromboembolic disease after total joint replacement, hip fracture surgery, and orthopedic trauma, far less attention has been directed to this problem in patients with disorders of the foot and ankle. This chapter focuses on the pathogenesis of DVT and pulmonary embolism, available diagnostic modalities, accepted prophylactic regimens, and treatment of established thromboembolism. In addition, a review of the foot and ankle surgery literature with respect to thromboembolic disease is also included.

THROMBOEMBOLIC DISEASE: OVERVIEW

Virchow initially described venous thromboembolism in 1856; however, the true morbidity and mortality in patients were not recognized for many years later. Approximately 90% of clinically important pulmonary embolisms arise from proximal DVT of the lower extremities, and it is estimated that pulmonary embolism may be fatal in 50,000 to 100,000 individuals a year. This statistic accounts for 5 to 10% of all hospital deaths in the United States annually. Venous thromboembolism is the third most common vascular disease, following acute ischemic attacks and cerebrovascular accidents. Unfortunately, pulmonary embolism is difficult to diagnose and has the potential to be rapidly fatal. Among the patients who will eventually die of a pulmonary embolism, two thirds will survive less than 30 minutes after the event, which is insufficient for most forms of treatment to be effective.[1] Certainly, preventing DVT is preferable to treating the condition after the diagnosis is established. Fortunately, the presence of clinical risk factors can be used to identify patients at greatest risk.[2] However, despite convincing evidence of the efficacy of a number of prophylactic agents, physicians have been slow to adapt these preventive regimens in patients at risk for thromboembolic disease.

Thromboembolic disease continues to pose a major threat for patients undergoing lower extremity surgery. A DVT occurs when one or more of the veins in the calf become obstructed to venous blood flow. In high-risk patients, such as those with total joint replacement of the hip and knee, the incidence of DVT without postoperative prophylaxis diagnosed by venography has been reported as high as 88%.[3–5] The majority of these thrombi occur in the deep veins of the calf; however, propagation of a calf thrombosis to a more proximal location in the popliteal or femoral veins is also known to occur. Using serial venous Doppler ultrasound, the rate of propagation after total knee replacement surgery has been documented at 23%.[6] Therefore, one must be cognizant of the fact that a DVT in the calf has the potential to propagate, and one should monitor these patients expectantly.

Pulmonary emboli result when a DVT in

the lower extremity or pelvis embolizes through the right side of the heart and into the pulmonary vasculature. As a result, a thromboembolism may lodge within the pulmonary artery, thus causing an obstruction of perfusion to the lung. Although many pulmonary emboli are asymptomatic, such an event may be fatal. The size and location of the pulmonary embolism are related to the morbidity and mortality of the event; a large saddle-type embolism has the greatest risk of mortality. After total joint replacement, the incidence of asymptomatic pulmonary emboli detected by routine lung scans has been reported to be between 10 and 20%, whereas the incidence of symptomatic pulmonary emboli is between 1 and 2%.[7, 8] Many surgeons may ignore the possibility of thromboembolic disease, because the occurrence of clinically significant pulmonary embolism is relatively uncommon, and the symptoms are easily confused with other medical conditions, such as cardiac or pulmonary problems.

Prevention of thromboembolic disease is essential to avoid the morbidity and mortality associated with this condition. A significant risk of hemorrhagic complications is associated with anticoagulation for thromboembolic disease in the immediate postoperative period. After total joint replacement surgery, Patterson and colleagues[9] from The Hospital for Special Surgery reported that anticoagulation with heparin within the first 5 postoperative days was associated with a complication rate greater than 50%. Unfortunately, the associated morbidity and mortality with untreated symptomatic thromboembolic disease are also significant.[8]

THROMBOEMBOLISM IN FOOT AND ANKLE SURGERY

Whereas much of our knowledge of thromboembolic disease is assimilated from the orthopedic literature, the risk after foot and ankle surgery is intuitively less common and has not been as thoroughly evaluated. Only recently has thromboembolism been evaluated in the foot and ankle literature. Mizel and coworkers[10] studied clinically apparent thromboembolic events in patients undergoing foot and ankle surgery. In their study of 2733 such patients, the authors noted only six calf or thigh DVTs and only

four nonfatal pulmonary emboli for a total prevalence of 0.22%. An interesting finding in the study was that patients who were non-weight bearing or immobilized after surgery of the foot and ankle had a 0.4% increase or a prevalence of 0.62%. Still, the rate of thrombosis in this cohort was quite low. The authors concluded that the routine use of postoperative prophylaxis for DVT after surgery of the foot and ankle might not be warranted.

In interpreting their conclusion, one must be cognizant of the fact that this was a multicenter retrospective study with 13 institutions and that routine screening for DVT or pulmonary embolism was not performed. We can assume, therefore, the true incidence of thromboembolic disease was grossly underreported. Whether this is clinically relevant, however, remains unanswered in this patient population.

RISK FACTORS FOR THROMBOEMBOLIC DISEASE

Multiple risk factors have been identified that increase a patient's predisposition to thromboembolism. Although these factors are discussed individually, one should recognize that patients may have multiple risk factors, which may further increase their propensity for a thromboembolic event. As such, patients should be classified as to their relative level of risk (Table 16–1).

History of Thromboembolism

Patients with a history of thromboembolic disease are at significant risk for repeat thromboembolism. Hospitalized patients who have a history of thromboembolic disease have an increase of acute thromboembolism of almost eightfold compared with patients without such a history. As such, this is one of the more important risk factors for thromboembolic disease. Patients with a history of thromboembolic disease who undergo major surgery, immobilization, or a protracted hospitalization for serious medical illness must be considered to be at very high risk. Thromboembolic disease prophylaxis is mandatory in this cohort of patients.

Table 16–1. Classification of Level of Risk

Thromboembolic Event	Low Risk*	Moderate Risk†	High Risk‡	Very High Risk§
Calf vein thrombosis	2%	10–20%	20–40%	40–80%
Proximal vein thrombosis	0.4%	2–4%	4–8%	10–20%
Clinical pulmonary embolism	0.2%	1–2%	2–4%	4–10%
Fatal pulmonary embolism	0.002%	0.1–0.4%	0.4–1.0%	1–5%

*Uncomplicated minor surgery in patients younger than 40 with no risk factors.
†Major surgery in patients older than 40 with no other risk factors.
‡Major surgery in patients older than 40 with additional risk factors.
§Major surgery in patients older than 40 with history of thromboembolism, malignancy, major orthopedic surgery, cerebrovascular event, or spinal cord injury.
Adapted from Clagett GP, Reisch JS. Prevention of venous thrombosis in general surgical patients: results of meta-analysis. Ann Surg 208:227–240.

Elective Lower Extremity Surgery

Orthopedic surgery of the lower extremity is well appreciated as one of the most significant risk factors for development of thromboembolic disease. Without prophylaxis, DVT may develop in more than 50% of patients undergoing elective total joint replacement surgery.[11] More than 90% of proximal thrombi occur on the operated side in hip replacement. Twisting and kinking of the common femoral vein during the surgical procedure have been shown to occlude femoral venous return and also damage venous endothelium.

Fractures of the Pelvis, Hip, and Long Bones

Fractures of hip joint, pelvis, and long bones of the lower extremity have a significant association with the development of thromboembolic disease. Historically, patients with such fractures were recognized as high risk and used as a model to study the efficacy of various prophylactic regimens. A reduction in mortality from pulmonary embolism was noted with systemic anticoagulation. The mortality rate secondary to pulmonary embolism in patients with hip fractures who do not receive prophylaxis may be as high as 10%.[12] Patients with a long bone fracture of the lower extremity that require cast immobilization are also considered at increased risk.

Multiple Trauma

It is now accepted that patients who sustain multiple trauma are at a significantly increased risk for the development of thromboembolic disease. Studies have established an independent and significant risk for such patients, especially when the primary site of injury includes the face, chest, or abdomen. In this group, the incidence of DVT may be as high as 40%.[13] Patients with pelvic and acetabular fractures are especially prone to thromboembolic disease. Thromboembolic disease prophylaxis is mandatory in this cohort of patients.

General Surgery

Abdominal operations that require general anesthesia for greater than 30 minutes result in a significantly increased risk for thromboembolic disease.[14] An increased risk of thromboembolic disease is also associated with neurosurgery, coronary artery bypass surgery, major urological surgery, and surgery for gynecological malignancy. Of note, the risk for thromboembolic disease may be reduced with new surgical techniques that use endoscopic methods compared with open surgical procedures.

Patient Age

The incidence of thromboembolic disease increases exponentially between ages 20 and 80 years of life.[15] Although a 40-year-old patient has traditionally been used as an indication for an age-related increase in thromboembolic disease, the risk continues to increase after age 40 and nearly doubles with each successive decade. Thromboembolic disease is rare in children and usually occurs with high-risk situations, such as multiple trauma and lower extremity fractures.

Malignancy

Patients with malignancy are at increased risk for thromboembolic disease because of the hypercoagulable state that many of these patients experience. Advanced pancreatic cancer, gynecologic cancer, lung cancer, breast cancer, gastrointestinal cancer, and brain tumors are particularly linked to this increased risk.[16] The hypercoagulant state is known to result from both an increase in procoagulant activity and a reduction in fibrinolysis. Chemotherapy has a toxic effect on the endothelium and may produce an additional thrombotic effect. Surgery for malignant disease results in a two- to threefold increase in the risk for thromboembolism compared with surgery for nonmalignant ailments.

Immobility

It is widely accepted that immobilization results in an increased risk for thromboembolic disease. An autopsy study noted a 15% incidence of thrombosis in patients at bedrest for less than 1 week compared with 80% in patients at bedrest for greater than 1 week.[17] Early mobilization of all patients after surgery or trauma is necessary to prevent thromboembolism. Immobilization secondary to traumatic spinal cord injury and paralysis of lower extremities has an associated risk of thromboembolic disease that approaches 40%.

Obesity

Although obesity is usually cited as a risk factor for the development of thromboembolism, the actual risk is unclear. It is possible that obese patients with other risk factors may have an additive or synergistic risk for thromboembolism; however, this is speculation and has not been scientifically established. Furthermore, the term obesity is subjective and open to interpretation. One should use a percentage over ideal body weight to truly study obesity.

Oral Contraceptives and Estrogen Therapy

Although historically oral contraceptives were associated with an increased risk of thromboembolism, current preparations use less estrogen and are associated with a significantly lower risk of thromboembolic disease. Currently, mortality from oral contraceptives is considered to be less than the risk of pregnancy itself. Although estrogen therapy may increase incidence of thromboembolism in patients with prostate cancer, estrogen replacement therapy in women appears not to be an additional risk factor.[18, 19]

Hypercoagulable States

More attention has been directed to systemic hematologic abnormalities that may predispose patients to thromboembolism. The presence of a lupus anticoagulant as well as deficiencies of protein S, protein C, and antithrombin III all reduce the fibrinolytic activity and put the patient at increased risk of thromboembolism.

PATHOGENESIS

The formation of DVT is multifactorial and was best described by Virchow in 1846.[20] Virchow's triad established the basis of our understanding of the pathogenesis of DVT and includes hypercoagulability, endothelial injury, and venous stasis.[21] In the human vascular system, there is a delicate balance between thrombosis and fibrinolysis, and either surgery or trauma to the lower extremity affects all three aspects of Virchow's triad. Hypercoagulability occurs as a result of activation of clotting factors with a decrease in antithrombin III levels and changes in platelet activity. Also, bone surgery produces the release of thromboplastins, which further activate the clotting cascade. Surgery may also lead to endothelial injury of the vessels. Venous stasis occurs by two mechanisms: the use of a tourniquet or by postoperative immobilization, thus inhibiting the normal venous return in the low extremity. Postoperative swelling and limited ambulation further contribute to venous stasis and the establishment of a milieu that facilitates the formation of DVT.

Other comorbidities are factors in the formation of DVT or subsequent pulmonary embolism, and the surgeon should be aware of these risk factors preoperatively. Such risk factors include advanced age (older than 40 years), female gender, obesity, immobilization, oral contraceptive use, superficial thrombophlebitis, a history of DVT or pulmonary embolism, and cardiac disease. If one considers the fact that most patients undergoing knee replacement are elderly and many have comorbid conditions, it is obvious that these patients are at extremely high risk for DVT.

DIAGNOSIS OF THROMBOEMBOLISM

It must be understood that the majority of DVTs are asymptomatic and, therefore, not grossly apparent on physical examination. However, when the clinical suspicion of thrombosis in the lower extremity does exist, the accuracy of the physical examination for the diagnosis of DVT (e.g., Homans' sign, cords, edema) is notoriously unreliable. Therefore, screening tests, such as a venogram or an ultrasound imaging study, are often used to establish whether a DVT exists.[22] In addition, many current treatment protocols rely on the location and the extent of a DVT in the lower extremity, as determined by the screening test.

Routine postoperative screening for DVT is performed in many institutions; however, the type of screening test varies considerably.[22–36, 82, 97, 98] In addition, the efficacy of such tests is dependent on the technician who performs the study as well as the radiologist who interprets the findings.[22–36] This has become so variable that some authors have recommended that each institution perform an internal validity study to assess the sensitivity, specificity, predictive values, and accuracy of the screening test that is used within that institution.[37, 38] In addition, a learning curve has been noted with such techniques that warrant initial study and then subsequent study to document improvement in the reliability of the screening test.[39] Some centers use routine DVT screening with duplex ultrasonography before discharge. The sensitivity of duplex ultrasound scanning varies widely and has been shown to be extremely operator dependent.[40] Because sensitivity is lowest for calf thrombi, a follow-up duplex study may be beneficial for detecting distal thrombi that may propagate.

At the Hospital for Special Surgery, we evaluated the efficacy of color Doppler imaging for the detection of calf, popliteal, and femoral thrombosis compared with ascending venography in a prospective blinded trial.[99] Ascending venography was considered the gold standard with which all ultrasound studies were compared. Overall, the sensitivity of color Doppler ultrasound was 67.4% and the specificity, 99.2%. In the latter 6 months of the study in which the ultrasound technician had gained considerable experience, significant improvement was noted, with a sensitivity of 83.3% and a specificity of 100%. Our initial assessment of color Doppler imaging for the detection of thrombosis in postoperative total joint replacement patients was less than satisfactory but improved significantly after the technician gained experience. Because of the limitations of duplex ultrasound screening and its associated cost, we have almost eliminated routine screening after major orthopedic procedures and now routinely provide secondary postdischarge prophylaxis for 6 weeks postoperatively.

PROPHYLACTIC REGIMENS

The ultimate goal of any prophylactic regimen is to prevent not only the formation of a DVT but also the occurrence of symptomatic or fatal pulmonary emboli. However, the incidence of symptomatic and fatal pulmonary emboli is low. As a result, a definitive evaluation of the various prophylaxis regimens would require many thousands of patients. Therefore, most studies have focused on the prevention of DVT. Although there are limitations in this methodology, studies have shown that a DVT places a patient at risk for pulmonary emboli.[11, 14] Proximal thrombi represent the greatest risk; however, calf thrombi have also been shown to propagate to the proximal veins in approximately 23% of patients, and have been correlated with the occurrence of both symptomatic and asymptomatic pulmonary emboli.[13, 16] Numerous prophylactic regimens have been studied in orthopedic surgery and include pharmacologic agents such as warfarin, low-molecular-weight heparins (LMWHs) and aspirin as well as mechanical devices such as compression stockings and foot pumps.

Warfarin

Warfarin has become a popular form of prophylaxis after orthopedic surgery.[77, 83] Warfarin is an oral anticoagulant that inhibits the blood coagulation cascade by affecting the synthesis of active vitamin K–dependent coagulation factors (factors II, VII, IX and X as well as protein C). Because warfarin inhibits synthesis of active coagulation factors, it has no effect on existing circulating coagulation factors. Therapeutic anticoagulation is reached 24 to 72 hours after the initial dose of warfarin. Most commonly, 5 or 10 mg of warfarin (Coumadin) is started the night before or the night of surgery and then dosing is adjusted to maintain an INR (international normalized ratio) of 2.0 to 2.5.

Risks for using warfarin include bleeding and, less frequently, warfarin-induced skin necrosis. Bleeding complications have been reported in 0 to 4% of patients receiving warfarin prophylaxis.[41–43] Another pitfall associated with the use of warfarin is the need to monitor the prothrombin time. The advantages of warfarin are that it is administered orally and can be continued as treatment if DVT is detected.

Like most prophylactic regimens, the incidence of DVT using low-dose warfarin varies considerably depending on the patient population at risk. Although warfarin appears to be an effective agent in reducing the incidence of DVT after total hip replacement, its efficacy in knee replacement surgery is not clear. Warfarin may limit propagation and embolization of a thrombus after total knee arthroplasty, but it has not clearly been shown to decrease the occurrence of DVT. Warfarin has also been shown to be effective after orthopedic trauma; however, multiply injured patients may not be candidates for anticoagulation because of head or major organ involvement.

Low-Molecular-Weight Heparin

LMWHs comprise a relatively new form of prophylaxis that has been popularized in Europe and is currently being evaluated in the United States.[79, 84, 94] LMWH was developed in the 1970s and has been shown to have very good antithrombotic activity. Compared with standard heparin, the LMWHs have less bleeding per unit of equivalent antithrombotic effect. LMWHs are the fractionated forms of heparin with a molecular weight ranging from 4000 to 6000 D. Several LMWH compounds are produced by various pharmaceutical companies, each differing in its fractionation technique and dosing schedule. However, all LMWHs contain a specific tetrasaccharide that binds antithrombin III. Because of their smaller size, they can bind antithrombin III, and this complex can inactivate coagulation factor Xa to a greater extent than factor IIa. Its small size also inhibits their combining with heparin cofactor II, a specific mediator that inactivates factor IIa. These compounds have a high bioavailability at low doses, unlike standard heparin, because they only bind to one circulating protein. LMWHs are administered in a fixed dose without daily monitoring of partial thromboplastin time.

Currently, only enoxaparin is approved by the Food and Drug Administration (FDA) for DVT prophylaxis in patients undergoing orthopedic surgery or trauma. Dalteparin is approved by the FDA for general surgical use, but has not been approved for orthopedic surgery at this time. The advantages of LMWHs are that they are easily administered in the hospital with subcutaneous injection and do not require monitoring with partial thromboplastin times. Risks associated with using LMWHs include bleeding and heparin-induced thrombocytopenia. Major bleeding complications have been reported in 0 to 2.8% of patients. Other disadvantages are that they are relatively expensive, require self-injection or help with injection (if administered after discharge), and have a known associated risk of bleeding.

Aspirin

Aspirin (acetylsalicylic acid) is a nonsteroidal anti-inflammatory agent that irreversibly inhibits cyclooxygenase of platelets, thereby inhibiting the synthesis of thromboxane A2.[44] Thromboxane A2 causes platelet aggregation and vasoconstriction. Aspirin has been reported to be an effective antithrombotic agent in patients with ischemic heart disease and cerebrovascular disease. It gained popularity as a prophylactic modality in orthopedic patients after early reports of success in total hip replacement.[44] Follow-up reports and further evaluation revealed that aspirin is not an effective agent in preventing DVT in patients who had total joint replacement surgery or trauma.

Some authors recommended the continued use of aspirin after hospital discharge as a secondary prophylactic agent.[45] These authors noted that aspirin is safe and is associated with a low rate of pulmonary emboli and that most thrombi that occur with the use of aspirin are found in the calf veins. Risks of using aspirin include the development of gastritis, gastric erosions, and gastric ulcers. These side effects appear to be dose related. Most regimens use aspirin by mouth, 325 to 650 mg twice daily.

We do not routinely use aspirin as a single prophylactic agent after major orthopedic surgery; however, we have noted that when aspirin is combined with routine venographic screening and treatment of detected thrombi, it is associated with a low rate of symptomatic and fatal pulmonary emboli.

Mechanical Devices

Mechanical devices and physical agents have been used for the prophylaxis of DVT after a variety of surgical procedures or trauma. Early mobilization, continuous passive motion machines, and graded compression stockings have all been advocated. A number of studies have demonstrated that mechanical devices designed to reduce venous stasis are effective in reducing the rate of DVT after total joint arthroplasty.[13, 16, 23, 25, 27–29, 35, 36, 38, 39, 46–61] Currently, marketed devices incorporate different parameters such as foot pumps, foot-calf pumps, calf pumps, and calf-thigh pumps, whereas some are singe chamber yet others provide sequential chambers with a number of chambers. Although the optimal characteristics of these pumps to reduce DVT and pulmonary embolism are not yet known, it has been proposed that pneumatic compression devices are effective by two mechanisms: decreased stasis (accelerated venous emptying) and increased fibrinolysis.[1, 13, 23, 25, 27, 35, 36, 38, 39, 46–52, 54–56, 58, 60, 61] However, the relative contribution of these two mechanisms is unknown. Newer devices that produce impulse pumping, as opposed to a slow rise in venous return, have been introduced. Although some of these devices are thought to produce an increased peak venous velocity, the optimal contribution of increased venous velocity or increased venous volume necessary to provide adequate DVT prophylaxis in the lower extremity is unclear.[13, 27, 39, 46, 48–52, 54, 56, 58, 60–62] In addition, the fibrinolytic effect of such impulse pumping devices has not been elucidated.

Intermittent pneumatic devices include polyvinyl boots or leggings, stockings with inflatable bladders, multicompartment vinyl leggings, and more recently foot pumps.[63, 64, 85–88] Generally, pressures reach 35 to 55 mm Hg and inflate in cycles of 60 to 90 seconds. The devices are intended to decrease stasis by augmenting venous flow in the lower extremities. In addition, studies have shown stimulation of the fibrinolytic system with the intermittent compression.[65]

The boot or stockings can be applied to the nonoperative leg preoperatively and the operative extremity postoperatively. The pneumatic devices are continued until the patient is ambulating independently. The pneumatic devices can also be used in conjunction with continuous passive motion.

The incidence of DVT with the use of calf and thigh-length devices has been reported to be between 7.5 and 33% after unilateral total knee arthroplasty.[13, 66–71] We evaluated the efficacy of a multichamber thigh-length pneumatic compression stocking compared with aspirin in a randomized, prospective study and found that the incidence of DVT was reduced to 22% with pneumatic stockings compared with 47% with aspirin.[13] The greatest reduction was seen in large thrombi (> 6 cm), which were reduced from 31% with aspirin to 6% with the pneumatic stockings. Patients undergoing simultaneous bilateral total knee arthroplasty are at even higher risk for DVT. Despite the use of pneumatic compression stockings, a DVT developed in 48% of patients.

More recently, there has been interest in the use of foot pump devices. These devices increase venous circulation by applying a rapid increase in pressure to the plantar plexus. Studies have shown that these devices can lead to a significant increase in venous flow in the lower extremity.[52] Two studies have evaluated foot pumps in knee replacement. Westrich and Sculco evaluated the efficacy of the PlexiPulse (NuTech, San Antonio, TX) device combined with aspirin compared with aspirin alone.[72] The authors found a significant reduction in DVT with the use of a PlexiPulse; a DVT developed in 27% of patients using the Plexipulse compared with 59% using aspirin alone. Although no patient using Plexipulse experienced proximal thrombi, 14% of the patients using aspirin alone were found to have proximal thrombi. Westrich and Sculco also evaluated compliance and found a relationship between DVT and the duration for which the device was used. Wilson and associates evaluated the efficacy of foot compression after knee arthroplasty.[64] They found a significant reduction in proximal thrombi; 19% in the control group compared with 0% using foot pumps.

Pneumatic devices have been shown in numerous studies to lower the incidence of both proximal and distal thromboses after total joint replacement. Additionally, these devices have been associated with an extremely low rate of complications. Generally, however, they are not recommended for use in patients with severe peripheral vascular disease. The devices are relatively inexpensive, but compliance problems have been noted by some. The foot pump devices appear to be well tolerated, and we are now using them routinely on our knee replacement patients at The Hospital for Special Surgery. The use of foot pumps or other mechanical compression devices after surgery or trauma of the foot and ankle may be difficult, because most of these patients are immobilized in a splint or cast. Although under-cast pads are available for mechanical compression, these devices have not been studied for their clinical efficacy.

RECOMMENDED PROPHYLAXIS

It is well accepted that patients undergoing major orthopedic surgery are at very high risk for thromboembolic disease, and they should receive an effective primary prophylactic agent to prevent this predicament.[78, 80, 81, 90–93, 95] The type of prophylactic regimen, however, is dependent not only on the patient's relative risk factors for the development of thromboembolism but also the type and duration of surgical intervention. The ideal type of prophylaxis inhibits all thrombus formation and allows healing of the sur-

gical site without bleeding or other complications. Unfortunately, no such prophylaxis regimen is currently available. As discussed in the previous section, the several prophylactic regimens that are commercially available and would satisfy the necessity for prophylaxis do not inhibit all thrombus formation and also have some associated risks.

Patients undergoing foot and ankle surgery are at less risk for thromboembolism than from major orthopedic surgery such as total joint replacements. However, such patients are still at risk for the development of thromboembolic disease, albeit with less relative risk than those undergoing more extensive orthopedic surgery. As such, one needs to assess the relative risk for thromboembolism, and compare this with the potential risks of the prophylactic treatment. Is it justifiable to use heparin or warfarin in a young healthy patient after an elective foot operation to prevent thromboembolism? What is the relative risk, and what prophylaxis, if any, should be used in patients who undergo foot and ankle surgery?

To answer this question, one should evaluate the literature and establish criteria for such patients. However, there are few data regarding the incidence of thromboembolism after foot and ankle surgery. Mizel and coworkers[10] studied clinically apparent thromboembolic events in patients undergoing foot and ankle surgery, with a prevalence of only 0.22%. Although they also noted that patients who were non-weight bearing or immobilized were at increased risk (with a prevalence of 0.62%), the rate of thrombosis in this cohort of patients was still quite low. As such, they concluded that the routine use of postoperative prophylaxis for DVT after surgery of the foot and ankle is not warranted. Because the authors did not routinely screen their patients, the study grossly under-reported the true incidence of thromboembolism, and the authors' conclusions may be debatable.

I maintain that the surgeon is obliged to discuss the possibility of thromboembolism with any patient who plans to have surgery of the foot and ankle and especially evaluate patients to determine who may be at increased risk. In patients with known risk factors, such as previous thromboembolism, age greater than 40 years, history of malignancy or obesity, postoperative prophylaxis is strongly encouraged. Because random-

Table 16–2. Suggested Prophylactic Regimens

Regimen	Low Risk*	Moderate Risk†	High Risk‡	Very High Risk§
Prophylaxis	None or aspirin (3–6 weeks)	Aspirin (3–6 weeks) or warfarin (3–6 weeks)	Warfarin (3–6 weeks) or pneumatic compression device and warfarin or LMWH	Warfarin (3–6 weeks) or pneumatic compression device and warfarin or LMWH
Screening	Not indicated	Not indicated	If no screening, continue prophylaxis for 3 to 6 weeks or routine screening with ultrasonography	If no screening, continue prophylaxis for 3 to 6 weeks or routine screening with ultrasonography

LMWH = low-molecular-weight heparin.
*Uncomplicated foot and ankle surgery in patients younger than 40 with no risk factors for thromboembolic disease.
†Uncomplicated foot and ankle surgery in patients older than 40 with no other risk factors for thromboembolic disease.
‡Complicated foot and ankle surgery in patients older than 40 years with other known risk factors for thromboembolic disease.
§Foot and ankle surgery in patients with a history of thromboembolic disease.

ized, prospective studies evaluating different types of prophylactic regimens have not been performed in this patient population, we have to extrapolate the recommendation from other studies (Table 16–2).

TREATMENT OF ESTABLISHED THROMBOEMBOLISM

Treatment of DVT in the postoperative patient is not without potential complication, and the goals for treatment must be clearly defined. Preventing embolization of the clot is the primary concern because of the possibility of fatal pulmonary embolism. Morbidity from postphlebitic syndrome and pulmonary hypertension are also concerns. Numerous factors must be taken into consideration when deciding on the appropriate treatment, including location of the thrombi, patient age, underlying medical status, history of thromboembolism, and time interval since surgery.

Treatment regimens for DVT include anticoagulants, vena cava interruption devices, and, in the case of calf thrombosis, serial clinical or ultrasound monitoring.[96]

Anticoagulants

The most commonly used anticoagulants are heparin and warfarin; however, more recently LMWHs are being investigated for treatment of DVT. Medical patients without contraindication to anticoagulation are gen-

erally treated with initial administration of intravenous heparin along with the initiation of warfarin therapy. When the warfarin dosage is therapeutic with an INR between 2.0 and 2.5 (prothrombin time at 1.3–1.5 × normal), the heparin is discontinued. Warfarin is generally continued for a period of approximately 6 weeks to 3 months.

Unfortunately, intravenous heparin therapy in the postoperative period has been shown to be associated with a high incidence of complications, including bleeding at the operative sight, gastrointestinal bleeding, thrombocytopenia, venous thrombosis, and arterial thrombosis. Patterson and colleagues found that when intravenous heparin therapy was administered within the first 5 days after joint replacement surgery, bleeding from the wound occurred in 50% of patients.[9] The occurrence of wound bleeding dropped to 15% when heparin was started more than 1 week after surgery. Overall, heparin therapy had to be discontinued in 35% of patients because of local or systemic complications related to heparin therapy.

The use of warfarin therapy appears to be associated with less complication than intravenous heparin. The risk of bleeding is, however, related to the intensity of the therapy. Hull and associates reported a decrease in bleeding complications from 22.4% to 4.3% when a moderately intense regimen of warfarin (prothrombin time between 16–18) was used.[73]

LMWHs administered subcutaneously have been advocated for use in the treatment of DVT. The LMWH compounds are generally administered with subcutaneous injection twice daily. Numerous studies indicate that the LMWHs are at least as effective as intravenous heparin. Although not yet FDA approved for the treatment of DVT, LMWHs may prove to be a simpler and safer method of treatment.

Vena Cava Filter Devices

Numerous vena cava filters are available in the United States.[84] These devices are generally placed by interventional radiologists or vascular surgeons. The filters are placed percutaneously in the inferior vena cava and stop the migration of emboli from the distal venous system to the lungs. These devices have been shown to be effective in reducing pulmonary embolism while maintaining adequate blood flow. Long-term follow-up of the Greenfield filter revealed a recurrent embolism rate of 4% and a patency rate of 98%.[74] Indications for vena cava filter include recurrent embolism despite anticoagulation and DVT with a contraindication to, or complication of, anticoagulation therapy. Vena cava filters have also been advocated as prophylaxis in high-risk patients undergoing total joint replacement surgery.

The filters have no effect on the dissolution of thrombi and, therefore, no effect on the risk of postphlebitic syndrome. Complications are unusual but can occur. At insertion, there is a risk of filter misplacement (2.6%) and a risk of bleeding at the insertion site. Although rare, migration of the vena cava filter can occur over time as can bleeding secondary to perforation of the vena cava.

Thrombolytics

Thrombolytics, such as streptokinase and urokinase, dissolve thrombi and are used mainly for massive pulmonary emboli. Complete clot lysis occurs in 30 to 40% of patients medicated with these agents.[75] Because of the extremely high risk of bleeding, there is almost no indication for thrombolytics in the postoperative orthopedic patient.

Surgical Intervention

Surgical intervention (i.e., venous thrombectomy or pulmonary embolectomy) is per-

formed only in extreme cases: (1) patients with venous obstruction that leads to cerulea dolens and limits the viability of the leg and (2) patients with massive pulmonary embolization who have not responded to other therapy.

RECOMMENDED TREATMENT

There is a general agreement that large proximal thrombi and symptomatic pulmonary emboli should be treated aggressively (Table 16–3). In addition to medical treatment (i.e., intravenous fluids, oxygen, possible ventilation support), these patients require a vena cava filter or anticoagulation with heparin followed by long-term warfarin therapy. The choice of whether to use a vena cava filter or anticoagulation must be individualized. If heparin is chosen in the early postoperative period, one must be cautious not to give large boluses of heparin, which may transiently raise the partial thromboplastin time to greater than 100 seconds. We generally use vena cava filters for patients in whom proximal thrombi or symptomatic pulmonary emboli develop within the first 5 days after major orthopedic surgery. Warfarin should be continued for 3 to 6 months. Patients who are identified with large proximal thrombi or symptomatic pulmonary emboli after the first 7 days are generally treated with intravenous heparin, followed by 3 to 6 months of low-dose warfarin therapy.

There continues to be controversy concerning the treatment of calf thrombi in the postoperative patient. At The Hospital for Special Surgery, we have previously demonstrated that patients in whom calf thrombi

Table 16–3. Suggested Treatment Regimens

Disease	Regimen
Calf thrombi	Low-dose warfarin therapy for 6 weeks or follow-up duplex ultrasonography (to evaluate propagation)
Proximal thrombi	Anticoagulation with heparin–warfarin for 3 to 6 months or vena cava filter
Symptomatic pulmonary emboli	Anticoagulation with heparin–warfarin for 3 to 6 months or vena cava filter or both

developed are at increased risk for pulmonary embolism. We recommend that patients who are identified postoperatively as having calf thrombi should be treated with low-dose warfarin therapy for 6 weeks after surgery. We do not believe that calf thrombi detected in the early postoperative period should be treated routinely with heparin because of the risk of complication with intravenous anticoagulation therapy. Lotke recommended that patients identified as having calf vein thrombosis should be continued on aspirin therapy for 6 weeks postoperatively.[45] Because the primary risk of isolated calf thrombi is through proximal propagation, Oishi advocated serial duplex ultrasound scanning without the use of anticoagulants to detect for proximal migration.[100] Anticoagulation therapy is only initiated if propagation of a calf thrombi to a more proximal thrombi occurs.

CONCLUSION

Thromboembolic disease in any patient population is potentially life threatening. As a result, the diagnosis of DVT should be considered in any patient who sustained trauma to the foot and ankle, who has undergone foot and ankle surgery, or who has been immobilized in a cast or splint. In this patient population, pain in the lower extremity can arise from a DVT, and this potential diagnosis warrants further evaluation. If one suspects thrombophlebitis, then noninvasive, ultrasonographic monitoring is necessary to evaluate the deep venous system. Whereas the diagnosis of a proximal DVT mandates treatment, the management of a calf thrombosis is controversial. DVT of the calf can be treated with anticoagulation or monitored with serial ultrasound examinations to exclude propagation.

Prophylaxis of DVT should be considered in this patient population and should be based on the relative risks of the specific patient. Although minimal data exist on the incidence of thromboembolism in patients with foot and ankle maladies, we must follow some guidelines until further information is available and definitive. Classification of the level of risk and classification of the type of prophylaxis based upon the level of risk is available in Tables 16–1 and 16–2. We are certainly in need of randomized prospective studies with solid methodology to evaluate further thromboembolism and its prophylaxis in patients with foot and ankle disorders.

Acknowledgment

I thank Steven B. Haas, M.D., Ph.D., for his assistance with this chapter.

REFERENCES

1. Donaldson GA, Williams C, Scannell JG, et al. A reappraisal of the application of the Trendelenburg operation to massive fatal embolism: report of a successful pulmonary-artery thrombectomy using a cardiopulmonary bypass. N Engl J Med 268:171–174, 1963.
2. Anderson FA, Wheeler HB. Venous thromboembolism risk factors and prophylaxis. Clin Chest Med 16:235–251, 1995.
3. McKenna R, Bachmann F, Kullshal SP, Galante JO. Thromboembolic disease in patients undergoing total knee replacement. J Bone Joint Surg Am 58:928–932, 1976.
4. Lotke PA, Ecker ML, Alavi A, Berkowitz H. Indications for the treatment of DVT following total knee replacement. J Bone Joint Surg Am 66:202–208, 1984.
5. Stulberg BN, Insall JN, Williams GW, Ghelman B. Deep vein thrombosis following total knee replacement. J Bone Joint Surg Am 66:194–201, 1984.
6. Grady-Benson JC, Oishi CS, Hannson PB, et al. Postoperative surveillance for deep venous thrombosis with duplex ultrasound after total knee arthroplasty. J Bone Joint Surg Am 76:1649–1657, 1994.
7. Haas SB, Insall JM, Scuderi GR, et al. Pneumatic sequential compression boots compared with aspirin prophylaxis of deep vein thrombosis after total knee arthroplasty. J Bone Joint Surg Am 72:27–31, 1990.
8. Lotke PA, Wong RY, Ecker ML. Asymptomatic pulmonary embolism after total knee replacement. Orthop Trans 10:490, 1986.
9. Patterson BM, Marchand R, Ranawat C. Complications of heparin therapy after total joint arthroplasty. J Bone Joint Surg Am 71:1130–1134, 1989.
10. Mizel MS, Temple HT, Michelson JD, et al. Clinically apparent thromboembolism following foot and ankle surgery. Presented at the Annual Meeting of Foot and Ankle, 1996.
11. Paiement GD, Bell D, Wessinger SJ, et al. New advances in the prevention, diagnosis, and cost effectiveness of venous thromboembolic disease in patients with total hip replacement. In The Hip, Proceedings of the Fourteenth Open Scientific Meeting of the Hip Society. St. Louis: C. V. Mosby, 1987, pp. 94–119.
12. Sevitt S, Gallagher NG. Prevention of venous thrombosis and pulmonary embolism in injury patients: a trial of anticoagulant prophylaxis with phenindione in middle-aged and elderly patients with fractured necks of femurs. Lancet ii:981–989, 1959.

13. Geerts W, Code KI, Jay RM, et al. A prospective study of venous thromboembolism after major trauma. N Engl J Med 331:1601–1606, 1994.

14. Clagett GP, Reisch JS. Prevention of venous thrombosis in general surgical patients: results of meta-analysis. Ann Surg 208:227–240, 1988.

15. Anderson FA Jr, Wheeler HB, Goldberg RJ, et al. A population-based perspective of the hospital incidence and case-fatality rates of deep vein thrombosis and pulmonary embolism: the Worcester DVT Study. Arch Intern Med 151:933–938, 1991.

16. Rahr HB, Sorensen IV. Venous thromboembolism and cancer. Blood Coagul Fibrinolysis 3:451–460, 1992.

17. Gibbs NM. Venous thrombosis of the lower limbs with particular reference to bedrest. Br J Surg 45:209–236, 1957.

18. Lundgren R, Sundin T, Colleen S, et al. Cardiovascular complications of estrogen therapy for nondisseminated prostatic carcinoma. Scand J Urol Nephrol 20:101–105, 1986.

19. Devor M, Barrett-Connor E, Renvall M, et al. Estrogen replacement therapy and the risk of venous thrombosis. Am J Med 92:275–282, 1992.

20. Kraritz E, Karino T. Pathophysiology of deep vein thrombosis. In Leclerc JR, ed. Venous Thromboembolic Disorders. Philadelphia: Lea and Febiger, 1991:54–64.

21. Virchow R. Neuer fall von todlicher emboli der kungerarteries. Arch Path Anat 10:225, 1856.

22. Britt LD, Zolfaghari D, Kennedy E, et al. Incidence and prophylaxis of deep vein thrombosis in a high risk trauma population. Am J Surg 172:13–14, 1996.

23. Ziomek S, Read RC, Tobler HG, et al. Thromboembolism in patients undergoing thoracotomy. Ann Thorac Surg 56:223–227, 1993.

24. Nurmohamed NIT. Verhaeghe R, Haas S, et al. A comparative trial of a low molecular weight heparin (enoxaparin) versus standard heparin for the prophylaxis of postoperative deep vein thrombosis in general surgery. Am J Surg 169:567–571, 1995.

25. Kakkar VV, Cohen AT, Edmonson RA, et al. Low molecular weight versus standard heparin for prevention of venous thromboembolism after major abdominal surgery. Lancet 341:259–265, 1993.

26. Caprini JA, Arcelus JI, Hoffman K, et al. Prevention of venous thromboembolism in North America: results of a survey among general surgeons. J Vasc Surg 20:751–758, 1994.

27. Janku GV, Paiement GD, Green HD. Prevention of venous thromboembolism in orthopaedics in the United States. Clin Orthop 325:313–321, 1996.

28. Bergqvist D, Benoni G, Bjorgell O, et al. Low-molecular-weight heparin (enoxaparin) as prophylaxis against venous thromboembolism after total hip replacement. N Engl J Med 335:696–700, 1996.

29. Warwick D, Williams MH, Bannister GC. Death and thromboembolic disease after total hip replacement. J Bone Joint Surg Br 77:6–10, 1995.

30. Pellegrini DV, Laghans MJ, Totterman S, et al. Embolic complications of calf thrombosis following total hip arthroplasty. J Arthroplasty 8:449–457, 1993.

31. Imperiale TF, Speroff T. A meta-analysis of methods to prevent venous thromboembolism following total hip replacement. JAMA 271:1780–1785, 1994.

32. Leclerc JR, Geerts WH, Desjardins L, et al. Prevention of deep vein thrombosis after major knee surgery—a randomized, double-blind trial comparing a low molecular weight heparin fragment (enoxaparin) to placebo. Thromb Haemost 67:417–423, 1992.

33. Fauno P, Suomalainen AO, Rehnberg V, et al. Prophylaxis for the prevention of venous thromboembolism after total knee arthroplasty. J Bone Joint Surg 12:1814–1818, 1994.

34. Frim DM, Barker FG, Poletti CE, et al. Postoperative low-dose heparin decreases thromboembolic complications in neurosurgical patients. Neurosurgery 30:830–833, 1992.

35. Green D, Chen D, Chmiel JS, et al. Prevention of thromboembolism in spinal cord injury: role of low molecular weight heparin. Arch Phys Med Rehabil 75:290–292, 1994.

36. Hamilton MD, Hull RD, Pineo GF. Prophylaxis of venous thromboembolism in brain tumor patients. J Neurooncol 22:111–126, 1994.

37. Warlow C, Terry G, Kenmure ACF, et al. A double-blind trial of low-dose subcutaneous heparin in the prevention of deep vein thrombosis after myocardial infarction. Lancet ii:934–937, 1973.

38. Keith SL, McLaughlin DJ, Anderson FA, et al. Do graduated compression stocking and pneumatic boots have an additive effect on the peak velocity of venous blood flow? Arch Surg 127:727–730, 1992.

39. Gardlund B. Randomised, controlled trial of low-dose heparin for prevention of fatal pulmonary embolism in patients with infectious diseases. Lancet 347:1357–1361, 1996.

40. Garino J, Lotke P, Kitziger K, Steinberg M. Deep venous thrombosis after total joint arthroplasty: the role of compression ultrasonography and the importance of experience of the technician. J Bone Joint Surg Am 78:1359–1365, 1996.

41. Bern MM, Lokich JJ, Wallach SR, et al. Very low doses of warfarin can prevent thrombosis in central venous catheters: a randomized prospective trial. Ann Intern Med 112:423–428, 1990.

42. Wells PS, Lensin AWA, Hirsh J. Graduated compression stockings in the prevention of postoperative venous thromboembolism. Arch Intern Med 154:67–71, 1994.

43. Knight MTN, Dawson R. Effect of intermittent compression of the arms on deep venous thrombosis in the legs. Lancet ii:1265–1267, 1976.

44. Hirsh J, Salzman EW, Harker L, et al. Aspirin and other platelet active drugs: relationship among dose, effectiveness and side effects. Chest 95(Suppl 2):12S–16S, 1989.

45. Lotke PA. Aspirin prophylaxis for thromboembolic disease. In Instructional Course Lectures, The American Academy of Orthopedic Surgeons, vol 44. St. Louis: C. V. Mosby, 1995.

46. Agnelli G. Anticoagulation in the prevention and treatment of pulmonary embolism. Chest 107 (Suppl):39S–44S, 1995.

47. Jorgensen LN, Willie-Jorgensen P, Hauch O. Prophylaxis of postoperative thromboembolism with low molecular weight heparins. Br J Surg 80:689–704, 1993.

48. Carter CA, Skoutakis VA, Spiro TE, et al. Enoxaparin: the LMWH for prevention of postoperative

thromboembolic complications. Ann Pharmacother 27:1223–1230, 1993.

49. Noble S, Peters DH, Goa KL. Enoxaparin: a reappraisal of its pharmacology and clinical applications in the prevention and treatment of thromboembolic disease. Drugs 49:388–410, 1995.

50. Frampton JE, Faulds D. Pamaparin: a review of its pharmacology, and clinical application in the prevention and treatment of thromboembolic and other vascular disorders. Drugs 47:652–676, 1994.

51. Collignon F, Frydman A, Caplain H, et al. Comparison of the pharmacokinetic profiles of three low molecular mass heparins—dalteparin, enoxaparin and nadroparin—administered subcutaneously in healthy volunteers (doses for prevention of thromboembolism). Thromb Haemost 73:630–640, 1995.

52. Friedel HA, Balfour JA. Tinzaparin: a review of its pharmacology and clinical potential in the prevention and treatment of thromboembolic disorders. Drugs 48:638–660, 1994.

53. Nicolaides AN, Fernandes JF, Pollock AV. Intermittent sequential pneumatic compression of the legs in the prevention of venous stasis and postoperative deep venous thrombosis. Surgery 87:69–76, 1980.

54. Keane MG, Ingenito FP, Goldhaber SZ. Utilization of venous thromboembolism prophylaxis in the medical intensive care unit. Chest 106:13–14, 1994.

55. Cade JF. High risk of the critically ill for venous thromboembolism. Crit Care Med 10:448–450, 1982.

56. Halkin H, Goldberg J, Modan M, et al. Reduction of mortality in general medical in patients by low-dose heparin prophylaxis. Ann Intern Med 96:561–565, 1982.

57. Knudson MM, Collins JA, Goodman SB, et al. Thromboembolism following multiple trauma. J Trauma 32:2–11, 1992.

58. Geerts WH, Jay RM, Code KI, et al. A comparison of low-dose heparin with low-molecular-weight heparin as prophylaxis against venous thromboembolism after major trauma. N Engl J Med 335:701–707, 1996.

59. Flinn NVR, Sandaraer GP, Silva MB, et al. Prospective surveillance for perioperative venous thrombosis. Arch Surg 131:472–480, 1996.

60. Grady-Benson JC, Oishi CS, Hanson PB, et al. Postoperative surveillance for deep venous thrombosis with duplex ultrasonography after total knee arthroplasty. J Bone Joint Surg Am 76:1649–1657, 1994.

61. Howell R, Fidler J, Letsky E, et al. The risks of antenatal subcutaneous heparin prophylaxis: a controlled trial. Br J Obstet Gynaecol 90:1124–1128, 1983.

62. Barbour LA, Pickard J. Controversies in thromboembolic disease during pregnancy: a critical review. Obstet Gynecol 86:621–633, 1995.

63. Tarnay TJ, Rohr PR, Davidson AG, et al. Pneumatic calf compression, fibrinolysis, and the prevention of deep venous thrombosis. Surgery 88:489–96, 1980.

64. Wilson NV, Das SK, Kakkar VV, et al. Thromboembolic prophylaxis in total knee replacement: evaluation of the A-V impulse system. J Bone and Joint Surg Br 74:50–52, 1992.

65. Knight MTN, Dawson R. Effect of intermittent compression of the arms on deep venous thrombosis in the legs. Lancet 2:1265–1267, 1976.

66. Lynch JA, Baker PL, Polly RE, et al. Mechanical measures in the prophylaxis of post-operative thromboembolism in total knee arthroplasty. Clin Orthop 260:24–29, 1990.

67. Hodge WA. Warfarin and sequential calf compression in the prevention of deep vein thrombi following total knee replacement. Presented at the meeting of the Knee Society, Las Vegas, NV, 1989.

68. Kaempffe FA, Lifeso RM, Meinding C. Intermittent pneumatic compression versus Coumadin: prevention of deep vein thrombosis in lower-extremity total joint arthroplasty. Clin Orthop 269:89–97, 1991.

69. Graor RA, Davis AW, Borden LS, Young J. Comparative evaluation of deep vein thrombosis prophylaxis in total joint replacement patients. Presented at the meeting of American Academy of Orthopaedic Surgeons, Las Vegas, NV 1989.

70. Hood RW, Flawn LB, Insall JN. The use of pulsatile compression stockings in total knee replacement for prevention of venous thromboembolism: a prospective study. Presented at the meeting of the Orthopaedic Research Society, New Orleans, LA, 1982.

71. Hull R, Delmore TJ, Hirsh J, et al. Effectiveness of intermittent pulsatile elastic stockings for the prevention of calf and thigh vein thrombosis in patients undergoing elective knee surgery. Thromb Res 16:37–45, 1979.

72. Westrich GH, Sculco TP. Prophylaxis against deep vein thrombosis after total knee arthroplasty: pneumatic plantar compression and aspirin compared to aspirin alone. J Bone Joint Surg Am 78:826, 1996.

73. Hull R, Hirsh J, Jay R, et al. Different intensities of oral anticoagulant therapy in the treatment of proximal-vein thrombosis. N Engl J Med 307:1676–1681, 1982.

74. Greenfield LJ, Michna BA. Twelve year clinical experience with the Greenfield vena caval filter. Surgery 104:706–712, 1988.

75. Emerson RH, Cross R, Head WC. Prophylactic and early therapeutic use of the Greenfield filter in hip and knee joint arthroplasty. J Arthroplasty 6:129–135, 1991.

76. Mohan CR, Hoballah JJ, Shari WJ, et al. Comparative efficacy and complications of vena caval filters. J Vasc Surg 21:235–246, 1995.

77. Barritt DW, Jordan SC, Brist MB. Anticoagulant drugs in the treatment of pulmonary embolism: A controlled trial. Lancet 18:1309–1312, 1960.

78. Clagett GP, Anderson FA Jr, Levine MN, et al. Prevention of venous thromboembolism. Chest 102:391S–407S, 1992.

79. Green D, Lee Y, Ito VY, et al. Fixed- vs adjusted-dose heparin in the prophylaxis of thromboembolism in spinal cord injury. JAMA 260:1255–1258, 1988.

80. Nicolaides AN, Irving D. Clinical factors and the risk of deep venous thrombosis. In Nicolaides AN, ed. Thromboembolism Etiology, Advances in Prevention and Management. Baltimore, MD: University Park Press, 1975:193–204.

81. Carter C, Gent M. The epidemiology of venous thrombosis. In Coleman RW, Hirsh J, Marder VJ, et al, eds. Hemostasis and Thrombosis: Basic

Principles and Clinical Practice. Philadelphia: J. B. Lippincott, 1987:805–819.

82. Stewart WP, Youngswick FD. Deep vein thrombosis: diagnosis, treatment, and prevention. J Foot Surg 20:232–238, 1981.

83. Menzin F, Colditz GA, Re-an MM, et al. Cost-effectiveness of enoxaparin vs low-dose warfarin in the prevention of deep-vein thrombosis after total hip replacement surgery. Arch Intern Med 155:757–764, 1995.

84. Warkentin TE, Levine MN, Hirsh J, et al. Heparin-induced thrombocytopenia in patients treated with low-molecular-weight heparin or unfractionated heparin. N Engl J Med 273:1032–1038, 1995.

85. Fordyce MJF, Ling RSM. A venous foot pump reduces thrombosis after total hip replacement. J Bone Joint Surg Br 74:45–49, 1992.

86. Ramos R, Salem BI, De Pawlikowski MP. The efficacy of pneumatic compression stockings in the prevention of pulmonary embolism after cardiac surgery. Chest 109:82–85, 1996.

87. Fisher CG, Blachut PA, Salvian, et al. Effectiveness of pneumatic leg compression devices for the prevention of thromboembolic disease in orthopaedic trauma patients: a prospective, randomized study of compression alone versus no prophylaxis. J Orthop Trauma 9:1–7, 1995.

88. Jacobs DG, Piotrowski JJ, Hoppensteadt, et al. Hemodynamic and fibrinolytic consequences of intermittent pneumatic compression: preliminary results. J Trauma 4:710–717, 1996.

89. Alexander JJ, Yuhas JP, Piotrowski JJ. Is the increasing use of prophylactic percutaneous IVC filters justified? Am J Surg 168:102–106, 1994.

90. Clagett GP, Anderson FA Jr, Heit J, et al. Prevention of venous thromboembolism. Chest 108 (Suppl):312S–334S, 1995.

91. Hirsh DR, Ingenito EP, Goldhaber SZ. Prevalence of deep venous thrombosis among patients in medical intensive care. JAMA 274:335–337, 1995.

92. Keaton C, Hirsh J. Starting prophylaxis for venous thromboembolism postoperatively. Arch Intern Med 155:366–372, 1995.

93. Knudson MM, Lewis FR, Clinton A, et al. Prevention of venous thromboembolism in trauma patients. J Trauma 37:480–487, 1994.

94. Upchurch GR, Demling, RH, Davies J, et al. Efficacy of subcutaneous heparin in prevention of venous thromboembolic events in trauma patients. Am Surgeon 61:749–755, 1995.

95. Eriksson BI, Ekman S, Kalebo P, et al. Prevention of deep-vein thrombosis after total hip replacement: direct thrombin inhibition with recombinant hirudin, CGP 39393. Lancet 347:635–639, 1996.

96. Cole CW, Shea B, Bormanis J. Ancrod as prophylaxis or treatment from thromboembolism in patients with multiple trauma. Can J Surg 38:249–254, 1995.

97. Wells PS, Lensina AW, Davidson BL, et al. Accuracy of ultrasound for the diagnosis of deep venous thrombosis in asymptomatic patients after orthopedic surgery: a meta-analysis. Ann Intern Med 122:47–53, 1995.

98. Pederson OM, Aslaksen A, Vik-Mo H, et al. Compression ultrasonography in hospitalized patients with suspected deep venous thrombosis. Arch Intern Med 151:2217–2220, 1991.

99. Westrich GH, Schneider R, Ghelman B, et al. The incidence of deep venous thrombosis with color Doppler imaging compared to ascending venography in total joint arthroplasty: a prospective study. Contemp Surg 54:225–234, 1997.

100. Oishi CS, Grady-Benson JC, Otis SM, et al. The clinical course of distal deep venous thrombosis after total hip and total knee arthroplasty as determined with duplex ultrasonography. J Bone Joint Surg Am 76:1658–1663, 1994.

17

Knee Pathology and Pain Related to Rearfoot and Heel Dysfunction

Thomas L. Wickiewicz
Peter T. Simonian

There is a scarcity of orthopedic literature on the effect of pathologic rearfoot mechanics on knee function. This relationship has not been clearly established or described. The majority of information on this association can only be implied from gait analysis and other indirect studies. Gait analysis has helped establish the timing and relationships of normal joint motions and the role of the neuromuscular system. Anterior knee pain and the relation to subtalar pronation has been described; however, the relationship has not been clearly delineated. The rheumatoid foot with the characteristic valgus deformity may impact the already susceptible knee to increased valgus force. Several studies have evaluated the use of heel wedges as a conservative treatment for knee osteoarthritis. These results can be extrapolated to aid in understanding forces on the knee from the rearfoot with varus or valgus deformity. Further, studies evaluating the effect of tibial torsion and ankle foot orthoses on the knee may provide some additional insight.

GAIT ANALYSIS

The pattern of normal femur, knee, tibia, ankle, and subtalar joint motion during the gait cycle can aid in understanding their relationships. Normal gait is dependent on the normal relationships and timing of the joint motions described next.

Motions of the femur and tibia together define knee rotation, flexion-extension, and varus-valgus. Rotation of the femur is maximally internal at the end of weight acceptance and maximally external at the early swing phase of the gait cycle. Internal rotation of the tibia is maximal at opposite toe-off, and external rotation is maximal between toe-off and foot strike. Structural changes in hindfoot position, with particular attention to varus-valgus and pronation-

supination, might impact these relationships.

The knee is in about 10° of flexion at heel strike. This will increase to approximately 15° at weight acceptance and then extend to 0° during single-limb stance. Flexion begins before and during weight release. Rapid and maximal knee flexion is seen in early swing and decreases in the remainder of the swing phase.[1] Structural changes in hindfoot position, with particular attention to limited dorsiflexion and plantar flexion, might impact these relationships.

The ankle motion ranges from 5° of plantar flexion at heel strike to a maximum of 10° of plantar flexion during weight acceptance. At the beginning of single-limb stance, the ankle is neutral. With the progression of the tibia over the foot, dorsiflexion is seen during single-limb stance. The ankle returns to neutral at the beginning of weight release, and maximal plantar flexion is seen at the start of the swing phase.[1] Again, structural changes in hindfoot position, with particular attention to limited dorsiflexion and plantar flexion, might impact these relationships.

The subtalar joint is a uniaxial joint behaving similar to a mitered hinge. The talocalcaneal joint allows further rotation of the proximal leg to occur over the foot because of the orientation of the axis of rotation.[1] Again, structural changes in hindfoot position, with particular attention to varus-valgus and pronation-supination, might impact these relationships.

In addition to joint motion, appropriate and timely neuromuscular control of limb motion may play an important role in the preservation of the joints of the lower extremity. Radin and associates[2] found that patients with mild knee pain, possibly consistent with early osteoarthritis, had a 37% higher loading rate of the vertical ground reaction force associated with heel strike.

Knee pain patients struck the ground faster and had a more violent follow-through.

ANTERIOR KNEE PAIN

Abnormal mechanics of the foot may contribute to patellofemoral pain. Increased or prolonged subtalar pronation results in compensatory internal rotation of the lower extremity. This may cause a functional increase in the Q-angle as the patella is displaced medially relative to the anterosuperior iliac spine.[3, 4] However, the exact nature of this link between the foot and anterior knee has not been clearly described. The failure to provide an adequate explanation may be due in part to some confusion regarding the in vivo kinematics of the knee joint complex. Some have also stated that the role of the Q-angle on patellar tracking may be overemphasized.[5] There are many causes of abnormal pronation of the subtalar joint, including subtalar varus, forefoot varus, tibial varus, and limited ankle joint dorsiflexion. Patients with patellofemoral pain that is related to abnormal pronation of the subtalar joint require a detailed assessment of the foot to determine the cause of the abnormal foot mechanics. For example, foot orthotics with appropriate posting may be useful for controlling abnormal pronation that is related to varus alignment. Abnormal pronation that is secondary to inadequate ankle joint dorsiflexion requires stretching of the gastrocnemius and soleus muscles.[6]

RHEUMATOID FOOT

Valgus deformity of the hindfoot is a common and disabling defect in patients who have rheumatoid arthritis. Keenan and associates[7] reported the only clinical study directly evaluating this specific foot deformity and its effect on the knee. They found a radiographic association between the valgus deformity of the feet and valgus deformity of the knees in patients with rheumatoid arthritis. Two groups of patients were evaluated clinically, radiographically, and with gait analysis. Group 1 consisted of 7 patients with rheumatoid arthritis and normal alignment of the feet. Group 2 consisted of 10 patients who had rheumatoid arthritis and valgus deformity of the hindfoot. In

Group 2, the disease was of longer duration and, as expected because of the deformity, the feet were more painful than in Group 1. There was no evidence of muscular imbalance, equinus contracture, valgus deformity of the tibiotalar joint, or isolated deficiency of the tibialis posterior that could have contributed to the development of the valgus deformity.

The results of this study suggest that valgus deformity of the hindfoot in rheumatoid patients results possibly from exaggerated pronation forces on the subtalar joint. These forces are likely the result of alterations in gait as a result of muscular weakness and the effort of the patient to minimize pain in the feet. As mentioned, radiographs suggested an association between the valgus deformity of the feet and valgus deformity of the knees in these patients.[7]

HEEL WEDGES FOR KNEE ARTHRITIS

Several studies have also evaluated the effect of heel wedges as a treatment for unicompartmental knee arthritis (Fig. 17–1A, B). These results, although not completely consistent, might be extrapolated to the varus or valgus foot and the resulting effects on the knee.

Tohyama and associates[8] concluded that the lateral heel wedge is useful for patients with early medial compartment osteoarthritis provided it is used with an understanding of the indications and limitations. In this study, as expected, the lateral heel wedge had no effect on the progress of the radiographic changes. Sixty-two patients with early medial compartment osteoarthritis of the knee were treated with lateral heel wedges and monitored for 7 to 12 years. Those who were treated with heel wedges and analgesics showed a significantly greater improvement in pain score than those treated with analgesics only. However, their walking ability score did not improve.

Keating and coworkers[9] analyzed the use of lateral heel wedges in the treatment of medial osteoarthritis in 121 knees. They concluded that there was a place for lateral wedges in the conservative treatment of medial osteoarthritis. However, follow-up was an important limitation of the study, with an average of 12 months follow-up after the insertion of the wedge. Overall, 38% of pa-

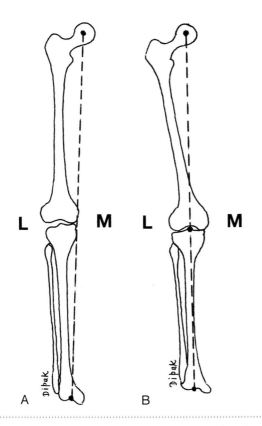

Figure 17–1. *A*, Diagram demonstrating the alignment of the knee with medial joint arthritis (L = lateral; M = medial). *B*, Diagram demonstrating the theoretical decrease in medial joint forces through correction of the varus deformity with the use of a lateral heel wedge.

tients improved to a Hospital for Special Surgery pain score of 25 to 30, corresponding to an excellent result after total knee arthroplasty. Fifty percent of patients improved to a pain score of 20 or higher, corresponding to a good result after total knee arthroplasty. The patients with milder osteoarthritis achieved greater pain relief. However, the authors claimed that even patients with complete loss of joint space and bony erosion showed some improvement.

These results may be extrapolated to understand the forces on the knee from the foot with varus or valgus deformity. One might assume that a hindfoot with varus or valgus deformity will act similar to the respective heel wedge and decrease force in one knee compartment while increasing it in the other. Aside from the concern for knee osteoarthritis, these respective foot deformi-

ties may also result in symptomatic varus or valgus ligamentous laxity about the knee.

TIBIAL TORSION AND ANKLE-FOOT ORTHOSES

Implications can also be made on the basis of studies evaluating the effect of tibial torsion and ankle-foot orthoses on knee function. One can assume that internal or external rotation of the hindfoot, for whatever reason, would have a similar effect on knee mechanics, as would internal or external tibial torsion. Similarly, stabilization of the hindfoot with an ankle-foot orthosis may simulate a hindfoot fusion or coalition. Again, one can assume that stabilization of the hindfoot with an orthosis would have a similar effect on knee mechanics as would a hindfoot fusion or coalition.

Turner and coworkers[10] studied the association of tibial torsion with knee joint pathology. They concluded that abnormal torsion causes a gait adaptation that changes the physiologic loading of the knee, which may lead to osteoarthrosis. Measurements in several diagnostic groups were compared with those of a control group. Two of the groups differed significantly from the controls. Those patients with patellofemoral instability had greater than normal external tibial torsion, whereas patients with panarticular osteoarthrosis of the knee had reduced external torsion or true internal torsion. Again, they concluded that this abnormal torsion creates a gait adaptation, changing loads across the knee, leading to osteoarthritis.

Lindgren and associates[11] studied the influence of mediolateral deformity, tibial torsion, and different centers of foot support with a three-dimensional computer model that incorporated the significant muscles of the lower extremities needed for quasistatic walking. The model avoided the variability in gait pattern secondary to pain and discomfort associated with deformity. Internal torsion and varus deformity resulted in the highest loads in the medial compartment of the knee. Interestingly, the peak load for each deformity occurred in different phases of the gait cycle. Both external torsion and valgus deformity generally decreased the load in the medial compartment, but early in the gait cycle external torsion increased the loads on the medial side. The study also illustrated the possible importance of the muscle force on the load across the knee and ankle. High strains in the medial gastrocnemius and the medial hamstring created particularly high loads in the medial compartment of the knee. In addition, when the center of support of the body was in the forefoot, the loads through the knee were lower than when foot support was at the heel. As expected, if the center of support was on the lateral foot line, the lateral compartment was subjected to more load, and, conversely, when the center of support was on the medial part of the foot, the medial compartment of the knee was more loaded.

The relationship between subtalar motion and tibial torsion has been studied.[12–14] Lundberg[14] found that internal rotation of the tibia gave rise to considerably less motion at the foot and ankle compared with external tibial rotation. Lundberg also found that the entire foot contributes pronation and supination, particularly the talonavicular joint. This demonstrates the importance of the whole foot rather than primarily the hindfoot regarding the association between excessive pronation and knee pain.

This relationship is also underscored in the clubfoot literature. In the patient with a clubfoot deformity, it has been recommended that severe internal tibial torsion also be addressed after correction of the clubfoot deformity. Otherwise, as the patient walks, the internally rotated foot is dynamically adducted and inverted, resulting in the possible recurrence of adduction of the forefoot, inversion of the heel, and cavus deformity.

On another topic, Lehmann and coworkers[15] found that the use of an ankle-foot orthosis can cause instability of the knee joint. Forces and moments seen during ambulation were compared with those generated with the use of an ankle-foot orthosis with an adjustable double stop. The major effect on total knee moment occurred during the midstance phase and was most affected by the moment arm of the brace.

SUPRAPATELLAR PLICA

Treatment of synovial plica is controversial, and no definitive studies exist relating this problem to foot pathology; however, extrapolations can be posed. Any foot abnormality

will result in a gait adaptation. This may result in increased irritation of a previously asymptomatic plica. The synovial linings of the knee joint and the suprapatellar bursa freely communicate in most knees. It has been estimated that in less than 20% of knees a fold or plica of synovial tissue persists in the suprapatellar region. The fold extends along the medial aspect of the patella to the medial surface of the synovial covering of the patellar fat pad. Any foot pathology that results in a gait adaptation may produce chronic irritation of this fold of synovium and may resemble symptoms of an internal derangement of the knee; however, careful examination should allow differentiation of these problems. A pathologic plica produces popping and catching in the knee by snapping across the patella or medial femoral condyle. Palpation along the medial side of the patella as the patient flexes and extends the knee often will localize the abnormal plica as it flips over the medial femoral condyle, which may produce a momentary catching of the patella.

The first line of treatment should be conservative, including restriction of activities, administration of anti-inflammatory agents, and implementation of an isometric exercise program. This treatment should also include addressing foot pathology as a possible contributor.

CONCLUSION

There seems to be a logical relationship between hindfoot deformity and resulting knee pathology. Any patient with knee pathology requires careful and complete evaluation, including abnormalities of the leg and foot. This will provide insight and allow determination of the true cause of the problem. Despite the logical relationship between hindfoot and knee pathology, clinical studies demonstrating this association are clearly lacking. Further trials objectively evaluating these associations are indicated.

REFERENCES

1. Tylkowski CM. Assessment of gait in children and adolescents. In Morrissy RT, ed. Lovell and Winter's Pediatric Orthopaedics, vol 1. Philadelphia: J. B. Lippincott, 1990:57–90.
2. Radin EL, Yang KH, Riegger C, et al. Relationship between lower limb dynamics and knee joint pain.

J Orthop Res 9:398–405, 1991. Erratum J Orthop Res 9:776, 1991.

3. Larson RL. Subluxation–dislocation of the patella. In Kennedy JC, ed. The Injured Adolescent Knee. Baltimore, MD: Williams & Wilkins, 1979:161–195.

4. Paulos L, Rusche K, Johnson C, Noyes FR. Patella malalignment: a treatment rationale. Phys Ther 60:1624, 1980.

5. Tiberio D. The effects of excessive subtalar joint pronation on patellofemoral mechanics: a theoretical model. J Orthop Sports Phys Ther 9:160, 1987.

6. Irrgang JJ. In Fu FH, Harner CD, Vince KG, eds. Knee Surgery, vol 1. Baltimore, MD: Williams & Wilkins, 1994:485–502.

7. Keenan MA, Peabody TD, Gronley JK, Perry J. Valgus deformities of the feet and characteristics of gait in patients who have rheumatoid arthritis. J Bone Joint Surg Am 73:237–247, 1991.

8. Tohyama H, Yasuda K, Kaneda K. Treatment of osteoarthritis of the knee with heel wedges. Int Orthop 15:31–33, 1991.

9. Keating EM, Faris PM, Ritter MA, Kane J. Use of lateral heel and sole wedges in the treatment of medial osteoarthritis of the knee. Orthop Rev 22:921–924, 1993.

10. Turner MS. The association between tibial torsion and knee joint pathology. Clin Orthop 302:47–51, 1994.

11. Lindgren U, Seireg A. The influence of mediolateral deformity, tibial torsion, and foot position on femorotibial load. Prediction of a musculoskeletal computer model. Arch Orthop Trauma Surg 108:22–26, 1989.

12. Benink RJ. The constraint mechanism of the human tarsus: a roentgenological experimental study. Acta Orthop Scand (Suppl), 215:1, 1985.

13. Van Langelaan EJ. A kinematical analysis of the tarsal joints. Acta Orthop Scand (Suppl) 54:1, 1983.

14. Lundberg A. Patterns of Motion of the Ankle/Foot Complex. Stockholm: Karolinski Hospital, 1988.

15. Lehmann JF, Ko MJ, de Lateur BJ. Knee moments: origin in normal ambulation and their modification by double-stopped ankle-foot orthoses. Arch Phys Med Rehabil 63:345–351, 1982.

18 Reflex Sympathetic Dystrophy: Complex Regional Pain Syndrome of the Ankle and Foot

Jeffrey Y. F. Ngeow
David Y. Wang

Throughout medical history, clinicians who treat foot and ankle ailments, like their colleagues of all other disciplines, have seen patients who complained of severe pain so disabling that they became social or emotional cripples. When the medical history included what amounted to trivial injuries and routine or even extensive investigations failed to reveal significant underlying causes, the natural reactions of the vexed practitioners were to suspect that the patients exaggerated their symptoms and sufferings. It was little wonder then that many of such mysterious complainers were labeled neurotics and promptly referred to psychologists for "pain management." Patients with reflex sympathetic dystrophy (RSD) affecting their lower extremities have often suffered such fates, and many have languished in dark corners of psychiatric centers.

Recent change in attitudes and interests has given rise to research that focuses on pain as a disease state in and by itself. An area that has received much scrutiny is neuropathic pain; symptoms include spontaneous burning and hypersensitivity to noxious stimuli that arise subsequent to nerve injury. Neuropathic symptoms often play a prominent part in RSD. Although the clinical picture is far from clear, results of animal studies have shed new light on the pathophysiology of the RSD-related group of conditions. Our knowledge base has expanded sufficiently to demand a change in the very name of the condition itself. RSD will henceforth be known as complex regional pain syndrome-I (CRPS-I). It is our intention to discuss some of the foot and ankle conditions that we have seen in a pain unit at an orthopedic center that have been associated with CRPS-RSD and to review their treatment in light of current understandings.

BRIEF HISTORIC REVIEW

In 1864, Mitchell and colleagues first described, in victims of the American Civil War who sustained bullet injuries to their peripheral nerves, the syndrome of severe lancinating, burning pain in a limb that showed features of dystrophy.[1] Later, Mitchell also named the condition "causalgia," from the Greek *kausis* (burning) and *algos* (pain).[2] Since then, several similar conditions, not necessarily the result of penetrating injuries but sharing the common features of burning pain with dystrophy, have been recognized. In many of them, evidence of sympathetic hyperactivity such as vasospasm, hyperhidrosis, and decreased skin temperature are also present. These causalgia conditions were given different names such as posttraumatic pain dysfunction syndrome, shoulder-hand syndrome, reflex neurovascular dystrophy, algoneurodystrophy, Sudeck's atrophy, and others. These labels make long, interesting lists, but they merely served to emphasize differences and reflect the disagreement regarding their underlying mechanisms. There was general agreement, however, that the sympathetic nervous system was somehow involved, and excessive activity in this autonomic system brought about the dystrophic changes. This led to the gradual adoption of the term reflex sympathetic dystrophy.

As RSD implies, physicians are apt to believe that blocking the sympathetic pathway would result in resolution of the neuropathic symptoms and dystrophy. Sympathetic blockade, either with local anesthetics or with drugs, became the preferred treatment modality. Disappointment soon set in, however, when it was found that many of the RSD cases simply did not respond to sympatholysis and, therefore, could not have been sympathetically mediated.

By 1986, the term sympathetically maintained pain (SMP) as proposed by Roberts[3] was accepted for those cases labeled RSD that responded to sympathetic blockade. True RSD was naturally a member of SMP. Other cases that might not show much sympathetic overactivity but yet responded to sympathetic blockade were also included here. Conversely, pain conditions that showed features of sympathetic overactivity and even dystrophy but yet failed to respond to sympathetic blocks were labeled sympathetic independent pain (SIP). It was later recognized that SMP and SIP could represent the two ends of the spectrum for a single disease process.[4]

Despite improved nomenclature, much debate still continued as more underlying mechanisms were proposed for the SMP-SIP syndromes. Further attempts to reduce the confusion brought forth another revision in the terminology. A special Consensus Workshop in 1993 chose the umbrella name complex regional pain syndromes.[4] To emphasize the distinction of the original causalgia, CRPS was subdivided into two categories:

- CRPS-I covers a syndrome that develops after an initiating noxious event. Spontaneous pain or allodynia-hyperalgesia occurs. It is not limited to the territory of a single peripheral nerve and is disproportionate to the inciting event. There is or has been evidence of edema, skin blood flow abnormality or abnormal sudomotor activity in the region of the pain since the inciting event. This diagnosis is excluded by the existence of conditions that would otherwise account for the degree of pain and dysfunction. RSD thus falls into this category.
- CRPS-II is a syndrome similar to CRPS-I except that it develops after a known nerve injury. Traditionally, these injuries involve large named nerves, such as the median or sciatic nerve.

PATHOPHYSIOLOGY

Our understanding of the pathophysiology of RSD (or CRPS) is still very sketchy. As more knowledge is gained from clinical observations and experimental studies, there is less agreement in a single common mechanism. Because the manifestations of the somatosensory and motor disorders, coupled with autonomic dysfunction and tissue structural changes, are so variable, clinicians and scientists alike are loath to accept any one animal model or hypothesis that purports to explain them all.[5]

Given the aforementioned caveat, there is now generally accepted experimental evidence that suggests that partial injury to a mixed peripheral nerve may be responsible for at least some of the features found in CRPS. Under normal conditions, sympathetic nerve stimulation does not excite the nociceptors (pain receptors) at the endings of an uninjured somatic nerve. Within days after partial nerve injury, however, changes occur that render the nociceptors excitable by sympathetic stimulation. The nociceptors now also respond to intra-arterially injected norepinephrine. If tissue injury and inflammation have already sensitized these nociceptors, their responses can be further augmented by sympathetic activities.

Some of the proposed hypotheses that link this local event of nociceptor sensitization to the generalized manifestation of sympathetic hyperactivity, are as follows:

- Activated sympathetic system mechanism. Local tissue factors, including sensitized nociceptors and neurotransmitter mediators, may activate the sympathetic system. In a vicious cycle, the noxious stimuli activate segmental and suprasegmental sympathetic discharges, producing vasoconstriction, ischemia, and further nociceptor activation. Impaired perfusion eventually leads to dystrophic changes.[6]
- Abnormal connection—"cross-talk" mechanism. After tissue injury, abnormal connections between the sympathetic and somatic nervous systems are established. This results in cross-talk between sympathetic efferents and somatosensory afferents. It explains the sympathetic component of the pain in causalgia.[7] In 1983, Devor presented the finding that inflamed or damaged peripheral nerve twigs formed abnormal synapses in the same manner as injured nerve trunks. Such connections allowed cross-talk between the two systems, leading to increased signal input into the spinal cord, increased activity of the internuncial neuronal pool, and further stimulation of the sympathetic efferent and sensory afferents.[8]
- Spinal mechanism. The neuronal turbu-

lence hypothesis proposed by Sunderland[9] in 1976 suggested that injury to the post-ganglionic sympathetic ganglia and transynaptic degeneration in the spinal cord would impair the function of spinal neuron groups. These groups of neurons could then form self-sustaining reverberating circuits.[9]

- Central mechanism. In 1965, when Melzack and Wall proposed the gate control theory of pain transmission in the spine, they also suggested a central biasing mechanism mediated through a system of descending fibers.[10] The descending fibers arise from the brain stem reticular system, and they exert a tonic inhibition on the somatic sensory system at all levels. Reduced sensory input after somatic nerve injury (especially when the nerve is severed) would result in a decrease in the descending tonic inhibition and thus allow an increase in the transmission of self-sustaining neuronal activities generated either in the periphery or within the spinal cord. In this situation, they postulated that prolonged pain may leave "memory traces" in the somesthetic system, making an individual more susceptible to recurrent pain. The practical application of this theory becomes relevant in the treatment of patients with phantom limb pain.[11, 12]

- Neuronal plasticity mechanism. This proposed theory, which has become more commonly accepted, suggests that the perpetuation of abnormal firing pattern in the internuncial neuron pool in the spinal cord is responsible for the abnormal pain perception. At the spinal cord level, a class of dorsal horn neurons that are multireceptive, the so-called wide-dynamic-range (WDR) neurons, usually do not contribute to painful sensations under normal conditions. Chronic stimulation of the WDR by nociceptors, however, causes hyperexcitability and plasticity of the WDR, resulting in expansion of their receptive fields. This may explain why innocuous stimulations are now perceived as painful (hyperalgesia).[13] Roberts and Foglesong demonstrated that WDR neurons are the only spinal nociceptive neurons activated by sympathetic efferent activity. Therefore, WDR neurons (i.e., the high-threshold neurons) are most likely those that mediate the spinal component of SMP. Sympathetic activation of WDR neurons is abolished by subcutaneous injection of local anesthetic, cooling of the receptive field with ice, and intravenous injection of the α-adrenergic blocker phentolamine.[14]

- Psychologic predisposition. Because none of the proposed mechanisms offers any predictability to who will fall victim to RSD, the existence of a particular diathesis or personality predisposition toward developing RSD or CRPS has often been raised. The patient's exaggerated response to mild stimulation naturally led the physician to suspect psychologic disorders. There is literature on both adults and children that hypothesizes the presence of psychologic disorders, particularly anxiety and depression, which predispose one to RSD. Alternatively, it is obvious that any chronic pain and suffering, particularly that with dubious origins, will produce a host of psychologic complications of its own.

CLINICAL FEATURES OF THE RSD (CRPS I)

History

RSD may be associated with minor (e.g., sprains or bruises, skin irritation) or major (e.g., fractures, thermal or chemical burns, wound or joint infections, ischemic necrosis) injuries. In these conditions, involvement of peripheral nerves is common. Its association with other diseases in which direct nerve damage is not so apparent, such as metastatic malignancy, Lyme borreliosis, diabetes, hyperthyroidism, hyperlipoproteinemia, lumbar radiculopathy resulting from lateral disc fragment, previous lumbar laminectomy, tarsal tunnel syndrome, and so on, has been reported.

Without history of significant trauma, the patient may appear disproportionately disabled, frequently with startling loss of range of motion if an extremity is affected. If the patient had undergone an operation, a protracted recovery period during which the patient poorly tolerated all rehabilitative efforts is a common feature. Stories such as these when elicited should raise a high index of suspicion and should prompt the search for more specific RSD features.

Symptoms and Signs

The outstanding feature of RSD pain is a spontaneous superficial burning sensation

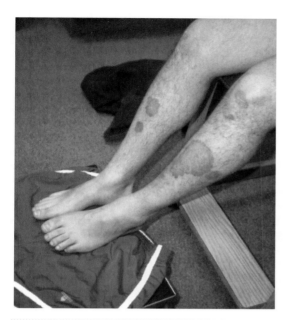

Figure 18–1. Patient with history of psoriasis suffering from reflex sympathetic dystrophy caused by blunt trauma to the left foot showing vasomotor instability. Note erythematous patch over dorsum of foot that is distinct from the pre-existing scaly skin on leg.

superimposed on a continuous deep, often described as crushing, tearing, or throbbing pain. Exacerbation with movement is usual, but many patients notice worse pain when resting at night. There is often increased pain with weather changes as well as heat or cold intolerance. Patients usually shy away from bright sunshine and cold wind or even air conditioners. Peculiar signs in the affected parts include allodynia (pain resulting from nonpainful stimuli such as light pressure), dysesthesia (unpleasant abnormal sensation such as stinging when lightly scratched), and hyperesthesia (increasing pain sensation to mild noxious stimuli such as a pinprick or a heat lamp). Other findings may be more extensive, not limited to the territory of a single nerve. Vasomotor (Fig. 18–1) and sudomotor disturbances may be found in more than just the affected limb. In more advanced or chronic cases, structural changes of the skin appendages and deeper tissues may be present.

Varied symptoms and signs may be grouped according to their severity. In 1953, Bonica proposed a continuum of the RSD syndrome using stages I to III.[15] Later

Schwartzman[16] redefined the stages as acute, dystrophic, and atrophic, respectively.

Stage I (Acute)

This stage may occur immediately or within days of the inciting event. It is characterized by spontaneous pain with dysesthesia and warm skin with localized edema. There is a reluctance to touch and move the affected body part as a result of tenderness and muscle spasm. Increased hair and nail growth may be seen. In early stage I, the pain is usually limited to the distribution of the principle nerves involved. The skin is usually warm, dry, and red, sometimes showing vasomotor instability. In late stage I, however, the pain spreads beyond the involved dermatomes, and the skin becomes cyanotic or mottled (Fig. 18–2), cold, and clammy. In some patients, friction from clothing or light air movement on the skin may cause excruciating pain. There are usually no radiographic bone changes at this time.

Stage II (Dystrophic)

Stage II usually sets in 3 to 6 months from the onset but may appear sooner in rapidly progressing cases. This stage is heralded by a gradual increase in the area of pain, extent of the edema, degree of joint stiffness, extent of soft tissue, and muscle wasting.

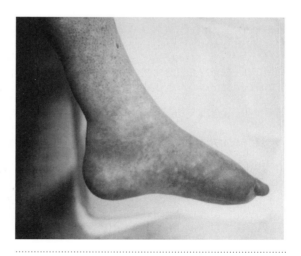

Figure 18–2. Patient with reflex sympathetic dystrophy resulting from ischemic necrosis, which required toe amputation. Patchy erythema and pallor produced a mottled appearance.

The edema changes from a soft to a brawny type with glazed overlying skin. More advanced changes in the skin appendages are present. The hair becomes scant, and the nails become brittle, cracked, and grooved. Disturbance of motor functions such as tremors or dystonia may be present. Radiographic changes appear in this stage.

Stage III (Atrophic)

This stage is characterized by advanced trophic changes that are mostly irreversible. The skin is smooth, almost glossy. It may be pale or cyanotic and feels cold as the temperature further decreases. The hair becomes sparse and coarse. Subcutaneous tissue turns brawny as it becomes atrophic with marked loss of fat. The digits are thin with severe atrophy of muscles, particularly the interossei. The interphalangeal and other joints of the extremity become stiff with decreased range of motion. They eventually result in ankylosis. Pain symptoms may have spread proximally or to other parts of the body. The affected parts are almost always aggravated by passive motion or touching. Emotional disturbance and visual or auditory stimuli can also cause marked sudden aggravation.

It should be noted that in any individual case there is usually some overlapping of the features described in the different stages because the changes are seldom clear-cut. For example, when the initial injury includes bone or joint trauma, osteoporotic changes may appear within a few weeks in a limb that otherwise appears completely normal. Furthermore, vasomotor instability and trophic changes, disparate though they may seem, are thought to be manifestations of a progressive pathophysiologic process.[17]

DIAGNOSIS

A complete history and physical examination with high index of suspicion is crucial for diagnosis of RSD and CRPS-I in the early stages. Often disproportionate pain is the only abnormal feature. Differentiation from other conditions may be difficult. Neuropathic pain caused by an injured or entrapped peripheral nerve or a neuroma anywhere from its root to the terminal branches, may present similar symptoms, such as burning pain with hyperpathia. They are, however, usually limited to the territory of the involved nerve and associated with little sympathetic activities.

Inflammatory processes not involving nerves, such as tenosynovitis and bursitis, may produce burning pain which persists for months.[17] They do not, however, show Tinel's sign, which is specific to nerves. Vascular diseases that cause decreased circulation such as Raynaud's phenomenon or disseminated lupus erythematosus may mimic RSD, although they usually affect more than one extremity at once. Therefore, the diagnosis is not infrequently made by exclusion, especially in cases of early SIP. Little wonder that there are still many clinicians who do not even accept that there is a pathologic state called RSD!

Several investigative tools may help to consolidate the diagnosis of RSD. Quantitative sweat test may show excessive sweating, and thermography can demonstrate a disorder in heat regulation. Heat loss from the skin surface is mainly regulated by sudomotor activity on the sweat gland and the dermal microcirculation.[18] An affected hand or foot may at times be hyperthermic, but relative coldness is the most common finding. These changes allow the observation of vasomotor instability. They have been related to sympathetic vasoconstriction and to compensatory or rebound vasodilatation of skin capillaries, which are, in turn, influenced by irritation of peripheral nerve fibers.[19]

Radiographic studies may reveal characteristic though not pathognomonic changes. Patchy osteoporosis is the primary roentgenographic manifestation of early stage II RSD.[20] Other features such as patchy epiphyseal demineralization of the short bones with soft tissue swelling; subperiosteal resorption; striation and tunneling in the cortex; as well as large excavation and tunneling of the endosteal surfaces may also be present. One must be aware, however, that similar pictures may also be seen in hyperparathyroidism, thyrotoxicosis, and other conditions with increased bone turnover.[21] In later stage II, when dystrophy borders on atrophy, severe and diffuse osteoporosis is the usual finding.

Triple-phase bone scan using technetium-99 may demonstrate increased periarticular uptake in the involved extremity (Fig. 18–3).[20] A positive bone scan in a patient with

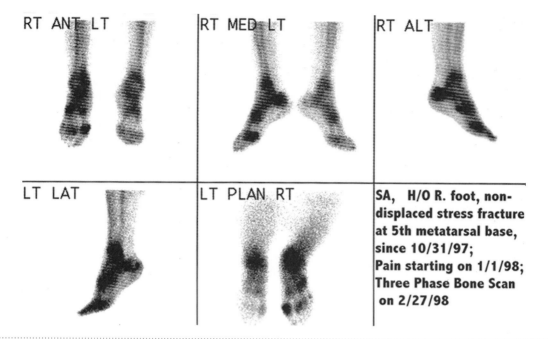

Figure 18–3. Bone scan from a patient 4 months after right fifth metatarsal fracture. Clinical reflex sympathetic dystrophy developed within 8 weeks of injury.

clinical signs and symptoms of RSD helps to confirm the diagnosis. Conversely, a negative scan in a patient with clinical RSD does not rule out the condition because some patients will present with initial negative scans that become positive later.[60]

Each finding, be it thermographic, radiographic, or scintigraphic, despite their sensitivity, when present in isolation, tends to be nonspecific and impossible to distinguish from other metabolic or inflammatory conditions. Taken together, they greatly strengthen the diagnosis. The diagnostic gold standard has been pain relief from a sympathetic nerve block. Clearly, RSD can be confirmed after positive responses to diagnostic sympathetic blocks only in patients with SMP. When evaluating the result, care must be taken that somatic nerves are not anesthetized during the sympathetic block, or the outcome cannot be interpreted. Even when done properly, there is still the unavoidable confounding placebo effect. To circumvent this, an α-adrenergic receptor blocker, phentolamine, has been used intravenously as a predictor agent before invasive lumbar sympathetic blockade.[22, 23] Of course, for patients with SIP, negative response to sympathetic blocks does not rule out RSD.

TREATMENT

Any treatment must be targeted toward relief of suffering, avoidance of disuse atrophy, and ultimately a return to normal function. Many patients, especially those with early stages of RSD, do recover gradually with physiotherapy and analgesic drugs alone. In more advanced or chronic cases, more aggressive treatments are needed to break the vicious cycle of pain, immobility, disuse atrophy, and suffering, which lead to more pain. For any patient, treatment should follow a preplanned algorithm to effect minimum time lost between each chosen method. Psychologic evaluation with ongoing counseling for the patients and their immediate family members must be an integral part of the treatment regimen. The emphasis is toward a multidisciplinary approach, which ensures that important aspects of the patient's care are not overlooked.

Noninvasive Modalities
Physical Therapy

Physical therapy is the mainstay of overcoming disuse atrophy. To minimize fear of painful motion, patients should be given only active or actively assisted therapy within limits of tolerance. Aggressive physical therapy without adequate pain management usually leads to patient noncompliance with the treatment program and delayed recovery. Therefore, passive exercise may be undertaken only when both the patient and the therapist thoroughly understand and accept the risk of more pain, swelling, and stiffness by forcing motions beyond the point of discomfort.[24]

Transcutaneous Electrical Nerve Stimulation

Transcutaneous electrical nerve stimulation became popular after the gate theory, proposed by Melzack and Wall, became generally accepted. When delivered at levels that produce skin tingling, it has been postulated to activate both large (Aβ, B) and small (Aδ, C) fibers.[25] The large-fiber signals close the "gate" and block the small-fiber signals. Alternatively, activation of small fibers may facilitate the descending inhibitory system.[24, 25] Using this modality, Robaina and colleagues reported excellent results in 25% and good results in 45% of RSD patients.[26]

Nonsteroidal Anti-Inflammatory Drugs

Although often used as the first-line analgesics for most chronic conditions, nonsteroidal anti-inflammatory drugs may be helpful during the acute stage when inflammatory changes and tissue edema are present. Their efficacy in established RSD has not been documented.

Tricyclic Antidepressants

Tricyclic antidepressants block norepinephrine and serotonin reuptake. They also block the α_1-adrenergic receptors, hence reducing sympathetic efferent activity. In animal models, they have been shown to block the hyperalgesia induced by intrathecally injected N-methyl-D-aspartate.[27, 28] It has been shown effective in reducing some of the neuropathic symptoms such as burning sensation.

Opioids

Opioid analgesics have been shown to block neuropathic pain less effectively than nociceptive pain. Although opioids are not very effective in treating RSD pain symptoms, they do improve the quality of pain control. They are especially helpful to patients getting over severe acute episodes. Because tolerance inevitably builds up, chronic use will result in escalating doses, with increasing potential for side effects. These medications should, therefore, be given judiciously.

Corticosteroids

Steroids have been used since 1953, when favorable results were reported in the treatment of shoulder-hand syndrome.[29] The pharmacodynamics remain largely unknown. Kozin and coworkers observed a chronic perivascular inflammatory infiltrate in synovial biopsy specimens from involved extremities.[30] Hence, the potent anti-inflammatory properties of the corticosteroids may partially account for their therapeutic effects. By stabilizing basement membranes, they reduce capillary permeability and decrease plasma extravasation commonly associated with early stages of RSD.[24] One potential advantage of systemic corticosteroids over the regional beneficial effects of sympathetic block becomes apparent when multiple body parts are involved. A 1997 review by Kingery confirmed consistent support in the literature for use of corticosteroids, which showed long-term effectiveness.[28]

Gabapentin

Gabapentin, an anticonvulsant, has been used for partial seizures with or without secondary generalization. Recently, it has been used for neuropathic pain with notably good results, as reported by Rosner and associates.[31] When given to patients with RSD, dramatic pain relief was observed and, in some cases, reversal of early trophic changes. Mellick and Mellicy reported corrections in skin temperature and color and lessening of and eventual relief from allodynia, hyperalgesia, and hyperpathia.[32] A major advantage of gabapentin is its low toxicity and side effect profile. It is generally well tolerated by most patients.

Carbocalcitonin

When bone scans show increases in blood flow and uptake of the tracer in the involved area, both porcine and salmon calcitonin have been reported to reduce local blood flow and decrease local clinical signs with relief from pain.[33] Nuti and others demonstrated similar improvements in the feet of RSD patients.[34] Salmon calcitonin is now available as a nasal spray, which significantly increases patient acceptance over the previous injectable formulation.

Clonidine Transdermal Application

Clonidine has a dual mode of action. In the central nervous system it acts as an α_2 agonist, and in the peripheral nervous system it inhibits the release of norepinephrine from sympathetic terminals. Thus, centrally it has analgesic effects, whereas peripherally it reduces the ongoing activity of nociceptors, hence decreasing the central sensitization and relieving hyperalgesia.[35] It is available as a transdermal patch, which is easy to use. In some patients, however, it may cause unacceptable hypotension or sedation.

Invasive Modalities

Intermittent sympathetic nerve blocks done in the early stages can be effective in achieving remission. Even in established cases, they are valuable as an option in offering to the patients periodic "breaks" from the vicious cycle. The procedure is not without risk, and repeated blocks tend to lose efficacy. When judiciously done at the crest of periods of exacerbation, intermittent sympathetic block can usually abort the need to resort to opioid medication. Of course, this is applicable only to those who respond to sympathetic blockade (SMP).

Sympathetic nerve blocks with local anesthetics can either be done at the lumbar sympathetic chain or as a regional perfusion in the limb with an α-adrenergic blocker such as reserpine, guanethidine, or bretylium. Currently, only bretylium is available in the intravenous form in the United States.

Lumbar Sympathetic Block

The purpose of sympathetic blockade in patients with CRPS is to interrupt the abnormal reflexes mediated by the autonomic nervous system. Sympathetic blockade can be

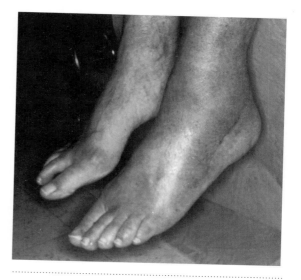

Figure 18–4. View 3 months postoperatively of patient with history of peroneal tendon repair who developed left foot reflex sympathetic dystrophy. Note shiny skin with subcutaneous edema.

both diagnostic and therapeutic.[24] In the early stage of SMP, a prolonged remission may be obtained from a single sympathetic block (Figs. 18–4, 18–5). Far more commonly, however, multiple blocks are required for prolonged pain control.[5] Typically, blocks are done closely, up to three times per week for 2 weeks in early cases, and then are tapered off to once weekly or less when symptoms subside or responses are stabilized.[36] When the condition is bilateral, lumbar sympathetic blockade (LSB) can be

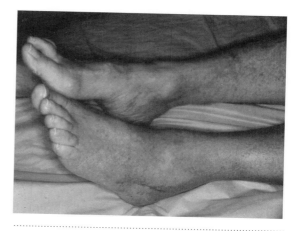

Figure 18–5. The same patient as in Figure 18–4 after one lumbar sympathetic block. Note significant improvement with reduced edema.

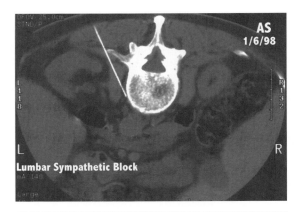

Figure 18–6. Lumbar sympathetic block under computed tomography guidance showing correct location of needle.

achieved bilaterally with epidural infusions for inpatients.[37] To maximize benefit from the nerve block, it should be followed by a course of physical therapy to improve range of motion.

NEUROLYTIC LSB WITH INJECTABLE CHEMICALS. Chemical agents such as concentrated alcohol or phenol can produce longer duration blocks lasting from a few weeks to several months. Haynsworth and Noe reported that 89% of patients in the phenol group showed signs of sympathetic blockade after 8 weeks (Figs. 18–6 and 18–7).[38] Some controversy surrounds the use of these agents, however, such as a high incidence (5–40%) of postsympathectomy neuralgia resulting from inadvertent damage to so-

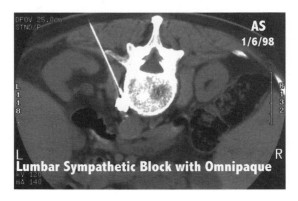

Figure 18–7. Lumbar sympathetic block under computed tomography guidance with contrast showing proper spread over lateral aspect of vertebral body.

matic nerves (e.g., genitofemoral neuralgia).[39, 40]

SURGICAL LUMBAR SYMPATHECTOMY. Because of the relative extensive area involved, surgical lumbar sympathectomy is usually not recommended, except when definitely indicated. The sympatholytic effect can be transient as a result of incomplete denervation.

INTRAVENOUS REGIONAL SYMPATHOLYSIS WITH GUANETHIDINE AND RESERPINE. As described by Hannington-Kiff in 1977,[41] it is essentially a modification of the Bier block procedure for local anesthesia. Pharmacologically, guanethidine acts as a false transmitter. It is taken up by sympathetic nerve endings and displaces norepinephrine from its storage sites. Thus, there is an initial release of norepinephrine followed by depletion. Excellent pain relief lasts from 12 to 36 hours but may be as long as a few weeks. Wahren and colleagues demonstrated that patients with SMP benefited considerably for 2 weeks or more, whereas no significant pain relief was achieved in patients with SIP.[42]

Reserpine acts by reducing reuptake of catecholamines, thereby slowly depleting norepinephrine stores in sympathetic nerve endings. Pain relief lasting from weeks up to a few months has been reported.[43]

Although reported complications from these drugs have been few, prolonged orthostatic hypotension with dizziness, somnolence, nausea, and vomiting can occur. Neither of these two agents has been approved by the U.S. Food and Drug Administration for intravenous infusion.

Studies such as that by Blanchard and associates[44] have thrown doubt on the efficacy of these drugs when used in this fashion. Saline infusion was observed to produce comparable results. This led some to contend that tourniquet ischemia was actually the active ingredient.

Intravenous Bretylium and Lidocaine Regional Block

Similar to guanethidine in structure, bretylium accumulates in postganglionic adrenergic neurons and inhibits their conduction by preventing norepinephrine release. In high concentrations, it also has local anesthetic and neuromuscular blocking properties. Poplawski and others reported good results with 1% lidocaine and methylprednisolone.[45] Hord and coworkers used the combination of lidocaine and bretylium, which resulted in longer relief than lidocaine alone.[46] Hypertension and tachycardia are the primary immediate side effects, followed by orthostatic hypotension resulting from the chemical sympathetic block.

Electroacupuncture

Electroacupuncture is claimed to release endogenous opioids, endorphins, and enkephalins in the central nervous system, thereby achieving pain reduction. The electric current during electroacupuncture may also act locally to relax the postcapillary sphincters, thus reducing the local edema and swelling.[47] Needle stimulation may also increase large-fiber transmission and close the gate to small-fiber pain signals according to the gate control theory of Melzack and Wall.[10]

New Invasive Modalities

Radiofrequency Lumbar Sympathectomy

This technique uses a heat-generating radiofrequency directed through an insulated wire at the nerve or ganglion. It offers a limited, controlled thermal lesion, thus avoiding significant neurologic deficits that may occur with injected chemicals. Also, less scar is produced, making repeated procedures possible.[48] Kantha reported that the duration of relief from radiofrequency sympathectomy appears to be longer than that from chemical neurolytic agents and may be as long as that from open surgery.[59] On the other hand, Rocco concluded that despite early successful lumbar sympathetic block, long-lasting pain relief was difficult to obtain.[49] Comparing incidence of postsympathectomy neuralgia, Haynsworth and Noe's study showed 11% in the radiofrequency group versus 33% in the phenol group.[38]

Epidural Clonidine

Clonidine is an α_2-adrenoreceptor agonist, which binds both pre- and postsynaptic neurons. It decreases anesthetic requirement during surgery[50, 51] and postoperative morphine requirement.[52] Clonidine administered epidurally produces analgesia that is not reversed by opiate antagonist. Rauck and colleagues[53] demonstrated extensive analgesia with epidural clonidine. The proposed mechanisms include reduced norepinephrine release peripherally, reduction of sympathetic outflow centrally, and the postsynaptic action of hyperpolarization of dorsal horn WDR neurons.[53]

Spinal Cord Stimulation

Electrical stimulation of the spinal cord for analgesia was proposed soon after publication of the gate control theory.[10] Technically simplistic, it involves insertion of an electrode-tipped catheter into the epidural space at the appropriate spinal segment. This allows a variety of currents to stimulate the spinal cord directly (Fig. 18–8). Many different theories have been proposed to explain how it works.[54] Experience has shown that, in addition to pain relief, spinal cord stimulation has been successful to some degree in reversing the "inability" to move injured extremities.[55] It was also found helpful in patients who suffer recurrent pain after surgical sympathectomy.[56]

PROGNOSIS

Two important factors that influence long-term patient outcome regardless of etiology are (1) early recognition with appropriate treatments and (2) vigorous rehabilitation therapies. If diagnosed early, the majority

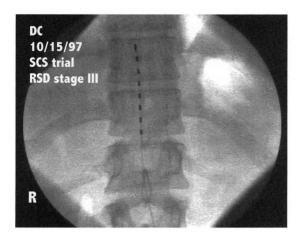

Figure 18–8. Spinal cord stimulator inserted at T10-11 with eight electrodes. (RSD = reflex sympathetic dystrophy; SCS = spinal cord stimulation.)

of patients with RSD–CRPS-I will respond to a course of prudent physical therapy and adequate analgesia. With delayed treatment, the RSD syndrome may spread proximally from one extremity or even to the other extremities. It is potentially devastating to patients in whom the disease progresses to the dystrophic-atrophic stages. Evaluation of any particular treatment regimen must be tempered by the awareness that a certain number of cases will show spontaneous resolution, whereas certain others will continue down a road of relentless progression despite maximum and timely therapeutic efforts.

Any surgery performed in or close to the RSD affected area may lead to acute and prolonged exacerbation of pre-existing symptoms. In other words, to an RSD patient, there is no minor surgery. A simple arthroscopy can lead to loss of ground gained by months of hard work. Therefore, adequate pain control by epidural anesthetic and opiate infusion for a period of time perioperatively to create a pain-free window for regaining or maintaining range of motion is of utmost importance.[5]

PATIENT HISTORIES

Patient A

S.A. is a 59-year-old woman who had a nondisplaced right fifth metatarsal fracture in October 1997. She was treated with cast stabilization for 8 weeks. She was referred to pain consultation 5 months after the injury. S.A. reported that she had suffered from throbbing, aching, and occasional shooting pain while wearing the cast. Symptoms escalated since cast removal. The pain was aggravated by movement and weather changes. She could not tolerate wearing sock and walked with a cane. Her pain score (visual analogue score) was 8/10. Bone scan revealed diffuse increased vascularity and uptake in the right lower leg, ankle, and foot (see Fig. 18–3). The right plantar skin temperature was 29.7°C versus 28.7°C on the left. Patient history and symptoms and signs were consistent with RSD early stage I. Diagnostic LSB resulted in 2 to 3 days of significant pain relief. Thereafter, three more lumbar sympathetic blocks were performed with concomitant physical therapy. Gabapentin (Neurontin) was also pre-scribed. Within 3 weeks, she reported improvement of 70 to 80%. She could wear shoes and walk without a cane.

Patient B

D.C. is a 30-year-old man who has suffered a right foot and ankle injury after falling through an improperly covered manhole. There was no fracture, but he had progressive debilitation and pain in the right lower extremity. He described his pain as spreading from the tips of the toes to the groin. Other symptoms included constant sharp and burning pain. Physical findings included cold skin with atrophic changes, limited range of motion, and inability to weight bear. He could not tolerate wearing a shoe on the injured side. He had undergone treatments, including several kinds of medication (amitriptyline, tramadol [Ultram], and gabapentin), diagnostic study (phentolamine infusion), physical therapy, and invasive treatment LSB as well as 5 days of epidural catheter infusion with local anesthetics. He had no long-term relief. About 20 months after the injury, spinal cord stimulation trial (Fig. 18–8) produced immediate improvement. One week later, the permanent stimulator was implanted. D.C. continues to do well at 5 months follow-up with 70% less pain medication, and he can tolerate aggressive physical therapy.

SUMMARY

Despite voluminous literature, many aspects of the treatment of these disorders are still based on empiricism. For example, it is not yet clear why sympathetic interruption in a warm, edematous, and vasodilated extremity does not produce further relaxation of arteriolar smooth muscle and subsequently an increase in swelling and pain.[24] Hypotheses have been proposed, but they lack experimental support.[57] The precise role of steroids also remains to be settled. There is no explanation either for the phenomenon that LSBs become less effective with repetition. Part of the difficulty in studying these patients has been the ubiquitous confounding effect of the placebo response.[58] Establishing a rationale for the treatments requires further careful investigation.

To the physician, the ultimate goal is restoration of complete functional and anatomic integrity of the extremities at the earliest possible time and by the simplest therapeutic procedure. Selecting the treatment best suited to the individual at the earliest moment will increase the chances of remission and reduce intractability. Long, continued vascular disturbances and disuse because of pain are the major cause of permanent disability.[35] Early diagnosis and specific, goal-directed treatments buttressed by a supportive social structure offer the best chance of returning the patient to a meaningful existence.

REFERENCES

1. Mitchell SW, Morehouse GR, Kean WW. Gunshot Wounds and Other Injuries of Nerves. Philadelphia: J. B. Lippincott, 1864:164.
2. Mitchell SW. On the diseases of nerves, resulting from injuries. In Flint A, ed. Contributions Relating to the Causation and Presentation of Disease, and to Camp Diseases. New York: U.S. Sanitary Commission Memoirs, 1867:412–468.
3. Roberts W. A hypothesis on the physiological basis for causalgia and related pains. Pain 24:297–311, 1986.
4. Stanton-Hicks M, Janig W, Hassenbusch S, et al. Reflex sympathetic dystrophy: changing concepts and taxonomy. Pain 63:127–133, 1995.
5. Ngeow J. Reflex sympathetic dystrophy of the knee. In Scuderi G, ed. The Patella. New York: Springer-Verlag, 1995:333–339.
6. Kuntz A. Afferent innervation of blood vessels through sympathetic trunks. JAMA 44:673–678, 1951.
7. Doupe J, Cullen CR, Chance CQ. Post-traumatic pain and the causalgia syndrome. J Neurol Neurosurg Psychiatr 7:33–38, 1944.
8. Devor M. Nerve pathophysiology and mechanism of pain in causalgia. J Auton Nerv Syst 7:371–384, 1983.
9. Sunderland S. Pain mechanism in causalgia. J Neurosurg 39:471–448, 1976.
10. Melzack R, Wall PD. Pain mechanisms: a new theory. Science 150:971–979, 1965.
11. Melzack R. Phantom limb pain: implication for treatment of pathologic pain. Anesthesiology 35:405–419, 1971.
12. Melzack R, Leser J. Phantom body pain in paraplegics: evidence for a central "pattern-generating mechanism" for pain. Pain 4:195–210, 1978.
13. Woolf C, King A. Dynamic alterations in the cutaneous mechanoreceptive fields of dorsal horn neurons in the rat spinal cord. J Neurosci 10:2717–2726, 1990.
14. Roberts W, Foglesong M. Spinal recordings suggest that wide-dynamic range neurons mediate sympathetically maintained pain. Pain 34:289–304, 1988.
15. Bonica J. The Management of Pain. Philadelphia: Lea & Febiger, 1953.
16. Schwartzman RJ. Reflex sympathetic dystrophy. Arch Neurol 44:555–559, 1987.
17. Butler SH. Reflex sympathetic dystrophy: clinical features. In Stanton-Hicks M, Janig W, Boas RA, eds. Reflex Sympathetic Dystrophy. Boston: Kluwer Academic Publishers, 1990:1–8.
18. Brelsford K, Uematsu S. Thermographic presentation of cutaneous sensory and vasomotor activity in the injured peripheral nerve. J Neurosurg 62:711–715, 1985.
19. Pochaczevsky R. Thermography in posttraumatic pain. Am J Sports Med 15:243–250, 1987.
20. Kozin F, Genant H, Berkerman C, McCarty D. The reflex sympathetic dystrophy syndrome: roentgenographic and scintigraphic evidence of bilaterality and periarticular accentuation. Am J Med 60:332–338, 1976.
21. Genant HK, Kozin JS, Bekerman C, McCarty DJ. The reflex sympathetic dystrophy syndrome. Radiology 117:21–32, 1975.
22. Arner S. Intravenous phentolamine test: diagnostic and prognostic use in reflex sympathetic dystrophy. Pain 46:17–22, 1991.
23. Raja S, Treede R-D, Davis K, Cambell J. Systemic alpha-adrenergic blockade with phentolamine: a diagnostic test for sympathetically maintained pain. Anesthesiology 74:691–698, 1991.
24. Schutzer S, Gossling H. Current concepts review—the treatment of reflex sympathetic dystrophy syndrome. J Bone Joint Surg Am 66:625–629, 1984.
25. Melazck R. Prolonged relief of pain by brief, intense transcutaneous somatic stimulation. Pain 1:357–373, 1975.
26. Robaina FJ, Rodriguez JL, de Vera JA, Martin MA. Transcutaneous electrical nerve stimulation and spinal cord stimulation for pain relief in reflex sympathetic dystrophy. Stereotact Funct Neurosurg 52:53–62, 1989.
27. Eisenach JC, Gebhart GF. Intrathecal amitriptyline acts as an NMDA receptor antagonist in the presence of inflammatory hyperalgesia in rats. Anesthesiology 83:1046–1054, 1995.
28. Kingery W. A critical review of controlled clinical trials for peripheral neuropathic pain and complex regional pain syndromes. Pain 73:123–139, 1997.
29. Steinbrocker O. The shoulder-hand syndrome: present perspective. Arch Phys Med Rehabil 49:388–395, 1968.
30. Kozin F, Ryan LM, Carerra GF, et al. The reflex sympathetic dystrophy syndrome (RSDS): III. Scintigraphic studies, further evidence of the therapeutic efficacy of systemic corticosteroids, and proposed diagnosis criteria. Am J Med 70:23–30, 1981.
31. Rosner H, Rubin L, Kestenbaum A. Gabapentin adjunctive therapy in neuropathic pain states. Clin J Pain 12:56–58, 1996.
32. Mellick G, Mellicy L. Gabapentin in the management of reflex sympathetic dystrophy (letter). J Pain Symptom Manage 10:265–266, 1995.
33. Caniggia A, Gennari C, Vattimo A, et al. Effetti terapeutici della calcitonina sintetica di salmone nel morgo di Paget e nelle osteoporosi. Clin Terap 82:213, 1981.
34. Nuti R, Vattimo A, Martini G, et al. Carbocalcitonin treatment in Sudeck's atrophy. Clin Orthop Rel Res 215:217–222, 1987.
35. Davis KD, Treede RD, Raja SN, et al. Topical application of clonidine relieves hyperalgesia in patients with sympathetically maintained pain. Pain 4:309–317, 1991.

36. O'Brien S, Ngeow J, Gibney M, et al. Reflex sympathetic dystrophy of the knee: etiology, diagnosis and treatment (abstract). Orthop Trans 15;747, 1991.

37. Betcher A, Casten D. Reflex sympathetic dystrophy: criteria for diagnosis and treatment. Anesthesiology 16:994–1003, 1995.

38. Haynsworth R, Noe C. Percutaneous lumbar sympathectomy: a comparison of radiofrequency denervation versus phenol neurolysis. Anesthesiology 74:459–463, 1991.

39. Cousins MJ, Reeve TS, Glynn JA, et al. Neurolytic lumbar sympathetic blockade: duration and relief of rest pain. Anesth Intensive Care 7:121–133, 1979.

40. Sayson SC, Ramamurthy S, Hoffman J. Incidence of genitofemoral nerve block during lumbar sympathetic block: comparison of two lumbar injection sites. Reg Anesth 22:569–574, 1997.

41. Hannington-Kiff JG. Relief of Sudeck's atrophy by regional intravenous guanethidine. Lancet 1:1132–1133, 1977.

42. Wahren L, Torebjork E, Nystrom B. Quantitative sensory testing before and after regional guanethidine block in patients with neuralgia in the hand. Pain 46:23–30, 1991.

43. Benzon H, Chomka C, Brunner E. Treatment of reflex sympathetic dystrophy with regional intravenous reserpine. Anesth Analg 59:500–502, 1980.

44. Blanchard J, Ramamurthy S, Walsh N, et al. Intravenous regional sympatholysis: a double-blind comparison of guanethidine, reserpine, and normal saline. J Pain and Symptom Manage 5:357–361, 1990.

45. Poplawski ZJ, Wiley AM, Murray JF. Post-traumatic dystrophy of the extremities: a clinical review and trial of treatment. J Bone Joint Surg Am 65:642–655, 1983.

46. Hord A, Rooks M, Stephens B, et al. Intravenous regional bretylium and lidocaine for treatment of reflex sympathetic dystrophy: a randomized, double-blind study. Reg Anesth Pain Manage 74:818–821, 1992.

47. Chan CS, Chow SP. Electroacupuncture in the treatment of post-traumatic sympathetic block (Sudeck's atrophy). Br J Anaesth 53:899, 1981.

48. Kline M. Stereotactic Radiofrequency Lesions as Part of the Management of Pain. Delray Beach, FL: St. Lucie Press, 1996:75.

49. Rocco A. Radiofrequency lumbar sympatholysis: the evolution of a technique for managing sympathetically maintained pain. Reg Anesth 20:3–12, 1995.

50. Bloor BC, Flacke WE. Reduction in halothane anesthetic requirement by clonidine, an alpha-adrenergic agonist. Anesth Analg 61:741–745, 1982.

51. Richard MJ, Skues MA, Jarvis AP, Prys-Roberts C. Total IV anesthesia with proprofol and alfentanil: dose requirements for proprofol and the effect or premedication with clonidine. Br J Anesth 65:157–163, 1990.

52. Park J, Forrest J, Kolesar R, et al. Oral clonidine reduces postoperative PCA morphine requirements. Can J Anest 43:900–906, 1996.

53. Rauck R, Eisenach J, Jackson K, et al. Epidural clonidine treatment for refractory reflex sympathetic dystrophy. Anesthesiology 79:1163–1169, 1993.

54. Krames E. Mechanism of action of spinal cord stimulation. In Waldman S, Winnie A, eds. Interventional Pain Management. Philadelphia: W. B. Saunders Company, 1996:407–411.

55. Barolat G. Current status of epidural spinal cord stimulation. Neurosurg Qu 5:1995.

56. Kumar K, Nath RK, Toth C. Spinal cord stimulation is effective in the management of reflex sympathetic dystrophy. Neurosurgery 40:503–508, 1997.

57. Blumberg H, Hoffmann U, Mohadjer M, Scheremet R. Clinical phenomenology and mechanisms of reflex sympathetic dystrophy: emphysis on edema. In Gebhart GF, Hammond DL, Jensen TS, eds. Proceedings of the 7th World Congress on Pain, Progress in Pain Research and Management, vol 2. Seattle: IASP Press, 1994:455–481.

58. Ochoa JL, Verdugo RJ, Campero M. Pathophysiological spectrum of organic and psychogenic disorders in neuropathic pain patients fitting the description of causalgia or reflex sympathetic dystrophy. In Gebhart GF, Hammond DL, Jensen TS, eds. Proceedings of the 7th World Congress on Pain, Progress in Pain Research and Management, vol 2. Seattle: IASP Press, 1994:483–494.

59. Kantha Sri R. Techniques of Neurolysis. Boston: Kluwer Academic Publishers, 1989.

60. Holder LE, Cole LA, Myerson MS. Reflex sympathetic dystrophy in the foot: clinical and scintigraphic criteria. Radiology 184:531–535, 1992.

Treatment of Bone and Soft Tissue Tumors of the Ankle and Foot

Ralph C. Marcove

As an introduction to this chapter, tables of both bone and soft tissue tumors are provided: Tables 19–1 to 19–5 from Arlen and Marcove,[1] Table 19–6 from Marcove and Arlen,[2] and Tables 19–7 and 19–8, which are based on my own personal experience.

Levels of amputation can range from phalangeal, ray, Lisfranc's, Chopart's, and Syme's to below-knee amputations. In advanced situations, when groin and iliac nodes are proven positive for cancer but the disease is still regionally localized, even a hemipelvectomy may be considered, along with the usual decision of performing groin and iliac node resections.

Radiation therapy (RT), especially for the small round cell tumors, may be indicated and even curative.[3–6] Radiation may also be given preoperatively to make a large inoperable lesion become operable. RT may be used postoperatively to improve the chance of cure of an otherwise marginal resection. Repeat postradiation biopsies may be of prognostic value. Late repeat biopsies may be necessary to rule out recurrence or secondary radiation sarcoma when the suspicion arises.

Similarly, cryosurgery may be useful instead of more radical surgery. This can also be used before resection or after marginal resection to achieve cure, which otherwise would not be possible. No late secondary sarcomas have been seen or reported in more than 30 years of experience in several thousand cryosurgery cases. Cryosurgery is especially useful in radioresistant lesions when a more limited level of amputation is desired. A prerequisite, of course, is that the area is small enough to freeze adequately: about 2 to 3 inches around the heat sink area. For best results, the eutectic point should be reached several times. Cryoimmunity, especially when repeated three times, has caused regression of limb-skipping lesions in satellite melanoma spread (A Gage, personal communication). Other suggestions of cryoimmunity have been seen

in several metastatic carcinoma cases (i.e., kidney and breast lesions). This has also been reported by Soanes et al.[7] for metastatic carcinoma of the prostate. Very little effort has been made by the medical community to duplicate these most important reports, even though literature on this subject has been in existence for up to 30 years!

Preoperative chemotherapy may similarly be used. Marcove and Rosen[8–27] and colleagues were the first to initiate preoperative (adjuvant) chemotherapy to shrink the tumor. Later resections can evaluate the resected specimens for adequacy of chemotherapy effectiveness.[8–27] (Preoperative chemotherapy also gives time to have custommade prostheses manufactured.) Marcove was also the first to evaluate multiple pulmonary resections to obtain cure rates that are now well known.[28–32] The published cure rates were later confirmed by the Mayo Clinic.

Prostheses for foot-ankle resections may not be needed for multiple-ray resections, Lisfranc's and Chopart's resections, and even Syme's resections as long as a distally filled high-top shoe can be worn. This may give a remarkably good gait. Below-knee resections can be performed even if only 1 cm of tibia and tibial tubercle can be saved. Postoperative flexion contractures, which would cause this level to fail, can be avoided if a Steinmann pin is inserted intraoperatively to maintain the functional position until spasms and healing are no longer a problem.

Prophylactic chemotherapy, radiation, and cryosurgery have been well discussed in many of our articles.

Vaccine trials for osteogenic sarcoma (autogenous lysed cell) have been tried in the past with an increase in "cure rate" from 17 to 38%.[33–38] This rate excludes the increased additional cure rate of 20% when multiple pulmonary resections are subsequently performed. Unfortunately, confirmatory trials were not done elsewhere. If chemotherapy
Text continued on page 237

Table 19–1. Classification of Somatic Soft Tissue Tumors

Area	Benign Tumors	Malignant Tumors
Fibrous tissue	Fibroma Keloid Dupuytren's contracture; palmar and plantar fibromatosis Peyronie's disease of penis; chronic fibrosing cavernitis Desmoid tumor of abdominal wall (desmoma) Progressive fibrosing myositis (Meyenburg's disease) Dermatofibrosarcoma protuberans	Fibrosarcoma Myxosarcoma
Undifferentiated mesenchyme	Myxoma Mesenchymoma (hamartoma)	Myxoma Malignant mesenchymoma
Heterotopic bone and cartilage	Myositis ossificans	Osteogenic sarcoma Chondrosarcoma
Adipose tissue	Lipoma (solitary and multiple) Congenital diffuse lipomatosis	Liposarcoma (well differentiated; myxoid) Pleomorphic (anaplastic)
Blood and lymph vessels	Hemangioma Systemic angiomatosis Rendu-Osler-Weber disease Lymphangioma Cystic hygroma Glomus tumor Hemangiopericytoma	Angiosarcoma Lymphangiosarcoma Angioendothelioma Kaposi's idiopathic sarcoma Hemangiopericytoma
Histiocytes	Fibrous histiocytoma xanthoma Giant cell tumor (soft tissue)	Dermatofibrosarcoma protuberans; fibroxanthosarcoma Malignant fibrous histiocytoma; malignant giant cell tumor
Synovial tissue	Giant cell tumor of tendon sheath Synovial xanthoma Hypertrophic arborescent synovitis of joints	Malignant synovioma (synovial sarcoma)
Smooth muscle	Leiomyoma Leiomyoblastoma	Leiomyosarcoma
Striated muscle	Rhabdomyoma	Rhabdomyosarcoma
Peripheral nervous system		
Non-neoplastic neuroectodermal tumors	Traumatic and amputation neuroma	
Peripheral nerve supportive tissues	Neurilemoma Neurofibroma Multiple neurofibromatosis (Recklinghausen's disease)	Malignant schwannoma (malignant neurilemoma; malignant neuroepithelioma)
Secondary neoplasms		Direct invasion into nerve sheath Intraneural metastasis Tumors of ganglia lying within nerves
Sympathetic ganglia	Ganglioneuroma (differentiated)	Partly differentiated ganglioneuroma; sympathicoblastoma (neuroblastoma)
Paraganglionic cells	Pheochromocytoma Paraganglioma Carotid bodies Ganglion nodosum of vagus nerve	Malignant pheochromocytoma Malignant paraganglioma
Miscellaneous	Granular cell myoblastoma	Alveolar soft part sarcoma

Modified from Arlen M, Marcove RC. Surgical Management of Soft Tissue Sarcomas. Philadelphia: W. B. Saunders, 1987.

Table 19–2. Soft Tissue Sarcomas
Evaluated by the American
Joint Committee Task Force

Alveolar soft part sarcoma	Liposarcoma
Angiosarcoma	Malignant fibrohistiocytoma
Extraskeletal chondrosarcoma	Malignant mesenchymoma
Extraskeletal osteosarcoma	Malignant schwannoma
Fibrosarcoma	Rhabdomyosarcoma
Leiomyosarcoma	Synovial sarcoma

Modified from Arlen M, Marcove RC. Surgical Management
of Soft Tissue Sarcomas. Philadelphia: W. B. Saunders, 1987.

Table 19–3. TNM Classification and Staging of Soft Tissue Sarcoma

TNM Classification		**Stage Grouping**	
Primary Tumor (T)		Stage I	G1, T1, N0, M0
Tx	Minimum requirements cannot be met	IA	Grade 1 tumor, < 5 cm in diameter, no regional lymph node or distant metastases
T0	No demonstrable tumor		
T1	Tumor < 5 cm in diameter	IB	G1, T2, N0, M0
T2	Tumor ≥ 5 cm in diameter		Grade 1 tumor, ≥ 5 cm in diameter, no regional lymph node or distant metastases
T3	Tumor that grossly invades bone, major vessel, or major nerve	Stage II	
Nodal Involvement (N)		IIA	G2, T1, N0, M0
Nx	Minimum requirements cannot be met		Grade 2 tumor, < 5 cm in diameter, no regional lymph node or distant metastases
N0	No histologically verified metastases to lymph nodes	IIB	G2, T2, N0, M0
N1	Histologically verified regional lymph node metastases		Grade 2 tumor, ≥ 5 cm in diameter, no regional lymph node or distant metastases
Distant Metastasis (M)		Stage III	
Mx	Not assessed	IIIA	G3, T1, N0, M0
M0	No (known) distant metastasis		Grade 3 tumor, < 5 cm in diameter, no regional lymph node or distant metastases
M1	Distant metastasis present	IIIB	G3, T2, N0, M0
			Grade 3 tumor, ≥ 5 cm in diameter, no regional lymph node or distant metastases
		IIIC	Any G, T1,2, N1, M0
			Tumor of any histologic grade or size (no invasion) with regional lymph node metastases but without distant metastases
		Stage IV	
		IVA	Any G, T3, any N, M0
			Tumor of any histologic grade of malignancy that grossly invades bone, major vessels, or major nerves, with or without regional lymph node metastases, but without distant metastases
		IVB	Any G, any T, any N, M1
			Tumor with distant metastases

Modified from Arlen M, Marcove RC. Surgical Management of Soft Tissue Sarcomas. Philadelphia: W. B. Saunders, 1987.

Table 19–4. Histologic Types of Lower Extremity Sarcomas

Type	All Stages	Stage I	Stage II	Stage III	Stage IV
All types*					
No. of cases	1215	177	86	329	110
Survival rate (%)†	41	75	(55)	29	7
Fibrosarcoma					
No. of cases	231	65	15	36	12
Survival rate (%)	48	(73)	5/15	(43)	1/12
Malignant fibrohistiocytoma					
No. of cases	128	15	29	45	7
Survival rate (%)	46	11/13	(72)	(22)	1/7
Liposarcoma					
No. of cases	221	57	18	48	13
Survival rate (%)	55	(78)	10/17	(35)	0/12
Angiosarcoma					
No. of cases	33	2	2	9	4
Survival rate (%)	24	2/2	1/2	0/9	1/4
Synovial sarcoma					
No. of cases	84	5	6	25	6
Survival rate (%)	(43)	4/5	4/6	(16)	2/5
Rhabdomyosarcoma					
No. of cases	234	1	0	97	35
Survival rate (%)	23	0/1	0/0	(30)	0
Leiomyosarcoma					
No. of cases	79	14	5	12	11
Survival rate (%)	(32)	8/14	1/5	3/11	1/11
Malignant schwannoma					
No. of cases	60	11	7	7	1
Survival rate (%)	(45)	8/10	1/6	—	0/1
Unclassified					
No. of cases	121	4	4	41	18
Survival rate (%)	36	4/4	2/4	(31)	0/17

*There were 24 cases of nine other types, each of which occurred too infrequently to warrant a separate listing. The specific diagnoses for these types were as follows: extraskeletal osteosarcoma (6), alveolar soft part sarcoma (5), extraskeletal chondrosarcoma (4), malignant mesenchymoma (4), malignant embryonal mesenchymal tumor (1), epithelioid sarcoma (1), fibrosarcoma with areas of chondrosarcoma (1), mesothelioma (1), and malignant hemangiopericytoma (1).

†Rates in parentheses have standard errors between 5 and 10%. When there were too few cases to calculate a reliable rate, a fraction is given with respect to the status of the group at the end of the 5 years. The numerator equals the denominator (the total number of cases in the group) minus losses to follow-up or patients diagnosed too recently to be observed for 5 years.

Modified from Arlen M, Marcove RC. Surgical Management of Soft Tissue Sarcomas. Philadelphia: W. B. Saunders, 1987.

Table 19–5. Distribution of the More Common Sarcomas

Sarcoma	Shoulder	Abdomen	Chest	Back	Head and Neck	Arm	Thigh, Buttock, and Groin	Leg	Hands	Feet
Dermatofibrosarcoma	15	19	17	17	11	7	20	6	—	2
Desmoid tumor	9	13	20	22	29	14	30	18	2	3
Fibrosarcoma	6	4	10	6	11	28	51	10	3	—
Fibrous histiocytoma	5	7	7	6	10	16	28	14	1	3
Liposarcoma	4	3	8	35	7	119	—	29	1	1
Pleomorphic rhabdomyosarcoma	11	6	8	5	8	9	58	10	1	2
Synovioma	11	1	—	3	5	12	49	14	10	25
Neurogenic sarcoma	2	3	9	13	17	8	21	2	1	1
Angiosarcoma	1	2	4	2	12	4	9	1	—	—

Modified from Arlen M, Marcove RC. Surgical Management of Soft Tissue Sarcomas. Philadelphia: W. B. Saunders, 1987.

Table 19–6. Tumors Involving the Osseous System

Origin	Benign	Malignant	Grade
Fibrous tissue	Fibromyxoma	Malignant fibromyxoma	Low grade High grade

	Subperiosteal desmoid
	Desmoplastic fibroma
		Low-grade fibrosarcoma
		High-grade fibrosarcoma
		Types
		  Central
		  Juxtacortical
		  Soft tissue	

	Benign fibrous
	histiocytoma
		Malignant fibrous histiocytoma
		Types
		  Myxoid
		  Giant cell storiform pattern
		  Fibrous type
			Low grade
			High grade

Bone	Enostosis (bone island)
	Ivory exostosis (no
	  cartilage cap)
		Osteogenic sarcoma (most common
		  malignant bone tumor of
		  childhood)
		Types
		  Central (low-grade type is rare)
		  Intracortical
		  Juxtacortical
		    Fibrous types
		    Cartilagenous type
		    Osteogenic type
		    Rule out myositis ossificans
		  Soft tissue osteogenic sarcoma
			Grade I
			Grade II
			Grade III

Cartilage	Osteochondroma
	  Solitary
	  Multiple
		Chondrosarcoma
		Types
		  Peripheral chondrosarcoma (on
		    an old osteochondroma)
		  Juxtacortical chondrosarcoma
		  Central type chondrosarcoma
		  Mesenchymal chondrosarcoma,
		    types A and B
		    A. 1. Hemangiopericytoma
		        (cells in periphery)
		      2. Ewing's (cells in
		        periphery)
		    B. 1. Osteogenic sarcoma
		        (probably best called a
		        variety of osteogenic
		        sarcoma)
			Grade I
			Grade II
			Grade III
			(keratin
			negative)

	Enchondroma
	  Solitary
	  Multiple
		Types
		  Chondrosarcoma central type
		  Soft tissue chondrosarcoma
			Grades I, II, III

Blood vessel	Hemangioma	Hemangiopericytoma	Low grade High grade
		Hemangioendothelioma	Low grade High grade
	Maffucci's syndrome with enchondromatosis	Chondrosarcoma	

Notocord
  Mesoderm
  Ectoderm
  Endoderm
		Chordoma (keratin positive)	Low grade
			High grade

Myeloid elements	Pseudomyeloma (infection)	Myeloma	Low grade High grade

Table continued on following page

Table 19–6. Tumors Involving the Osseous System *Continued*

Origin	Benign	Malignant	Grade

Primitive reticulum		Ewing's sarcoma
		  A. Differentiate Ewing's from neuroblastoma or sympathicoblastoma, which can mature into ganglioneuroma
		  B. With or without primitive neuroectodermal cells
		  C. Soft tissue Ewing's rare
		Malignant lymphoma
		Types
		  Reticulum cell sarcoma
		  Hodgkin's disease
		  Lymphosarcoma
		Leukemia
		Di Guglielmo's disease (acute erythemic myelosis)	

Nerve	Neurofibromatosis	Neurosarcoma	Low grade High grade
Fat	Lipoma	Liposarcoma	Low grade (rare) High grade (rare)
Mixed fibroelastic connective tissue series	Hyperparathyroidism ("brown tumor") Giant cell reparative granuloma		
Osteitis fibrosa group or giant cell variants or fibrocystic disease	Giant cell tumor, grade 1	Malignant giant cell tumor (rate may increase with radiation therapy)	Grade II (low grade) Grade III (high grade)
	Benign chondroblastoma, grade 1	Malignant chondroblastoma	Grade II (low) Grade III (high)
	Benign osteoblastoma Osteoid osteoma Unicameral bone cyst Aneurysmal bone cyst Fibrocortical defect (nonossifying fibroma)		
	Fibrous dysplasia	Malignant fibrous dysplasia (fibrosarcoma) (very rare malignant change; rate may increase with radiation therapy)	

	Ossifying fibroma (usual tibia)
	Chondromyxoid fibroma
	Eosinophilic granuloma
	  Solitary
	  Disseminated
		Disseminated eosinophilic granuloma (malignant form is rare)
		Letterer-Siwe disease (sarcoma; younger than age 4)	

	Paget's disease of bone Giant cell tumor in Paget's disease	Paget's sarcoma (high grade)	

Modified from Marcove RC, Arlen M. Atlas of Bone Pathology. Philadelphia: J. B. Lippincott, 1992.

Table 19–7. Foot, Ankle, and Distal Tibia-Fibula Lesions (N = 186)

Benign	No. Cases	Malignant	No. Cases
Aneurysmal bone cyst	9	Basal cell carcinoma	1
Chondroblastoma	2	Chondrosarcoma	13
Chondroma	2	Dermatofibrosarcoma protuberans	1
Chondromyxoid fibroma	2	Desmoid tumor	3
Enchondroma	1	Epithelioid sarcoma	2
Fibroma	2	Ewing's sarcoma	9
Fibromatosis	2	Fibrosarcoma	5
Fibromyxoma	4	Hemangiopericytoma	1
Giant cell tumor	10	Hodgkin's disease	1
Hemangioma	8	Kaposi's sarcoma	1
Neurilemoma	1	Leiomyosarcoma	1
Neurofibromatosis	1	Liposarcoma	3
Nonossifying fibroma	5	Lymphoma	4
Osteochondroma	11	Malignant fibrous histiocytoma	9
Osteoid osteoma	5	Melanoma	4
Osteomyelitis	10	Metastatic disease	2
Schwannoma	1	Myxoma	1
Unicameral bone cyst	3	Osteogenic sarcoma	12
Vascular leiomyoma	1	Plasmacytoma	1
Xanthoma	1	Renal cell carcinoma	2
	81	Reticulum cell sarcoma	1
		Rhabdomyosarcoma	1
		Small cell tumors	1
		Spindle cell sarcoma	2
		Sweat gland carcinoma	2
		Synovial cell sarcoma	22
			105

Age range: 5–84 years; no. females: 86; no. males: 100.

is given at the time of pulmonary metastases, it may delay the actual pulmonary resection. The surgical cure rate seems to fall to 15% from 20%, especially if the chemotherapy is similar to the previous treatment that was obviously not effective.

The benefit of Chopart's amputation with anterior tibial transfer into the head of the talus and held at 90° ankle position with a Steinmann pin intraoperative fixation (until healing is completed) is illustrated. Harold Dick has even successfully used os calcis allografts with good results in three cases, even though one graft was lost (personal communication). Cryosurgery of the talus and os calcis lesions has worked well in the author's cases. Illustrated cases are shown and personal tables of survival rates discussed.

PATIENT HISTORIES

PATIENT I

A 17-year-old boy presented with a swollen left ankle resulting from a sports injury. X-ray films were consistent with osteochondroma (Fig. 19–1A,B). The patient underwent excision of a mass from the left fibula, and pathology confirmed osteochondroma. Seven months later, left ankle x-ray films showed possible recurrent disease, and the patient underwent re-excision. Pathology was reported as recurrent osteochondroma (probable low-grade chondrosarcoma). This illustrates the need for fibula removal for good exposure and adequate margin of re-

Table 19–8. Treatments

Low-dose radiation therapy (i.e., eosinophilic granuloma)
High-dose radiation therapy (i.e., Ewing's sarcoma)
Excision alone
Incision with cryosurgery (i.e., aneurysmal bone cyst, giant cell tumor, and low-grade chondrosarcoma)
Preoperative chemotherapy and limited excision or limited ablation
Preoperative chemotherapy, preoperative radiation therapy, and then excision
Amputation
Pulmonary resections (preoperative chemotherapy?)
Limitations of radiotherapy to lungs (1500 rads, less with doxorubicin [Adriamycin], heart problems)

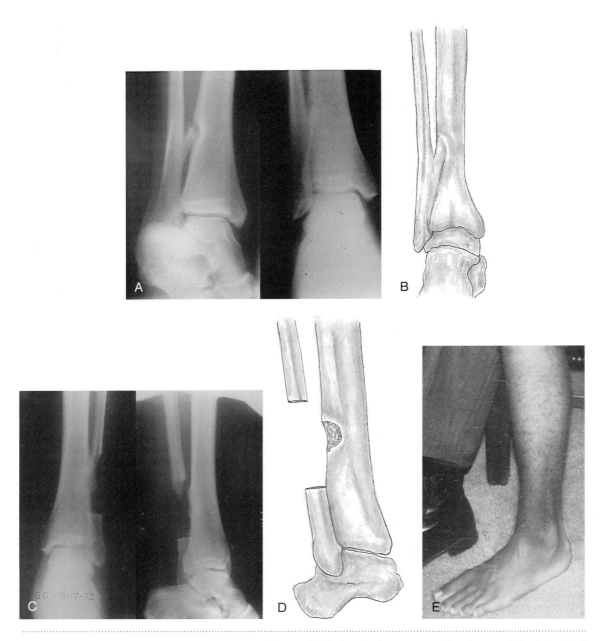

Figure 19–1. Patient 1. *A,* Preoperative x-ray films and *(B)* sketch showing osteochondroma of the left distal fibula. *C,* X-ray films and *(D)* sketch after excision of mass. *E,* Postoperative results show healed incision. Removal of the fibula is necessary for good wide excision of primary tumors in either the fibula or adjacent tibia.

section of a tumor in this area (and also adjacent primary tibia lesion). The patient is doing well 23 years later (Fig. 19–1C–E).

PATIENT 2

A 24-year-old black woman presented with a lesion of the left lower leg. A biopsy of the lesion had been previously performed at a local hospital, and pathology indicated low-grade chondrosarcoma (Fig. 19–2A,B). Three months after the initial biopsy, the patient underwent repeat biopsy, curettage, cryosurgery, and insertion of cement to prevent fracture of the left distal tibia. Pathology showed low-grade chondrosarcoma (Fig. 19–2C,D). Note the depigmentation of skin after cryosurgery (Fig. 19–2E,F). A repeat biopsy was performed 2 years after cryosurgery, and pathology showed some necrotic bone with no tumor identified (Fig. 19–2G). Eight years after the cryosurgery, the skin pigmentation began to return. Twelve years after the repeat biopsy, computed tomography (CT) and magnetic resonance imaging (MRI) showed fractures within the postsurgical bone. The patient underwent insertion of fibula bone grafts to the left distal tibia. Pathology showed bone with fibrous nonunion and no tumor (Fig. 19–2H,I). A circumduction fusion of the left tibia was performed 2 months later (Fig. 19–2J,K). The patient is doing well 19 years later, walking with full weight bearing and a normal gait (Fig. 19–2L).

PATIENT 3

A 20-year-old woman presented with a history of four recurrences of fibromatosis of the right foot. The mass was located on the dorsal area of the foot, and the second and third toes were involved with tumor. Her previous pathology slides were confirmed at our medical center. The patient was admitted to the hospital and underwent en bloc resection of the mass, dorsum of the right foot, including resection of the second, third, and fourth metatarsals, and insertion of a stabilizing transverse Steinmann pin. Pathology indicated a diagnosis of desmoid tumor (low-grade fibrosarcoma) (Fig. 19–3A–F). One and one-half years later, the patient underwent a below-knee amputation for multifocal disease. An above-knee amputation was performed 1 year later, and recurrent multifocal disease was found in the specimen. A follow-up MRI scan 2 years later revealed an expansive process involving the posterior compartment of the right thigh. A biopsy was done and showed fibromatosis (low-grade fibrosarcoma). We administered 5400 rads to the right proximal thigh. The patient is monitored yearly with CT scans and, aside from restricted flexion of the right hip, she is alive with no evidence of disease 15½ years later. Because we have seen one case of pulmonary metastasis of a "desmoid," we prefer to call these low-grade fibrosarcomas.

PATIENT 4

A 9-year-old boy presented with a history of lymphoma with secondary deformity of the left distal fibula. The ankle was treated with 600 rads. Because of ulceration and secondary infection, a distal fibulectomy was done (Fig. 19–4A–E). One year later, he underwent osteotomy of the left distal tibia with insertion of stabilizing pins (Fig. 19–4F). Pins were removed later (Fig. 19–4G–I). Eight months later, the patient underwent right tibial and fibular epiphysiodesis, and bilateral testicle biopsies were taken. Pathology showed that the right testicle was densely infiltrated by immature mononuclear cells consistent with lymphoma/leukemia; the left testicle was negative. We administered 1500 rads to the right testicle. The patient presented again 6 years later for foot deformity and poor ankle function; he underwent left ankle fusion with exostectomy of the medial malleolus. Pathology showed no evidence of tumor. Deformity can be seen on x-ray films (Fig. 19–4J–L). The patient is alive with no evidence of disease 25 years later. His leg lengths are satisfactory, and he walks well.

PATIENT 5

A 51-year-old woman presented with malignant lesions of both lower extremities (Fig. 19–5A). The patient underwent unsuccessful right foot disarticulation through the ankle. Pathology showed basal cell carcinoma and squamous cell carcinoma of the right foot involving the margin of resection. The patient subsequently underwent a right below-knee amputation. Margins of resection were negative.

The left ankle mass was resected with excision of the lateral two toes, part of the fibula, lateral tibia, lateral talus, os calcis, and cuboid with bone grafting across the

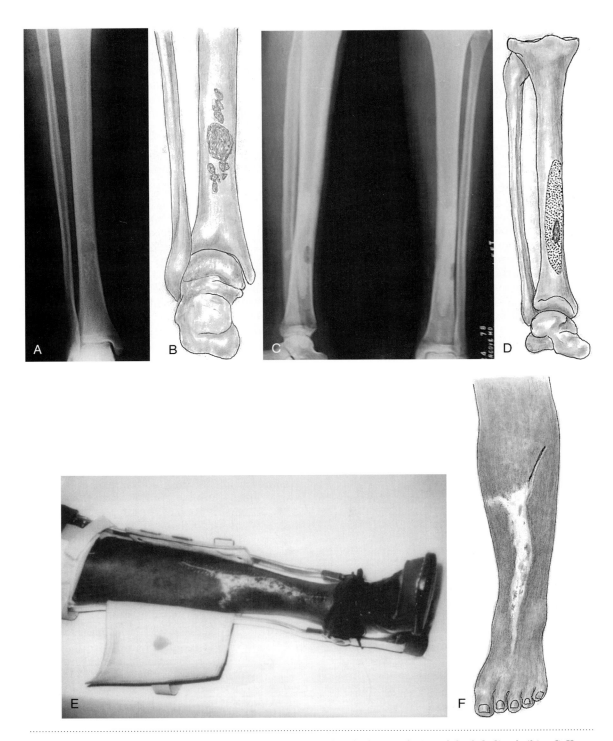

Figure 19–2. Patient 2. *A,* Preoperative x-ray film and *(B)* sketch showing lesion of the left distal tibia. *C,* X-ray films and *(D)* sketch after biopsy, curettage, cryosurgery, and insertion of cement to prevent fracture. Biopsy-derived diagnosis was grade I chondrosarcoma. *E,* Photograph and *(F)* sketch showing local depigmentation of skin after cryosurgery. Pigmentation began to return 8 years later.

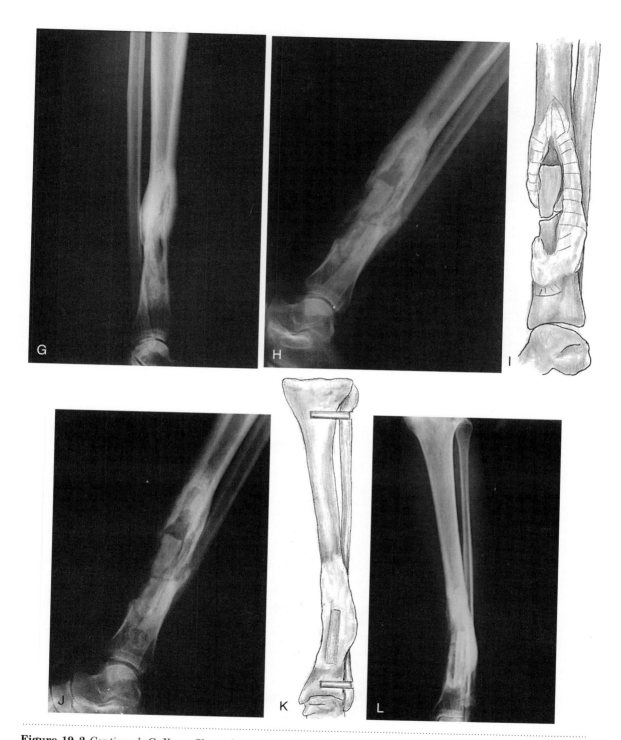

Figure 19–2 *Continued. G,* X-ray films after second-look biopsy. No tumor was identified. *H,* X-ray film and *(I)* sketch showing nonunion fracture of the distal tibia. Fibula bone grafts were inserted. *J,* X-ray film and *(K)* sketch after circumduction fusion (upper and lower tibia-fibula areas). *L,* Long-term follow-up x-ray showing healing of fracture after circumduction fusion.

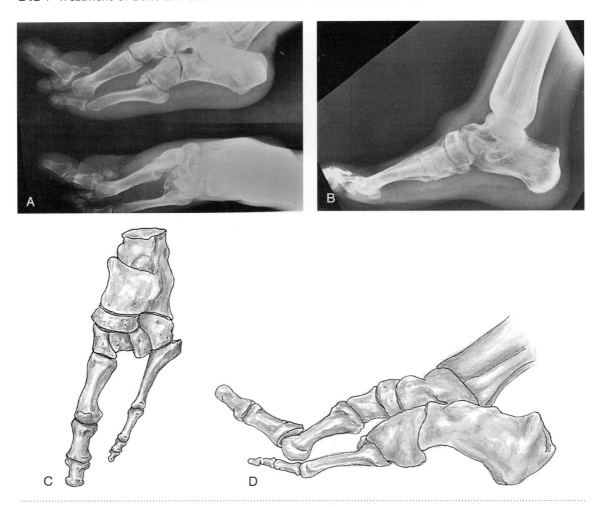

Figure 19–3. Patient 3. *A* and *B,* X-ray films after resection of the second, third, and fourth metatarsals and resection of mass at the dorsum of foot. Pathology was reported as desmoid tumor (low-grade fibrosarcoma). *C* and *D,* Sketches of anteroposterior and lateral x-ray films, respectively.

tibia to the remaining talus and os calcis. Pathology showed malignant fibrous histiocytoma of the lateral aspect of the left foot arising from subcutaneous soft tissue; the margins of resection were negative, as were soft tissue, skin, and bone from two resected toes on the left foot. One month later, the patient underwent debridement of soft tissue and bone of the left leg. Pathology showed necrotic skin and subcutaneous tissue with fibrous and marked inflammation. Two weeks later, she underwent open reduction of the deformed left lower extremity with insertion of a Steinmann pin through the heel into the residual tibia (Fig. 19–5*B–E*). Two years later, a local recurrence was seen; a left groin mass was also noted, and the patient underwent inguinal node dissec-

tion. Pathology was reported as basosquamous carcinoma. The patient underwent RT to the left leg. Approximately 4 years later, the patient underwent a left above-knee amputation as a result of radiation necrosis problems. She is alive without evidence of disease and is chairbound but otherwise doing well 10 years later.

PATIENT 6

A 12-year-old boy presented with a lesion of the left distal tibia. X-ray films were suggestive of aneurysmal bone cyst (ABC) (Fig. 19–6*A–D*). The patient underwent curettage and cryosurgery of the left distal tibia. Pathology identified a benign fibromyxoma lesion with cyst formation, osseous repair,

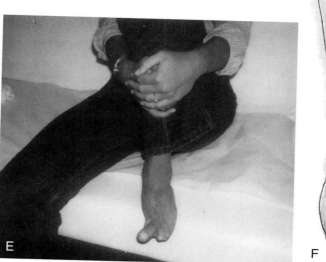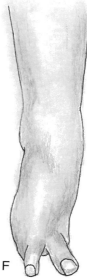

Figure 19–3 *Continued. E,* Photograph and *(F)* sketch after resection of toes. Multifocal disease later occurred. This occasionally is seen with abnormal metaphyseal tubulation.

and foci of giant cells in the area of hemorrhage (ABC with fibromyxoma). No lobulation was present (lobulation *must* be seen in chondromyxoid fibroma) (Fig. 19–6E,F). The patient is well healed and asymptomatic 25 years later and walks with full weight bearing (Fig. 19–6G–I). It is noteworthy that a large midwestern medical center has illustrated many chondromyxoid fibromas without lobulation. By Jaffe's original description, these could be fibromyxomas but not chondromyxoid fibromas, which need microscopic lobulation to fit Jaffe's criteria.[2]

PATIENT 7

A 16-year-old girl presented with a 3-month history of swelling over the right distal tibia, causing her to walk with a limp. She underwent open biopsy, curettage, cryosurgery, and insertion of fibula bone grafts to the right distal tibia. Pathology was reported as fibromyxoma of bone with secondary ABC (Fig. 19–7A–D). Again, no lobulation was present (as must be seen in all chondromyxoid fibromas). Approximately 3 years later, x-ray films showed the lesion to be recurring, and the patient was advised to undergo repeat curettage, cryosurgery, and bone grafting (Fig. 19–7F,G). The patient underwent exploration, curettage, and repeat cryosurgery to the right distal tibia

with insertion of left fibula bone grafts into the right distal tibia. Pathology showed fibromyxoma of bone with secondary reactive ossification. Follow-up x-ray films showed good solid healing, and the patient walks with full, normal weight bearing without pain 10 years later (Fig. 19–7H–M).

PATIENT 8

This patient presented with a lytic lesion in the distal tibia. Biopsy showed hyperparathyroidism. Note the mature fatty marrow dissecting fibrosis with new immature bone formation within the fibrosis (Fig. 19–8). This is a classic and pathognomonic finding.

PATIENT 9

A 23-year-old woman presented with a 3-month history of a constant dull ache in the left medial malleolus region. X-ray films showed a round cystlike lesion in the distal tibia. The patient underwent open biopsy and curettage of the distal tibia mass. Pathology showed dense fibrous tissue with a few scattered aggregates of lymphocytes. Cultures grew out *Debaryomyces hansenii.*[39] The patient's fungal bone lesion healed, and she continues to do well (Fig. 19–9A,B) without further treatment 16¼ years later.

Text continued on page 253

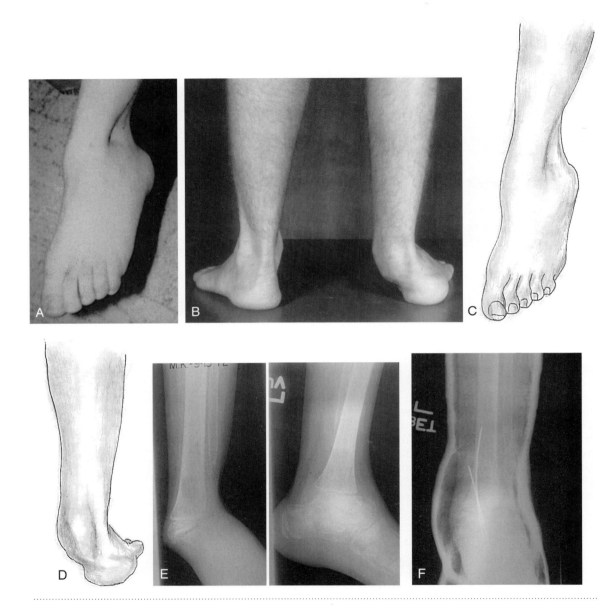

Figure 19–4. Patient 4. *A* and *B,* Preoperative photographs and *(C* and *D)* sketches showing deformity of the left distal fibula, secondary to lymphoma, local infection, and distal fibulectomy. *E,* X-ray films showing left ankle after being treated with 600 rads. *F,* X-ray film after osteotomy of left distal tibia with insertion of a stabilizing pin. G–I, Follow-up x-ray films after removal of stabilizing pin. J–L, Follow-up x-ray films after ankle fusion with exostectomy of the medial malleolus showing deformity of the ankle. (Patient walks well in spite of deformed foot).

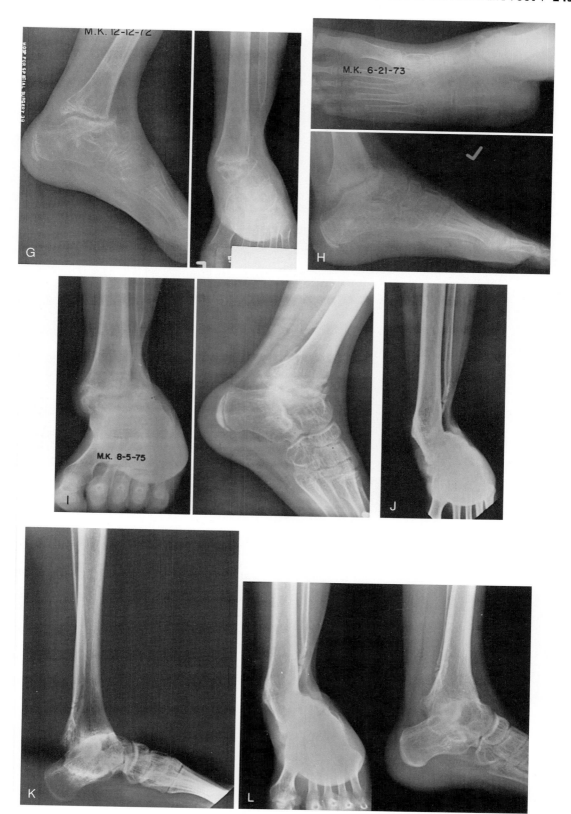

Figure 19–4 *Continued. See legend on opposite page.*

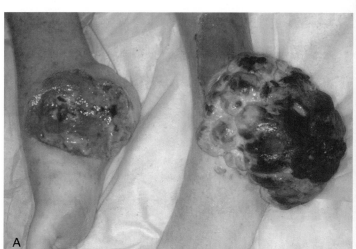

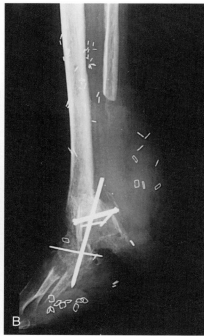

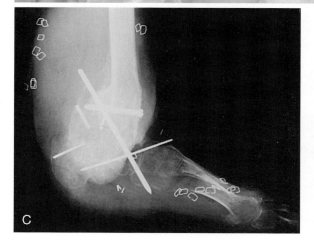

Figure 19–5. Patient 5. *A,* Malignant lesions of both lower extremities: basal cell carcinoma and squamous cell carcinoma of right foot and malignant fibrous histiocytoma of the left foot. A right below-knee amputation was subsequently performed. *B–E,* X-ray films of the left leg after amputation of two toes and excision of lateral tibia, talus, os calcis, and cuboid with bone grafting. Stabilizing Steinmann pin was inserted. A left above-knee amputation was subsequently performed.

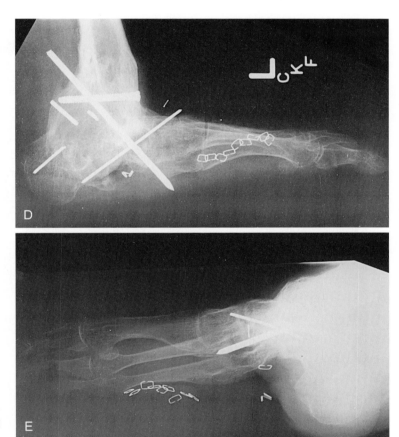

Figure 19–5 *Continued. See legend on opposite page.*

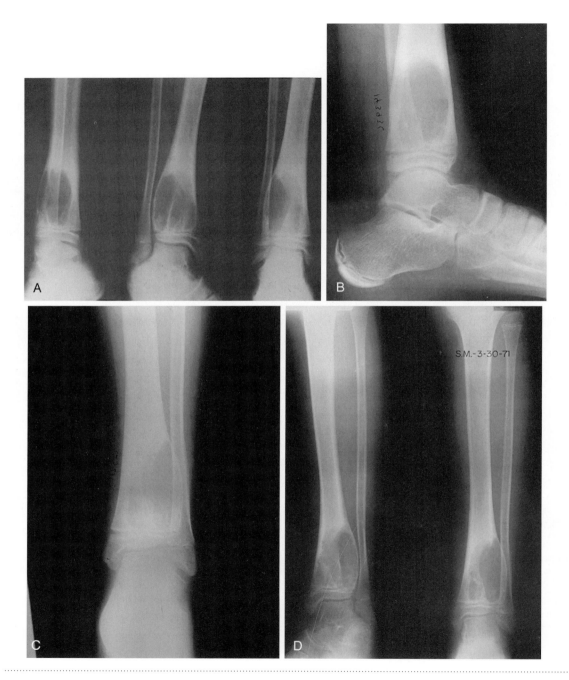

Figure 19–6. Patient 6. *A–D,* Preoperative x-ray films suggestive of aneurysmal bone cyst (ABC) of the left distal tibia.

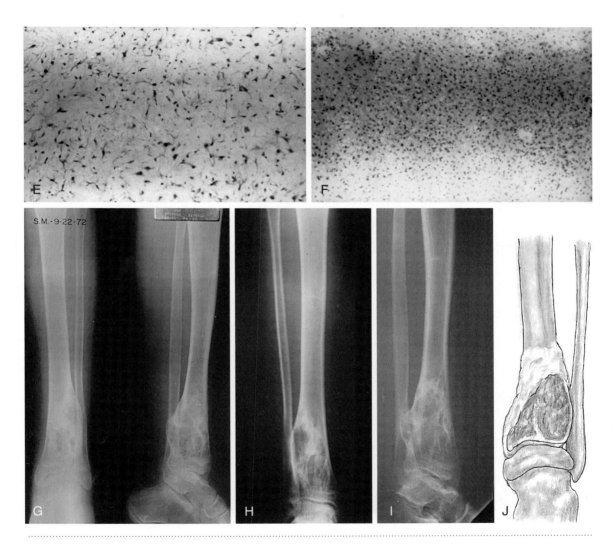

Figure 19–6 *Continued. E* and *F,* Specimen photograph showing ABC with fibromyxoma. Note that no lobulation is present, in contrast to a true chondromyxoid fibroma. *G–I,* Follow-up x-ray films and *(J)* sketch after curettage and cryosurgery. The patient is doing well 25 years later.

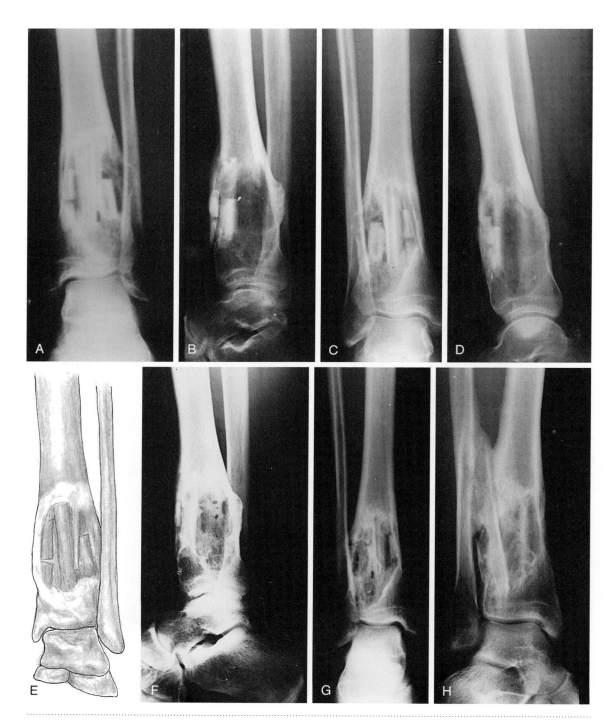

Figure 19–7. Patient 7. *A–D,* X-ray films and *(E)* sketch after biopsy, curettage, cryosurgery, and insertion of fibula bone grafts to the right distal tibia. Pathology showed fibromyxoma of bone with secondary aneurysmal bone cyst (ABC). Early peripheral new bone formation is present. *F* and *G,* Follow-up x-ray films showing recurrent disease 2 years later. *H, See legend on opposite page.*

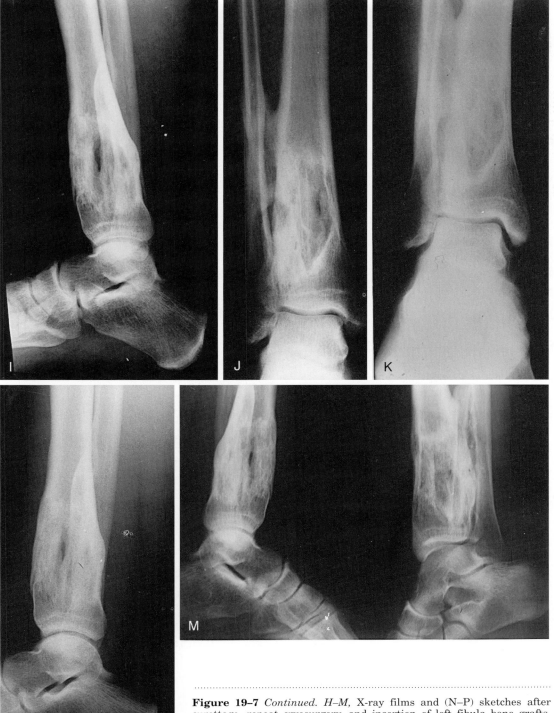

Figure 19–7 *Continued. H–M,* X-ray films and (N–P) sketches after curettage, repeat cryosurgery, and insertion of left fibula bone grafts. X-ray films show good solid healing 4 years later.

Illustration continued on following page

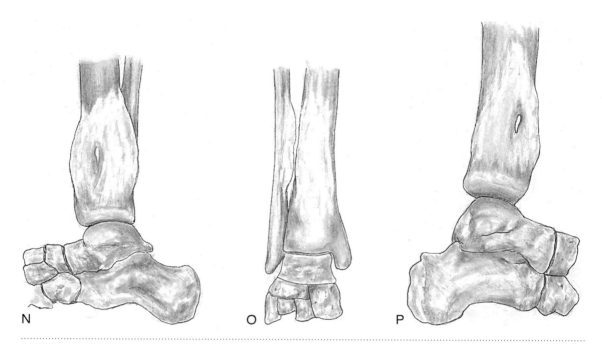

Figure 19–7 *Continued. See legend on page 251.*

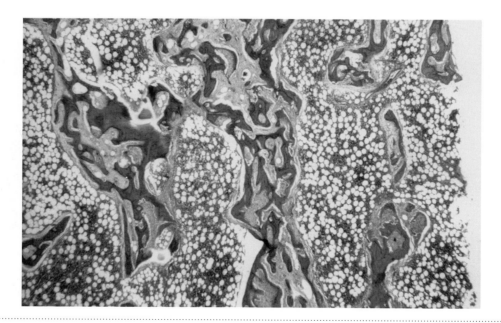

Figure 19–8. Patient 8. Specimen photograph showing hyperparathyroidism. Note mature fatty marrow dissecting fibrosis with new immature bone formation.

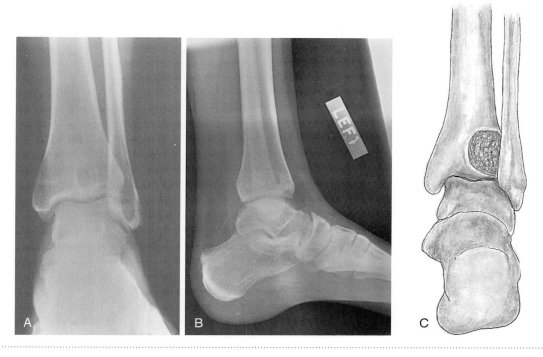

Figure 19–9. Patient 9. *A* and *B*, X-ray films and *(C)* sketch after biopsy and curettage of the left distal tibia mass. Cultures grew out *Debaryomces hansenii*.

PATIENT 10

An 8-year-old boy presented with a constant dull pain in the left foot lasting for 1½ years. X-ray films showed a lytic lesion in the left fifth metatarsal, and a biopsy was performed at a local hospital. Pathology indicated Ewing's sarcoma, and slide results were confirmed at our institution (Fig. 19–10*A*–*C*). The patient was admitted to the hospital and underwent a lateral forefoot amputation. Pathology showed Ewing's sarcoma with extension into adjacent soft tissue medially. Margins were free of tumor (Fig. 19–10*D*–*F*). Chemotherapy was then given. Seven years after amputation, a chest CT scan showed a lesion in the right middle lung lobe. A thoracotomy was performed, and pathology showed metastatic Ewing's sarcoma. Chemotherapy was recommended, but the patient refused treatment. He was alive with no local disease present for 7½ years. He died subsequently of pulmonary disease.

PATIENT 11

A 37-year-old man presented with a lump on the left forefoot of 2½ years duration after an accident. Biopsy of the mass was performed at a local hospital, and pathology indicated intermediate-grade fibrosarcoma (Fig. 19–11*A*). Slide results were confirmed at our medical center, and 1 month after the biopsy the patient underwent Chopart's amputation of the left forefoot with insertion of a Steinmann pin into the ankle to hold the foot at 90° for 2 months. The anterior tibial tendon was inserted into the talar neck at the time of the forefoot amputation. Pathology of the forefoot amputation showed foci of residual fibrosarcoma with negative bone and soft tissue margins (Fig. 19–11*B*–*H*). The patient continues to do well 18½ years later and ambulates well with a high-top shoe with a leather insert (Fig. 19–11*I*–*M*). He walks, runs, and dances normally.

PATIENT 12

A 40-year-old woman presented with a lump on the top part of the left foot of 3 months duration. An MRI scan showed a mass involving almost the entire cuboid, lateral cuneiform, and the third to fifth metatarsal base (Fig. 19–12*A,B*). The mass was

Text continued on page 260

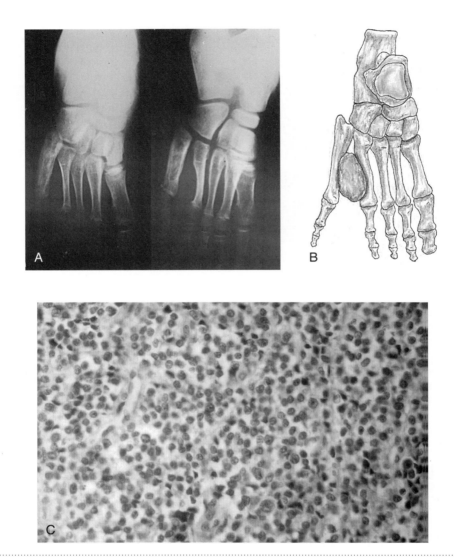

Figure 19–10. Patient 10. *A,* Preoperative x-ray films and *(B)* sketch showing lytic lesion in the left fifth metatarsal. *C,* Specimen photograph showing Ewing's sarcoma.

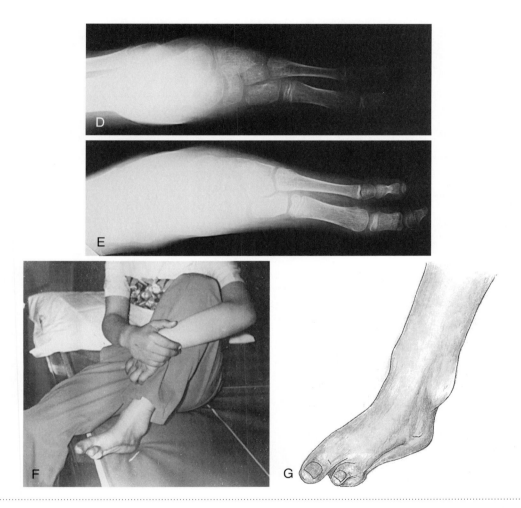

Figure 19–10 *Continued.* *D* and *E*, X-ray films after lateral forefoot amputation. *F*, Photograph and *(G)* sketch after partial forefoot amputation. The patient walks without a limp.

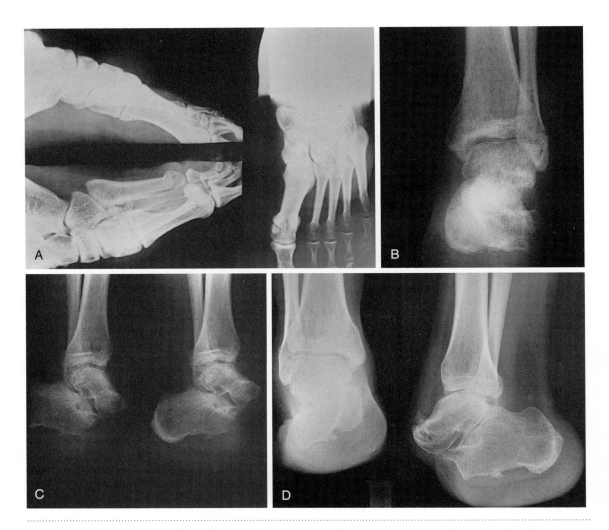

Figure 19–11. Patient 11. *A*, X-ray films after open biopsy of the left forefoot mass. Pathology showed intermediate-grade fibrosarcoma. *B–G*, X-rays after Chopart's amputation.

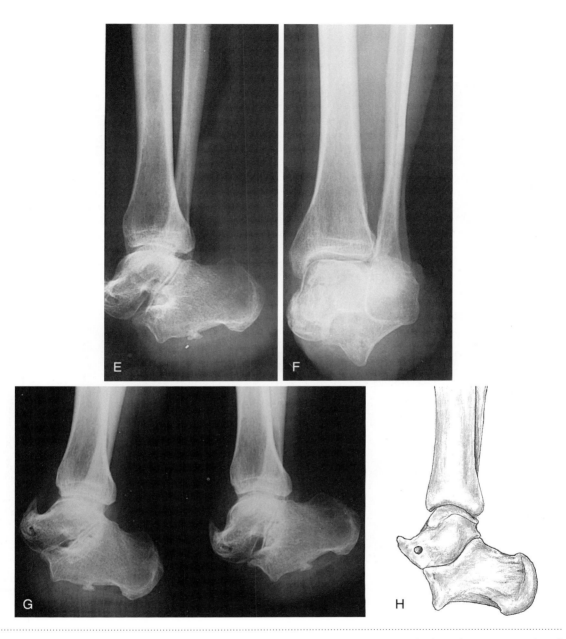

Figure 19–11 *Continued. H,* sketch after Chopart's amputation. The anterior tibial tendon was transferred through a drill hole in the talar neck.

Illustration continued on following page

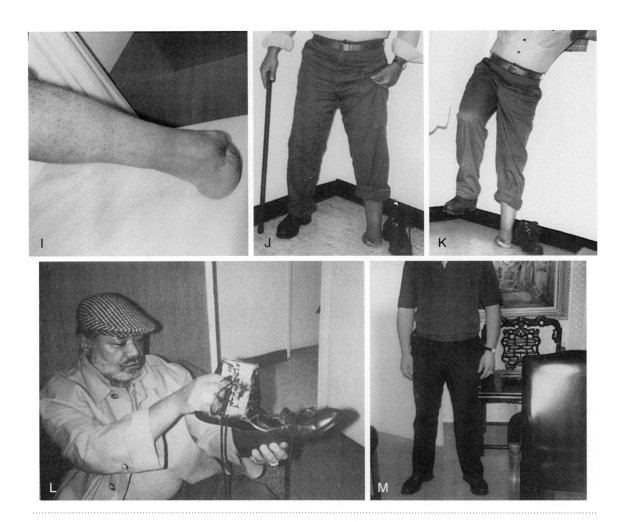

Figure 19–11 *Continued. I,* View after Chopart's amputation. *J–M,* Photographs showing that patient ambulates well with a high-top shoe with leather insert. Figure 19–11*L* shows the patient inserting his soft leather support into a regular shoe.

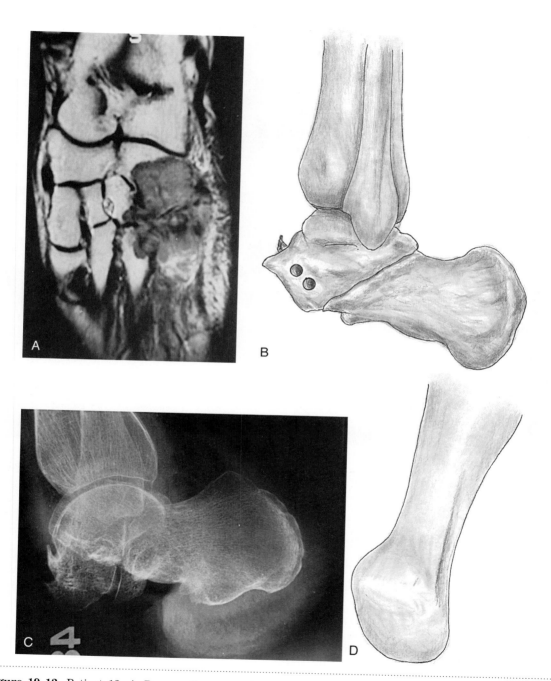

Figure 19–12. Patient 12. *A*, Preoperative magnetic resonance image and *(B)* sketch of lytic foot high-grade lesions (multifocal). *C*, X-ray film and (D) sketch after a high Chopart's amputation as a result of a high-grade sarcoma of bone.

Illustration continued on following page

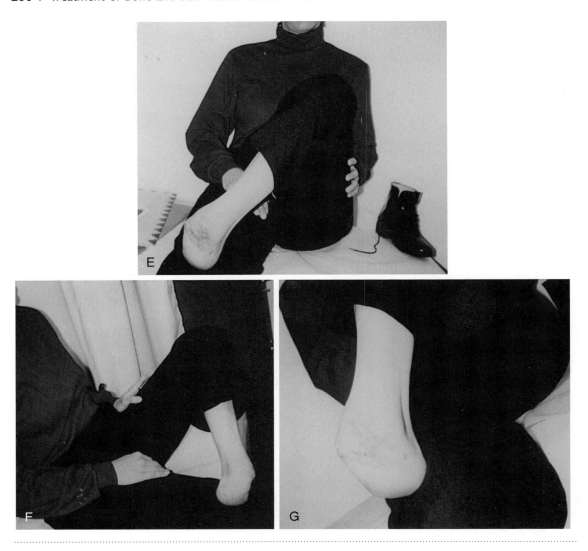

Figure 19–12 *Continued. E–G,* Views after amputation. Patient ambulates with a high-top shoe with leather insert.

multifocal and infiltrative with the appearance of an aggressive neoplastic process. The patient underwent an open biopsy and resection of the fore and midfoot. Pathology indicated high-grade sarcoma of bone. One month later, because of the close margin of resection, she underwent a higher Chopart's amputation of the left foot, including part of the distal os calcis. Two months after the amputation, the patient underwent surgical debridement of the left foot because of poor wound healing. Pathology was negative for tumor. Two months later, she underwent ex-

cision of the margin and deep surface of the left stump; split-thickness skin grafts were taken from above the knee. Again, no tumor was identified on pathologic evaluation. The patient continues to do well 2½ years later and ambulates with a high-top shoe (Fig. 19–12C–G).

PATIENT 13

A 46-year-old man presented with an 8-month history of a right ankle mass. The patient underwent excision of the mass from

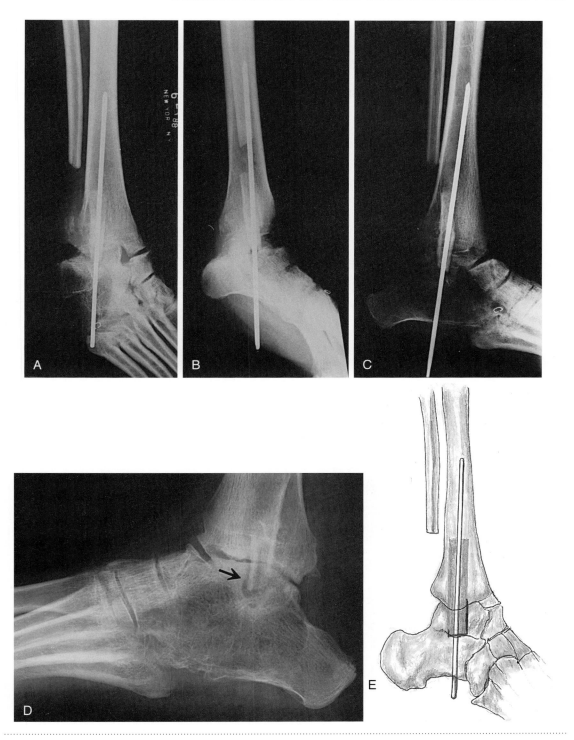

Figure 19–13. Patient 13. *A–D,* X-ray films and (E) sketch after wide excision of right lateral ankle mass, distal fibula, lateral tibia, talus, and os calcis with insertion of a stabilizing Steinmann pin. Bone graft from the fibula above the resection is seen.

Illustration continued on following page

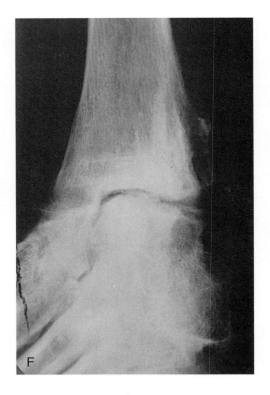

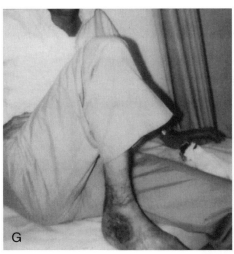

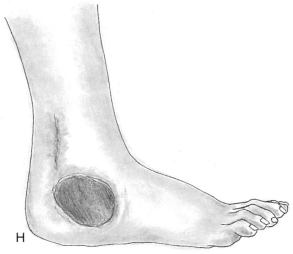

Figure 19–13 *Continued. F,* X-ray film after removal of Steinmann pin. The fibula graft has a fibrous painless union. *G,* Photograph and *(H)* sketch of the split-thickness skin graft onto the cancellous bone below. The patient walks well in a high-top laced shoe.

the lateral aspect of the right foot, and pathology indicated malignant mesodermal tumor. Slides were reviewed at our medical center and were reported as grade III leiomyosarcoma. The patient was then admitted and underwent a wide excision of the right lateral ankle mass, including the dis- tal fibula and lateral tibia, talus, and os calcis. A split-thickness skin graft was placed directly onto cancellous bone from the left thigh; a Steinmann pin was inserted in the heel into the tibia to maintain firm right-angle fixation (Fig. 19–13A–E). Pa- thology of the resection specimen showed residual viable leiomyosarcoma within bone underlying scar at the previous biopsy site. Margins of resection were negative. The Steinmann pin was later removed (Fig. 19–13*F*). The skin healed onto this cancellous bone, and the patient continues to do well 5 years later. The ankle has a fibrous union, and the patient walks well with a high-top shoe. He has no limp or pain (Fig. 19–13*G*).

REFERENCES

1. Arlen M, Marcove RC. Surgical Management of Soft Tissue Sarcomas. Philadelphia: W. B. Saunders, 1987.
2. Marcove RC, Arlen M. Atlas of Bone Pathology. Philadelphia: J. B. Lippincott, 1992.
3. Tefft M, Lattin PB, Jereb B, et al. Acute and late effects on normal tissues following combined chemo- and radiotherapy for childhood rhabdomyosarcoma and Ewing's sarcoma. Cancer 37:1201, 1976.
4. Marcove RC, Rosen G. Radical en bloc excision of Ewing's sarcoma. CORR 153:86, 1980.
5. Rosen G, Caparros B, Nirenberg A, et al. Ewing's sarcoma: ten-year experience with adjuvant chemotherapy. Cancer 47:2204, 1981.
6. Marcove RC. The treatment of Ewing's sarcoma. Arch Putti 35:317, 1985.
7. Soanes WA, Gonder MJ, Albin RJ, et al. Clinical and experimental aspects of prostatic cryosurgery. J Cryosurg 2:23, 1969.
8. Marcove RC. New trends in the treatment of osteogenic sarcoma. Orthop Digest 3:11, 1975.
9. Rosen G, Murphy ML, Huvos AG, et al. Chemotherapy, en bloc resection, and prosthetic bone replacement in the treatment of osteogenic sarcoma. Cancer 37:1, 1976.
10. Huvos AG, Rosen G, Marcove RC. Primary osteogenic sarcoma. Arch Pathol Lab Med 101:14, 1977.
11. Marcove RC. En bloc resection for osteogenic sarcoma. Can J Surg 20:521, 1977.
12. Marcove RC. En bloc resections for osteogenic sarcoma. Cancer Treat Rep 62:225, 1978.
13. Rosen G, Marcove RC, Caparros B, et al. Primary osteogenic sarcoma: the rationale for preoperative chemotherapy and delayed surgery. Cancer 43:2163, 1979.
14. Marcove RC. En bloc resection for osteogenic sarcoma. Bull N Y Acad Med 55:744, 1979.
15. Marcove RC. En bloc resection for osteogenic sarcoma. In Kumar S, ed. Advances in Medical Oncology, Research and Education. Oxford, England: Pergamon Press, 1979:197.
16. Marcove RC, Rosen G. En bloc resections for osteogenic sarcoma. Cancer 45:3040, 1980.
17. Marcove RC, Huvos AG, Meyers PA, et al. Conspectus—en bloc surgery for osteogenic sarcoma: analysis and review. Compr Ther 14:3, 1988.
18. Marcove RC, Rosen G. En bloc resections for osteogenic sarcoma. NCI Monograph 56:165, 1981.
19. Rosen G, Caparros B, Huvos AG, et al. Preoperative chemotherapy for osteogenic sarcoma: selection of postoperative adjuvant chemotherapy based on the response of the primary tumor to preoperative chemotherapy. Cancer 49:1221, 1982.
20. Rosen G, Marcove RC, Huvos AG, et al. Primary osteogenic sarcoma: eight-year experience with adjuvant chemotherapy. J Cancer Res Clin Oncol (Suppl)106:55, 1983.
21. Marcove RC, Abou-Zahr K. En bloc surgery for osteogenic sarcoma: analysis and review of ninety operative cases. Bull N Y Acad Med 60:748, 1984.
22. Marcove RC. Limb-sparing resections for osteogenic sarcoma. Clin Trials Cancer Med 81:75, 1985.
23. Bertermann O, Marcove RC, Rosen G. Effect of intensive adjuvant chemotherapy on wound healing in 69 patients with osteogenic sarcoma of the lower extremities. Recent Results Cancer Res 98:135, 1985.
24. Rosen G, Huvos AG, Marcove RC, et al. Telangiectatic osteogenic sarcoma: improved survival with combination chemotherapy. Clin Orthop 207:164, 1986.
25. Marcove RC, Huvos AG, Meyers PA, et al. En bloc surgery for osteogenic sarcoma: analysis and review of 180 cases. In Ryan JR, Baker O, eds. Recent Concepts in Sarcoma Treatment. Norwell, MA: Kluwer Academic, 1988:245.
26. Glasser DB, Lane JM, Huvos AG, et al. Survival prognosis, and therapeutic response in osteogenic sarcoma. Cancer 69:698, 1992.
27. Marcove RC, Sheth DS, Healey H, et al. Limb-sparing surgery for extremity sarcoma. Cancer Invest 12:497, 1994.
28. Martini N, Huvos AG, Mike V, et al. Multiple pulmonary resections in the treatment of osteogenic sarcoma. Ann Thorac Surg 12:271, 1971.
29. Marcove RC, Lewis MM. Prolonged survival in osteogenic sarcoma with multiple pulmonary metastases: a case report and review of the literature. J Bone Joint Surg Am 55:1516, 1973.
30. Marcove RC, Martini A, Rosen G. The treatment of pulmonary metastasis in osteogenic sarcoma. Clin Orthop 111:65, 1975.
31. Rosen G, Huvos AG, Mosende C, et al. Chemotherapy and thoracotomy for metastatic osteogenic sarcoma: a model for adjuvant chemotherapy and the rationale for the timing of thoracic surgery. Cancer 41:841, 1978.
32. Beattie EJ, Harvey JC, Marcove RC, et al. Results of multiple pulmonary resections for metastatic osteogenic sarcoma after two decades. J Surg Oncol 46:154, 1991.
33. Marcove RC, Mike V, Huvos AG, et al. Autogenous lysed cell vaccine in the treatment of osteogenic sarcoma—a preliminary report on fifteen cases. Colston Papers 24:313, 1972.
34. Marcove RC, Mike V, Huvos AG, et al. Vaccine trials for osteogenic sarcoma. CA Cancer J Clin 23:74, 1973.
35. Marcove RC, Southam CM, Levin AG, et al. Autogenous vaccines in the treatment of osteogenic sarcoma. Contemp Surg 2:54, 1973.
36. Southam CM, Marcove RC, Levin AG, et al. Clinical trial of autogenous tumor vaccine for treatment of osteogenic sarcoma. Proc Natl Cancer Conf 91, 1973:91.
37. Marcove RC. A clinical trial of autogenous vaccines in the treatment of osteogenic sarcoma. Beitr Pathol 153:65, 1974.
38. Marcove RC. A clinical trial of autogenous vaccines in the treatment of osteogenic sarcoma. Recent Results Cancer Res 67:488, 1974.
39. Wong B, Kiehn TE, Edwards F, et al. Bone infection caused by *Debaryomyces hansenii* in a normal host: a case report. J Clin Microbiol 16:545, 1982.

20 Stress Fractures of the Rearfoot, Midfoot, Distal Tibia, and Fibula

Lisa R. Callahan

Stress fractures are an easily recognized, less easily understood group of injuries. Defined as "a partial or complete fracture of a bone resulting from its inability to withstand nonviolent stress that is applied in a rhythmic, repeated, subthreshold manner,"[1] stress fractures were first reported by Breihaupt, a Prussian military physician who in 1855 described the painful, swollen feet of soldiers after long marches as "march fractures." Since that time, with the advent of roentgenography, many such fractures have been recognized in both military and civilian populations.[2–4] As our knowledge of bone health has expanded, so has our understanding of the different factors contributing to the development of stress fractures. It now appears that, similar to other disease processes, stress injury to bone occurs along a continuum, from normal physiologic bone remodeling to pathophysiologic stress fracture.[1]

Stress fractures generally fall into one of two categories: *fatigue fractures,* caused by the application of abnormal stress to a "normal" bone, and *insufficiency fractures,* caused by the application of normal stress to an "abnormal" bone. The term *pathologic fracture* should be restricted to fracture occurring in a bone that has already been weakened by disease (infection or neoplasm).[5] Determining the type of stress fracture and elucidating the factors contributing to its occurrence are critical not only to treat the acute fracture successfully but also to optimize attempts at prevention of recurrence.

BONE PHYSIOLOGY

Wolff's law states that every change in the form and function of a bone is followed by certain changes in its internal architecture and secondary alterations in its external conformation. A corollary to Wolff's law is that skeletal loading produces fatigue damage in the calcified matrix of bone, which is continually repaired by remodeling.[6] This is supported by substantial evidence that, although fatigue-related microdamage occurs in the living skeleton, this microdamage does not accumulate with age.[7] Understanding, then, that bone is a dynamic tissue, one must consider the factors that affect "form and function," thereby determining the point at which the skeleton's ability to repair microdamage is exceeded by the rate or degree of microdamage incurred. Basically, this is a function of both mechanics and bone biology.

BIOLOGY

The primary biologic determinant of bone integrity is the process of bone remodeling, which is an intricate, cyclic process of bone resorption and bone formation. Regulation of this process is complex and is governed by intrinsic as well as extrinsic factors. Bone is composed of distinct cell types that produce various proteins. Most of the protein production is controlled at the level of messenger ribonucleic acid (mRNA) transcription,[8] which to date is not well studied in human bone tissue. However, it is known that, during bone formation, synthesis of the major proteins of the bone matrix, type I collagen and osteocalcin, is regulated through various growth factors, including transforming growth factor, insulin-derived growth factors I and II, platelet-derived growth factor, and heparin-binding fibroblast growth factor.[1] Vitamin D then plays a significant role in the mineralization of this new bone, a process that takes months to complete. (The fundamentals of the mineralization process are beyond the scope of this chapter, but are well detailed in other works).[9] Interestingly, the vitamin D receptor appears to have at least one structural similarity to the receptors for estrogen, retinoic acid, and glucocorticoid: the structure of each of these receptors includes a "finger" containing an atom of zinc. Although vitamin D–resistant rickets is apparently caused by a deletion in one of these "zinc fingers" of the vitamin D receptor, it is not yet known whether other disorders of bone integrity have similar associations.[8]

Bone resorption occurs when osteoclasts release protons, which demineralize bone. Proteolytic enzymes then degrade the remaining matrix. Again, this process is hormonally controlled by local factors as well as systemic hormones, including parathyroid hormone, calcitonin, and 1,25-dihydroxy-vitamin D.[1] Of note, the rate at which each phase of the remodeling process occurs has a significant impact on bone strength at any given point. Although remodeling appears to be continuous, repairs are not instantaneous. Full mineralization can take several months to achieve, whereas the resorption phase can be completed in 1 to 2 weeks, leaving the fragile new tissue susceptible to injury.[1] Additional factors contributing to the material strength of remodeling bone include porosity, histology, and collagen fiber orientation.[6]

MECHANICS

The primary mechanical determinants of bone remodeling are applied tensile and compressive forces. Tensile forces are resisted by the collagen component of bone, whereas compressive forces are opposed by the mineral component. According to Wolff's law, an increasing amount of stress on a bone correlates with an increasing deformity throughout its elastic range. When the stress is removed, the bone will return to its original shape, provided the stress load did not cause the bone to exceed its elastic range. In addition to the amount of applied stress, the number of repetitions and frequency of loading affect the bone's reaction to stress. This reaction may be to become either weakened or strengthened, and is affected by a variety of additional factors, detailed throughout this chapter.

The force actually transmitted to bone tissue depends largely on muscular action. Several variations of current theories, based on ability of muscle to either produce or withstand force, seek to explain the role of muscle in the development of stress fractures. It is widely accepted that muscle responds to exercise training more quickly than does bone; this allows the athlete to progress training at a pace or intensity level that is tolerable for the muscles but too aggressive for the bone, resulting in a stress fracture. Alternatively, some blame muscle weakness for inadequate "shock absorption," requiring the redistribution of force to bone, again resulting in a stress fracture. Additionally, imbalance of opposing muscle groups (with one fatiguing more rapidly than its antagonist) may contribute to bone stress and subsequent bone failure. It is likely that each of these theories plays some role in the genesis of a stress fracture.

STRESS FRACTURE EPIDEMIOLOGY

As mentioned, stress fractures fall into two categories: fatigue and insufficiency type. Fatigue-type fractures generally occur in bone with adequate mineralization and normal elasticity (i.e., normal bone). Insufficiency fractures occur in bone that has decreased mineralization and lowered elasticity (i.e., abnormal bone). Insufficiency fractures may occur in bone that is affected by a variety of disease processes such as those outlined in Table 20–1. Osteoporosis has traditionally been associated with classic insufficiency-type fractures[10]; however, the clinician should be aware that some young female athletes presenting with apparent fatigue-type fractures are at risk for premature osteoporosis. Such an athlete should receive appropriate evaluation and intervention (as detailed in the following section on risk factors for stress fracture).

Fatigue fractures are commonly seen in the bones of the lower extremity, including the fibula, tibia, and calcaneus, although they may also occur in bones of the upper body such as the humerus and ribs. The

Table 20–1. Conditions Predisposing to Insufficiency Fractures

Generalized osteopenia
Osteoporosis
Hyperparathyroidism
Osteomalacia
Arthritis
Radiation therapy
Paget's disease

majority of reported fatigue stress fracture studies have been in athletes and military populations; little or no information is available about this type of stress fracture in the general population.[11] Because there is no standardized definition of a stress fracture and most of the athletic stress fracture literature is composed of case reports, it is not possible to define the entirety of stress fracture epidemiology. Nevertheless, a review of the available information allows one to constitute an approximate profile of patients most at risk for these overuse injuries.

Review of the literature confirms that stress fractures in athletes seem to occur most commonly in runners and other track and field athletes.[11, 12] Several studies have also documented an increased incidence in ballet dancers.[13, 14] Although few studies have systematically documented repeat injury, there are multiple reports in both the athletic and military literature attesting to recurrence of stress fracture. Clinically, recurrence at a different site seems especially common. It is unclear whether age and ethnicity are independent risk factors for stress fracture; more data are needed to help elucidate these issues.

Clinically, there is a propensity to consider stress fractures an injury more common in women than in men. Review of the military literature supports this: multiple studies consistently show that female recruits have a relative risk of fracture up to 10 times greater than male recruits.[11] In the athletic population, however, the difference is much less dramatic; overall fracture risk is reported as no more than 3.5 times greater in female athletes.[11] It is important to be aware, however, that in certain populations, such as runners and gymnasts, stress fractures seem to occur at significantly higher rates in women than in their male counterparts.[1, 11] Because of the dependence of these statistics on case series, it is impossible to determine the true incidence of fracture in the various populations from the currently available data. From a clinical perspective, it seems likely that stress fractures do occur more commonly in female athletes. Certainly, the tibia is the most common site of fracture in both sexes in the civilian population, and women sustain more stress fractures of the metatarsals, pelvis, and femur than men. Conversely, fibular stress fractures are more common in

men.[1] In military populations, the calcaneus and metatarsals are the most common sites of stress fractures.[15]

STRESS FRACTURE RISK FACTORS

It has been postulated that a number of variables, including conditioning, bone density and geometry, anatomy and biomechanics, and nutritional and hormonal factors, play a role in the development of a stress fracture. This section provides a review of the current understanding of some of these factors.

Bone Density

Bone mineral density clearly plays a role in insufficiency fractures and likely is a factor in the development of some fractures suspected of being fatigue type, especially in female athletes. Bone mineral density may be determined easily through several radiographic techniques, including single- or dual-photon absorptiometry, computed tomography, and dual-energy x-ray absorptiometry (DEXA). Measurements of the proximal radius, lumbar spine, and femoral neck obtained by DEXA provide the current "gold standard" for evaluation. The results of these measurements can be compared with data base averages for age-matched normal bone mineral density established by the World Health Organization.

Peak bone mass is generally thought to be achieved somewhere between the ages of 18 and 30; most bone mass is attained during the adolescent growth spurt. Generally, the peak bone mass attained by males is greater than that achieved by females. After the age of 30, bone loss occurs at the rate of 0.5% per year in both sexes. However, after menopause, the rate accelerates to 2% per year for approximately 10 years and then slows again to 0.5% to 1% per year.[16] Although genetics are thought to account for more than half the peak mass attainable, nutrition (specifically regarding calcium and vitamin D) and endocrine status clearly play an important role in maximum bone density achieved.

A variety of growth factors and hormones affect bone metabolism and bone density (Table 20–2). A complete review of these

Table 20–2. Regulation of Bone Remodeling

Systemic Factors	Local Factors
Parathyroid hormone	Transforming growth factor
Thyroid hormone	
Calcitonin	Insulin-derived growth factor
Insulin	
1,25-dihydroxyvitamin D	Platelet-derived growth factor
Sex steroids	
Glucocorticoids	Heparin-binding fibroblast growth factor

factors is beyond the scope of this text. However, a great deal of attention has focused on the role of the sex steroid hormones, specifically estrogen. For women to achieve peak bone mass, adequate quantities of estrogen (manifested by normal menstrual cycles) are required. During periods of amenorrhea or oligomenorrhea, young women lose 2% of their bone mass per year instead of gaining the normal 2 to 4%.[17] Unfortunately, it appears that at least some, if not all, of this lost bone mass is not recovered even when normal menses resume.[1, 16] Estrogen receptors have been found in osteoblast-like cells,[17] and have been shown to play a role in prevention of bone loss, although the exact mechanisms of action have not been clearly delineated. It is evident, however, that hypoestrogenemia—whether in the young woman who has not achieved peak bone mass or in the peri- or postmenopausal woman—contributes to decreased bone mineral density. Additionally, some scientists postulate that low progesterone levels also contribute to low bone density,[18] although this has not been well studied.

In addition to an optimal hormonal environment, nutritional factors play a critical role in achieving a healthy bone density. Calcium requirements vary with age (Table 20–3), depending on the body's needs. Absorption of calcium from the intestine depends on multiple factors. Calcium absorption is decreased by age, gastrointestinal disorders such as sprue and achlorhydria, renal disease, and many medications, such as corticosteroids. Adequate absorption and transport of calcium also require a normal level of vitamin D. This sterol hormone is formed in the skin from 7-dehydrocholesterol by ultraviolet light stimulation, which is then converted to 25-hydroxyvitamin D in the liver and finally hydroxylated to 1,25-dihydroxyvitamin D in the kidney. Vitamin D plays a complex role in bone metabolism by increasing calcium transport and stimulating bone resorption.[19] The role of vitamin D has become of even greater interest in osteoporosis research with twin studies of vitamin D receptor alleles that may predict differences in bone density and account for some of the variability of genetic expression.[1]

Although little is known about the role of other nutritional factors, inadequate total caloric intake is thought to contribute to an energy-deficit state[1] that can lead to bone loss and, therefore, place one at risk for bone injury, including stress fractures. Most studies of low bone mineral density in the setting of caloric restriction have been in young, underweight, female athletes, whose inadequate nutrition and vigorous exercise habits have been implicated in contributing to menstrual dysfunction, with the subsequent hypoestrogenemia contributing to loss of bone mineral density. The interrelatedness of disordered eating, amenorrhea, and osteoporosis in the female athlete has become known as the "female athlete triad."

Female Athlete Triad

The female athlete triad[20, 21] was described in the early 1990s by a task force of the American College of Sports Medicine after several sports medicine specialists began to see a pattern of abnormal eating behaviors, menstrual dysfunction, and low bone mineral density in young female athletes (Fig. 20–1). Although the prevalence of the triad is not known, its components individually and collectively are probably underrecognized. Recreational athletes as well as elite

Table 20–3. Daily Calcium Requirements

Group	Calcium Requirements (mg/day)
Childhood	800–1000
Adolescent, young adult	1200
Premenopausal woman	1000
Postmenopausal woman	1500
Pregnancy	1500
Lactation	>1500

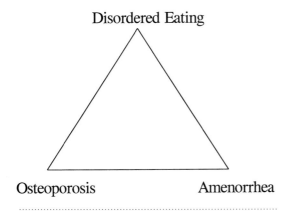

Figure 20–1. The female athlete triad.

athletes may be at risk for this syndrome. Female athletes at particular risk include those in individual sports; participants in sports in which low body weight or lean physique is thought to be an advantage (distance running); one in which judging may be influenced by aesthetics (gymnastics, ballet, figure skating); or sports that require "making weight" (judo, rowing). Female athletes seem to be especially vulnerable during adolescence and young adulthood, perhaps related to cultural as well as biologic factors.

Disordered eating refers to a spectrum of abnormal eating patterns, including food restriction, prolonged fasting, bingeing, purging, and use of diet pills, diuretics, or laxatives. Thought patterns such as preoccupation with food, fear of gaining weight or becoming fat, and dissatisfaction with one's body or distorted body image often accompany these eating patterns. It is important to recognize that disordered eating represents a spectrum of abnormal behaviors. At the extreme end are anorexia nervosa and bulimia nervosa, true eating disorders with specific psychiatric criteria for diagnosis. Although the majority of young female athletes do not meet these criteria, their abnormal eating habits put them at risk for some of the same medical complications experienced by patients with anorexia and bulimia.[21]

Similarly, one should view menstrual irregularities in the female athlete as a spectrum, ranging from luteal phase suppression to hypoestrogenic amenorrhea. Although it is not clear whether all phases of this continuum contribute to low bone mass, it is certain that any menstrual abnormality associated with low estrogen states can do so. As discussed previously, hypoestrogenism places the athlete at risk for premature osteoporosis, manifested by premature bone loss and inadequate bone formation. Obviously, not all female athletes with bone injuries such as stress fractures will be at risk for the triad. However, in light of the research that suggests that this bone loss may not be reversible, even with calcium supplementation and estrogen replacement therapy or resumption of menses,[1, 16, 21] it seems prudent to review risk factors for the triad carefully in all female athletes with stress fractures.

Anatomy and Biomechanics

Multiple additional factors have been suggested as contributing to the development of stress fractures, including biomechanic and anatomic influences. The influence of muscle on bone has been postulated as one such factor. For example, poor posture has been blamed for shifting the center of gravity, thereby altering muscular pull, contributing to the muscle fatigue and imbalance that has often been suspected as a culprit in the production of lower extremity stress injury.[5] However, the relationship between bone and muscle is complex, and the exact roles muscle mass and function play in stress fracture development is unclear. For instance, it has been postulated that the relatively low muscle mass around the tibia decreases the ability of the lower extremity to absorb force, contributing to the high number of tibial stress fractures.[15] What is unclear is how muscle mass interfaces with other anatomic variables. For instance, a narrow tibia[1, 15] has been positively correlated with an increased risk for stress fracture.[22, 23] Interestingly, a study of ballet dancers[13] found a striking pattern of cortical hypertrophy in the tibia as well as the other bones of the lower extremity, which may represent a protective response by the bone to repetitive stress. Current research at the University of California, Los Angeles[1] measuring area moments of inertia of the tibia may help to delineate how critical factors such as bone width are in the development of stress fractures.

Another intrinsic anatomic factor to consider is the structure of the foot, which has been implicated in several studies as a contributor to stress fractures in specific anatomic sites. It has long been thought that a cavus foot with a high, rigid arch absorbs force poorly, whereas a flexible flatfoot with greater ligamentous laxity and joint mobility absorbs energy more readily. This concept has been explored by studies of athletes and of military personnel. Matheson and colleagues[12] found that cavus feet were most likely to be found in athletes with metatarsal and femoral stress fractures, whereas pronated feet were most common in tarsal bone and tibial stress fractures. Because excessive pronation has been found to increase tibial torsion[24] during the support phase of running, it is not surprising that pronated feet are a common finding in athletes with tibial and fibular stress fractures. Additionally, varus alignment[12] and increased external rotation of the hip[15] have been accused of predisposing to stress fractures, although there is some controversy in the literature regarding the true contribution of each of these variables.

Training Errors

Although training errors are often cited as a cause of stress fractures, it can be difficult to define accurately exactly what constitutes a training error. Generally, the accepted definition, at least as applies to runners, is a significant increase in mileage or speed or a change in running surface. Muscular pull can also be altered by training conditions. For instance, changes in terrain for running or marching can change the muscular force on the bones of the lower leg. Similar significant alterations can occur simply by changing running surface or shoes. In Matheson's review of 320 stress fractures in athletes, running accounted for the vast majority (221) of the reported stress fractures; identifiable training errors occurred in 22.4% of the injured runners.[12] Similarly, military reports of stress fractures have identified the traditional style of training of recruits—marching on hard (cement or asphalt) surfaces and emphasizing heel strike while wearing hard combat boots—as factors contributing to stress fractures. One study of marine recruits found that changing to tennis shoes and a grass surface for training reduced the incidence of

calcaneal stress fractures from 20.5% to 7%.[25] A study of Israeli recruits found that a shock-absorbing orthotic reduced the incidence of stress fractures by 16.9%.[12] Finally, lower levels of fitness at the commencement of a training program have been found in various studies to correlate positively with the development of stress fractures.

LOWER EXTREMITY STRESS FRACTURES

As mentioned throughout this chapter, the distal lower extremity contains many of the sites most commonly affected by stress fractures. With a few specific exceptions that are noted, fatigue stress fractures of the distal tibia, fibula, rearfoot, and midfoot are generally similar in clinical presentation, diagnosis, and treatment. The following comments are, therefore, applicable to fatigue-type stress fractures of the lower extremity in general. The reader is reminded that, although every patient requires individualized evaluation and treatment, one must be especially vigilant in the case of the patient with an insufficiency fracture because of the likelihood of underlying bone disease.

Clinical Presentation

A patient presenting with foot or ankle pain secondary to a stress fracture classically complains of pain associated with a particular activity (e.g., running or marching). Often, there has been a nagging ache in the area of injury for weeks or even months that has become progressively more severe. Occasionally, the patient reports a sudden "snap" or acute increase in pain. The common description is of pain that initially occurs at some point during the activity but resolves with rest. Eventually, this may progress to constant pain that becomes so severe as to preclude the desired activity. This is frequently the catalyst that brings the patient in for evaluation. As alluded to previously in this chapter, history taking should include questions regarding changes in training and footwear and review of the nutrition status. Additionally, in the female athlete, menstrual history should be recorded.

On physical examination, there may or

may not be mild swelling at the site of pain. The patient's gait is often affected by hesitancy to bear weight fully on the injured extremity. Almost always there is exquisite point tenderness at the site of the fracture. Percussion distal or proximal to the fracture site may cause "transmission pain."[26] There may be diffuse tenderness around the site of the fracture as a result of accompanying soft tissue overuse such as tendinitis. The examiner should make note of any of the biomechanic or anatomic variables (e.g., pronated feet) reviewed previously in this chapter.

The differential diagnosis depends to some degree on the site of the fracture, but can include other stress syndromes (such as medial tibial stress syndrome or periostitis), bone tumor, arthritis, plantar fasciitis, osteomyelitis or soft tissue infection, and injury to or inflammation of ligaments, tendons, or bursae. A high index of suspicion is helpful in making the correct diagnosis expeditiously.

Imaging

When stress fracture is suspected, radiographs should be obtained. In addition to standard views, one might consider an over-penetration technique, which provides better definition within dense sclerotic area of bone[27] or coned-down view ("spot film"). Although stress fractures have been described as compression (usually in cancellous bone) or distraction (usually in compact bone),[27] the radiographic appearance depends largely on the amount of elapsed time from onset of symptoms to presentation (Figs. 20–2 to 20–4). If imaged in the early phase, the fracture may appear as a lucency in compact bone in contrast to a more radiopaque appearance in cancellous bone. Generally, stress fractures affect only one cortex[27] and are frequently associated with periostial reaction. However, one should keep in mind that radiographs frequently show no sign of fatigue fracture for several weeks, and further imaging may be necessary. Options include repeating the radiographs after 2 to 3 weeks, radionuclide bone scanning, magnetic resonance imaging (MRI), and computed tomographic (CT) scan.[28, 29] Generally, a bone scan is considered the gold standard of diagnosis, although one must remember that there is a

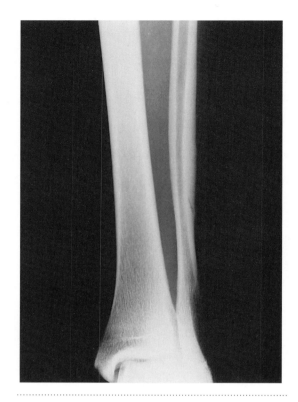

Figure 20–2. Radiographic appearance of stress fracture of fibula.

period for several days after the onset of symptoms during which even the bone scan may not be positive. Additionally, although very sensitive, a bone scan is not very specific. For further information, the reader is referred to the chapters on radiographic techniques provided elsewhere in this text.

Treatment

Development of a general treatment plan for most uncomplicated stress fractures can be guided by a few simple concepts. The first principle is to stop the causative activity, thereby eliminating the repetitive stress on the fracture site, allowing bone healing to occur. Once the offending activity has been stopped, pain control can often be achieved with nonsteroidal anti-inflammatory medications and ice massage or, additionally, physiotherapy modalities. Especially in an athlete, a non-weight-bearing alternative activity such as stationary biking or exercise in a pool often encourages compliance

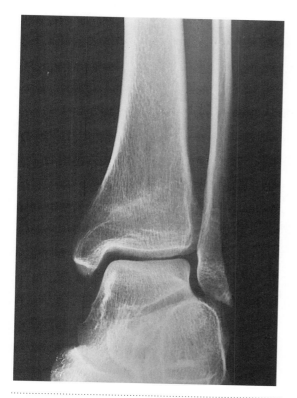

Figure 20–3. Radiographic appearance of stress fracture of tibia.

with the treatment protocol while preventing loss of aerobic conditioning. Additionally, this may present an opportunity for the athlete to engage in strength training exercises because inadequate muscle mass and muscle imbalance have been implicated by some as contributing to stress fracture development. This recovery phase offers the occasion to improve general muscle flexibility. It is also an excellent opportunity to address relevant issues of nutrition and, in the female athlete, menstrual irregularities.

According to the guidelines established by Clement,[30] the second phase of the treatment plan should begin when the athlete has been pain free for 10 to 14 days. At this point, gradual resumption of sport can commence. It is recommended that this occur on a schedule of alternate days to allow for periods of rest. Also at this time, any other identified risk factors (e.g., training surface, footwear) should be addressed and modified. It should be noted that some have advocated a delay in return to sport until radiographic evidence of fracture healing is present, although many physicians believe that clinical examination and elimination of pain are sufficient criteria for reintroducing sport.

These are general guidelines, applicable to most stress fractures. However, there are some instances in which these will not be adequate. The reader is reminded that in the case of a stress fracture with a propensity toward displacement, such as the tarsal navicular, aggressive management with non-weightbearing and immobilization is warranted. Stress fractures that are displaced, occurring in multiple, or not responding to conservative therapy as outlined previously need to be reassessed on an individual, case-by-case basis for treatment modifications. Possibilities for additional treatment include prolonged decrease in weight bearing, more aggressive immobilization, and surgery.

SPECIFIC LOWER EXTREMITY STRESS FRACTURES

Rearfoot

In the rearfoot, the most common site of stress fracture is the calcaneus; the fracture

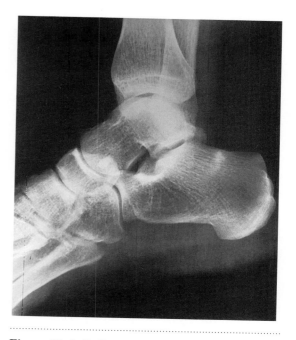

Figure 20–4. Radiographic appearance of stress fracture of calcaneus.

is frequently in a posterosuperior location. The patient with this injury often complains of heel pain; physical examination reveals swelling and tenderness to palpation on both the medial and lateral aspects of the heel. This location is a frequent one for stress fracture in military populations but has also been reported in dancers and other athletes. Repetitive compression loads from heel strike (such as seen with marching) and forces from the gastrocnemius-soleus complex have been implicated in this fracture.[31] This fracture rarely becomes displaced and responds to reduction in activity, often requiring immobilization and decreased weight bearing until symptoms resolve. Regarding insufficiency fractures of the calcaneus, there seems to be a unique pattern of fracture seen in diabetics, especially in the setting of distal neuropathy.[32]

Although less common, stress fractures of the talus have also been described, most often involving the dome.[31]

Midfoot

Although not common, fatigue fractures have been reported in the bones of the midfoot, especially of the tarsal navicular. This fracture deserves special attention because it is often missed, with potentially debilitating results. The patient with this stress fracture often complains of vague midfoot pain of insidious onset. The pain is often described as a cramp, worsened by activity and relieved with rest. Tenderness to palpation along the medial longitudinal arch or the dorsum of the foot, with mild swelling near the navicular, are the hallmarks of the physical exam. Additionally, pain may be elicited when the forefoot is either inverted or everted or when the patient stands on the toes. Pronated feet are a familiar finding in athletes with tarsal stress fractures. An additional consideration in the differential diagnosis is posterior tibial tendon injury.

When obtaining radiographs in the patient with midfoot pain, be aware that the navicular may be bipartite, causing it to be mistaken for a stress fracture. In this case, a bone scan may help to differentiate the anatomic variant from an injury. Classically, the radiographic appearance of a navicular stress fracture is linear and sagittal, occurring in the central third of the bone.[33]

Although a tarsal stress fracture is often difficult to diagnose, it is an especially important one to identify because of its tendency to displace if activity is not curtailed. Once displacement occurs, internal fixation is required. If nondisplaced, treatment with immobilization and non-weight bearing for several weeks under careful observation is usually sufficient. Especially careful attention to return to activity is recommended.

Although uncommon, stress fractures of other bones of the midfoot, including the cuboid, have been reported. It is wise for the clinician to note that, generally, stress fractures of the midfoot are symptomatic and require longer periods of decreased activity than similar fractures in the hindfoot.

Distal Tibia and Fibula

Activities requiring repetitive impact loading, such as running, dancing, and gymnastics, place the participant at risk for stress fracture about the ankle. Although the tibia is often cited as the most frequent site of stress fracture in athletes, it is important to consider that a large number of these injuries occur at sites proximal to the ankle. The region of the tibia affected seems to correlate with the participant's specific activity: classically, runners experience stress fractures at the junction of the middle and distal thirds, whereas military recruits and dancers sustain fractures at the proximal and middle thirds, respectively.[34] Stress fractures about the ankle are usually seen proximal to the malleoli, although stress fractures of the malleoli have been reported, often complicated by delayed healing.[15] Typically, the athlete with a stress fracture of the distal tibia will complain of insidious onset of pain in the lower anterior tibia, which worsens with impact loading activity. Physical examination commonly reveals point tenderness, often with palpable soft tissue swelling or fracture callus formation. Especially important to consider in the differential diagnosis of tibial stress fracture is exertional compartment syndrome, the presentation of which often mimics a stress fracture. Once the diagnosis is confirmed, tibial stress fractures generally respond to relative rest and correction of any identifiable contributing factors.

Stress fractures of the distal fibula are not as common, although they have often been described in runners and dancers. Again, the physical examination is usually significant for point tenderness and often mild swelling at the site of fracture. Relative rest in addition to a supportive ankle brace or walking cast is usually sufficient treatment of these fractures as long as there is no displacement. Displacement of the fracture requires evaluation for internal fixation.

SUMMARY

Stress fractures of the rearfoot, midfoot, distal tibia, and fibula are common overuse injuries, especially in athletes such as runners, who are exposed to repetitive application of force. The clinician should have a high index of suspicion for this injury when an athlete presents with insidious onset of pain that is aggravated by activity and relieved by rest. Radiographs, bone scan, CT scan, and MRI all may be useful in confirming the diagnosis. Conservative treatment is usually successful, although one must be especially vigilant in treating a stress fracture in a site prone to complications, such as in the tarsal navicular. Identifying risk factors for susceptibility to stress fracture development may help to avoid recurrence of the injury and, especially in the case of the young female athlete, may allow for interventions to avoid chronic conditions such as osteoporosis.

Acknowledgment

I thank Helene Pavlov, MD, for providing Figures 20–2 to 20–4.

REFERENCES

1. Nattiv A, Armsey TD Jr. Stress injury to bone in the female athlete. Clin Sports Med 16:197, 1997.
2. Mandelbaum BR, Knapp TP. Stress fractures. Clin Sports Med 16:179, 1997.
3. Devas MB. Stress Fractures. Edinburgh: Churchill Livingstone, 1975.
4. Milgrom C, Giladi M, Stein M, et al. Stress fractures in military recruits: a prospective study showing an unusually high incidence. J Bone Joint Surg Br 67:732, 1985.
5. Daffner RH, Pavlov H. Stress fractures: current concepts. AJR Am J Roentgenol 159:245, 1992.
6. Martin B. Aging and strength of bone as a structural material. Calcif Tissue Int 53 Suppl 1:S34, 1993.
7. Burr DB. Remodeling and the repair of fatigue damage. Calcif Tissue Int 53 Suppl 1:S75, 1993.
8. Young MF: Transcription and aging of human bone tissue. Calcif Tissue Int 56 Suppl 1:S39, 1995.
9. Boskey A. Mineral-matrix interactions in bone and cartilage. Clin Orthop 281:244, 1992.
10. Cooper KL. Insufficiency stress fractures. Curr Probl Diagn Radiol 23:30, 1994.
11. Bennell KL, Brukner PD. Epidemiology and site specificity of stress fractures. Clin Sports Med 16:179, 1997.
12. Matheson GO, Clement DB, McKenzie DC, et al. Stress fractures in athletes. Am J Sports Med 15:46, 1987.
13. Schneider HJ, King AY, Bronson JL, et al. Stress injuries and developmental change of lower extremities in ballet dancers. Radiology 113:627, 1974.
14. Kadel NJ, Teitz CC, Kronmal RA. Stress fractures in ballet dancers. Am J Sports Med 20:445, 1992.
15. Leach RE, Zecher SB. Stress fractures. In Guten GN, ed. Running Injuries. Philadelphia: W. B. Saunders, 1997, p. 30.
16. Wirganowicz PZ, Lane JM. Postmenopausal osteoporosis: an update for the clinician. J Musculoskeletal Med 10:29, 1996.
17. Lane JM, Riley EH, Wirganowicz PZ. Osteoporosis: diagnosis and treatment. J Bone Joint Surg Am 78:618, 1996.
18. Prior JC, Vigna YM, Barr SI, et al. Cyclic medroxyprogesterone treatment increases bone density: a controlled trial in active women with menstrual cycle disturbances. Am J Med 96:521, 1994.
19. Fauvus MJ. Primer on the Metabolic Bone Diseases and Disorders of Mineral Metabolism. New York: Raven Press, 1993.
20. Putukian M. The female triad. Sports Med 78:345, 1994.
21. Nattiv A, Agostini R, Drinkwater B, et al. The female athlete triad. Clin Sports Med 13:405, 1994.
22. Frankel VH, Burstein AH. Orthopedic Biomechanics: The Application of Engineering to the Musculoskeletal System. Philadelphia: Lea and Febiger, 1970.
23. Giladi M, Milgrom C, Simkin A, et al. Stress fractures and tibial bone width: a risk factor. J Bone Joint Surg 69:326, 1987.
24. McKenzie DC, Clement DB, Taunton JE. Running shoes, orthotics, and injuries. Sports Med 2:334, 1985.
25. Greaney RB, Gerber FH, Laughlin RL, et al. Distribution and natural history of stress fractures in US Marine recruits. Radiology 146:339, 1983.
26. Knapp TP, Garrett WE Jr. Stress fractures: general concepts. Clin Sports Med 16:339, 1997.
27. Pavlov H, Torg JS, Hersh A, et al. The roentgen examination of runners' injuries. Radiographics 1:17, 1981.
28. Deutsch AL, Coel MN, Mink JH. Imaging of stress injuries to bone: radiography, scintigraphy, and MR imaging. Clin Sports Med 16:275, 1997.
29. Arendt EA, Griffiths HJ. The use of MR imaging in the assessment and clinical management of stress reactions of bone in high-performance athletes. Clin Sports Med 16:29, 1997.
30. Clement DB. Tibial stress syndrome in athletes. J Sports Med 2:81, 1974.
31. Eisele SA, Sammarco GJ. Fatigue fractures of the foot and ankle in the athlete. J Bone Joint Surg Am 75:290, 1993.

32. Kathol MH, El-Khoury GY, Moore TE, et al. Calcaneal insufficiency avulsion fractures in patients with diabetes mellitus. Musculoskeletal Radiol 180:725, 1991.
33. Pavlov H, Torg J, Freiberger RH. Tarsal navicular stress fractures: radiographic evaluation. Radiology 148:641, 1983.
34. Maitra RS, Johnson DL. Stress fractures: clinical history and physical examination. Clin Sports Med 16:259, 1997.

Calcaneal Fractures: Etiology, Diagnosis, and Classification

Craig S. Bartlett III
David L. Helfet
Steven S. Louis

The calcaneus (os calcis) is the tarsal bone most often fractured and accounts for 2% of all fractures in the body.[1-3] It has been a common, often disabling, injury since humans have assumed the erect posture and began to test the laws of gravity by climbing trees, ladders, and scaffolding. Climbing out of second-story windows on hearing the footsteps of an approaching husband ("lover's heel") or law enforcement agent has proven to be hazardous to the calcaneus as well. Boehler pointed out that any "fall of greater than one meter should suggest this fracture."[4] Interestingly, the incidence of calcaneal fractures has not increased with the advent of mechanized industry, automobile travel, and even war.[1]

The most simple classification system divides calcaneal fractures into two main groups: intra-articular and extra-articular fractures of the subtalar joint. Intra-articular fractures make up 70 to 80% of all calcaneal fractures.[3, 5-11] Of the patients suffering from a calcaneal fracture, 7% will have bilateral injuries, 10% will have associated fractures of the spine, and 26% will have an associated extremity injury. Fortunately, less than 2% will be open fractures of the calcaneus.[3, 9, 11-15]

Intra-articular fractures of the calcaneus have and still represent a true challenge to any orthopedic surgeon (Fig. 21–1). In 1916, Cotton and Henderson wrote "the man who breaks his heel bone is done."[7] In 1942, Bankart wrote "the results of the treatment of crush fractures of the os calcis are rotten,"[16] and in 1963, Cave wrote "once the subastragalar joint is markedly distorted, it is unlikely that any form of treatment will bring about a result that will not be followed by permanent disability of a varying degree."[1] Because the outcomes after comminuted intra-articular fractures of the calcaneus have been much worse than desired, the management has been much more diffi-cult and controversial. Extra-articular fractures, on the other hand, are usually much more benign and treatable and lead to far less disability.[1, 3, 4, 7, 9, 14]

The economic importance of calcaneal fractures is glaringly apparent when one understands that they occur most often in middle-aged industrial workers. In fact, 90% of them occur in men between 25 and 50 years of age.[3, 9, 13] The economic impact is even more serious when one realizes that 20% of patients may be totally incapacitated for up to 3 years, and many are still partially incapacitated 5 years or longer.[1, 3, 6, 13, 15, 17]

ANATOMY

The identification, classification, and treatment of calcaneal fractures require a strong working knowledge of normal and pathologic anatomy. In general, the uninjured calcaneus is shaped like an irregular rectangular box with relatively thin cortical walls. It presents six surfaces with three facets that articulate with the talus and one that articulates with the cuboid.

The superior surface of the calcaneus consists of the posterior, middle, and anterior subtalar articulating facets and the top of the tuberosity (Fig. 21–2). The posterior facet is the largest and most independent, and it occupies the middle third of the calcaneus. It supports the body of the talus and is separated from the anterior and middle facets by the calcaneal sulcus. The anterior and middle facets are located on the sustentaculum tali and are often confluent. They provide the bony support to the neck of the talus. The three facets all lie at different angles to one another and have different surface topography, but they act in perfect concert to provide smooth subtalar motion.

The medial surface is deeply concave be-

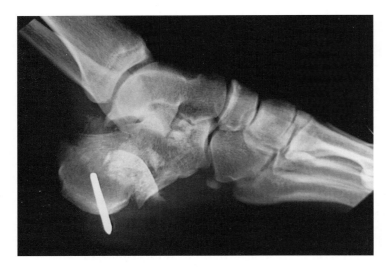

Figure 21–1. An open calcaneal fracture from an 8-foot fall off a ladder. Patient was initially treated in calcaneal traction.

cause of the sustentaculum tali. The underside of the sustentaculum tali is arched to form a groove for the flexor hallucis longus (FHL) tendon (Fig. 21–3). The bone here is relatively dense and is rarely fractured in a calcaneal injury. This bone then becomes the keystone to reduction and a strong anchor for internal fixation.

On the lateral surface, there is a shallow groove just posterior and inferior to the lateral malleolus for the peroneal tendons. The groove is bordered by a ridge termed the *peroneal tubercle*. Otherwise, the lateral surface is nearly flat, making it a perfect surface for internal fixation plates (Fig. 21–

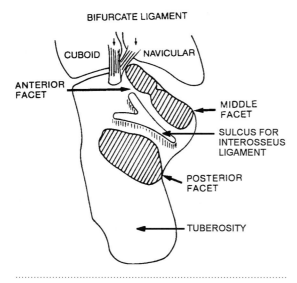

Figure 21–2. Superior surface of the calcaneus.

4). The bone on the lateral surface is essentially subcutaneous, and when fractured can cause tremendous injury to the overlying skin. Surgical intervention through this area can be quite hazardous[18] (Fig. 21–5).

The calcaneus has a very thin cortical shell, except at the posterior edge of the tuberosity and directly under the posterior facet. Inside the cortical margins, there is a simple pattern of trabecular bone that reflects the internal stresses to which it is repeatedly subjected. On the lateral x-ray view, traction trabeculae radiate from the inferior cortex toward the posterosuperior corner of the tuberosity. Compression trabeculae converge to support the articular facets. The thickening of the compression trabeculae under the posterior facet was identified as "the thalamic portion of the calcaneus" by Soeur and Remy.[11] There is a triangle of relatively sparse trabecular bone just inferior to the "thalamic" condensation that has been coined the *neutral triangle*. This area is fairly weak and is commonly impacted in compression-type injuries (Fig. 21–6).

Medially, the soft tissues covering the calcaneus include the neurovascular and musculotendinous units of the posterior compartment of the leg. The neurovascular bundle travels within the tarsal tunnel, coursing directly under the posteromedial edge of the sustentaculum tali.[19] The FHL runs under the sustentaculum just posterior to the neurovascular bundle, whereas the flexor digitorum longus (FDL) courses just anterior to the neurovascular bundle and

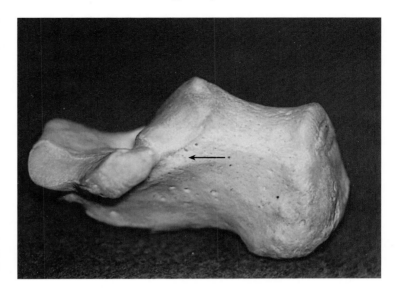

Figure 21–3. Medial surface of the calcaneus. Note the groove for the flexor hallucis longus *(arrow)*.

directly over the sustentaculum (Fig. 21–7). Anterior to the FDL is the tibialis anterior. The deltoid ligament is deep to all these structures and usually remains intact in fractures of the calcaneus. With the "key to and anchoring of reduction" being the

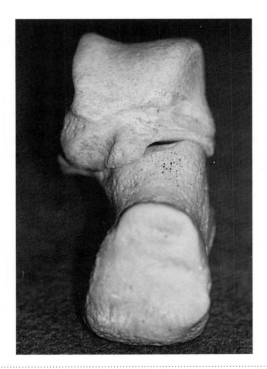

Figure 21–4. Posterior view of the talocalcaneal relationship. Note the flatness of the lateral surface of the calcaneus.

sustentacular fragment, any breach of the medial cortex runs the risk of damaging some of the structures just described.[20]

Inferiorly, the calcaneal heel pad helps cushion and dissipate the load seen at heel strike of the gait cycle. It is a complex structure made up of fatty tissue held firmly to the bottom of the calcaneus by innumerable fibrous septa. This structure can be disrupted with an axial load–type injury, causing permanent damage and atrophy of the tissues. This may represent a cause of pain late after a calcaneal fracture.[9, 12]

Radiographically, two anatomic angles have been described and are used consistently in the evaluation of calcaneal fractures. The Boehler tuberosity joint angle[4] and the crucial angle of Gissane[7, 21] are seen on the lateral x-ray film (Fig. 21–8). The Boehler angle is measured at the intersection of two lines: one line drawn from the most superior point of the tuberosity to the highest point on the posterior articular facet; the second drawn from the highest point of the posterior facet to the highest point on the anterior process. Normal ranges from 25 to 40°. Gissane's angle measures the difference between the two cortical struts seen on x-ray film just inferior and anterior to the posterior facet. The first strut follows the subchondral bone under the posterior facet, whereas the second strut follows the subchondral bone of the middle and anterior facets and runs to the beak of the anterior process. This obtuse angle normally varies between 120 and 145°.

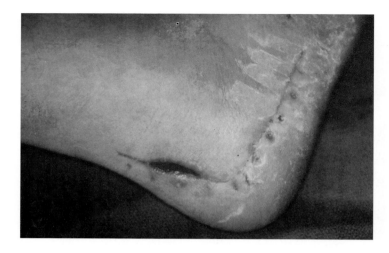

Figure 21–5. Minor wound sloughs after open reduction and internal fixation of a calcaneal fracture.

CLINICAL AND RADIOGRAPHIC DIAGNOSIS

With a history of a fall directly on the heel or a direct traumatic or twisting event to the hindfoot, acute pain and swelling are usually noted. If (1) a patient is unable to bear weight, (2) there is evidence of ecchymosis around and below the heel, and (3) pain accompanies any subtalar motion, one should suspect a calcaneal fracture and proceed to radiographic evaluation. Ecchymosis that extends to the sole of the foot is considered virtually pathognomonic for calcaneal fractures and is referred to as Mondor's sign.[22] If the swelling goes unchecked, it often becomes quite severe, and blistering of the skin may develop around the foot and heel (Fig. 21–9).

Correct radiographic visualization is essential for proper evaluation, classification, and treatment of calcaneal fractures. Both the radiology technician and the treating physician should be very familiar with positioning the foot for proper standard plain film and computed tomography (CT) views.

Plain Films

The initial x-ray examination of the patient suspected of having a fractured calcaneus should consist of (1) the lateral projection of the hindfoot, (2) the anteroposterior (AP) view of the foot, and (3) the posterior axial view of the heel.

With intra-articular fractures being much more common, the lateral projection of the hindfoot will confirm the diagnosis in most cases. The lateral projection will demonstrate nicely the loss of calcaneal height and the amount of superior displace-

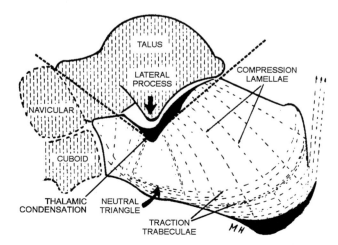

Figure 21–6. Lateral projection of an uninjured calcaneus demonstrating the bony trabeculae, neutral triangle, and "thalamic" condensation.

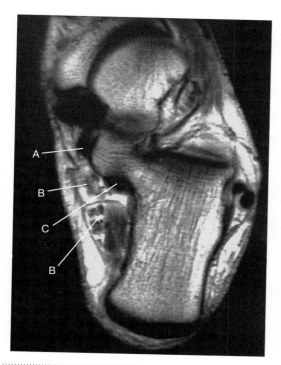

Figure 21–7. A magnetic resonance coronal image demonstrating *(A)* flexor digitorum longus, *(B)* posterior tibialis neurovascular bundle, and *(C)* flexor hallucis longus.

rior facet joint surface. With intra-articular fractures, this view clearly shows the widening of the heel and the varus malalignment of the tuberosity (Fig. 21–12), and if the x-ray beam is correctly aligned, the posterior facet joint surface can be visualized. Unfortunately, this view is extremely difficult to obtain properly in the acute setting because of excessive pain to the patient. Fortunately, the imperfect view is of some informative value. An extra-articular fracture of the medial process is demonstrated best with this view (Fig. 21–13).

In addition to the standard three views listed previously, other views are indicated in different situations. The lateral oblique projection is the best view to see an anterior process fracture.[23] To obtain this view, the medial border of the foot is placed on the cassette and the sole is inclined 45°. The beam is centered 1 inch below and 1 inch anterior to the lateral malleolus (Fig. 21–14). A CT scan may be required to define the extent of injury more accurately.

Because fractures of the calcaneus are bilateral in many cases, radiographs of both feet may be indicated. An anteroposterior view of the ankle may be helpful in differ-

ment of the tuberosity (decreased Boehler tuberosity joint angle and increased critical angle of Gissane). If only the lateral half of the posterior facet is fractured and depressed, one will often see a "double density" within the body of the calcaneus (Fig. 21–10*A, B*). This is the subchondral bone of the lateral half of the posterior facet and can be rotated up to 90° from horizontal. The avulsion-type extra-articular fractures of the tuberosity are well demonstrated in this view. Some extra-articular fractures of the anterior process can be seen as well.

The AP view of the foot will help demonstrate involvement of the calcaneocuboid joint and the spread of the lateral calcaneal wall. It may also demonstrate medial subluxation of the talus at the talonavicular joint. The spread of the lateral wall of the calcaneus is also well visualized on the AP view of the ankle (Fig. 21–11). Extra-articular fractures of the anterior process can sometimes be seen on this view.

The Harris axial heel view will show the medial and lateral cortical walls, the axial alignment of the tuberosity, and the poste-

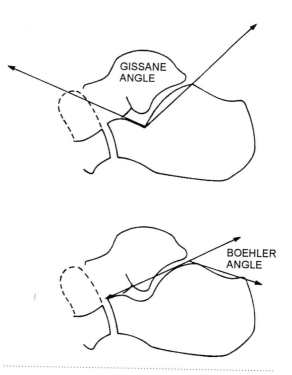

Figure 21–8. Measurement of the Boehler angle and the crucial Gissane angle.

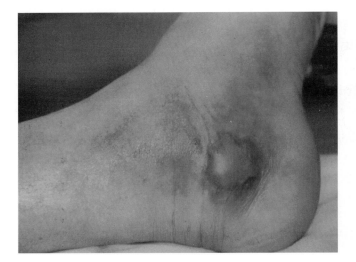

Figure 21–9. Blistering of skin after an injury to the hindfoot.

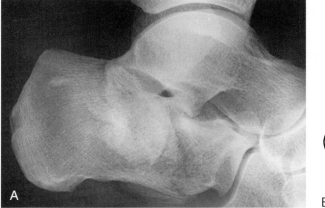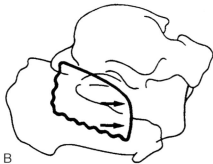

Figure 21–10. "Double density" is easily seen on x-ray film *(A)* and demonstrated on the line drawing *(B)*. Note the decrease in the Boehler angle.

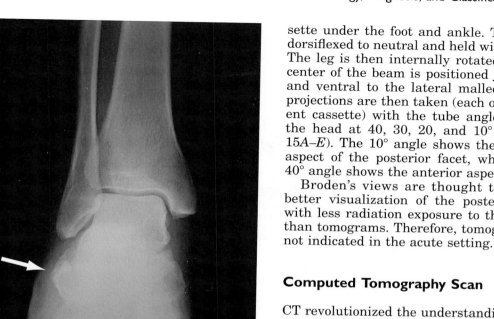

Figure 21–11. Lateral spread of the calcaneal wall seen on anteroposterior view of the ankle *(arrow)*.

entiating an ankle versus tarsal injury. Given the incidence of associated lumbar spine fractures, some authors recommend routine lumbar spine films on all patients with intra-articular fractures of the calcaneus.[13]

Should these radiographs reveal an intra-articular fracture of the subtalar joint, a CT scan of the hindfoot should be obtained. Some believe a CT scan is an absolute necessity.[24, 25] If unavailable, the oblique plain x-ray views of Broden[26] are most useful. Isherwood[8] and Anthonsen[13] have described alternate oblique views to help assess the subtalar joint, but these are not used as often as Broden's views.

Broden's Views

Broden described two x-ray projections that can be used to evaluate subtalar joint incongruity.[26] Projection 1 is more commonly used and is obtained in the following manner. The patient is supine with the x-ray cas-

sette under the foot and ankle. The foot is dorsiflexed to neutral and held with a strap. The leg is then internally rotated 45°. The center of the beam is positioned just distal and ventral to the lateral malleolus. Four projections are then taken (each on a different cassette) with the tube angled toward the head at 40, 30, 20, and 10° (Fig. 21–15A–E). The 10° angle shows the posterior aspect of the posterior facet, whereas the 40° angle shows the anterior aspect.

Broden's views are thought to provide better visualization of the posterior facet with less radiation exposure to the patient than tomograms. Therefore, tomograms are not indicated in the acute setting.

Computed Tomography Scan

CT revolutionized the understanding of calcaneal fractures and has become an essential component in the evaluation and preoperative planning of all such injuries. A calcaneal CT scan is also used for the postoperative evaluation of surgical correction

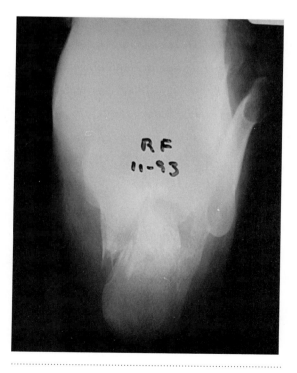

Figure 21–12. Axial heel view demonstrating widening of the calcaneus and varus alignment of the tuberosity. The depressed lateral half of the posterior facet is seen.

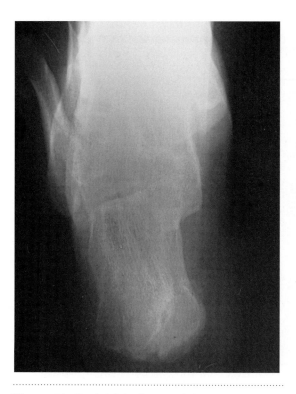

Figure 21–13. Axial heel view of the calcaneus with fracture of the medial process.

and to confirm the late sequelae of subtalar arthrosis. Two different scans (semicoronal and transverse) are required to assess fully the size and number of fragments, degree of subtalar joint incongruity, degree of calcaneocuboid joint involvement, amount of calcaneal widening, and extent of lateral wall expansion and peroneal impingement. Both feet are scanned for comparison, and plaster splints *do not* preclude an adequate evaluation.[27]

To maximize the usefulness of CT scanning, the positioning of the patient is critical.[28] Improperly obtained CT scans are nearly useless.[29] For the semicoronal views, the patient must lie in the scanner supine with both hips and knees flexed 30 to 45°. Both ankles should be maintained in approximately 30° of plantar flexion (normal splinting position for calcaneal fractures). A 30° wedge can be used to assist the unaffected foot. If the gantry is oriented 90° to the table, the proper 60° semicoronal view will be obtained of the calcaneus (Fig. 21–16). This particular view ends up perpendicular to the plane of the posterior facet of

the subtalar joint. Three-millimeter cuts are obtained from the posterior calcaneus to the navicular. The legs are then straightened so that the second set of 3-mm images would be obtained parallel to the long axis of the foot.[28]

In the semicoronal views, the articular surface of the posterior facet is analyzed for the number of major articular pieces, anatomic location of the fracture lines, and degree of displacement (Fig. 21–17). The body may show widening, shortening, lateral wall displacement, and impingement. In the transverse (axial) cuts, fractures into the calcaneocuboid joint and of the sustentaculum tali can be determined (Fig. 21–18).

CLASSIFICATION AND PATHOANATOMY (MECHANISM OF INJURY)

In 1916, Cotton wrote "attempts to classify these fractures are about as useful as trying to classify a walnut shell after the nutcracker is through with it."[30] Despite this comment, numerous classification systems for calcaneal fractures have been devised and include those of Boehler,[4] Palmer,[31] Widen,[15] Rowe and associates,[14] Essex-Lo-

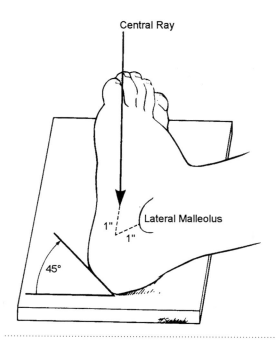

Figure 21–14. Proper technique for the lateral oblique projection of the foot.

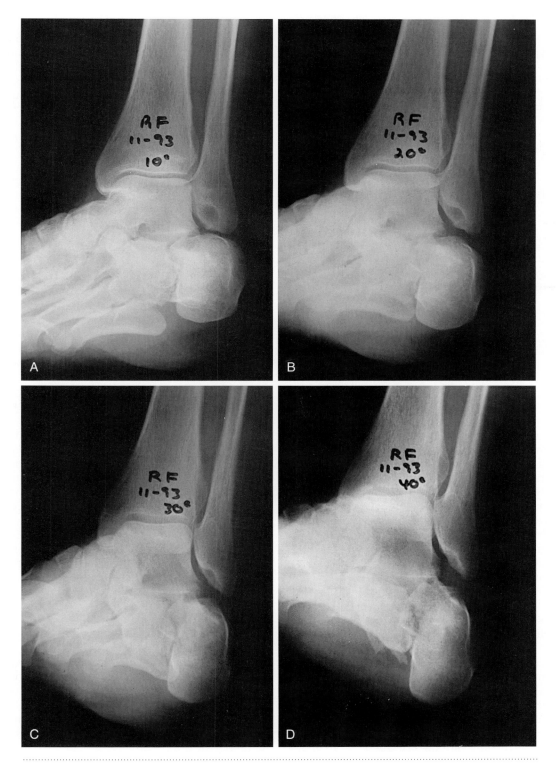

Figure 21–15. *A–E*, Broden's views of the fractured calcaneus (projection 1).

Illustration continued on following page

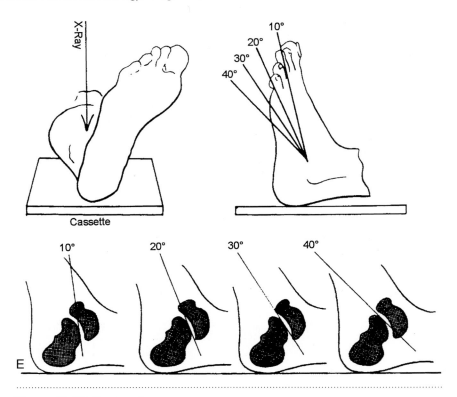

Figure 21–15 *Continued*

presti,[7] Warrick and Bremner,[32] Nade and Monahan,[3] Stephenson,[33] Soeur and Remy,[11] Lindsay and Dewar,[9] and Sanders.[34] The development and advancement of all these systems seem to have followed clinical experience and radiologic advances as demonstrated by the CT classification of Sanders being a "natural progression of the classification by Soeur and Remy."[35]

All the classification systems start by separating those that tend to have a good prognosis from those that tend to fair worse and may need more aggressive treatment. Essex-Lopresti was one of the first to emphasize the difference between extra-articular fractures, which tend to fair well, and those that involve the subtalar joint that generally have a worse prognosis.[7] In general, extra-articular and intra-articular fractures are the result of different mechanisms of injury; tension versus axial compression loads. The major differences in the classification systems are seen when dealing with the intra-articular fractures of the calcaneus.

Extra-articular fractures of the calcaneus occur infrequently (20–30%) and are caused most commonly by torsional or traction strain forces that avulse fragments of bone, leaving the ligamentous and the tendinous structures intact.[1, 23] These extra-articular fractures have been grouped by anatomic sites: (1) anterior process, (2) tuberosity, and (3) medial process.

There are two different types of anterior process fractures: avulsion and compression.[13, 23, 36] The avulsion type is more common and thought to be caused by a pull from either the bifurcate ligament or the extensor digitorum brevis muscle after an inversion stress to an adducted and plantar flexed foot (Fig. 21–19). It is often misdiagnosed as an ankle sprain.[13, 23] Hunt described the compression fracture as a larger fragment that is usually displaced superiorly and posteriorly. Significant calcaneocuboid joint involvement and incongruity can occur[37] (Fig. 21–20A, B). The mechanism of injury is thought to be forced abduction causing an impaction of the calcaneocuboid joint, thereby creating a compression-type fracture of the anterior process.

Tuberosity fractures result from a violent contraction of the gastrocnemius-soleus

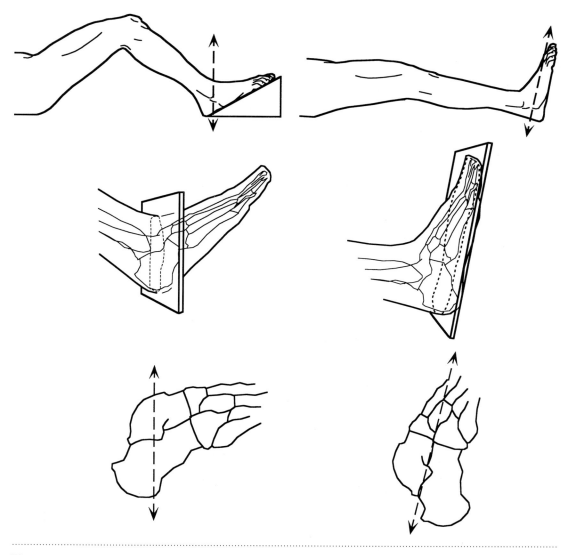

Figure 21–16. Proper leg position for computed tomographic scanning of the hindfoot (see text).

muscle group. The fracture involves the posterosuperior aspect of the calcaneus and stops short of the subtalar joint. Two sub-types were identified in the older literature, "break" and "avulsion."[4] They are now con-sidered to be the same entity because the insertion of the tendo-Achilles can vary so much that a break fracture is simply a high avulsion fracture.[38] Older patients (average age of 63 in reported cases) seem to be more prone to this injury.[8] The mechanism of in-jury is usually a fall or misstep down a short height (e.g., a street curb or a stair).

The medial calcaneal process is the origin of the abductor hallucis and the medial por-tion of the flexor hallucis brevis and plantar fascia. A fracture of this portion of the calca-neus is rare. Postulated mechanisms range from abduction or adduction force applied to the heel while it strikes the ground in eversion (Boehler) to the heel receiving a glancing blow from below while the foot is held in a valgus position (Watson-Jones).[13]

Isolated fractures of the sustentaculum tali and fractures of the body that do not involve the subtalar joint used to be catego-rized in the extra-articular group because they did not involve the subtalar joint. The current understanding of the pathoanatomy and pathomechanics of intra-articular cal-

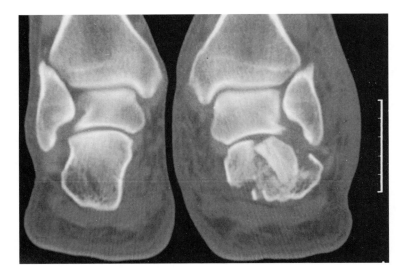

Figure 21–17. Semicoronal computed tomographic scan image at the level of the posterior facet. The number of main fragments, their displacement, and the amount of widening or lateral wall blow-out is well demonstrated.

caneal fractures (axial loading) places these two "extra-articular" fractures at the extremes of the "intra-articular" category. They should be thought of as intra-articular fractures with a better prognosis.

Intra-articular fractures of the calcaneus are usually the result of an axial load to the heel that surpasses the energy dissipation capabilities of the calcaneus and soft tissue systems of the foot. A fall from a height is the usual scenario, but a significant force can be inflicted from below, as in a motor vehicle accident or via a land mine in war.

In the sagittal plane, the center of the tuberosity of the calcaneus is situated just lateral to the center of the talus. As a result, when an axial load is applied to the heel, as in a fall, the posterolateral edge of the talus is driven into the posterior facet, causing an oblique shearing-type fracture through the calcaneus. The anterior extent of the fracture line exits on the superolateral side of the calcaneus. Sometimes this line extends into the calcaneocuboid joint. Posteriorly, the fracture line moves medially and exits on the inferomedial corner of the sustentaculum. This has been coined the primary fracture line and is nearly consistent in all axial loading–type fractures[7, 25, 31, 39] (Fig. 21–21A, B). This separates the calcaneus into two main pieces, the medial or constant fragment, which includes the sustentaculum tali, and the posterolateral or tuberosity fragment. Low impact injuries result in

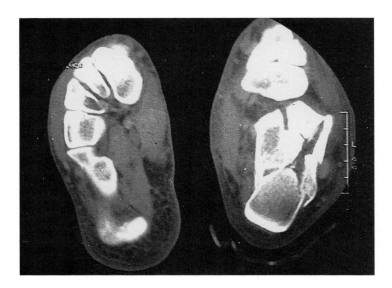

Figure 21–18. Transverse computed tomographic scan image of a calcaneal fracture with extension into the calcaneocuboid joint.

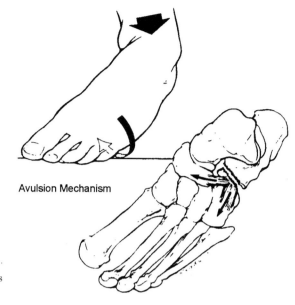

Avulsion Mechanism

Figure 21–19. The mechanism of an anterior process fracture of the calcaneus.

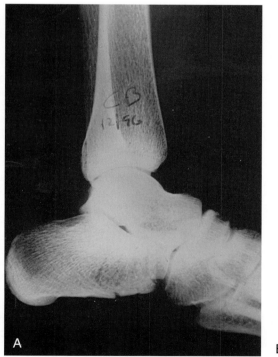

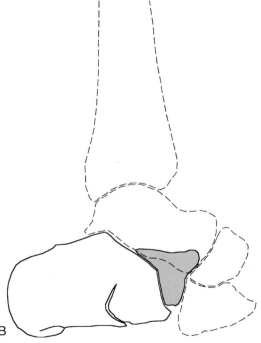

Figure 21–20. A and B, Compression-type anterior process fracture secondary to an eversion and dorsiflexion mechanism.

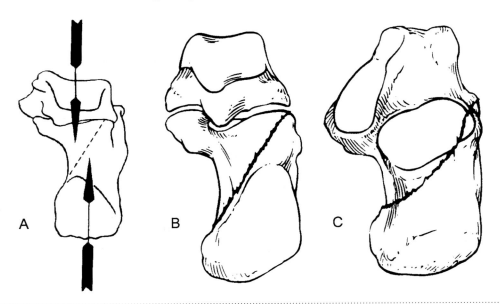

Figure 21–21. *A,* The pathomechanics and shear forces involved in an axially loaded calcaneal fracture. Posterior *(B)* and superior *(C)* views of the primary fracture line.

simple two-part minimally or nondisplaced fractures. There is minimal or no articular impaction, the lateral portion of the posterior facet is intact with the tuberosity piece, and the lateral wall remains intact. The fracture is basically a result of shearing forces.

Higher energy injuries usually add more compression forces and lead to more comminution. As described by Palmer,[31] Essex-Lopresti,[7] Warrick and Bremner,[32] and Burdeaux,[40] a secondary fracture line that exits posteriorly can be identified beneath the posterior facet. If the fracture extends horizontally and exits posteriorly in the tuberosity, the result is the "tongue-type" fracture. If it exits just posterior to the facet, the result is the "joint depression" fracture, and the piece has been termed the "thalamic portion," the "semilunar fragment," or the "superolateral fragment" (Fig. 21–22*A, B*).

Continued downward force drives the sustentacular fragment inferiorly and medially, shortening and widening the heel. The posterolateral side of the talus will drive the semilunar fragment down through the neutral triangle and into the body of the tuberosity. The end result of such a force can be a posterior facet articular surface rotated up to 90° from horizontal. As this piece is being driven down, the lateral wall is violently pushed outward to the extent of impingement on the fibula. Greater force leads to marked osteochondral comminution and collapse of the calcaneus (Fig. 21–23).

The standard mechanism of injury (a fall) will lead to a pattern of deformity that is relatively constant but of varying severity. The heel becomes widened, shortened, and malaligned into varus. The arch of the foot is flattened, and the lever arm of the tendo-Achilles is shortened. The subtalar joint becomes incongruous, and the function of the peroneal tendons is impaired.

Before the advent of the CT scanner, classification schemes were based on the assessment of plain radiographs described previously. No single classification system was found to be completely satisfactory because the limitations of plain film technology made it difficult to assess fully the degree of intra-articular damage. Prognosis, treatment, and assessment of results, therefore, varied for similar injuries. This has lead to often misleading and inconsistent evaluation of the results reported in the literature.

Essex-Lopresti[7] contributed significantly to the understanding of intra-articular fractures when he classified them into joint depression and tongue type. These designations produced a clearer mental image of the fractures and are still used today by many in the initial categorization and decision making regarding treatment.

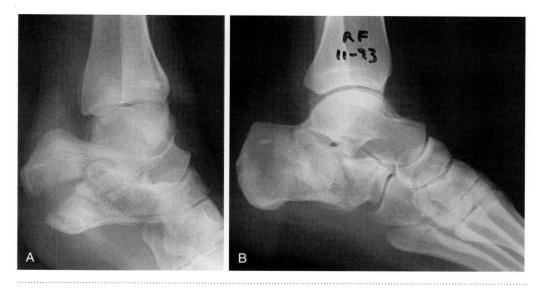

Figure 21–22. Examples of *(A)* tongue-type and *(B)* joint depression–type calcaneal fractures.

Stephenson[33] modified a classification scheme of Warrick and Bremner's[32] that was based on conclusions derived from experimentally created calcaneal fractures. The following factors were considered: (1) major force of injury (shear, compression, or both), (2) location of the primary fracture line in regards to the posterior facet, (3) number of major fragments, and (4) configuration of the posterolateral fragment (tongue or joint depression). Although the use of CT scan-

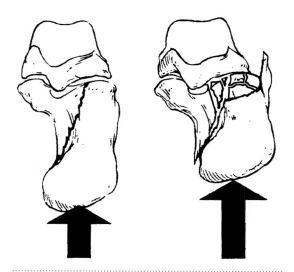

Figure 21–23. Increased axial force leads to greater shortening, widening, and osteochondral comminution.

ning was briefly discussed, most of Stephenson's work was based on plain films.

In 1986, Gilmer and colleagues,[41] using Warrick and Bremner's[32] classification system as a base, studied 32 acute fractures using CT scan images. They compared this modality with plane films in evaluating the displacement of the medial cortex as well as the disruption of the lateral weight-bearing surface. Although the CT scans verified that each fracture had the expected components, there was significant variability in the degree to which they were present. They concluded that the precise understanding of the fracture anatomy provided by the CT scans could predictably dictate surgical treatment.

In 1990, Crosby and Fitzgibbons[42] evaluated the results of nonoperative treatment in 30 intra-articular fractures. These fractures were classified by CT scans as having (1) a nondisplaced fracture of the posterior facet, (2) a displaced fracture, or (3) a comminuted fracture of the posterior facet. Their conclusions were that all type I and some type II fractures did well, but all type III fractures did poorly with closed treatment. Although this retrospective review had some inherent bias,[42–44] in general it did anticipate the expected outcome depending on fracture type, using nonoperative methods of treatment.

In 1992, Sanders[29, 34, 35] reported on a relatively simple classification system based on

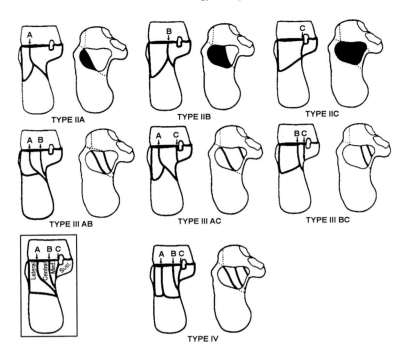

TYPE IIA   TYPE IIB   TYPE IIC

TYPE III AB   TYPE III AC   TYPE III BC

TYPE IV

Figure 21–24. Sanders' classification of calcaneal fractures.

the semicoronal section CT scans (Fig. 21–24). He believed it was a natural progression of the system proposed by Soeur and Remy.[11] Both studies associated the number and location of the articular fracture fragments with the prognosis. Soeur and Remy's series was based on intra-operative findings, whereas Sanders used the preoperative CT scans for classification and evaluation. As a result, Sanders hoped to develop an accurate preoperative prognostic scale and treatment guidance system.

Sanders concluded that the treatment of calcaneal fractures should be tailored to the "personality" of the injury (Fig. 21–25). Best determined via good clinical judgment and a prognostic fracture classification system.

He wrote, "CT scanning is the only accurate method of analyzing this complex fracture and therefore only a CT scan classification can be prognostic."[36] Recently, however, the prognostic capabilities for Sander's classification have been put into question by Buckley and colleagues, who found no statistical link between the initial Sander's classification and the patient outcome, as assessed at the 2-year follow-up point.[45]

With the Sanders classification, all nondisplaced articular fractures, irrespective of the number of fracture lines, are considered type I and do well with nonoperative treatment and early motion.[36] The overwhelming majority of intra-articular fractures are type II and should undergo surgical correc-

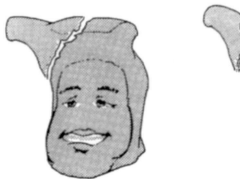
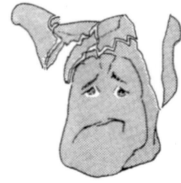

Figure 21–25. The personality of the fracture must always be considered when determining ultimate treatment.

tion and stabilization. Type III fractures are less frequent and should undergo surgical correction, but both the surgeon and the patient need to understand that these have a worse prognosis. Type IV fractures are rare, and surgical correction is based on restoring calcaneal shape, not articular congruence. Many have poor outcomes, and primary arthrodesis should be considered at the time of surgery.

CONCLUSION

The diagnosis of a fractured calcaneus is relatively easy to make with the history of direct trauma to the heel or a fall from a height of more than 1 meter onto the foot and the clinical signs of ecchymosis, tenderness around the heel, and an inability to bear weight. The standard radiologic evaluation of plain x-ray films and CT scans will confirm the diagnosis and allow, at least, a classification of the fracture. Currently, the most accepted classification scheme is that of Sanders,[34] which is based on anatomic findings.

To treat the fractured calcaneus most effectively, one must understand the mechanism of injury and appreciate the degree of damage to the cartilage, bone, and soft tissues. The pathomechanics and pathoanatomy of calcaneal fractures have been extensively researched over the past 90 years. At this point, a good understanding of the osteology of these fractures has been developed and published. There is, however, less known and published about the degree of injury to the cartilage and soft tissues around the hindfoot and how to best manage these portions of the injury.

With all the technologic advancements in the past few decades, only the diagnosis and classification of calcaneal fractures have been made easier. The management of the fracture and soft tissue injury is still a significant challenge and should not be taken lightly.

REFERENCES

1. Cave EF. Fracture of the os calcis—the problem in general. Clin Orthop 30:64–66, 1963.
2. Eastwood DM, Gregg PJ, Atkins RM. Intra-articular fractures of the calcaneum. Part I: pathological anatomy and classification. J Bone Joint Surg Br 75:183–188, 1993.
3. Nade S, Monahan PRW. Fractures of the calcaneus: a study of the long-term prognosis. Injury 4:200–207, 1973.
4. Boehler L. Diagnosis, pathology, and treatment of fractures of the os calcis. J Bone Joint Surg Am 13:75–89, 1931.
5. Anglen JO. Advances in the treatment of calcaneus fracture. Mod Med 90:183–187, 1993.
6. Crosby LA, Kamins P. The history of the calcaneal fracture. Orthop Rev 20:501–509, 1991.
7. Essex-Lopresti P. The mechanism, reduction technique, and results in fractures of the os calcis, 1951–52. Clin Orthop 290:3–16, 1993.
8. Heckman JD. Fractures and dislocations of the foot. In Rockwood CA, Green DP, Bucholz RW, eds. Fractures and Dislocations of the Foot. Philadelphia: J. B. Lippincott, 1991:2041–2182.
9. Lindsay WRN, Dewar FP. Fractures of the os calcis. Am J Surg 95:555–576, 1958.
10. Sanders R, Hansen ST, McReynolds IS. Trauma to the calcaneus and its tendon: fractures of the calcaneus. In Jahss MH, ed. Disorders of the Foot and Ankle: Medical and Surgical Management. Philadelphia: W. B. Saunders, 1991:2326–2354.
11. Soeur R, Remy R. Fractures of the calcaneus with displacement of the thalamic portion. J Bone Joint Surg Br 57:413–421, 1975.
12. Carr JB. Mechanism and pathoanatomy of the intraarticular calcaneal fracture. Clin Orthop 290:36–40, 1993.
13. Mann RA, Coughlin MJ. Surgery of the Foot and Ankle. St. Louis, MO: C. V. Mosby, 1992.
14. Rowe CR, Sakellarides HT, Freeman PA, Sorbie C. Fracture of the os calcis. JAMA 184:920–923, 1963.
15. Widen A. Fractures of the calcaneus. Acta Chir Scand Suppl 188:7–119, 1954.
16. Bankart ASB. Fractures of the os calcis. Lancet 2:175, 1942.
17. Buckley RE, Meek RN. Comparison of open versus closed reduction of intraarticular calcaneal fractures: a matched cohort in workmen. J Orthop Trauma 6:216–222, 1992.
18. Levin LS, Nunley JA. The management of soft-tissue problems associated with calcaneal fractures. Clin Orthop 290:151–156, 1993.
19. Hall RL, Shereff MJ. Anatomy of the calcaneus. Clin Orthop 290:27–35, 1993.
20. Albert MJ, Waggoner SM, Smith JW. Internal fixation of calcaneus fractures: an anatomical study of structures at risk. J Orthop Trauma 9:107–112, 1995.
21. Proceedings of the British Orthopaedic Association. J. Bone Joint Surg Br 29:254–255, 1947.
22. Tanke GM. Fractures of the calcaneus: a review of the literature together with some observations on methods of treatment. Acta Chir Scand Suppl 505:1–103, 1982.
23. Roesen HM, Kanat IO. Anterior process fracture of the calcaneus. J Foot Ankle Surg 32:424–429, 1993.
24. Giachino AA, Uhthoff HK. Intra-articular fractures of the calcaneus. J Bone Joint Surg Am 71:784–787, 1989.
25. Letournel E. Open treatment of acute calcaneal fractures. Clin Orthop 290:60–67, 1993.
26. Broden B. Roentgen examination of the subtaloid joint in fractures of the calcaneus. Acta Radiol 31:85–91, 1949.
27. Smith RW, Staple TW. Computerized tomography

(CT) scanning: technique for the hindfoot. Clin Orthop 177:34–38, 1983.

28. Segal D, Marsh JL, Leiter B. Clinical application of computerized axial tomography (CAT) scanning of calcaneus fractures. Clin Orthop 199:114–123, 1985.

29. Sanders R, Gregory P. Operative treatment of intra-articular fractures of the calcaneus. Orthop Clin North Am 26:203–214, 1995.

30. Cotton FJ, Henderson FF. Results of fractures of the os calcis. Am J Orthop 14:290, 1916.

31. Palmer I. The mechanism and treatment of fractures of the calcaneus. J Bone Joint Surg Am 30:2–8, 1948.

32. Warrick CK, Bremner AE. Fracture of the calcaneum: with an atlas illustrating the various types of fractures. J Bone Joint Surg Br 35:33–45, 1953.

33. Stephenson JR. Treatment of displaced intra-articular fractures of the calcaneus using medial and lateral approaches, internal fixation, and early motion. J Bone Joint Surg Am 69:115–130, 1987.

34. Sanders R, Fortin PD, Pasquale T, Walling A. Operative treatment in 120 displaced intraarticular calcaneal fractures. Results using a prognostic computed tomography scan classification. Clin Orthop 290:87–95, 1993.

35. Sanders R. Intra-articular fractures of the calcaneus: present state of the art. J Orthop Trauma 6:252–265, 1992.

36. Jahss MH, Kay BS. An anatomic study of the anterior superior process of the os calcis and its clinical application. Foot Ankle 3:268–281, 1983.

37. Hunt DD. Compression fracture of the anterior articular surface of the calcaneus. J Bone Joint Surg Am 52:1637–1642, 1970.

38. Protheroe K. Avulsion fractures of the calcaneus. J Bone Joint Surg Br 51:118–122, 1969.

39. Burns AE. Fractures of the calcaneus. Clin Podiatry 2:311–324, 1985.

40. Burdeaux BD. Reduction of calcaneal fractures by the McReynolds medial approach technique and its experimental basis. Clin Orthop 177:87–103, 1983.

41. Gilmer PW, Herzenberg J, Frank JL, et al. Computerized tomographic analysis of acute calcaneal fractures. Foot Ankle 6:184–193, 1986.

42. Crosby LA, Fitzgibbons T. Computerized tomography scanning of acute intra-articular fractures of the calcaneus. J Bone Joint Surg Am 72:852–859, 1990.

43. Sangeorzan BJ. (letter). J Bone Joint Surg Am 73:1430–1431, 1991.

44. Triffitt PD, Gregg PJ. (letter). J Bone Joint Surg Am 73:1429–1430, 1991.

45. Buckley RE, Aubin P, Connell D, Hildebrand K. Clinical and CT correlation of calcaneal fractures: a two year follow-up study. Presented at the meeting of the Orthopaedic Trauma Association, Boston, MA, 1996.

22 Calcaneal Fractures: Conservative and Surgical Management

Craig S. Bartlett III
Steven S. Louis
David L. Helfet

Fractures of the os calcis manifest over a broad spectrum of injury severity, with a variety of minor extra-articular and cortical avulsion fractures at one end and devastating high-energy intra-articular fractures at the other. Although the detrimental effects and poor functional outcomes accompanying the latter are well recognized, their optimal management strategy remains elusive. An understanding of the unique anatomy of this bone and of the fracture pattern is required to select the treatment plan most likely to maximize the patient's outcome while minimizing complications.

Over the past century, enthusiasm for surgical treatment of calcaneal fractures has waxed and waned.[1] In 1935 Böhler[2] remarked, "Fractures of the calcaneus should be treated like all other fractures, i.e., exact reduction must be made and the reduced fragments must be fixed in position until bony union has occurred, and during the period of fixation as many joints as possible should be exercised." More recently, Baumgaertel and Gotzen[3] wrote, "Why should the os calcis not be treated as any other load-sharing bone, where length and alignment, as well as joint congruency, have become main indications for surgery?"

Currently, most surgeons agree that anatomic reconstruction of a majority of comminuted intra-articular fractures of the calcaneus will afford patients their best chance for a good functional outcome.[1, 4–15] This sentiment is based on accepted principles of treatment of intra-articular fractures in weight-bearing joints, which include anatomic reduction of the articular surface and restoration of mechanical alignment. In further support of surgical treatment are the improved operative results over the past few decades, which can be attributed to improved understanding of fracture patterns from cross-sectional imaging, advanced surgical skills (Fig. 22–1), an appreciation of

osseous blood supply, atraumatic soft tissue handling, indirect reduction techniques, rigid internal fixation, modern antibiotics, and aggressive early rehabilitation. However, surgical treatment of these challenging fractures is not a panacea, since infection, wound problems, sural nerve injury, malreduction, and other complications occur in 10 to 20% of cases.[11]

ACUTE CARE

Management of the calcaneus fracture begins in the emergency room. Conditions that require rapid attention and surgical intervention include an open fracture, compartment syndrome, and impending posterior skin necrosis or acute tarsal tunnel syndrome secondary to a markedly displaced tongue-type fracture.[15] Otherwise, initial management should consist of the application of a bulky Robert Jones dressing splint and elevation on a Böhler frame.

It is imperative to reduce the marked, almost obligatory, swelling of the foot and ankle expeditiously, particularly before any attempts at open reduction. Admission to the hospital is usually prudent, because homebound patients rarely achieve adequate bedrest and elevation of their limb. Reliable patients who are discharged should return twice weekly for the next 10 to 14 days. After 5 to 7 days, the bulky dressing can be removed in lieu of a compressive stocking.[15]

Another promising adjunct, the intermittent compression foot pump, has reportedly effected a rapid and dramatic reduction of swelling in both the preoperative and postoperative setting.[16–18] Furthermore, evidence exists that dangerously high compartment pressures may be reduced to acceptable levels and fasciotomy avoided.[15, 18] Even for patients not undergoing surgery, the ap-

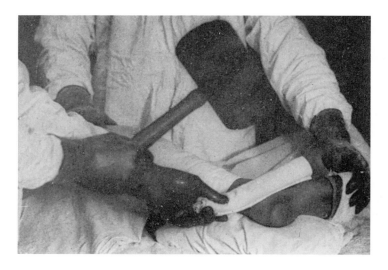

Figure 22–1. In the 1930s, the main reduction tool used by some surgeons was a weighted 7-pound mallet. (From Hermann OJ. Conservative therapy for fracture of the os calcis. J Bone Joint Surg Am 19:710, 1937.)

plication of a foot pump may lead to improved subtalar motion, reduced pain, and a shorter interval before returning to work.[19] Unfortunately, many patients find these devices painful and do not use them as directed on an outpatient basis.[15]

Blistering of the skin can be a difficult and controversial problem. Some authors ignore fracture blisters,[15] whereas others debride them under sterile conditions and provide coverage with a dressing or Tegaderm (3M Medical-Surgical Division. St. Paul, MN[13]) or institute whirlpool treatments.[5]

AVULSION, STRESS, AND EXTRA-ARTICULAR FRACTURES

The majority of small peripheral fractures can be treated simply with ice, elevation, a bulky Robert Jones dressing, early range of motion, and progressive weight bearing as tolerated. Among this group are minimally or nondisplaced fractures of the medial or lateral process, which, if widely displaced, may be considered for closed reduction to narrow the heel. Surgery, however, is rarely, if ever, required.[20] Another common entity, the anterior process fracture, is often misdiagnosed as a sprain of the ankle.[20] Although often extending into the calcaneocuboid joint, immobilization in a commercially available brace or removable short leg cast is acceptable for small fragments with minimal displacement or articular involvement. Range-of-motion exercises are begun when swelling and pain have diminished and weight bearing is advanced by 4 to 6 weeks.

In patients with large displaced intra-articular fractures, open reduction and internal fixation or excision should be considered.[20]

Stress fractures are treated by limitation of the causative activity, until symptoms subside, usually by 4 to 6 weeks.[20] For patients involved in rigorous activities, such as long-distance runners, a heel pad or arch support will help prevent recurrence.

Beak (distal to Achilles tendon insertion) and avulsion (at Achilles insertion) fractures of the posterosuperior aspect of the tuberosity are well recognized and are usually managed with a short-leg walking cast for 4 to 6 weeks. If continuity of the tendo-Achilles is in doubt, then non-weight bearing is preferable during this period.[20] For displaced beak fractures, in which the overlying skin is at risk, either a closed reduction and casting in plantar flexion or open reduction and internal fixation is required. Because of gastrocnemius-soleus involvement, most displaced avulsion-type fractures should be treated with open reduction and internal fixation, followed by protected weight bearing in a removable short leg cast or boot at 4 weeks.

Controversy exists as to the best method of treatment for extra-articular fractures of the body of the calcaneus. In most cases, treatment may consist of ice, elevation, a compressive dressing, early range of motion, and non-weight bearing for 4 to 12 weeks.[20] However, displaced fractures can result in widening and malalignment of the foot, with loss of the gastrocnemius-soleus lever arm. Therefore, closed reduction and immobilization in a short-leg cast or percutaneous fixation should be considered.[2, 20, 21]

INTRA-ARTICULAR FRACTURES: TREATMENT ALTERNATIVES AND RESULTS

The lack of a universally accepted protocol for the clinical and radiographic evaluation, classification, and treatment of calcaneal fractures has hampered efforts to compare the available literature precisely. Primary treatment strategies have included no attempts at reduction and early weight bearing; no reduction and immobilization or mobilization; closed reduction and immobilization in plaster; closed reduction and skeletal traction, percutaneous pin fixation, or external fixation; closed reduction and percutaneous screw fixation; open reduction and internal fixation from medial, lateral, or combined approaches; arthrodesis; and even amputation.

To simplify such confusion, it is best to consider management options as grouped into one of four broad categories: (1) nonoperative treatment; (2) open reduction and internal fixation; (3) limited open or closed reduction and percutaneous fixation; and (4) arthrodesis.

Results of Nonoperative Treatment

Natural history studies have shown that patients treated without surgery usually experience chronic, long-term symptoms.[11, 22] Four decades ago, Lindsay and Dewar[22] noted that 81% of their 83 patients with conservatively treated calcaneus fractures continued to have a painful foot at long-term follow-up. Interestingly, of the 48 fractures with marked persistent fracture displacement, 71% had good results, whereas only 29% had poor outcomes.

Kitaoka and colleagues[23] managed 27 patients suffering a unilateral displaced intra-articular fracture of the calcaneus with a cast instead of a reduction procedure or an operation. The clinical result after a mean of 6 years was excellent in 5 patients, good in 5, fair in 7, and poor in 10. Analysis of gait patterns revealed abnormalities in ground-reaction force with regard to vertical and temporal force factors. Motion was decreased in the sagittal, coronal, and transverse planes during walking on level ground, on a side-sloping surface, and especially when ambulating up and down stairs. Although complications were rare and these patients did not have a subsequent reconstructive procedure, most had persistent functional impairment.

In contrast, Pozo and coworkers,[24] in their study of 21 patients with severely comminuted fractures of the calcaneus, reported good results in 75% at an average follow-up of 14.6 years after nonoperative management. Their protocol included early active mobilization of the ankle, subtalar, and midtarsal joints. Although maximal recovery was obtained in 66% of patients by 2 to 3 years, 24% continued to improve after 6 years and no result deteriorated over time. These are not isolated findings. A review of the literature by Giachino and Uhthoff[25] found similar results with this management approach, although no report described a patient with an excellent outcome. This last detail hints at the limitations of nonoperative care.

The first report to stratify outcomes based on the fracture pattern was by Crosby and Fitzgibbons.[26] They evaluated 30 intra-articular calcaneal fractures with computed tomography (CT) before treatment with a variety of closed methods. Their type I fractures (less than 2 mm of displacement) recovered function and healed extremely well; good or better results were achieved in 92% of cases. Poor results were common after closed treatment of type II (40%) and III (100%) fractures; 50% of the former and 86% of the latter had or were considered for a subtalar arthrodesis.

Results of Open Reduction and Internal Fixation

Introducing his lateral approach, Palmer[27] was among the authors to report favorable results after open reduction and internal fixation of os calcis fractures. Although the majority of his patients regained only 25 to 50% of normal subtalar motion, this was usually painless, and all patients returned to their previous work between 4 and 8 months.

Stephenson[28] treated 22 displaced intra-articular fractures of the calcaneus by open reduction and internal fixation with a screw and one or two staples through a lateral and occasionally a supplemental medial approach. Even with a protocol of early motion, a nearly anatomic reduction was achieved and maintained in 86% of cases.

At a follow-up of 16 to 72 months, good or better clinical and radiographic results were achieved in 77%, with subtalar motion averaging 75% of normal. All but 1 patient returned to work within 6 months.

Melcher and associates reviewed 16 patients with intra-articular fractures of the calcaneus at 3 and 10 years after open reduction, internal fixation, and bone grafting.[8, 9] Typically, patients returned to work at 5 months. After 10 years, 75% demonstrated a good or better functional result. In no case was there an indication for a secondary arthrodesis. Despite most patients radiographically demonstrating a slowly progressing posttraumatic subtalar osteoarthritis, the subjective results (pain, capacity to work or sports) at 10 years were clearly better than those 3 years after surgery. In fact, several patients reported that their hindfoot function continued to improve for up to 5 years, suggesting the existence of an adaptive mechanism, which compensated for their functional disability. Although most patients seemed to benefit from open reduction and internal fixation, 31% were still forced to change their occupation.

Letournel[6] reviewed 99 patients with a follow-up of more than 2 years and found that 56% of his patients had no functional disability or, at most, occasional pain while walking on uneven ground. One half had subtalar mobility measuring 50% of the uninjured side.

Paley and Hal[29, 30] evaluated 52 calcaneal fractures at a follow-up between 4 and 14 years after open reduction and internal fixation through a medial approach. Factors associated with an unsatisfactory result included age greater than 50, increased weight, decreased height, increased time missed from work as a result of injury, heavy labor occupation, increased heel width, decreased fibulocalcaneal space, subtalar joint incongruity and osteoarthrosis, arthrosis of the talonavicular and tibiotalar joints, central depression-type fractures, and increased comminution. Surprisingly, heel alignment did not correlate with outcome. Function continued to improve for up to 2 years in 60% of the patients, 4 years in 20%, and 6 years in 11%. In only 9% of the patients did symptoms actually worsen. The most common primary clinical problems were subtalar joint pain, heel pad pain, and

fibulocalcaneal impingement. Böhler tuberosity joint angle, although not correlating well with excellent, good, or fair results, was significantly lower for patients with poor outcomes. Similarly, Dart and Graham[31] found that minor reductions of this angle were well compensated for, but that a significant decrease was associated with a painful flatfoot.

Benirschke and Sangeorzan[1] managed more than 100 calcaneal fractures with an extensile lateral approach, rigid internal fixation, and early motion, noting lower morbidity and improved outcome compared with previous published results. Although subtalar motion averaged 50% of the contralateral side, only 3 of 80 fractures required arthrodesis. At a more recent follow-up,[10] 70% reported satisfaction with their results, 65% were limited only in their ability to participate in vigorous activities and sports, more than 50% could walk comfortably on any surface, and 60% required no medications to control discomfort. Still, 40% were unable to return to their previous employment because of functional limitations.

Zwipp and others[32] reported 61% good or excellent results after osteosynthesis of 123 displaced intra-articular fractures of the calcaneus. In 68% of the cases, the sustentacular fragment was the key to open reduction, mandating a medial approach. For complex fractures, a lateral approach was added. In the presence of lateral wall blowout fractures or comminution of the sustentacular fragment, an extended lateral approach only was used.

Hutchinson and Huebner[33] treated 47 displaced intra-articular fractures of the os calcis with open reduction and internal fixation. Preoperative and postoperative CT was used to assess all fractures. At a follow-up of 1 year, 77% had satisfactory results. Langdon and colleagues[34] also stressed the importance of CT to facilitate understanding of fracture anatomy and subsequent surgical reconstruction. In reviewing 63 fractures, these authors observed a constant anterolateral fragment, which if unrecognized and unreduced, healed in a displaced position, thus limiting hindfoot eversion and disrupting the calcaneocuboid joint.

Bezes and others[12] reported on their 20-year experience of treating 257 intra-articular fractures of the calcaneus by open reduction and internal fixation with a one-third tubular plate through a lateral incision. Functional results were excellent or good in 85%. Although half of their patients demonstrated reduced subtalar mobility, pain and limited ambulation were rare. Only 6 patients required a late subtalar arthrodesis.

Sanders and associates[13, 14] monitored 120 displaced intra-articular fractures treated by open reduction and internal fixation via a lateral approach for an average of 29 months. Reduction in heel height, length, and width were respectively 98%, 100%, and 110%. In all but 3 cases, Boehler and Gissane angles were reduced to within 5° of normal. Of their type II fractures, 86% had a radiographic anatomic reduction and 73% had good or better function. For the type III and type IV fractures, these results, respectively, fell to 60% and 70%, and 0% and 9%. Type III fractures were more technically challenging than type II fractures, but outcomes for both improved over time. In contrast, outcomes for type IV fractures did not improve, even after 4 years.

Baumgaertel and Gotzen[3] reported moderate success with a two-stage reconstruction of 13 comminuted os calcis fractures. After an indirect reduction with medial external fixation, which improved alignment in every case, delayed lateral plate fixation completed the reconstruction. Residual widening was easily corrected during this second stage of the procedure, facilitated by the decreased edema and the restoration of alignment by the fixator. This technique appeared to reduce the incidence of blister formation, skin slough, postoperative edema, and venous thrombosis. Subtalar motion averaged 57% of the untreated side. Massive bone grafting was associated with a high occurrence of infection and soft tissue complications.

When reviewing the preceding reports of surgical treatment, there appears to be a consistent postoperative development of radiographic degenerative changes and a loss of subtalar motion of approximately 25 to 50%. However, this stiffness is usually not a problem except when walking on uneven ground.[6, 12, 15] In fact, many of these patients do quite well,[1, 8, 12, 15, 27, 35] indicating that subtalar arthrosis per se should not be viewed as a sign of fixation failure. Whether fractures of the os calcis are managed operatively or not, at least some subtalar motion

is lost.[15] However, retaining some subtalar motion is protective of the ankle.

Comparison of Open Reduction with Nonoperative Treatment

In reviewing much of the past literature, Paley and Hall[29] noted that nonoperative treatment of the calcaneal fracture typically resulted in unsatisfactory outcomes in 33 to 50% of cases compared with surgical treatment, which has led to unsatisfactory outcomes in 25 to 33% of cases. Unfortunately, very few studies have attempted to control variables to permit accurate and meaningful comparisons of these two treatment options.

At 2 to 12 years, Jarvholm and others[36] compared 20 patients with displaced intra-articular fractures of the calcaneus treated by open reduction and early postoperative motion with a similar group of 19 patients treated nonoperatively. Pain, residual symptoms, and disability were similar in both groups. Three patients in each group had marked complaints, and equally many had negligible symptoms. The operative group had greater subtalar motion (50% vs. 20%), a better ability to jump and run, greater endurance on uneven surfaces, less forward tilting of the lateral part of the posterior articular surface, but only a slightly improved Böhler angle, and more complications (two infections) than the nonoperative group. Radiographic signs of osteoarthrosis were noted in 45% of the operative group and 44% of the nonoperative group. These authors concluded that overall results of open and closed treatment are almost equal and that primary surgery is rarely indicated for a fracture of the os calcis. However, this was a poorly controlled, retrospective study in which the authors selected a control group based on roentgenograms of patients treated conservatively by other physicians. Also, their brief interval between injury and surgical intervention (average 3 days) may have been responsible for their two infections. Finally, compared with today's standards, their use of one screw for fixation is considered inadequate.

Parmar and colleagues[37] prospectively evaluated 56 displaced intra-articular fractures of the calcaneus, randomized into conservative or operative treatment groups.

Ten undisplaced fractures were treated conservatively. Their surgical protocol included open reduction of the posterior subtalar joint and fixation with Kirschner wires, no attempt to reduce and fix the tuberosity fragments, and immobilization of the foot for 6 weeks. At a mean review of 2 years, in the nonoperative group, undisplaced fractures had slightly better results than the displaced fractures. When comparing the results of treatment of displaced fractures, there was no significant difference in outcome between open reduction and nonoperative management. However, the correction of any heel widening was unlikely because of the failure to reconstruct the tuberosity fragments and the use of limited fixation. Also, immobilization does not permit early range of motion, one of the most beneficial effects of open reduction and internal fixation. It is not surprising then that their surgically treated fractures continued to have lateral impingement and pain in various areas. However, fewer patients in this group complained of pain at two or more sites. In the conservatively treated group, displaced fractures resulted in a greater degree of pain and more often required analgesia.

Buckley and Meek[38] reported on 17 displaced intra-articular calcaneal fractures treated operatively that were matched with a similar group of nonoperatively treated fractures. Although more of the former returned to work, the difference was not significant. At an average follow-up of 6 years, no significant differences existed between the two groups with regards to heel pain, subtalar motion, and return to work. However, in the operative group, the overall clinical result was better when an anatomic reduction of the subtalar joint had been achieved. A result less than perfect corresponded to an overall clinical score that was the same as if no surgery had been performed. The authors did not explore the possibility of a bias toward poor results by presence of workers' compensation status in all cases.

Leung and associates[39] compared the results of 44 displaced intra-articular fractures of the calcaneus 3 years after open reduction, internal fixation, and bone grafting through a lateral approach with those of 19 patients treated without surgery. Significantly better outcomes were noted in the former group with respect to pain, activity, range of movement, return to work, and swelling of the hindfoot. The operative group also demonstrated better radiographic scores for articular congruity and arthritic changes, with Böhler angle within 1.5°, Gissane angle within 1°, a height 96% of the normal side, and a width only 3% greater.

O'Farrell and coworkers[40] prospectively evaluated two groups of 12 patients with displaced intra-articular fractures of the os calcis. One group underwent open reduction and internal fixation through a lateral approach followed by early mobilization, whereas the second group was managed nonoperatively. At 15 months, patients treated by open reduction and osteosynthesis were more likely to have returned to work (67% vs. 25%), had greater walking endurance (4 km vs. 1 km), were less likely to have required a change in shoe size (8% vs. 67%), and had a greater range of subtalar motion (24° vs. 12°) than patients treated conservatively. Radiographically, partial or full restoration of Böhler angle was observed in the patients who underwent internal fixation.

Monsey and others[41] retrospectively studied 18 Crosby type II and III fractures at an average follow-up of 32 months after open reduction and internal fixation. Their findings suggested that Crosby type II fractures (displaced but simple intra-articular fractures) have a similar outcome when either operative or nonoperative treatment is used, but that type III fractures (severely comminuted) fared considerably better with operative intervention. However, the study group was small, and a large emphasis was placed on subtalar motion in their scoring system. Because no patient reported complaints of fibular impingement or peroneal tendon entrapment, these authors continue to recommend operative treatment for Crosby type II fractures. The most common symptom reported by their patients was heel pad pain.[41]

Results of Percutaneous Fixation

Although good results have been obtained after formal open exposures of os calcis fractures, indirect reduction techniques and percutaneous fixation, which have demonstrated utility for other intra-articular fractures, may be applicable in certain situations.[2, 30, 42-48] These more limited approaches have found increasing support because of concerns for possible serious soft tissue complications and the realization that anatomic restoration of the subtalar joint does not always lead to a good outcome.[4, 13, 14, 49]

In the 1930s, Böhler[42] popularized his technique of closed reduction, with pins placed into the tuberosity of the calcaneus and tibia, to allow traction and later maintenance of the reduction when they were incorporated into plaster. Two decades later, Essex-Lopresti[2] contributed his refined techniques of closed reduction and spike fixation. After a successful reduction, he reported that 80% of patients younger than 50 years had no pain or only trivial symptoms and returned to work within 6 months. In contrast, after successful reductions in an older age group, only 40% had trivial symptoms and returned to work. Of his unsuccessful reductions, 70% were disabled for work or play, and the majority of poor outcomes occurred in patients older than 50.

Improving on the original concepts of Böhler, Buch and associates[43] noted successful results 6 years after percutaneous wire fixation of 79 calcaneal fractures. Developing percutaneous wire techniques further, Pescatori and Fioriti[44] applied an Ilizarov external fixator below the ankle joint to treat 10 severe joint depression fractures. This resulted in the restoration of height and correction of alignment and permitted ankle joint motion. Postulating that early weight bearing might reduce soft tissue dystrophy and pain, Paley and colleagues[30, 45] used an Ilizarov device to achieve as anatomic a closed reduction as possible in seven patients, followed by limited open reduction and internal fixation of the depressed subtalar joint fragments. Weight bearing began within 24 hours of surgery, and all patients ambulated with partial to full weight bearing throughout treatment. Clinical results were excellent in five patients and good in two patients; four had greater than 50% subtalar motion. In the three patients with persistent pain, symptoms were mild and appeared related to the subtalar joint. There were no complaints of heel pain at follow-up.

Fernandez and Koella[46] combined a single extensile posterolateral approach, with open reduction and screw fixation of the posterior facet, bone grafting, percutaneous

pinning of the body, and early mobilization in 41 displaced intra-articular fractures of the calcaneus. An anatomic reduction was obtained in 28 cases and a residual displacement of less than 2 mm in 5. Of the 8 cases with greater residual displacement, 6 were comminuted fracture types. No fracture lost reduction and union occurred at an average of 8 weeks. At 4 years, a 76% rate of satisfactory results correlated with severity of articular comminution, restoration of articular congruency, and proper extra-articular alignment.

Combining the historic contributions of Böhler and Essex-Lopresti with modern techniques of indirect reduction and percutaneous fixation, Forgon[48] performed closed reduction and percutaneous screw fixation of 265 calcaneus fractures. Because of its minimal invasiveness, surgery was possible within several days of injury. Motion was begun immediately; limited protected weight bearing was permitted by the third or fourth postoperative day. At 1 year, good or excellent results had been achieved in 90% of cases, with an average interval of 6 months before return to work. Collapse of the fracture occurred in only 4% of patients, failure of fixation in 2%, lateral impingement in 5%, and wound complications in 3.7%.

Results of Arthrodesis

Early attempts at primary subtalar fusion for severely comminuted fractures of the calcaneus[22, 50-52] failed to restore precise hindfoot anatomy and lead to unpredictable outcomes. Although primary triple arthrodesis has also been advocated,[51, 53] new evidence indicates that this form of arthrodesis may have the worst results.[54] These findings, compounded with a fear of infection or nonunion, have led many physicians to avoid surgical treatment of comminuted calcaneus fractures.

In contrast, Myerson[16] reported good results after open reduction and primary subtalar arthrodesis of comminuted fractures of the calcaneus; 80% of patients returned to work within 9 months of injury. No patient required conversion to a triple arthrodesis at follow-up. Sanders and others[15] also reported success with this procedure, observing that 11 of their first 12 primary fusion patients were able to return to work, all within 5 months. The important difference between these two studies and earlier ones is their emphasis on the anatomic restoration of calcaneal height and width by open reduction and internal fixation, followed by primary subtalar arthrodesis when significant chondral loss or comminution is present.

Kusakabe and coworkers[55] described the successful use of a free vascularized fibular graft with a peroneal cutaneous flap to obtain simultaneous tibiotalocalcaneal fusion and skin coverage in a patient with severely comminuted open fractures of the talus and calcaneus.

SURGICAL INDICATIONS

Biomechanical Basis for Surgery

The function of the os calcis is to distribute the weight of the body from the subtalar joint to fore (calcaneocuboid joint) and aft (plantar surface) and from heel strike to foot flat during the gait cycle, and to act as a fulcrum between the plantar flexors and forefoot.[3] Superiorly, the subtalar joint functions as a torque converter to provide a cushioning effect on the foot and, by inversion and eversion, allows the foot to adapt to uneven surfaces.[10] A variety of anatomic and functional derangements accompany an intra-articular fracture of the calcaneus. Any of these can lead to chronic pain if not corrected:

1. Without free subtalar inversion and eversion, the subtalar joint is exposed to abnormally high stresses, which can ultimately result in arthrosis.[56] This is the likely outcome for a conservatively treated fracture, in which a reduction of the articular surface is never obtained.

2. The talus increasingly dorsiflexes as it falls into the collapsed calcaneus. This leads to anterior impingement of the talar neck on the tibial plafond, which limits dorsiflexion of the foot, and may result in tibiotalar arthrosis.[10, 15, 57]

3. Widening and varus collapse of the heel result in fibular or peroneal impingement, and increase tension on the lateral soft tissue structures, leading to chronic lateral ankle pain and an increased frequency of ankle sprains.[10, 15, 58]

4. Patients with more comminuted frac-

tures appear to have greater problems with stiffness, resulting in chronic ankle sprains as increased motion in the tibiotalar joint compensates for the motion lost in the subtalar area.[15]

5. Shortening of the lateral column and abduction of the forefoot and midfoot, especially when associated with a fracture of the anterior process, will increase tension on the posterior tibial tendon and may lead to lateral peritalar subluxation or frank dislocation and rupture of the tendon.[10]

6. Functional weakening of the gastrocnemius-soleus complex is produced by the reduction of heel height and length.

On the basis of this large volume of biomechanical evidence, the goal of surgery is to improve on the natural history of the injury by restoring the normal calcaneal anatomy (articular surfaces, height, width, length, and longitudinal axis) and stabilizing the construct well enough to allow early motion.[6, 11, 12] If the foot is immobilized in plaster, as is often required in conservative treatment protocols, any remaining subtalar motion is lost secondary to rapid fibrosis and stiffening of the damaged subtalar joint.[13, 15, 25] Reflex sympathetic dystrophy and nerve and soft tissue problems are also possible complications of plaster immobilization.[15]

Reduction of articular surfaces will restore the geometric relationships within the talocalcaneal and calcaneocuboid joints, diminishing stiffness, pain, and arthrosis. The restoration of height improves the tibiotalar position, which may diminish long-term articular degeneration. Achieving proper heel length and width will allow the patient to wear normal or slightly modified shoes and improve the gastrocnemius-soleus lever arm, while narrowing the heel will also relieve subfibular abutment, thus the observant comment by Letournel[6] that "patients may consider a postsurgical foot with a stiff subtalar joint to be ultimately better than a nonoperatively treated one with a stiff subtalar joint also, but a widened heel and lateral impingement [as well]." Paley and Hall[30] noted that, even in patients with unsatisfactory results, those treated surgically have fewer painful problem areas per foot than nonoperatively treated patients.

The exact reconstruction of the subtalar articular surface is the main prerequisite for a good clinical outcome.[6, 13–15, 38] Incongruity of the subtalar joint has been associated with poor clinical outcome secondary to loss of subtalar joint motion.[11] However, although the best outcomes appear to result from anatomic reduction and surgical stabilization of fractures of the os calcis, many of the worst functional results are obtained when there is failure to achieve an anatomic reduction.[2, 6, 38] In reporting his vast experience in more than 200 cases, Letournel[6] noted that the failure to restore the calcaneal anatomy perfectly was the major cause of postoperative stiffness of the subtalar joint. Essex-Lopresti[2] wrote that "unsuccessful or incomplete reduction gives the worst results."

These observations are substantiated by the finding that clinical results strictly correlate with the severity of articular comminution.[13, 14, 29, 46, 59] The more comminuted the fracture, the more likely is the failure to reduce the articular surface or restore Böhler angle. Failure to accomplish these goals will lead to poorer clinical results. In addition, surgery also carries the potential risk of catastrophic complications. Therefore, absolute indications for surgical stabilization have not yet been determined and are controversial.

Selection of an Optimal Treatment Strategy

Generally, nonoperative management is preferred for minimally displaced fractures (Crosby type I[60] and Sanders type I[14]), which do not significantly involve the weight-bearing surface of the subtalar joint or affect the biomechanical relationships of the foot.[1, 5, 10, 11, 13, 16, 25, 33, 61]

As much as 2 mm of displacement has been considered acceptable for closed treatment.[10, 15, 29, 33, 36, 46] However, Sangeorzan and associates[62] demonstrated that the contact area of the posterior facet is significantly decreased with even 2 mm of displacement. This is a significant finding because excessive contact pressure can harm articular cartilage and lead to joint degeneration.[4, 63] Furthermore, Buckley and Meek[38] demonstrated improved clinical scores of patients with anatomic reductions compared with those having a step malreduction of 1 to 2 mm. This correlation with reduction and final results was also confirmed in Sanders and others'[14] large series of operatively treated displaced intra-articular calcaneal fractures.

Therefore, open reduction and internal fixation is recommended for most displaced intra-articular calcaneus fractures (Sanders type II and III). Stable internal fixation will allow early active and passive mobilization of the subtalar and ankle joints. If this is not achieved, the functional outcome will be poor.[6] For a tongue-type fracture or simple two-part thalamic fracture (Sanders type II), consideration can also be given to percutaneous screw fixation, especially if concerns about soft tissue compromise are present. However, the surgeon must be well versed in these controversial techniques before considering their application. Also, many experienced fracture surgeons do not advocate their use[15]; Benirschke himself cautioned that "percutaneous reduction of a joint-depression injury isn't possible."

Although an anatomic articular reduction is necessary for a good outcome, it cannot guarantee it because of the possibility of cartilage necrosis resulting from the original injury.[4] Harding and Waddell[49] reported that patients with seemingly perfect intraoperative clinical and roentgenographic results were found to have disabling symptoms postoperatively. Sanders and others[13, 14] noted that a number of their anatomically reduced type II and III fractures ultimately required a subtalar fusion. Therefore, realistic goals must be set, and patients must be made aware of potential arthrosis, even in the face of successful surgical reconstruction.

For comminuted fractures, treatment must be individualized. Many three-part posterior facet fractures (Sanders type III) and a small number of the most severely comminuted fractures (Sanders type IV) may benefit from open reduction and internal fixation. However, the greater the comminution, the more difficult the management of the fracture and the more likely the prognosis to be poor.[5, 14–16, 29, 46, 54, 64]

In the presence of associated massive soft tissue swelling, the indications for open reduction and internal fixation of comminuted fractures becomes even more relative. If one cannot obtain an anatomic reduction, then the patient may be better off without surgery.[7, 65] Nonoperative treatment may also be reasonable when the deformity is not excessive and a later reconstructive procedure is possible.[5] However, when dealing with severely comminuted fractures of the os calcis, serious deformity is quite common, anatomic restoration of the joint surface is usually impossible, malunion is likely without treatment, and the specter of infection is eternally present. If conservative treatment is elected, these fractures rarely fail to unite but typically with poor alignment, which significantly complicates any future reconstructive efforts.[10, 54, 57] In addition, the longer the interval between injury and fusion, the longer is the subsequent interval until the patient returns to work.[15, 54]

These many factors have led several highly experienced surgeons[5, 13–16, 61] to manage (often successfully) the most severely comminuted fractures with open reduction and primary arthrodesis. Challenging this concept, however, is evidence that some patients do better than expected. After 4 years, only three of the eight patients with severely comminuted fractures in Fernandez and Koella's series[46] required a subtalar fusion for residual pain. Only 3.3% of Zwipp and colleagues'[32] patients experienced degenerative changes severe enough to require subtalar fusion. Although 50% of Bezes and coworkers'[12] patients demonstrated reduced subtalar motion, only 6 of 257 experienced posttraumatic arthritis severe enough to warrant a subtalar arthrodesis. Melcher and associates[8] noted that radiographic evidence of subtalar arthritis did not correlate with clinical outcome. Letournel[35] observed that a normal life and sports participation were possible with subtalar joint motion only half the normal amount, and that patients with only one-fourth their normal range still functioned better than those with an arthrodesis. Therefore, most surgeons still agree with Melcher and others,[9] who stated that "primary arthrodesis of the subtalar joint should remain an exceptional measure." Another opponent of primary fusion, Benirschke,[15] noted that "it is difficult to predict the degree to which a patient will become symptomatic despite the reconstruction of the posterior facet comminution. I agree that many patients have decreased pain following a fusion. My concern is that once a subtalar fusion is done, especially in a young patient, the clock has been set with respect to the development of arthrosis in the ankle joint."

Regardless of whether primary arthrodesis is performed or secondary arthrodesis is ultimately required, the results of Myerson[16] strongly support some form of primary reduction and fixation of the calcaneal fracture to prevent or lessen long-term disability. Should open reduction and internal fixation be contraindicated, then percutaneous screw fixation may still be an option to narrow the heel and improve alignment without excessive risk of soft tissue complications.

Contraindications to Surgery

Elderly patients and those with an inadequate soft tissue envelope, ischemic peripheral vascular disease, or peripheral neuropathy are unlikely to benefit from surgical treatment.[1, 11, 13, 15, 23] However, age is a controversial factor. While several studies have noted that patients older than 40 years[40] or 50 years[2, 29] are not optimal surgical candidates, others have failed to observe a relationship between age and long-term results.[22, 66, 67]

The presence of severe associated injuries or psychoaffective disorders must be factored into subsequent efforts to perform a difficult reconstruction.[13, 15, 23, 68] Patients with a sedentary lifestyle and those who are unable or unwilling to comply with the postoperative regimen should also be excluded from surgical consideration.[1, 11, 15, 68] In many cases, an individual with a low-demand foot will do better without surgery than with it.[15]

Open fractures may constitute a relative contraindication for internal fixation because of further devascularization and the risk of infection.[11, 13, 23, 68] These are best treated with irrigation and debridement alone or with external fixation, unless the risk of contamination is minimal and further incisions would not increase the likelihood of soft tissue complications.

NONOPERATIVE MANAGEMENT

Nonoperative management typically begins with a compression dressing and elevation of the leg for 2 to 7 days[36, 37] to allow edema to resolve. At this point, early active motion is instituted as pain permits, with delayed weight bearing for 6 to 12 weeks.[25, 36] Although a theoretical risk of fracture displacement exists with early motion, this does not appear to be a clinical problem,[20, 24] except in the case of the tongue-type fracture, in which less aggressive mobilization for 3 or 4 weeks has been recommended.[15]

When properly selected, nonoperative treatment yields a satisfactory functional result in 75 to 85% of cases, with an average return to work in labor-intensive occupations by 3 to 6 months.[5, 22, 24, 60]

SURGICAL MANAGEMENT

Timing of Surgery and Preoperative Planning

Proper timing and careful preoperative planning are essential to prevent complications and ensure the best possible outcome for the patient. In turn, these factors are dependent on the status of the soft tissues, particularly the amount of edema and the presence of fracture blisters. Fortunately, blisters are often not in the region of the standard lateral incision, occurring medially and posteriorly.[15] Ross[68] stated that if minimal swelling is present during the first 6 to 12 hours, then fracture fixation may be considered. However, this is rarely the case. Even should minimal edema be present to permit early surgical intervention, maximal swelling, which generally occurs by 48 to 72 hours, will jeopardize the surgical wounds.

Most surgeons consider from 6 to 10 days to be a sufficient period of time to allow the soft tissues to recuperate.[3, 6, 8–10, 14, 28, 42, 59, 69] Others noted that surgery can be delayed for up to 14 days without significantly compromising reconstructive attempts.[5, 13, 32, 46, 68] This is an important consideration because the soft tissue damage in cases of more severely comminuted fractures may preclude a surgical incision for 2 to 4 weeks.[5] After 3 weeks, early consolidation of the fracture has occurred beyond the point at which the fracture can easily be reduced and anatomically reconstructed.[8, 9, 13, 15] Regardless of the period of time required, hindfoot edema should be decreased before attempting surgical reconstruction, a state heralded when the tissue turgor allows the skin to wrinkle during eversion and dorsiflexion of the foot (wrinkle test)[13] or after the skin is subjected to gentle pressure.[10]

An open fracture or a severely deformed fracture, with shortening, lateral bulging, varus tilting, periarticular soft tissue compromise, contracture, and muscle spasm, produces a poor environment for venous outflow and soft tissue recovery. Thus, it may be advantageous to stage the reduction by initially applying an external fixator (Figs. 22–2 and 22–3),[3] with a Shantz pin into or through the tuberosity of the calcaneus, and pins in the anterior or medial border of the tibia. An articular reconstruction or arthrodesis can then be performed later, when the soft tissues pose less of a risk for a lateral approach.

While the decision to perform an open reduction and arthrodesis is usually made preoperatively, the intraoperative finding of excessive chondral damage may mitigate for fusion over a planned reconstruction. For this reason, the patient should be informed of this possibility before surgery.

Techniques of Open Reduction and Internal Fixation

Patients are usually positioned in the lateral decubitus position. For bilateral fractures, it has been suggested to position the patient prone, with the hips and knees flexed 30° and the legs internally rotated to allow the fractures to be addressed simultaneously.[16] Each leg should be prepared to the knee, with a tourniquet in place. The ipsilateral iliac crest should be prepared to allow autologous bone grafting. The indications and options for bone grafting are controversial. Some authors advocate routine bone grafting,[27, 36, 46, 70] others consider its use when the area beneath the posterior facet is vacuolated or a cortical defect must be bridged by a plate,[1, 11, 68] while others

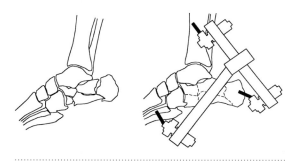

Figure 22–2. "Delta" configuration frame for treatment of open fractures or those with severe deformity and soft tissue compromise.

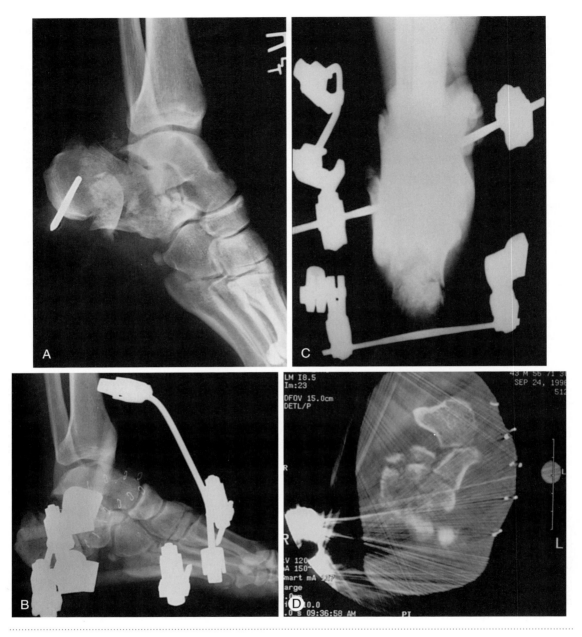

Figure 22–3. A 44-year-old man presented with a severely deformed grade IIIA open calcaneus fracture sustained during a 10-foot fall. After irrigation and debridement, a delta-style external fixator was used to correct the deformity; pins were placed into the tibia, across the tuberosity, and into the metatarsals (A–C). Because of evidence of severe comminution on a postoperative computed tomographic scan, it was believed that the risks of any open approach far outweighed the possibility of an anatomic reconstruction of the subtalar joint (D).

rarely find it beneficial.[6, 12, 14–16, 21, 29, 40, 59, 64, 71] Letournel[6] noted that "the speed of healing has not warranted the extra risk of a graft." In fact, massive bone grafting may increase the risk of deep infection.[3] In contrast, Leung and associates[70] noted that the biomechanical advantages of bone grafting have allowed early weight bearing by 6.5 weeks without fracture displacement. We believe there is no substitute for autologous graft. Compared with other options, it has the most biologic potential, is the most compatible, and appears to be the most resistant to infection.

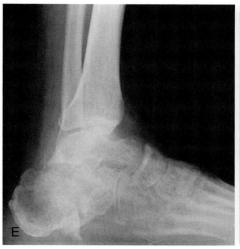
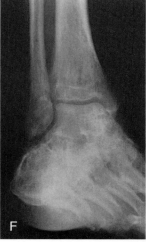
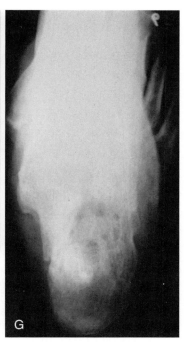

Figure 22-3 *Continued.* Six months later, lateral *(E)*, Broden's *(F)*, and Harris heel *(G)* views revealed a fused subtalar joint but a near-normal heel height, width, and alignment. The patient reported minimal pain and good function while walking on even ground, although a symptomatic plantar exostosis later required excision.

When planning the method and manner of fixation, the surgeon must appreciate that, because of the largely cancellous internal architecture of the calcaneus, there are few areas that will consistently support the placement of implants. These include

1. The thickened dense subchondral bone supporting the posterior facet (thalamic portion)
2. The dense cortical bone of the sustentaculum tali, which can reach 4 mm in thickness
3. The thick cortical bone in the region of the angle of Gissane, which functions as a strut between the cuboid and posterior facets[1, 15]
4. The area adjacent to the calcaneocuboid joint[12]
5. The area at the insertion of the Achilles tendon[1]
6. An area of intact cancellous bone inferomedially[12, 70]

An area of low bone density, where fixation is to be avoided, lies just below the critical angle of Gissane and is known as the "neutral triangle."[11]

The Lateral Approach

First advocated by Palmer in 1948,[27] the most common surgical approach for the op-

erative reduction and stabilization of calcaneal fractures is from the lateral aspect of the foot.[1, 6, 9–12, 46, 68] Although many versions exist, the most recent and popular modification by Benirschke[1, 10, 11] is advantageous for several reasons. It creates a thick flap based on the angiosome of the peroneal artery, which encompasses the sural nerve, peroneal tendons, and calcaneofibular ligament. There is no significant neurovascular risk, and mobilization of this flap permits an extensible exposure of the tuberosity, bulging lateral wall, subtalar joint, depressed thalamic fragments, and calcaneocuboid joint. Furthermore, the relatively flat lateral aspect of the os calcis provides a very accommodating site for internal fixation. However, this approach leads to significant dissection of a sparse soft tissue envelope,[1, 30] requires an indirect reduction of the tuberosity to the sustentaculum,[10] does not allow a facile evaluation of this reduction and alignment, and is more technically difficult in the presence of comminution.[30]

Beginning just anterior to the Achilles tendon and one to two fingerbreadths proximal to the tip of the fibula, an L-shaped incision is initiated (Fig. 22–4); care is taken not to injure the sural nerve, which crosses the surgical incision here. Next, the periosteocutaneous nature of this flap is ensured by incising straight down to the periosteum

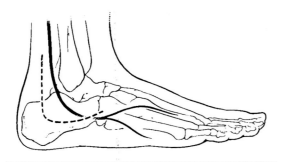

Figure 22–4. Incision for the lateral approach to the calcaneus. (From Benirschke SK, Sangeorzan BJ. Extensive intraarticular fractures of the foot: Surgical management of calcaneal fractures. Clin Orthop 292:131, 1993. Used with permission.)

of the lateral wall at the posterolateral corner of the calcaneus. The skin color and texture variation between the lateral and plantar skin now serves as a landmark for the distal plantar extension of the incision.[5] From this point, the incision curves distally and, staying plantar to the peroneal tendons, continues toward the base of the fifth metatarsal bone. Distally, the dissection must initially be superficial to avoid injuring the sural nerve, which once again crosses the surgical incision. Minimal handling of this flap is critical, and additional trauma should be avoided by refraining from the use of self-retaining retractors and intermittently relaxing the tension on other retractors.

The entire lateral wall, extending from the posterior aspect of the tuberosity, superiorly to the tip of the fibula and subtalar joint, and distally to the calcaneocuboid joint, is then exposed subperiosteally. The calcaneofibular ligament and peroneal tendon sheaths are stripped as a unit from the lateral wall and maintained with the skin flap.[6, 10, 46] Because of variable anatomy and fracture patterns, dissection is occasionally required above and below the peroneal tendons at the level of the calcaneocuboid joint.[1] The peroneal tendons are retracted dorsally, and Kirschner wires are placed into the shaft of the fibula, cuboid, and talus. These are then gently bent to retract the soft tissue flap and intermittently rotated to different positions to lessen the likelihood of flap necrosis. Exposure is complete when the blown-out portion of the lateral wall is retracted (or removed and marked to preserve its orientation) to reveal the depressed and hidden posterior facet (Fig. 22–5).

Because the malaligned tuberosity often interferes with the reduction of the posterior facet, several authors[1, 10, 11, 15] prefer to first reduce and provisionally fix the anterior process and tuberosity to the sustentaculum with .045-inch Kirschner wires. When this is required, Benirschke[15] recommends returning to the tuberosity to correct its reduction after reconstruction of the posterior facet. Alternatively, a medial two-pin external fixator has been advocated by Carr[15] to distract the tuberosity plantarward and posteriorly before reducing the posterior facet and anterolateral fragments.

We and other surgeons[6, 10, 13, 14] prefer to focus first on the reduction of the posterior facet to the sustentaculum tali, because the restoration of the articular surface is the most critical portion of the procedure. Because of the strong medial ligaments, the sustentaculum generally retains its ana-

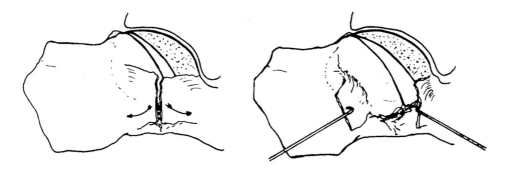

Figure 22–5. The depressed posterior wall is often obscured because it lies behind the blown-out lateral wall. Exposure is improved by swinging out or removing the lateral wall. (From Fernandez DL, Koella C. Combined percutaneous and "minimal" internal fixation for displaced articular fractures of the calcaneus. Clin Orthop 290:111, 1993. Used with permission.)

tomic relationship with the talus, thereby earning its designation as the "constant fragment."[15] This position makes it the ideal foundation for reconstruction of the fracture, because the undersurface of the talus will serve as a template for the reduction of the posterior facet to the sustentaculum.

The tuberosity is mobilized by forcing the heel into marked varus and wedging a periosteal elevator between the tuberosity and sustentacular fragment. A 4.0- or 5.0-mm Shantz pin is usually inserted laterally into the tuberosity for additional control. The posterior facet fracture line is identified and cleaned of hematoma and bone fragments, often through the coronal plane primary fracture line.[5] Next, the articular surface is reconstructed by rotating or elevating any depressed posterior facet fragments back into their proper positions under the talus (Fig. 22–6) and obtaining provisional fixation with Kirschner wires. For Sanders type III fractures, the intermediate fragment is generally reduced to the superomedial fragment, followed by closure of the lateral piece

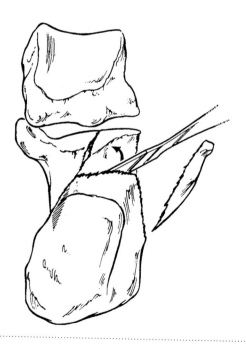

Figure 22–6. With the lateral wall opened outward to expose the depressed posterior facet fragments, the subtalar joint can be reconstructed. Fragments are elevated and rotated such that they are apposed to the medial sustentacular "constant" fragment. (From Benirschke SK, Sangeorzan BJ. Extensive intraarticular fractures of the foot: Surgical management of calcaneal fractures. Clin Orthop 292:133, 1993.)

onto this construct.[5] An alternative for this or more comminuted fracture types (as anticipated from the preoperative CT) is to identify and remove the fragments, assemble them on the back table with .045-inch Kirschner wires, and then reduce this construct to the medial fragment.[10]

Because adequate visualization of the posterior facet reduction is sometimes impossible, even with proper lighting, intraoperative fluoroscopic Broden's views are mandatory. After these have verified that proper height and rotational alignment of the fragments exist, two 3.5-mm cortical lag (or 4.0-mm partially threaded cancellous) screws are placed slightly anteriorly across the posterior facet into the sustentaculum. For additional stability in bone of suspect quality, these screws can be placed through a plate or washers.

The key to the anterior reduction is reconstitution of the critical angle of Gissane.[13] This is achieved when the anterolateral fragment is reduced to the properly derotated posterior facet fragments and sustentacular fragment at the apex of the angle. Working between the peroneal tendons and performing an occasional capsulotomy allows entry into the calcaneocuboid joint, whose articular surface might also require an anatomic reduction.[6, 30] Sanders and others[14] noted that problems associated with this joint are usually minimal, especially if reduction of the anterolateral wall is adequate. Isolated 3.5-mm screws are often helpful when obtaining fixation of any sagittal fracture lines.

Finally, the body is indirectly reduced to the sustentaculum and provisionally stabilized with axially directed .062-inch Kirschner wires, introduced from the heel into the sustentacular fragment.[10] The tuberosity is distracted distally to gain length and height (Fig. 22–7, arrow 1), into valgus to correct varus deformity (Fig. 22–7, arrow 2), and medially to narrow the heel (Fig. 22–7, arrow 3). A periosteal elevator through the fracture line, levering the body against the medial edge of the sustentacular fragment,[13] or a bone hook around the Achilles tendon insertion will provide additional distraction, if required.[6, 12] Reduction of tongue-type fractures can occasionally be complicated by the tremendous pull of the triceps surae. In these cases, Sanders and others[15] suggested that the fracture be converted into a joint-depression type by per-

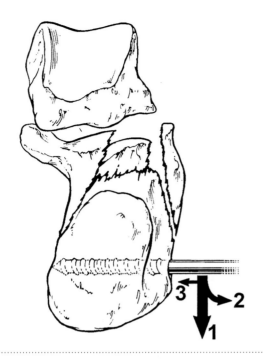

Figure 22–7. Three motions are required to reconstitute the anatomic position of the tuberosity fragments: 1 - distal distraction to gain length and height; 2 - valgus to correct varus deformity; 3 - medial translation to narrow the heel. (From Benirschke SK, Sangeorzan BJ. Extensive intraarticular fractures of the foot: Surgical management of calcaneal fractures. Clin Orthop 292:132, 1993.)

forming an osteotomy of the extra-articular fragment.

After intraoperative fluoroscopic lateral and Harris views have confirmed proper reduction and alignment of the hindfoot, a contoured plate is added to the construct (Fig. 22–8). A wide variety of plates are available, including the 3.5-mm (approximately seven to eight holes) or 2.7-mm reconstruction plates,[1, 11, 15] Y plate,[6, 15] one-third tubular plate (five to seven holes),[5, 12, 15] cervical H plate,[8, 9, 39, 41, 70] and low-profile H plate modified with a Y limb.[13] Regardless of the design used, the plate must bridge the bone, from the anterior process, to the most posterior aspect of the tuberosity (see Fig. 22-8A).[1] If the calcaneal surface at the calcaneocuboid joint cannot be reconstructed, a longer plate can be used to span the joint with one or two screws anchored into the cuboid.[6, 12] For this application, the stem of the Y plate usually has extra holes, which are removed if spanning of the joint is not required.[6]

Should the two sulci for the peroneal tendons and the trochlear process prevent the plate from lying flat against the lateral wall, then a rongeur can be used to contour this area and lessen the prominence of the plate. A minimum purchase of two screws is required for each of the tuberosity, sustentaculum, and anterior process fragments; the most anterior screw is placed into the subchondral bone adjacent to the calcaneocuboid articular surface and the most posterior screw into the thickened bone at the posterior aspect of the calcaneus. By fanning screws toward the medial plantar surface of the posterior tuberosity, thick sustentacular bone, and medial dorsal surface of the anterior process, purchase and stability are maximized (see Fig. 22–8B).[12] For comminuted fractures, supplemental Kirschner wires are occasionally useful. For an illustrative case, see Figure 22–9A–J.

Medial Approach

The medial approach, as advocated by McReynolds (Fig. 22–10)[21, 68, 69, 71] or combined with a lateral approach by Stephenson (Fig. 22–11),[28] offers direct visualization and anatomic reduction of the sustentaculum tali to the tuberosity. This may lead to more rapid healing and allow earlier weight bearing to stimulate the venous pump of the foot.[69]

However, the primary fracture line commonly exits near the tibial nerve, artery, and tendon,[1] increasing the risks of exposure, fixation, and later removal of implants. Furthermore, the sharp slope of the sustentaculum tali is an inhospitable location for implants. Finally, this approach fails to expose calcaneocuboid joint, visualize the posterior facet, bone graft easily, or achieve a direct reduction in the presence of comminution. Because of these problems and the present emphasis on the articular reduction, a medial approach rarely is indicated.

The standard medial operative approach (see Fig. 22–10)[21, 68, 69, 71] is begun behind the neurovascular bundle and parallel to the midportion of the tuberosity of the calcaneus. The length of the incision depends on the location of the primary fracture line. After the incision is carried through the skin, blunt dissection identifies and preserves the calcaneal sensory branches. The

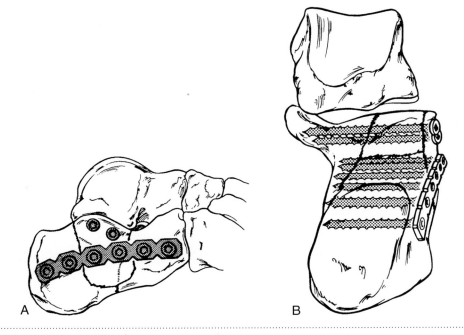

Figure 22–8. *A*, Lateral view of calcaneus after open reduction and internal fixation with posterior facet screws and a 3.5-millimeter reconstruction plate. *B*, Harris heel view demonstrating good orientation and spread of screws. (From Benirschke SK, Sangeorzan BJ. Extensive intraarticular fractures of the foot: Surgical management of calcaneal fractures. Clin Orthop 292:133, 1993.)

fascia is then incised longitudinally and the abductor hallucis bluntly stripped from the medial cortex. Finally, the neurovascular bundle is isolated and retracted anteriorly to expose the superomedial fragment. Fixation is usually performed with a staple[21, 68, 69, 71] or small H plate.[32]

Rarely, when reduction of the medial wall is insufficient after a lateral approach has been used, a limited medial approach may be required.[28, 46] Stephenson[28] recommended a 5-cm long posteromedial vertical incision (see Fig. 22–11). The flexor retinaculum is incised and the neurovascular bundle isolated and retracted to expose the superomedial fragment followed by fixation with a staple. This method offers the advantages of both approaches, but requires substantial soft tissue dissection and disruption of calcaneal blood supply.[10]

Percutaneous Screw Fixation

The techniques of percutaneous screw fixation are based on the original techniques introduced by Böhler[42] and Essex-Lopresti.[2] After allowing time for the soft tissues to

improve, Böhler[42] disimpacted fragments by placing the sole over a wooden wedge and forcing the foot into strong plantar flexion. A strong vise with padding, now coined the Böhler clamp, was also used to mobilize the tuberosity and narrow the heel (Fig. 22–12). Pins placed in the tibia and tuberosity were connected to a traction apparatus to achieve distraction and alignment. Essex-Lopresti[2] inserted a spike into the tuberosity fragment to manipulate, reduce, and align this fragment. In the more complicated joint depression fractures, he introduced an elevator through a limited open lateral approach and lifted the depressed thalamic fragment. The heels of his clasped hands were used to rock the fracture from side to side, thus reducing comminuted fragments, compressing the bulged out lateral wall, and aligning the tuberosity and sustentaculum.

Similarly, after positioning the patient in the supine position with a bump under the affected hip, we also achieve a closed reduction of the fracture (Fig. 22–13). A Shantz pin is drilled percutaneously through the posterior aspect of the tuberosity (Fig. 22–13F). This is used to vigorously disimpact the tuberosity (Fig. 22–13G, J). In a tongue-

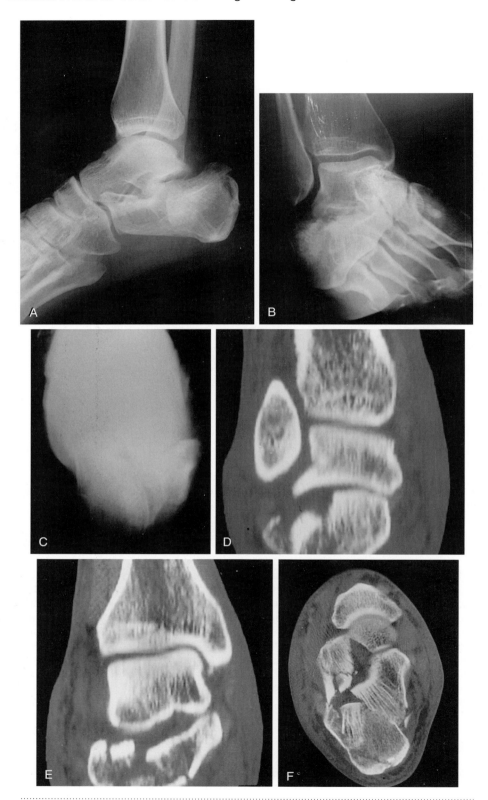

Figure 22–9 *See legend on opposite page*

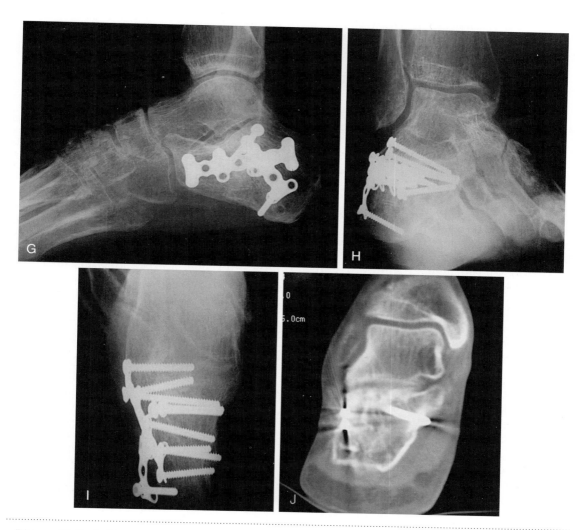

Figure 22–9. A 33-year-old man with calcaneus fracture after falling 5 feet on a scaffold. Lateral *(A)*, Broden's *(B)*, and Harris heel *(C)* views demonstrated a joint depression–type injury, with loss of length and height and a widened heel. Computed tomography (CT) revealed the extent of posterior facet depression *(D)*, a fracture pattern consistent with a Sanders type IIIAB fracture *(E)*, and involvement of the anterior process near the calcaneocuboid joint *(F)*. These findings mitigated for an open reduction and internal fixation. Postoperative lateral *(G)*, Broden's *(H)*, and Harris heel *(I)* views demonstrated the restoration of the articular surface, height, width, and alignment. A postoperative CT scan confirmed the articular reduction *(J)*. At 1 year, the patient continued to complain of weight bearing–related aching and paresthesias along the distribution of the sural nerve. Although having near-normal ankle range of motion, his subtalar motion was minimal.

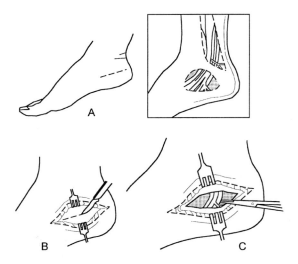

Figure 22–10. The medial approach to the calcaneus. *A*, The skin incision; *B*, the fascial incision; *C*, isolation of the neurovascular bundle (inset). (From Burdeaux BD. Reduction of calcaneal fractures by the McReynolds medial approach technique and its experimental basis. Clin Orthop 177:97, 1983. Used with permission.)

type injury, a 4-mm Shantz pin is also percutaneously inserted into the tongue fragment to allow its derotation into the remainder of the body and anterior process.[15] Next, narrowing of the heel is achieved using either a Böhler clamp or Essex-Lopresti's technique.

Any residual displacement or rotation of the depressed posterior facet is corrected with a small bone impactor inserted through a lateral stab incision (Fig. 22–13*G, H, I*). The often comminuted lateral wall usually provides little hindrance to its passage. This aspect of the reduction is technically demanding, must be performed using fluoroscopic Broden's views, and will rarely obtain an anatomic result in the presence of comminution. After an acceptable reduction of the posterior facet fragments to the sustentacular fragment has been obtained, fixation is achieved with one or two standard or cannulated 3.5-mm lag screws with or without washers (Fig. 22–13*I*).

The tuberosity is distracted distally to gain length and height, into valgus to correct varus deformity, and medially to narrow the heel. Provisional fixation is percutaneously obtained with two guide wires from a 4.5-mm cannulated screw set, placed axially from the heel on either side of the Achilles tendon, into the anterolateral fragment. Intraoperative fluoroscopic lateral and Harris views are then obtained to confirm proper hindfoot reduction and alignment before inserting screws over the guide wires (Fig. 22–13*J, K*).

Forgon[48] used a custom external fixator to obtain an indirect reduction of the frac-

ture, a Böhler clamp to narrow the heel, and Kirschner wires to correct the subtalar joint deformity. These steps are followed by percutaneous screw fixation through a small lateral incision, and stabilization of the tuberosity to the anterior fragment with two long cancellous screws placed through the heel.

Arthrodesis

For primary arthrodesis, the technique of Myerson[16] is suggested. The fracture should first be reduced and stabilized using the same techniques described for its reconstruction. After osteotomes and a high-speed bur have denuded any remaining cartilage from the calcaneus and undersurface of the talus, copious quantities of iliac crest bone graft are packed into the subtalar region. Myerson[16] warned that fusion of the posterior facet may be difficult because of large areas of bone loss, and that efforts be made to obtain both an intra-articular and extra-articular arthrodesis by also denuding cortical bone in the sinus tarsi corresponding to the neck of the talus and the calcaneus. If a large portion of the posterior facet is missing, this should be replaced with a matched-sized tricortical iliac crest graft. Finally, one or more large cannulated screws are directed from plantar to dorsal, across the subtalar joint, into the talus.

Closure and Postoperative Care

To prevent hematoma formation, wound closure should be performed over one or two

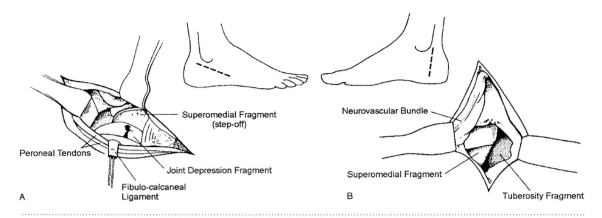

A

Superomedial Fragment (step-off)

Peroneal Tendons

Joint Depression Fragment

Fibulo-calcaneal Ligament

B

Neurovascular Bundle

Superomedial Fragment

Tuberosity Fragment

Figure 22–11. Combined lateral and medial approaches. *A*, The lateral exposure; *B*, the medial exposure. (From Stephenson JR. Surgical treatment of displaced intra-articular fractures of the calcaneus: A combined lateral and medial approach. Clin Orthop 290:71, 1993. Used with permission.)

deep suction drains. These are brought out dorsolaterally through the skin overlying the sinus tarsi.[10] The peroneal tendons should be sutured back to the bone or through holes in the plate.[6] Closure should consist of buried, interrupted periosteal subcutaneous 2-0 Vicryl sutures, and 3-0 nylon Allgower-Donati sutures for skin, placed with care to avoid any tension. A well-padded dressing and U-shaped plaster splint is then applied. Prophylactic cefazolin is recommended for at least 24 hours or until the drains are discontinued, usually by 24 to 48 hours.

Active range of motion of the toes begins immediately, as do active range-of-motion and isometric exercises of the ipsilateral knee and hip. Strengthening, isometric exercises, and active range of motion of the upper extremities and unaffected lower extremity should also be encouraged. The leg is strictly elevated for 2 to 3 days, at which time, the dressing is changed, crutch training begun, and toe-touch weight bearing allowed in a bivalved short leg cast. The advantage of early weight bearing is the activation of a powerful venous pump in the foot independent of muscular action.[18] Early

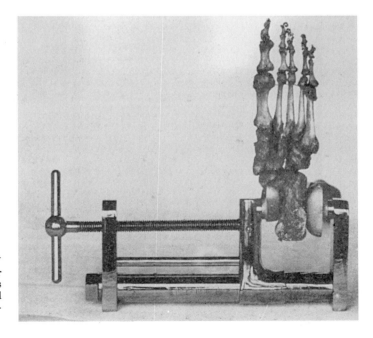

Figure 22–12. The original Boehler clamp, a device invented seven decades ago, may still have use when combined with today's techniques of indirect reduction and percutaneous fixation.

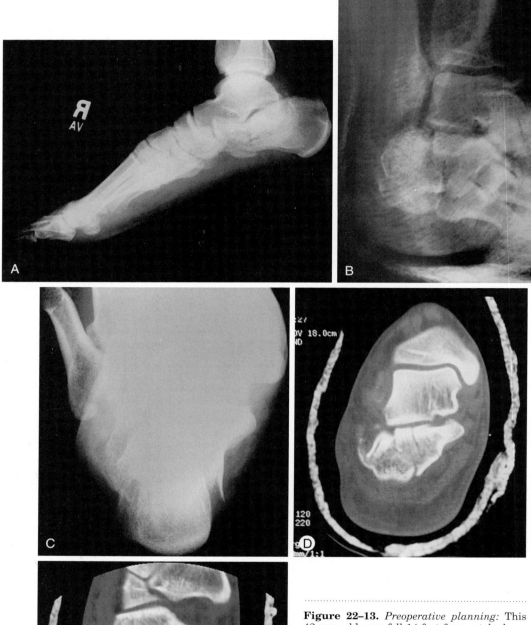

Figure 22–13. *Preoperative planning:* This 42-year-old man fell 14 feet from a telephone pole, fracturing his right calcaneus. Lateral *(A),* Broden's *(B),* and Harris heel *(C)* views demonstrated a joint depression–type injury. Computed tomography identified the fracture as a Sanders type IIIAB *(D).* However, the medial fracture line was nondisplaced *(D),* the depressed lateral fragment small *(D),* and the calcaneocuboid joint intact *(E).* The patient also demonstrated significant swelling 1 week after injury.

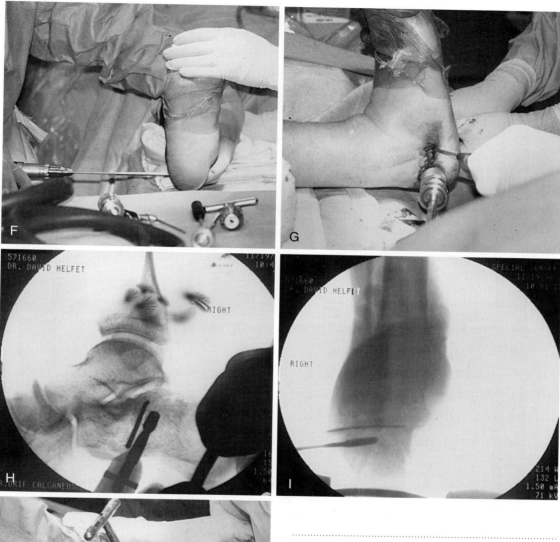

Figure 22–13 *Continued. Operating room: F*, A Shantz pin is drilled across the tuberosity, and two T-handle chucks are attached. *G*, After mobilization of the tuberosity fragment and narrowing of the heel, the assistant distracts the fracture while the surgeon places an elevator through a small lateral stab incision, disimpacts the posterior facet under fluoroscopic guidance, and obtains provisional fixation with a guide wire *(H). I*, After confirming that an acceptable reduction of the posterior facet has been achieved, a 3.5-mm cannulated screw is placed over the guide wire. *J*, Two 4.5-mm cortical screws are placed from the heel into the anteromedial and anterolateral areas.

Illustration continued on following page

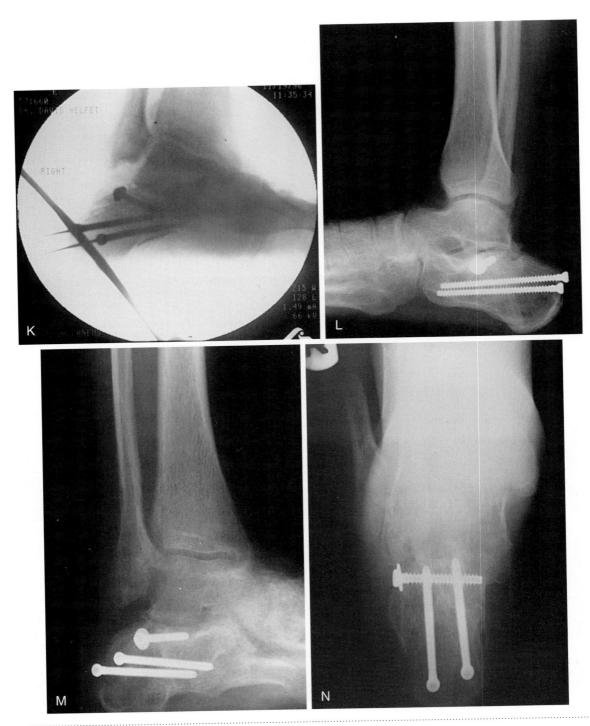

Figure 22–13 *Continued. K,* Intraoperative Broden's view delineating reduction posterior facet and placement of long cortical screws. *At 7-month follow-up:* Lateral *(L),* Broden's *(M),* and Harris heel *(N)* views demonstrate maintenance of joint space, height, width, and alignment. The patient notes occasional pain with ambulation, has not yet returned to work, and has subtalar motion one fifth that of the normal foot.

weight bearing also prevents loss of muscle tone and disuse changes of the bones and joints of the foot.[20]

Gentle ankle and subtalar range-of-motion exercises are instituted once the flap demonstrates uncomplicated healing and a sealed wound, usually by the fourth day. The forefoot and toes are mobilized with passive and active assisted range of motion. Other postoperative regimens begin ankle and subtalar motion exercises between 1 and 14 days.[1, 9, 10, 33] In the case of arthrodesis, a period of 2 weeks has been recommended before commencing range-of-motion exercises.[16]

Although the patient is usually discharged between the second and fifth postoperative days, swelling, atrophy, and weakness commonly persist for long periods. Therefore, formal rehabilitation and a carefully planned physical therapy program is required for approximately 1 to 3 months.[16] Depending on the condition of the wounds and the swelling of the extremity, the patient should return for suture removal and wound examination at 2 to 3 weeks. At this time, progressive strengthening and more aggressive range of motion involving the ankle and subtalar joints (unless an arthrodesis has been performed) is instituted. Desensitization techniques, soft tissue and scar immobilization, whirlpool, and ultrasonography may be commenced as appropriate. Over the next month, range of motion is gently increased.

By 6 to 10 weeks,[5, 12, 13, 16, 37] based on the appearance of callus (or trabeculation across a fusion mass) and the lack of warmth or swelling, weight bearing is usually advanced to 20 to 40 pounds. A soft heel or custom orthosis may be extremely beneficial for the many patients, whose heel remains hypersensitive after a long period of non-weight bearing. Emphasis is also placed on ankle and subtalar motion, progressive resistance therapy, stationary bicycle work, gait training, and linear walking (2 miles in 30 minutes). However, some authors have recommended limited or non-weight bearing for 8 to 12 weeks.[1, 10, 11, 30] This more conservative approach is especially important for patients with osteopenia, extensive comminution, or bilateral fractures.

Full weight bearing is usually achieved before 12 to 16 weeks.[6, 13, 16] During this time, ankle and subtalar joint active-as-sisted range of motion becomes more aggressive, with an additional emphasis on proprioceptive training. The patient should be gradually weaned from assisted devices and low-impact endurance training and strengthening begun. Exercises include single-leg weight lifting, plantar flexion resistance, and progressive strengthening of the entire extremity. Implant removal can be performed as early as 6 months later but is required only if the cuboid has been spanned[12] or if there is impingement.[10]

COMPLICATIONS

Soft Tissue Problems and Infection

Levin and Nunley[72] classified soft tissue problems into four categories: (1) closed fractures, (2) open fractures, (3) calcaneal osteomyelitis, and (4) reconstruction for unstable soft tissue.

Of the closed fractures, there are two groups. Group 1 problems involve the inability to close skin. A variety of options, including porcine allografts, Epigard (Synthese, Paoli, PA), split-thickness skin grafting, and delayed primary closure are available. Skin grafting alone in this region has been reported by some to be unsuccessful,[13] and, therefore, a free tissue transfer may be required. Group 2 problems involve postoperative wound breakdown, which may occur as late as 4 weeks.[13] The incidence of marginal wound necrosis is not insignificant, ranging somewhere between 0 and 10%.[8, 10–12, 32, 41, 46, 70, 73] This usually occurs near the apex of the flap and resolves with local wound care. Although Stephenson[28] reported a 27% rate of marginal necrosis in 22 patients, 4 of his 6 patients with necrosis had undergone surgery within 48 hours of injury. Dehiscence should be addressed by cessation of subtalar motion exercises, daily whirlpools, dressing changes, elevation of the extremity, and oral antibiotics. For partial-thickness defects, this treatment alone is usually successful.[13, 72] However, should any hardware become exposed, then a full-thickness defect exists, which requires early and aggressive soft tissue debridement. Subsequent coverage is obtained with local or distal flaps, depending on the presence of infection, size of the defect, presence of an adequate blood supply, and condition of the other areas of the foot.[72]

Open fractures are also separated into two groups: those with large soft tissue loss and adequate bone stock and those with traumatic loss of soft tissue and bone. In the former, early coverage is suggested if the wound environment is suitable.[72] In the latter, clean bone and tissue can occasionally be debrided and reattached. More likely, however, is a reconstruction with a free flap and structural bone block iliac crest, or osteocutaneous graft, and internal fixation.[72] Careful consideration must also be given to below-knee amputation, because this may ultimately offer the best outcome for the patient.

Of the superficial[1, 8, 10, 11, 41, 46, 70] and deep[1, 8, 11, 12, 32, 41, 70, 73] forms of infection, each generally occurs in 0 to 3% of cases. Fortunately, most of these tend to resolve with antibiotic treatment and fracture healing.[11] There is an inverse relationship between the experience of the surgeon and rate of deep infection. Bezes and colleagues[12] noted that the 6% rate of their earlier cases was reduced to less than 1% with more experience. The recommended treatment for calcaneal osteomyelitis is debridement, 6 weeks of intravenous antibiotics, and distant muscle flaps, if necessary. However, diffuse osteomyelitis warrants some consideration for amputation.[13, 72]

Problems associated with reconstruction of the heel pad resulting from lack of soft tissue support may require orthotics or bracing. Local or distal flaps are often required. However, patients who are treated with noninnervated flaps must be cared for in fashion similar to those with peripheral neuropathy.

Compartment Syndrome

Associated with falls from significant heights, crush injuries, and motor vehicle accidents,[74–76] compartment syndrome occurs in approximately 10% of os calcis fractures.[74] The most common symptom and sign are, respectively, pain and a tense plantar-medial swelling.[74–76] Other signs observed by Myerson[76] are numbness in 46% of cases, pain on passive dorsiflexion of the toes in 86%, impaired two-point discrimination in 64%, decreased light-touch sensation in 54%, motor deficits in 23%, and loss of pinprick sensation in 15%. Although pulses are difficult to palpate, secondary to swell-

ing, Myerson[76] was able to identify one with duplex ultrasonography in 12 of 14 feet with compartment syndrome.

Unfortunately, pain disproportionate to the injury, increased pain on passive dorsiflexion of the toes, and swelling are not reliable clinical findings of compartment syndrome in a patient who has sustained a massive injury to the foot.[75, 76] Therefore, multistick compartment pressure readings should be obtained if there is suspicion; pressures greater than 30 mm Hg are considered indications for fasciotomy by most authors.[75–77] Decompression is usually obtained via a medial approach of Henry, combined medial and dorsal approaches, or occasionally a lateral approach.[75, 76] In reviewing his experience and the literature, Myerson[76] noted that the end result of an untreated compartment syndrome in the foot is a painful, dysfunctional extremity characterized by sensory disturbances, stiffness, forefoot contracture, and clawing of the toes.

However, fasciotomy is not a panacea. We believe that some cases may best be treated expectantly, although this belief is controversial. In Myerson's[76] experienced hands, 14 cases of compartment syndrome lead to three primary split-thickness skin incisions, one of which sloughed; eight split-thickness skin grafts; and a free muscle transfer. Six patients continued to have occasional symptoms or minimal discomfort with walking, standing, or footwear. One of the 10 patients monitored continued to manifest signs of myoneural ischemia with mildly symptomatic claw toes and numbness. Fakhouri and Manoli[75] also observed patients with persistent paresthesias after fasciotomy for compartment syndrome secondary to a fracture of the calcaneus. Mittlmeier and colleagues[77] reported plantar muscle scarring and claw-toe formation in seven patients with a total of 11 fractures. These failures have been attributed to the failure to release a separate calcaneal compartment, which has been identified deep to the superficial compartment in the hindfoot area.[74, 77] This compartment contains the quadratus plantae muscle and is bounded by the plantar aponeurosis, which forms a constricting fascial envelope.

Salvage of the Painful Foot

Inadequate or inappropriate primary treatment of a calcaneus fracture results in persistent pain in the foot, especially when associated with a malunion of the fracture. This condition presents a formidable challenge, because in a substantial number of cases there is not just one source of pain.[10, 15, 30, 37, 57] In addition to the many biomechanical and structural causes of pain already discussed, other potential sources of pain include heel pad disruption (smashed heel pad syndrome), disruption of the plantar surface of the calcaneus, plantar exostoses, periarticular fibrosis, tarsal tunnel syndrome, flexor tendon entrapment beneath the medial malleolus, other sites of soft tissue impingement, tendinitis, arthritis in joints other than the subtalar area, prominent hardware, incisional neuromas, an unrecognized compartment syndrome, and reflex sympathetic dystrophy.[20, 22, 24, 30, 38, 54, 78] The therapeutic approaches to these conditions have included shoe modification, physiotherapy, operative reconstruction, neglect, sensory denervation of the heel, and even amputation.[54]

Subtalar arthritis most commonly results from a poor reduction of the subtalar joint, but may occur even in the presence of a normal radiograph and arthrogram, secondary to cartilage necrosis at the time of injury.[13, 14, 49] Often, modification of activities or footwear and anti-inflammatory medications are successful. Parmar and coworkers[37] noted that improvement, although common, is minor after the first year, and concluded that a decision regarding subtalar arthrodesis should be made at this time. In support of their recommendation is evidence that better results are obtained if fusion is performed within 1 year of injury.[15, 54, 79] However, Pozo and colleagues[24] and Lindsay and Dewar[22] reported continued subjective improvement at 6 and 10 years, respectively, after conservative treatment of os calcis fractures. Therefore, a careful evaluation is required when selecting patients likely to benefit from this procedure, including a subtalar steroid and local anesthetic injection to verify that the subtalar area is the major source of pain.[13] Braly and others[80] reported only a 46% satisfactory rate after late subtalar fusion for calcaneal malunion, but a 75% satisfactory rate when combined with excision of the lateral wall.

The limitation of a subtalar fusion in situ is that it does not address the other possible causes of pain in the posttraumatic foot. To this end, Carr and associates[57] advocated a salvage procedure known as subtalar distraction bone block arthrodesis, reporting satisfactory results in 13 of 16 patients with chronic pain. This procedure addresses the majority of calcaneal problem areas simultaneously through a single posterior approach to the subtalar joint. The calcaneus is distracted from the overlying talus, hinging on the anterior talocalcaneal articulations. A tricortical iliac crest bone block is wedged into this opening, which simultaneously increases the calcaneal height, eliminates the leg-length discrepancy, fuses the subtalar joint, alleviates the impingement in the fibulocalcaneal and anterior tibiotalar impingement areas, restores the longitudinal foot arch, and corrects heel malalignment.

Romash[81] presented another option in which a reconstructive osteotomy recreates the primary fracture, followed by internal fixation. This permits the repositioning of the tuberosity, narrowing of the heel, diminishment of impingement, and restoration of height. At the same time, a subtalar arthrodesis alleviates the symptoms of posttraumatic arthritis. The advantage of this technique is that bone grafts are not required for stability. His results were satisfactory in 9 of 10 feet treated in this fashion.

Myerson and Quill[54] retrospectively reviewed the results of secondary surgical treatment of 43 fractures of the calcaneus. Their procedures were performed a mean of 26 months after the injury, including an in situ subtalar arthrodesis in 15 patients, a subtalar distraction bone block arthrodesis in 14, a triple arthrodesis in 5, a lateral calcaneal ostectomy in 7, a transection and proximal transposition of the sural nerve in 7, and a release of the tibial nerve in 5. Thirty-two months after surgery, pain was partially relieved in 90% of patients, function improved in 83%, and 76% returned to work or their preinjury level a mean of 8 months after the operation. There was a trend that the longer the interval between the injury and the operation, the longer is the subsequent interval until the patient returned to full activities or work. The most successful results were in the patients who underwent a subtalar arthrodesis.

Miscellaneous Complications

Peroneal impingement and tendinitis are most commonly the result of either bulging of the lateral wall after nonoperative treatment or prominent hardware after surgery. Although its diagnosis is usually made by palpation, impingement can be confirmed by CT.[13] Occurring in 2 to 20% of postoperative patients,[10, 14, 15] symptoms are usually alleviated with the use of nonsteroidal anti-inflammatory agents. Should this treatment fail, as it usually will with retained hardware, impingement may consistently and successfully be treated by lateral wall resection or removal of hardware.[10, 13] Alternatively, Isbister[58] advocated the subperiosteal resection of the distal 1 cm of the fibula, reporting the relief of symptoms in 80% of patients. Another potential problem is mild peroneal subluxation, which has been noted in approximately 2 to 8% of cases.[22, 70]

Sural neuritis occurs in 2 to 10% of cases,[14, 46, 70] usually resulting from stretching, contusion, or laceration of the nerve during a lateral approach. Although symptoms usually resolve within several months,[11] should a symptomatic neuroma develop, proximal resection is advised.[13] More serious is a neuropraxia of the tibial nerve, which typically requires 8 months for resolution.[11]

Other problems appear to be rare but can be troublesome. Hematomas requiring decompression occur in 2 to 3% of cases.[32, 73] Essex-Lopresti[2] observed that in joint depression fractures, because the fragment hinges downward and backward on the posterior fracture line, along which the soft tissues remain intact, the risk of devascularization after reduction is low. Zwipp and others[32] noted that the incidence of nonunion is only 1.3%. Sudeck's atrophy may occur in 1.2% of cases.[12]

CONCLUSION

Sanders and colleagues[14, 15] noted that the learning curve for the surgical treatment of the os calcis fracture requires between 35 and 50 cases before results can become more predictable for Sanders type II and III fractures. Therefore, only a surgeon who is experienced in reduction techniques, soft tissue handling, and osteosynthesis should attempt operative treatment of this troublesome fracture, so that associated wound complications are prevented and optimal outcomes obtained.

REFERENCES

1. Benirschke SK, Sangeorzan BJ. Extensive intraarticular fractures of the foot. Surgical management of calcaneal fractures. Clin Orthop 292:128–134, 1993.
2. Essex-Lopresti P. The mechanism, reduction technique, and results in fractures of the os calcis. Br J Surg 39:395, 1951–1952.
3. Baumgaertel FR, Gotzen L. Two-stage operative treatment of comminuted os calcis fractures: primary indirect reduction with medial external fixation and delayed lateral plate fixation. Clin Orthop 290:132–141, 1993.
4. Borrelli J, Torzilli PA, Grigiene R, Helfet DL. Effect of impact load on articular cartilage: development of an intra-articular fracture model. J Orthop Traum 11:319–326, 1997.
5. Carr JB. Surgical treatment of the intra-articular calcaneus fracture. Orthop Clin North Am 25:665–675, 1994.
6. Letournel E. Open treatment of acute calcaneal fractures. Clin Orthop 290:60–67, 1993.
7. Ross SD, Sowerby MR. The operative treatment of fractures of the os calcis. Clin Orthop 199:132–143, 1985.
8. Melcher G, Degonda F, Leutenegger A, Ruedi T. Ten-year follow-up after operative treatment for intra-articular fractures of the calcaneus. J Trauma 38:713–716, 1995.
9. Melcher G, Bereiter H, Leutenegger A, Ruedi T. Results of operative treatment for intra-articular fractures of the calcaneus. J Trauma 31:234–238, 1991.
10. Macey LR, Benirschke SK, Sangeorzan BJ, Hansen ST. Acute calcaneal fractures: treatment options and results. J Am Acad Orthop Surg 2:36–43, 1994.
11. Sangeorzan BJ, Benirschke SK, Carr JB. Surgical management of fractures of the os calcis. Instr Course Lect 44:359–370, 1995.
12. Bezes H, Massart P, Delvaux D, et al. The operative treatment of intraarticular calcaneal fractures: indications, technique, and results in 257 cases. Clin Orthop 290:55–59, 1993.
13. Sanders R. Intra-articular fractures of the calcaneus: present state of the art. J Orthop Trauma 6:252–265, 1992.
14. Sanders R, Fortin P, DiPasquale T, Walling AK. Operative treatment in 120 displaced intra-articular calcaneal fractures: results using a prognostic computed tomography scan classification. Clin Orthop 290:87–95, 1993.
15. Sanders RW, Benirschke SK, Carr JB, et al. Symposium: the treatment of displaced intraarticular fractures of the calcaneus. Contemp Orthop 32:187–208, 1996.
16. Myerson MS. Primary subtalar arthrodesis for the treatment of comminuted fractures of the calcaneus. Orthop Clin North Am 26:215–227, 1995.
17. Myerson MS, Henderson MR. Clinical applications of a pneumatic intermittent impulse compression device after trauma and major surgery to the foot and ankle. Foot Ankle 14:198–203, 1993.
18. Gardner AM, Fox RH, Lawrence C, et al. Reduction of post-traumatic swelling and compartment pressure by impulse compression of the foot. J Bone Joint Surg Br 72:810–815, 1990.
19. Erdmann MW, Richardson J, Templeton J. Os

calcis fractures: a randomized trial comparing conservative treatment with impulse compression of the foot. Injury 23:305–307, 1992.

20. Mann RA, Coughlin MJ. Fractures of the Calcaneus. Surgery of the Foot and Ankle, vol 2. St. Louis: C. V. Mosby, 1992.

21. McReynolds IS. Trauma to the os calcis and heel cord. In Jahss MH, ed. Disorders of the Foot, vol 2. Philadelphia: W. B. Saunders, 1982, pp 1497–1542.

22. Lindsay WRN, Dewar FP. Fractures of the os calcis. J Bone Joint Surg Am 95:555, 1958.

23. Kitaoka HB, Schaap EJ, Chao EY, An KN. Displaced intra-articular fractures of the calcaneus treated non-operatively: clinical results and analysis of motion and ground-reaction and temporal forces. J Bone Joint Surg Am 76:1531–1540, 1994.

24. Pozo JL, Kirwan EO, Jackson AM. The long term results of conservative treatment of severely displaced fractures of the calcaneus. J Bone Joint Surg 66:386–390, 1973.

25. Giachino AA, Uhthoff HK. Current concepts review: intra-articular fractures of the calcaneus. J Bone Joint Surg Am 71:784–787, 1989.

26. Crosby LA, Fitzgibbons T. Intraarticular calcaneal fractures: results of closed treatment. Clin Orthop 290:47–54, 1993.

27. Palmer I. The mechanism and treatment of fractures of the calcaneus: open reduction with the use of cancellous grafts. J Bone Joint Surg Am 30:2, 1948.

28. Stephenson JR. Treatment of displaced intra-articular fractures of the calcaneus using medial and lateral approaches, internal fixation, and early motion. J Bone Joint Surg Am 69:115–130, 1987.

29. Paley D, Hall H. Intra-articular fractures of the calcaneus. J Bone Joint Surg Am 75:342–354, 1993.

30. Paley D, Hall H. Calcaneal fracture controversies: can we put Humpty Dumpty together again? Orthop Clin North Am 20:665–677, 1989.

31. Dart DF, Graham WP. The treatment of fractured calcaneum. J Trauma 6:362–367, 1966.

32. Zwipp H, Tscherne H, Thermann H, Weber T. Osteosynthesis of displaced intraarticular fractures of the calcaneus: results in 123 cases. Clin Orthop 290:76–86, 1993.

33. Hutchinson F III, Huebner MK. Treatment of os calcis fractures by open reduction and internal fixation. Foot Ankle Int 15:225–232, 1994.

34. Langdon IJ, Kerr PS, Atkins RM. Fractures of the calcaneum: the anterolateral fragment. J Bone Joint Surg Br 76:303–305, 1994.

35. Letournel E. Open reduction and internal fixation of calcaneus fractures. In Spiegel PG, ed. Techniques in Orthopaedics: Topics in Trauma. Baltimore, MD: University Park Press, 1984.

36. Jarvholm U, Korner L, Thoren O, Wiklund LM. Fractures of the calcaneus: a comparison of open and closed treatment. Acta Orthop Scand 55:652–656, 1984.

37. Parmar HV, Triffitt PD, Gregg PJ. Intra-articular fractures of the calcaneum treated operatively or conservatively: a prospective study. J Bone Joint Surg Br 75:932–937, 1993.

38. Buckley RE, Meek RN. Comparison of open versus closed reduction of intraarticular calcaneal fractures: a matched cohort in workmen. J Orthop Trauma 6:216–222, 1992.

39. Leung KS, Yuen KM, Chan WS. Operative treatment of displaced intra-articular fractures of the calcaneum: medium-term results. J Bone Joint Surg Br 75:196–201, 1993.

40. O'Farrell DA, O'Byrne JM, McCabe JP, Stephens MM. Fractures of the os calcis: improved results with internal fixation. Injury 24:263–265, 1993.

41. Monsey RD, Levine BP, Trevino SG, Kristiansen TK. Operative treatment of acute displaced intra-articular calcaneus fractures. Foot Ankle Int 16:57–63, 1995.

42. Böhler L. Diagnosis, pathology, and treatment of fractures of the os calcis. J Bone Joint Surg Am 13:75–89, 1931.

43. Buch J, Blauensteiner W, Scherafati T, et al. [Conservative treatment of calcaneus fracture versus repositioning and percutaneous bore wire fixation. A comparison of 2 methods.] Unfallchirurg 92:595–603, 1989.

44. Pescatori G, Fioriti M. The Ilizarov apparatus in the treatment of thalamic fractures of the calcaneus. Ital J Orthop Traumatol 15:302–314, 1989.

45. Paley D, Fischgrund J. Open reduction and circular external fixation of intraarticular calcaneal fractures. Clin Orthop 290:125–131, 1993.

46. Fernandez DL, Koella C. Combined percutaneous and "minimal" internal fixation for displaced articular fractures of the calcaneus. Clin Orthop 290:108–116, 1993.

47. Stockenhuber K, Seggl W, Feichtinger G, Szyszkowitz R. [Conservative and semiconservative treatment of calcaneus fractures]. Orthopade 20:43–54, 1991.

48. Forgon M. Closed reduction and percutaneous osteosynthesis technique and results in 265 calcaneal fractures. In Tscherne H, Schatzker J, eds. Major Fractures of the Pilon, the Talus, and the Calcaneus. New York: Springer-Verlag, 1993:207–213.

49. Harding D, Waddell JP. Open reduction in depressed fractures of the os calcis. Clin Orthop 199:124–131, 1985.

50. Hall MC, Pennal GF. Primary subtalar arthrodesis in the treatment of severe fractures of the calcaneum. J Bone Joint Surg Br 42:336–343, 1960.

51. Thompson KR, Friesen CM. Treatment of comminuted fractures of the calcaneus by primary triple arthrodesis. J Bone Joint Surg Am 41:1423–1436, 1959.

52. Harris RI. Fractures of the os calcis: treatment by early subtalar arthrodesis. Clin Orthop 30:100–110, 1963.

53. Knudsen HA, Sharon SM, Silberman J. A two-stage delayed surgical approach to salvaging Essex-Lopresti tongue type calcaneal fractures. J Foot Surg 23:231–234, 1984.

54. Myerson M, Quill GE Jr. Late complications of fractures of the calcaneus. J Bone Joint Surg Am 75:331–341, 1993.

55. Kusakabe N, Takagi M, Tsuzuki N. Tibio-talo-calcaneal fusion with a free vascularized fibular graft in comminuted open fractures of the talus and the calcaneus. J Orthop Trauma 6:386–390, 1992.

56. Angus PD, Cowell HR. Triple arthrodesis. J Bone Joint Surg Br 68:260–265, 1986.

57. Carr JB, Hansen ST, Benirschke SK. Subtalar distraction bone block fusion for late complications of os calcis fractures. Foot Ankle 9:81–86, 1988.

58. Isbister JF. Calcaneo-fibular abutment following crush fracture of the calcaneus. J Bone Joint Surg Am 56:274–278, 1974.

59. Prats DAD, Munoz SA, Llopis SF, et al. Surgery for fracture of the calcaneus: 5 (2–8) year follow-up of 20 cases. Acta Orthop Scand 64:161–164, 1993.

60. Crosby LA, Fitzgibbons T. Computerized tomography scanning of acute intra-articular fractures of the calcaneus: a new classification system. J Bone Joint Surg Am 72:852–859, 1990.

61. Lanfranco G, Gnemmi G, Bertuzzi B. Fractures of the calcaneum: when and how to operate. Ital J Orthop Traumatol 13:333–344, 1987.

62. Sangeorzan BJ, Ananthakrishnan D, Tencer AF. Contact characteristics of the subtalar joint after a simulated calcaneus fracture. J Orthop Trauma 9:251–258, 1995.

63. Repo RU, Finlay JB. Survival of articular cartilage after controlled impact. J Bone Joint Surg Am 59:1068–1076, 1977.

64. Romash MM. Calcaneal fractures: three-dimensional treatment. Foot Ankle 8:180–197, 1988.

65. Carr JB, Hamilton JJ, Bear LS. Experimental intra-articular calcaneal fractures: anatomic basis for a new classification. Foot Ankle 10:81–87, 1989.

66. Pennal GF, Yadav MP. Operative treatment of comminuted fractures of the os calcis. Orthop Clin North Am 4:197–211, 1973.

67. Gaul JS, Greenberg BG. Calcaneus fractures involving the subtalar joint: a clinical and statistical survey of 98 cases. South Med J 59:605–613, 1966.

68. Ross SDK. The operative treatment of complex os calcis fractures. Tech Orthop 2:55–70, 1987.

69. Burdeaux BD. The medial approach for calcaneal fractures. Clin Orthop 290:96–107, 1993.

70. Leung KS, Chan WS, Shen WY, et al. Operative treatment of intraarticular fractures of the os calcis—the role of rigid internal fixation and primary bone grafting: preliminary results. J Orthop Trauma 3:232–240, 1989.

71. Burdeaux BD. Reduction of calcaneal fractures by the McReynolds medial approach technique and its experimental basis. Clin Orthop 177:87, 1983.

72. Levin LS, Nunley JA. The management of soft-tissue problems associated with calcaneal fractures. Clin Orthop 290:151–156, 1993.

73. Tscherne H, Zwipp H. Calcaneal fractures. In Tscherne H, Schatzker J, eds. Major Fractures of the Pilon, the Talus, and the Calcaneus: Current Concepts of Treatment. Berlin: Springer-Verlag, 1993:153–174.

74. Myerson M, Manoli A. Compartment syndromes of the foot after calcaneal fractures. Clin Orthop 290:142–150, 1993.

75. Fakhouri AJ, Manoli A. Acute foot compartment syndromes. J Orthop Trauma 6:223–228, 1992.

76. Myerson MS. Management of compartment syndromes of the foot. Clin Orthop 271:239–248, 1991.

77. Mittlmeier T, Machler G, Lob G, et al. Compartment syndrome of the foot after intraarticular calcaneal fracture. Clin Orthop 269:241–248, 1991.

78. Miller WS. The heel pad. Am J Sports Med 10:19–21, 1983.

79. Johansson JE, Harrison J, Greenwood FAH. Subtalar arthrodesis for adult traumatic arthritis. Foot Ankle 2:294–298, 1982.

80. Braly W, Bishop J, Tullos H. Lateral decompression for malunited os calcis fractures. Foot Ankle 6:90, 1985.

81. Romash MM. Reconstructive osteotomy of the calcaneus with subtalar arthrodesis for malunited calcaneal fractures. Clin Orthop 290:157–167, 1993.

23

Ankle Sprain: Clinical Evaluation and Current Treatment Concepts

Dipak V. Patel
Russell F. Warren

Acute ankle sprain is one of the most common injuries seen in sports medicine practice. Sprains commonly involve the lateral ligamentous complex of the ankle. Injuries of the ankle syndesmosis or the medial ligament (deltoid ligament) are less common. It is estimated that there is approximately one inversion injury of the ankle per 10,000 persons per day.[1–3] Jackson and colleagues[4] noted ankle sprains to be the most common injury in cadets at West Point, New York. They found that 30% of the cadets had sustained one inversion sprain injury during the 4-year training period. In a 1-year follow-up study period, Sandelin[5] found that 21% of the sports injuries treated in the Casualty Department of Helsinki University Central Hospital (Finland) were acute ankle sprains. In a similar study performed in Oslo (Norway), acute ankle sprains accounted for 16% of all athletic injuries.[6]

The vast majority of ankle sprains occur in patients younger than 35 years (most common age range, 15–19 years).[7] Ankle sprains constitute approximately 25% of all sports injuries.[8] Acute ankle sprains occur in sports such as basketball, soccer, football, baseball, volleyball, cross-country running, dancing, and ballet.[6, 9–13] Garrick,[10] in a study of 1650 high school students, reviewed several sports and noted that ankle injuries occurred frequently in all sports, with the exception of tennis and swimming. Garrick[10] reported that 45% of basketball injuries, 25% of volleyball injuries, and 31% of soccer injuries involved the ankle. In other sports, ankle sprains constituted 10 to 20% of all injuries. Sandelin,[5] in a thesis on clinical and epidemiologic study of acute sports injuries, found that 29% of all injuries to the lower extremities in soccer involved the ankle; of these, 75% were distortions mostly involving the lateral ligamentous structures of the ankle joint.

Despite the high prevalence of ankle sprains, controversy still remains concerning the clinical and diagnostic evaluation, the criteria used for nonoperative and operative treatment, and rehabilitation program. Ankle sprains are not always simple injuries (as frequently believed) and may result in significant residual symptoms if a correct early diagnosis is not made and appropriate treatment measures not taken. The ultimate goal of treatment is to restore mobility, stability, and function of the ankle so that the patient can safely return to preinjury activity and sports at a preinjury level. The purpose of this chapter is to outline the clinical assessment, evaluation methods, and management of patients with acute ankle sprains. The clinical features and treatment of patients with chronic ankle sprains with instability are also discussed.

FUNCTIONAL ANATOMY OF THE LATERAL LIGAMENTS OF THE ANKLE

Most textbooks on foot and ankle disorders have described the anatomy of the lateral ligaments of the ankle in detail. A few important points deserve a mention. The lateral ligamentous complex of the ankle is composed of three ligaments: anterior talofibular ligament (ATFL), calcaneofibular ligament (CFL), and posterior talofibular ligament (PTFL) (Fig. 23–1).

The ATFL is approximately 2 to 2.5 mm thick, 6 to 8 mm wide, and 10 mm long. It originates from the anterior border and tip of the lateral malleolus and runs anteriorly to insert on the neck of the talus. It runs almost parallel to the long axis of the foot when the foot is in neutral position. However, when the foot is in plantar flexion, the ATFL assumes a course parallel to the long axis of the leg, thus functioning as a collateral ligament[14, 15] (Fig. 23–2A and B). The ATFL is the most commonly injured liga-

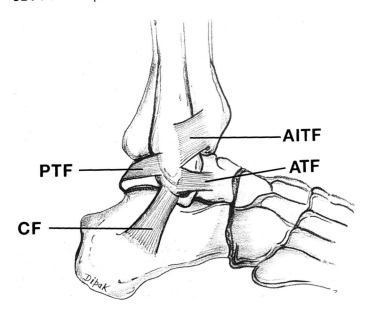

Figure 23–1. The lateral ligaments of the ankle consist of anterior talofibular ligament (ATF), calcaneofibular ligament (CF), and the posterior talofibular ligament (PTF). AITF, anterior inferior tibiofibular ligament.

ment after a plantar flexion-inversion injury to the ankle. The CFL is approximately 3 to 5 mm thick, 4 to 8 mm wide, and 25 mm long. The CFL is an extracapsular ligament that originates from the tip of the lateral malleolus and runs, with a slight backward inclination, to the lateral surface of the calcaneum. It forms the floor of the peroneal tendon sheath. This relationship between the CFL and the peroneal tendon sheath is important for interpretation of the results of ankle arthrography and peroneal tenography in patients with suspected rupture of the CFL. The PTFL is approximately 5 to 8

mm thick, 5 mm wide, and 25 to 30 mm long. It originates from the posteromedial aspect of the lateral malleolus and runs posteromedially to the posterior process of the talus.

The primary function of the ATFL and PTFL is to restrain anterior and posterior displacement, respectively, of the talus in relation to the fibula and tibia. The CFL restrains inversion of the calcaneum with respect to the fibula. The extent of normal dorsiflexion-plantar flexion movement varies depending on various measurement techniques in the literature. Rasmussen[16]

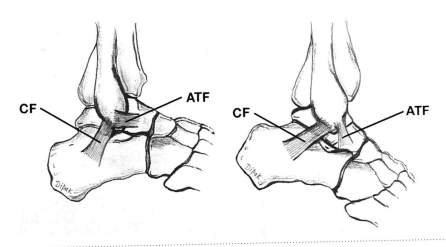

Figure 23–2. *Left,* The anterior talofibular ligament (ATF) runs parallel to the long axis of the foot when the foot is in neutral position. *Right,* The ATF assumes a course almost parallel to the long axis of the tibia and fibula when the foot is in plantar flexion. CF, calcaneofibular ligament.

reported that the dorsiflexion at the ankle ranges from 10 to 51°, and the plantar flexion ranges from 15 to 56°. The total mobility in the sagittal plane is evaluated to be 62°. The functional range of motion (ROM) of the ankle (as seen in walking) is on the order of 10° of dorsiflexion and 50° of plantar flexion.

MECHANISM OF INJURY

Clear elucidation of the mechanism of injury is helpful to make an appropriate diagnosis. The lateral ankle sprain usually occurs as a result of plantar flexion-inversion injury. For example, the basketball player landing on another player's foot after a jump may sustain lateral ankle sprain. The ATFL is the primary lateral stabilizer of the ankle in all positions of plantar flexion. Because the majority of ankle sprains occur during plantar flexion, adduction, and inversion of the foot, the ATFL is the first ligament to sustain rupture in patients with such injuries. If the tearing force continues, the CFL is injured next, followed by the PTFL.

Brostrom[17–19] found that isolated complete rupture of the ATFL was present in 65% of cases involving ankle sprain. A combined injury of the ATFL and CFL occurred in 20% of the patients in his series. The CFL was never ruptured alone. An isolated injury to the PTFL was rare. The anterior inferior tibiofibular ligament was injured in 10% of patients and the deltoid ligament in 3% of patients. Complete ruptures of the lateral ligaments of the ankle are usually midsubstance tears.[17] Approximately 15% of these ruptures occur at the insertion of the ligaments and sometimes may be associated with an avulsion of a bony fragment. Partial ruptures of the ligaments usually occur in midsubstance.

CLASSIFICATION OF ANKLE SPRAINS

Some surgeons tend to distinguish between grades of severity of ankle sprains for prognostic and treatment purposes, whereas others prefer not to. Various authors have classified ankle sprains as mild (grade I), moderate (grade II), and severe (grade III) injuries.[13–15, 20, 21] Grade I sprain involves stretch of the ligament without a macroscopic tear. Patients with grade I ankle sprain have mild swelling and tenderness, minimal or no functional loss, and no mechanical instability of the joint. Grade II ankle sprain is defined as a partial macroscopic tear of the ligament. Patients with grade II ankle sprain have moderate pain, swelling and tenderness, some restriction of joint motion, and mild to moderate joint instability. It is worth noting that patients with mild or moderate ankle instability have a "firm end point" on clinical stress testing. However, there are no well-defined, uniform criteria (in terms of millimeters of abnormal translation) to differentiate between mild and moderate instability of the ankle. A grade III ankle sprain indicates complete rupture of the ligament. Patients with such an injury have marked pain, swelling and tenderness, marked abnormal motion and joint instability, and severe restriction of ankle function. The ankle instability is classified as marked if "no end point" or a "soft end point" is felt on clinical stress testing.

CLINICAL ASSESSMENT

History

A thorough history and physical examination are important for establishing the diagnosis. It is important to determine whether the recent injury is the first ankle sprain or a recurrent injury. The following points should be considered in patients with a suspected ankle sprain:

1. Inquire about the details of the mechanism of injury: inversion sprain or eversion-external rotation sprain.

2. Did the patient hear a "pop" or "tear" or feel a "snap"?

3. Is the patient able to bear weight or walk on the injured ankle? One should ask whether the patient was able to continue his or her sport after the injury.

4. Determine the duration between the injury and the onset of symptoms such as pain, swelling, discoloration, and joint stiffness.

5. Does the patient have a history of injury to the affected ankle or to the opposite ankle?

6. How was the injury treated? Inquire

about the use of cold, compression, bandage or taping, crutches, ankle brace, high boot shoe, and physical therapy.

7. Does the patient have a history of surgery on the ankle?

8. Does the patient have residual symptoms (e.g., pain, swelling, giving-way or instability, weakness, stiffness)?

After sustaining an acute injury, patients often complain of intense pain localized to the lateral aspect of the ankle. The pain usually subsides after some time, especially with complete rupture of the ligament. The pain recurs after a few hours as a result of increased swelling. Most patients experience pain and discomfort when they try to bear weight on the injured leg. Some patients complain of a feeling of "giving way or instability" in the ankle, particularly while walking on an uneven surface.

Physical Examination

After 24 to 48 hours, the lateral side of the injured ankle is usually discolored, appearing blue and yellow as a result of organization and resorption of the hematoma. The discoloration is often noted more distally than the site of injury itself. On examination, the area of tenderness and swelling is usually localized over the ATFL, especially on its fibular insertion. Swelling and tenderness on the CFL are commonly seen at the calcaneal insertion of the ligament. In patients with a complete rupture of the ligament, a palpable defect along the course of the torn ligament may be felt. The best opportunity for examination of an injured ankle is immediately after the injury. Once swelling occurs, the specificity of palpable tenderness decreases. If the patient is seen after a delay of several hours after the injury, generalized swelling and increased pain often preclude a thorough evaluation of the severity of injury.

Injury to the anterior portion of the deltoid ligament may occur in patients with complete tears of the ATFL and PTFL. Therefore, medial tenderness (over the anterior aspect of the deltoid ligament) is a clue to a severe ankle sprain. If swelling and tenderness are located proximally over the anterior aspect of the ankle (between the tibia and the fibula), an injury to the anterior inferior tibiofibular ligament and

interosseous membrane should be suspected. This is seen after an external rotation type of injury, particularly on an artificial surface. In patients with severe ankle injuries, one must palpate the proximal fibula to rule out a Maisonneuve fracture. The midtarsal area should also be examined to rule out an associated fracture.

The ROM of the ankle is restricted in dorsiflexion, plantar flexion, and inversion. One should always examine the opposite, noninjured ankle to evaluate the normal mobility and stability of the joint. The findings of the normal ankle should then be compared with those of the injured ankle. The active and passive ROM at the ankle should be recorded within the limits of pain. The stability of the ankle should be tested by the anterior drawer test and the inversion stress (talar tilt) test. We acknowledge that in an acutely injured, painful, swollen ankle, it may be difficult to perform these tests. A repeat physical examination after few days (when the pain and swelling have decreased) is often helpful. Meticulous physical examination with fingertip palpation of the injured structures should lead the physician to a correct clinical diagnosis.

Clinical Tests for Ankle Stability

Several authors[20, 22, 23] believe that the anterior drawer test and the inversion stress (talar tilt) test should be performed to assess the stability of the ankle.

Anterior Drawer Test

A rupture of the ATFL may result in mechanical instability of the ankle. Clinically, this can be evaluated by anterior drawer test, which involves an anterior displacement of the talus in relation to the tibia. This test is performed with the patient sitting with the knee flexed to relax the calf muscles. The heel is grasped firmly with one hand and the foot is pulled forward while exerting a posterior force on the anterior aspect of the distal tibia with the other hand (Fig. 23-3). In a patient with a positive anterior drawer test, a visible dimpling over the anterolateral aspect of the ankle (the so-called suction sign) may be seen, indicating tear of the ATFL. In a patient with gross swelling of the ankle, the suction sign may not be apparent. The physician

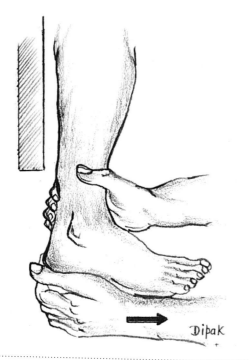

Figure 23–3. The anterior drawer test of the ankle.

Inversion Stress (Talar Tilt) Test

The inversion stress (talar tilt) test is considered to be a test for assessing the integrity of the CFL.[13, 22, 29] With the ankle in the neutral position, an inversion load places a high strain on the CFL, whereas with progressive plantar flexion of the ankle, an increased strain is exerted on the ATFL while the CFL is more relaxed.[26, 30, 31] The clinical application of this biomechanical finding is that if the CFL is of primary interest in the physical examination, the test should be performed with the foot in a neutral position or in 10° of dorsiflexion.[31] The talar tilt test should also be performed with the foot in plantar flexion for evaluation of the integrity of the ATFL.[16, 23, 27, 28]

In the inversion stress (talar tilt) test, the physician grasps the heel with one hand and holds the distal tibia with the other hand and then attempts to invert the talus and calcaneum on the tibia (Fig. 23–4). If the CFL is torn, the articular surfaces of the tibia and talus will separate, forming an angle that is referred to as the talar tilt.

should also record the quality of the end point when performing the anterior drawer test. The degree of anterior translation of the talus in relation to the tibia is recorded as mild, moderate, or severe. The just-mentioned distinction is based on subjective interpretation of the examining physician. The reproducibility of the anterior drawer test is debatable. Rasmussen[16] and Lahde and associates[24] found the anterior drawer test unreliable, whereas others[25–27] have found it valuable in assessing the integrity of the ATFL.

On physical examination, it is difficult to evaluate precisely the extent (in millimeters) of the anterior translation of the talus in relation to the tibia. Radiographic studies have shown that in normal ankles the mean anterior drawer translation of the talus is 3 to 4 mm.[25, 27] If the anterior talar translation is more than 6 mm with the foot in neutral position and 8 mm with the foot in plantar flexion, it is suggested that at least the ATFL is ruptured.[16, 23, 27, 28] However, it should be noted that these radiographic studies have varying criteria for measuring the anterior talar translation; therefore, it is difficult to obtain a valid comparison of the findings reported in these studies.

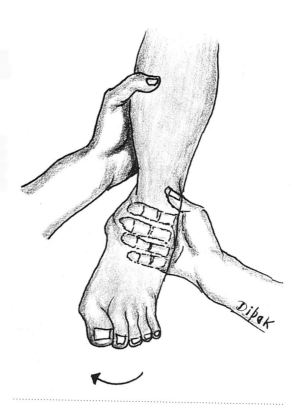

Figure 23–4. The inversion stress (talar tilt) test of the ankle.

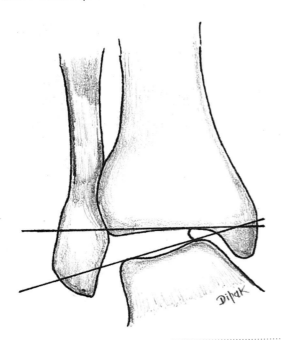

Figure 23–5. The inversion stress (talar tilt) radiograph is taken with the ankle in neutral position but internally rotated 10 to 20°. The talar tilt angle refers to the angle between two lines drawn tangential to the tibial plafond and the talar dome.

The talar tilt angle is the angle between the tibial plafond and the talar dome and can be measured on stress radiography, as shown in Figure 23–5. The degree of instability in the injured ankle is classified as mild, moderate, or severe. One must examine the opposite, noninjured ankle to assess the physiologic laxity and compare the findings with those of the injured ankle.

Radiographic Assessment

Plain Radiographs

In patients with clinically suspected grade II or grade III ankle sprain, routine anteroposterior (AP) and lateral views as well as an AP view with the foot in 15 to 20° of internal rotation (mortise view) should be obtained. The mortise view is helpful to exclude fractures of the distal tibia, fibula, and talus because the lateral malleolus does not overlap the tibia and the talus is equidistant from both malleoli. The plain radiographs should be carefully analyzed for avulsion fractures and osteochondral injuries.

Stress Radiography

Anterior drawer stress radiographs and talar tilt stress radiographs have been recommended for documentation of the degree of instability of the ankle. However, in clinical practice, a routine use of stress radiography for assessment of grade II and grade III ankle sprains is disputable.

Anterior drawer stress radiographs have been accepted as a sensitive indicator of instability of the ankle.[18, 26, 27] A 5-kg weight is applied to the distal tibia for 2 to 5 minutes to produce a steady posterior traction on the tibia, and then a lateral radiograph is taken. Some authors use a commercially available jig with specifically defined stresses. The stress can also be applied manually, but the manual test is less reliable. In patients with markedly painful ankle, local anesthesia is required to perform this test. An anterior talar translation of greater than 6 mm in the injured ankle or a talar displacement difference of greater than 3 mm between the injured and the noninjured ankles indicates a rupture of the ATFL.

It should be noted that the amount of anterior displacement in the injured ankle depends not only on the degree of injury to the lateral ligamentous complex of the ankle, but also on various factors such as general ligamentous laxity, magnitude and duration of the applied stress, type of anesthesia used, degree of muscle relaxation, and position of the foot. Moreover, there are various methods for measuring the anterior translation of talus in relation to tibia, and different criteria have been used to distinguish between normal (physiologic) and pathologic ankle laxity. For these reasons, it is difficult to establish the firm role of anterior drawer stress radiography in the evaluation of ankle instability.

Inversion stress (talar tilt) radiographs have also been used to assess lateral ligament ankle injuries. Inversion stress can be applied manually or by using a commercially available jig that applies a specific load. Various methods for measuring the talar tilt have been reported in the literature; the common one is the measurement of the talar tilt angle. Unfortunately, no universally accepted criteria exist that define an abnormal talar tilt. A talar tilt of greater than 20° or a side-to-side talar tilt difference of greater than 10° is suggestive of complete rupture of the ATFL and CFL. The inversion stress findings of the injured ankle must be compared with those of the opposite normal ankle. Some authors[28, 32, 33] suggested that the anterior drawer stress test and the inversion stress test should be used in combination to evaluate the injured ankle reliably.

Ankle Arthrography

Arthrography of the ankle has been used by several authors for assessing ligamentous injuries of the ankle.[17, 24, 33–36] However, it has several limitations:

1. It is an invasive procedure that requires a hospital environment.
2. It is difficult to quantify the amount of tear.
3. Arthrography is reliable only when performed within the first 24 to 48 hours after injury and not later than 1 week after an acute injury. Sealing of the rent by blood clots and fibrin has been noted as early as 48 hours after an injury, thus increasing the risk of a false-negative interpretation on an arthrogram.
4. Interpretation of arthrograms requires a precise understanding of possible variations and patterns of dye leakage along the tendon sheaths and into the adjacent subtalar joint. Normal communications of peroneal tendon sheaths and potential bursae with the ankle may be present, and give false-positive results.

Peroneal Tenography

The technique of peroneal tenography has been reported by Black and associates.[37] A radiopaque dye is injected into the peroneal tendon sheath as soon as possible after an acute injury. If the dye leaks from the peroneal sheath into the ankle joint, it indicates a tear of the CFL. It should be noted that if the dye is injected too far proximally (i.e., into the peroneal muscle instead of into the tendon sheath), a false-negative result may be obtained.

Bone Scan

Gallium and technetium-99m scans are highly sensitive for the diagnosis of acute ankle injuries but lack specificity. Bone scans are particularly useful for patients

with a suspected diagnosis of stress fracture, osteochondral fracture of the talar dome, infection, or an inflammatory lesion.

Ankle Tomography and Computed Tomography

In a patient with an acute ankle sprain, a tomogram or a computed tomography (CT) scan are not routinely needed. In the evaluation of patients with ankle sprains, ankle tomography may occasionally be helpful to rule out other conditions such as osteochondral fractures of the dome of the talus, sinus tarsi fractures, tarsal coalitions, and osteoid osteoma of the talus.

CT is useful for patients with complex fractures of the ankle. A CT scan may occasionally be needed for some patients in whom the diagnosis of ankle sprain is not clear on clinical grounds or when other diagnoses need to be considered.

Magnetic Resonance Imaging

Magnetic resonance imaging (MRI) of the ankle should not be routinely ordered for patients with ankle sprains. There is no doubt that MRI provides excellent visualization of the extent of soft tissue damage. MRI is helpful in identifying injury to various components of the lateral ligamentous complex (ATFL, CFL, and PTFL). The findings of MRI should be correlated with the degree of ankle instability. Lesions such as osteochondral fractures of the talar dome or the tibial plafond, osteochondritis dissecans of the talus, syndesmosis injury of the ankle, and tendon injuries around the ankle can be evaluated by MRI.

Ankle Arthroscopy

A detailed history and meticulous physical examination are essential for making an accurate clinical diagnosis of ankle sprain. Ankle arthroscopy should be neither routinely used for the diagnosis of acute ankle sprain nor used as a substitute for a good history and physical examination. Arthroscopy may be useful for the evaluation of patients with a chronic, symptomatic ankle lesion.

Differential Diagnosis

A list of lesions that should be considered in a patient with an acute ankle injury is given in Table 23–1. These conditions should be suspected, particularly when the patient has persistent symptoms. A high index of suspicion is needed to diagnose these entities.

Fractures of the ankle may occur in isolation or may be associated with ankle ligament injuries. One should look for fractures of the lateral, medial, and posterior malleolus; proximal fibula, lateral, or posterior process of the talus; anterior process of the calcaneum; and fifth metatarsal. Stress fractures of the distal fibula and the fifth metatarsal may mimic an ankle sprain. Osteochondral fractures of the talar dome or the tibial plafond, and osteochondritis dissecans may present with symptoms similar to those of lateral ligament injury. Radioisotope bone scan, tomography, CT scan, or MRI may be needed for a precise diagnosis.

Inflammation or rupture of the Achilles tendon and the peroneal tendon can sometimes mimic an acute ankle sprain. The integrity of the Achilles tendon should be tested by Thompson test. Thompson test is performed after positioning the patient prone with the foot off the examination table. Then the gastrocnemius-soleus complex is squeezed. In a patient with an intact Achilles tendon, on squeezing the gastrocnemius-soleus complex, passive plantar flexion of the foot occurs; absence of plantar flexion of the foot indicates rupture of the Achilles tendon. The peroneal tendon

Table 23–1. Conditions that Need to Be Differentiated from Ankle Sprain

1. Fractures of the ankle
2. Stress fractures
3. Osteochondral fractures of the talar dome or the tibial plafond
4. Osteochondritis dissecans of the talus
5. Inflammation and rupture of the tendons around the ankle
6. Subluxation or dislocation of the peroneal tendons
7. Sprain of the midfoot ligaments
8. Miscellaneous lesions
   Anterior or posterior tibiotalar impingement
   Posttraumatic synovitis
   Meniscoid lesion
   Loose bodies
   Sinus tarsi syndrome
   Diastasis of the ankle syndesmosis
   Subtalar joint instability
   Entrapment of the superficial or deep peroneal nerve

Table 23–2. Disorders that Mimic Ankle Sprain in Children and Adolescents

1. Epiphyseal fractures
2. Talar dome fractures
3. Osteochondritis dissecans of the talus
4. Fractures of the cuboid
5. Tarsal coalition
6. Pes planus
7. Juvenile rheumatoid arthritis
8. Osteomyelitis and pyogenic arthritis of the ankle

should be examined for subluxation or dislocation, which may occur in conjunction with ankle instability or simply mimic ankle instability. Sprains of the midfoot ligaments (in particular, dorsal calcaneocuboid ligament, bifurcate ligament, cervical ligament, and interosseous talocalcaneal ligament) may also simulate the symptoms of lateral ligament injury of the ankle.

Miscellaneous disorders (see Table 23–1) can also present with ankle pain, and physicians should be aware of these entities so that a precise diagnosis can be made and appropriate treatment provided.

In children and adolescents, many lesions (Table 23–2) can present with symptoms similar to those of an ankle sprain. A high index of suspicion, a careful history and physical examination, and, when needed, a detailed work-up should lead to an accurate diagnosis.

Treatment of Acute Ankle Sprain

With increasing participation in both recreational and competitive sports, there is an increasing need for early diagnosis and appropriate treatment of ankle sprain to enable the patients to return to sports at full capacity safely and predictably. The athletes are keen to return to their respective sports as soon as possible without compromising the ankle stability. With recent changes in the health care system with restricted economic resources, one also needs to consider the cost-benefit issue before selecting the treatment option. In general, nonoperative treatment is the mainstay of management for the vast majority of patients with ankle sprains, even in the athletically active patient population. It is now generally accepted that functional rehabilitation of the injured ankle provides the most rapid recovery, with earlier return to work and sports. If instability persists, late ligamentous reconstruction of the ankle can be undertaken and is quite successful.

Most authors agree that grade I and grade II ankle sprains can be satisfactorily treated by nonoperative measures[13–15, 21, 22] with an excellent or good prognosis.[2–4, 13–15, 21, 33, 38–40] The conservative treatment program for an acute ankle sprain consists of rest, ice, compression, and elevation. Early compression is critical to decrease bleeding. The goal is to decrease the acute swelling and pain and make the patient more comfortable. A short period of immobilization (1–3 weeks) using a tape, bandage, or a semirigid ankle orthosis may be needed. Some authors prefer to use a Cryocuff compression wrap, Aircast splint (Aircast, Inc., Summit, NJ), Unna boot, or a removable splint-walker and commence immediate rehabilitation.

Early ROM exercises are begun and early weight bearing is allowed within limits of pain. The range of dorsiflexion at the ankle can be improved by Achilles tendon stretching. Strengthening exercises of the ankle everters and dorsiflexors are undertaken in an isometric, eccentric, and concentric manner. Isometric exercises are performed by everting or dorsiflexing the ankle against a fixed point of resistance, such as a wall. TheraBand or surgical tubing is used for resistance when performing concentric and eccentric contractions. Peroneal muscle exercises[13–15, 23, 39] constitute an important part of the rehabilitation program. Stationary ergometer cycling can be used to improve the ROM and muscle strength.

The value of nonsteroidal anti-inflammatory drugs (NSAIDs) in the treatment of acute ankle sprains has been studied in prospective, randomized, double-blind trials.[3, 41, 42] With respect to ankle pain, swelling, tenderness, and function, NSAID treatment was found to be more effective compared with the placebo, although the differences were not striking and seemed to decrease over a period of time. In the initial 6 weeks after the injury, various supportive physical therapy modalities have been recommended to promote a speedy recovery. These include ultrasound, temperature-contrast baths, short waves, diadynamic or interference current therapy, and electrogalvanic stimulation. However, the efficacy of these modalities has been questioned by randomized controlled studies.[43, 44] The role of cryotherapy has been established by some studies.[45–47]

Proprioceptive training with a tilt board is commenced as soon as possible (usually after 4–8 weeks) to improve the balance and neuromuscular control of the ankle. The efficacy of tilt board training has been shown in prospective, randomized studies,[48–50] and such exercises should be continued for 3 to 4 months. Agility and endurance exercises are recommended to improve the functional performance of the ankle. Progression through the phases of rehabilitation depends on the extent of the ligament injury, resolution of pain and swelling, and weight-bearing ability of the patient. If pain or swelling develops during any phase of rehabilitation, the intensity of the program should be decreased and cryotherapy should be used to reduce the inflammation and swelling.

From this point onward, rehabilitation of the ankle depends on the desired activity level and athletic demands on the ankle. The most frequently used exercises are heel and toe raises, exercises with rubber tubes, rope skipping, climbing up and down stairs, straight-ahead jogging or running, backward running, running in circles, running in figure-eight patterns clockwise and counterclockwise, 90° cuts while running, and running zigzags at 45°.[13, 15] Progression through these activities occurs as confidence in the ankle increases.

Eversion-type sprains with pain along the syndesmosis are much slower to recover, and patients with such injuries return to activity at a slower rate. Patients with grade I or grade II ankle sprains may return to sports as early as 2 to 3 weeks after injury, whereas those with syndesmosis injuries may return to sports at 6 to 8 weeks.

The management of grade III ankle sprains of the lateral ligamentous complex is controversial. Many uncontrolled, non-randomized studies have suggested that primary repair is the treatment of choice because the majority of patients undergoing surgery seem to achieve a mechanically stable ankle and satisfactory subjective results.[1, 51–54] However, similar results with nonoperative treatment have also been reported by other authors.[4, 55–57]

Prospective, randomized studies comparing acute surgical repair and cast versus cast alone, with early controlled mobilization, or with both have been reported[18, 29, 33–36, 48, 58–61] Such studies eliminate the selection bias that is associated with nonrandomized, retrospective studies. On the basis of these studies, it is apparent that functional treatment (early controlled mobilization) of ankle sprain provides a quicker return of ankle mobility, and patients are predictably and safely able to return to full function and work without jeopardizing the mechanical stability of the ankle. After functional treatment of the ankle sprain, no increase in the incidence of residual symptoms (such as pain, swelling, giving way, stiffness, or muscle weakness) has been seen.

Various studies have shown that secondary surgical intervention (a delayed anatomic repair or tenodesis) of the ruptured ankle ligaments can be performed, if necessary, even years after the initial injury, and good results (comparable to those obtained with primary repair) have been obtained.[19, 62–68] Professional athletes can also be initially treated by nonoperative measures. If they have persistent symptoms despite nonoperative treatment, delayed surgery can be performed on an elective basis. Delayed anatomic repair of chronic lesions of the ATFL and CFL[19, 62, 68] is relatively a straightforward procedure that is often sufficient to stabilize the ankle. However, if the tissue is insufficient, then reconstruction of the ankle with an autogenous graft is appropriate. Although many reconstructive procedures[63–66, 69–72] have been developed, we prefer the Chrisman-Snook procedure[72] in this setting.

Although most ankle sprains can be satisfactorily treated by nonoperative methods, some cases (such as ankle injuries with a large bony avulsion, associated major osteochondral fracture of the talus, severe ligamentous damage on the medial as well as lateral side, and severe or recurrent grade III sprain) may require surgical intervention in the acute phase.

Chronic Lateral Ankle Sprain with Instability

Sequelae after acute ligamentous injuries of the ankle are frequently seen in clinical practice. These include persistent synovitis, pain, swelling, giving way, stiffness, and muscle weakness. In many patients with chronic ankle sprains, a feeling of giving way or "looseness" in the ankle is the chief complaint, and pain is rarely the presenting complaint. Many patients with chronic lateral ankle instability give a history of recurrent inversion injuries that occur when walking on uneven surfaces or descending stairs. The ankle instability should be differentiated into two types: mechanical and functional. Both types of instabilities may occur simultaneously, for instance, in a patient with a gross mechanical instability of the ankle.

A careful history and a detailed physical examination are vital for establishing a correct diagnosis. Mechanical instability can be confirmed by anterior drawer stress radiography and, in some cases, a talar tilt stress radiography. An anterior talar translation of 10 mm or more and a talar tilt of 10° or more reliably indicate mechanical instability of the ankle. These views are not routinely obtained because they may provide false-negative results. A careful physical examination (the anterior drawer test and the inversion stress [talar tilt test]) is usually sufficient.

Evaluation of patients with chronic ankle instability should include repeat radiographs. In some cases, a radioisotope bone scan may be needed to localize the disease. If the bone scan is positive, tomography or CT scan is required to clarify the disease more specifically. MRI is indicated if tendon injury, soft tissue impingement, or avascular necrosis of the talus is clinically suspected.

Mechanical Instability

Mechanical instability of the ankle is motion beyond the physiologic ROM. It indicates incompetence of the passive stabilizers of the ankle. This can be demonstrated by the anterior drawer test and the inversion stress (talar tilt) test. However, the amount of mechanical instability that is within the limits of normal variation is unknown, and it is unclear as to when the mechanical instability should be called pathologic. It is also unknown how much pathologic laxity can exist in the ankle without resulting in giving-way symptoms during activity. Various studies have shown that, after an acute injury, there is no correlation between radiographically proven (anterior drawer or talar tilt stress tests) mechanical instability of the ankle and the patient's symptoms of giving way, pain, or swelling.[49, 52, 60, 73] The active stabilizers of the ankle (i.e., muscles and tendons) are capable of compensating for ligamentous laxity of the ankle. The degree of varus opening of the ankle that is tolerated may relate to the heel position on heel strike. We have found that patients with valgus heel position may tolerate ankle instability better than those with varus heel position.

Treatment of Mechanical Instability

Before undertaking lateral ligament reconstruction, several points should be emphasized:

1. The patient's occupation, activity level, and sporting demands on the ankle should be taken into account.

2. The diagnosis of chronic mechanical instability of the ankle must be firmly established. A trial of supervised ankle rehabilitation program should be tried initially.

3. If the results of clinical instability tests are equivocal or doubtful, then stress radiography (anterior drawer stress or talar tilt stress or both) may be helpful to document the presence of mechanical instability. The findings of the injured ankle should be compared with those of the opposite, noninjured ankle. In patients with bilateral ankle instabilities, the absolute amount of the anterior talar displacement and the degree of talar tilt should be taken into account.

4. In patients with generalized ligamentous laxity, the results of surgery are less predictable and often less satisfactory. The patient should be carefully counseled and informed about the success rate of surgery in such circumstances. It is preferable to consider a tenodesis type of surgery (as opposed to anatomic reconstruction) in patients with generalized ligamentous laxity.

5. Patients with a chronic ligamentous instability (> 10 years) and those who have had previous tenodesis operations have been reported to do less well after reconstruction.[68] In such patients, osteoarthritis may occur with time and may compromise the result. If osteoarthritis is seen initially, it may indicate the need for early stabilization of the ankle.

The associated disease must be identified and addressed at surgery. An augmentation of the ligament repair may be indicated when the tissues are weak or the functional demands on the ankle are high. Care should be taken to preserve the ankle and subtalar motion while undertaking a reconstructive procedure. Once the subtalar motion is restricted beyond 50% of normal, there is an increasing likelihood that the patient's ability to return to sports will be significantly compromised.

Many surgical procedures have been described for the management of patients with chronic lateral instability of the ankle.[19, 62–72, 74, 75] These procedures can broadly be categorized into anatomic procedures and tenodesis procedures.

The most popular of the anatomic techniques is that described by Brostrom.[19] Anatomic reconstruction has two advantages. First, no normal tissue is sacrificed. Second, it does not create a tenodesis effect that may alter the ankle and subtalar joint biomechanics. Thus, no loss of motion at the subtalar joint results.

Althoff and associates[76] described their method of anatomic reconstruction (delayed repair) of the lateral ligaments for patients with chronic mechanical instability of the ankle. In this procedure, the lateral ligaments of the ankle are shortened and reinserted (or imbricated) (Fig. 23–6). It is

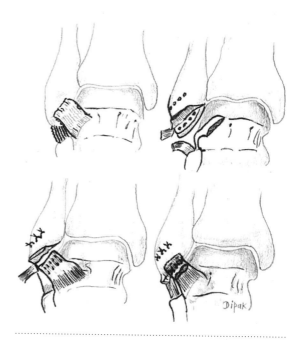

Figure 23–6. Anatomic reconstruction of the anterior talofibular and calcaneofibular ligaments of the ankle.

worth noting that with this technique, both the ATFL and the CFL are reconstructed, whereas using other reconstructive procedures, only the ATFL is reconstructed; the exception is the Elmslie procedure and its modification by Chrisman and Snook.[72] Technically, the anatomic reconstructions are relatively straightforward and easy to perform, whereas other reconstructive methods (tenodesis) are more time consuming and require experience and special skills.

After the anatomic reconstruction procedure, the ankle is immobilized in a below-knee cast for 7 to 10 days. Then, a walking boot is used for 6 weeks. A Cam-Walker will allow early ROM. After immobilization, plantar and dorsiflexion exercises are begun, passive at first, and then active ROM exercises are performed as tolerated. Proprioceptive training is also started immediately once the cast is removed. Sports are permitted at 3 months after surgery. An ankle brace may be required during sporting activities for 6 to 9 months postoperatively.

The clinical results of anatomic reconstruction have been reported by various authors.[19, 67, 68] Gould and associates[62] reported a slightly different method of anatomic reconstruction of the lateral ligaments of the ankle with excellent clinical results. In his technique, after repair of the ATFL or CFL,

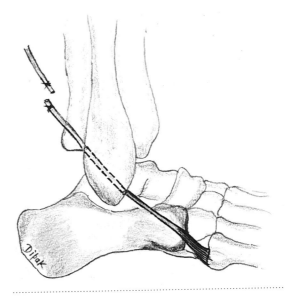

Figure 23–8. The Evans procedure for reconstruction of chronic ankle instability.

reinforcement using the lateral talocrural ligament and ankle retinaculum is made.

The commonly used tenodesis procedures include the Watson-Jones procedure,[70] the Evans procedure,[71] the Elmslie procedure,[69] and Chrisman and Snook's modification of the Elmslie procedure.[72] Basically, these techniques use either a split portion or complete section of the peroneus brevis tendon to reconstruct the lateral ligaments of the ankle.

The Watson-Jones procedure[70] is performed by sectioning the peroneus brevis tendon and directing it from posterior to anterior through a tunnel in the distal fibula, then through a tunnel in the neck of the talus, and back through a second drill hole in the fibula (Fig. 23–7). This technique reconstructs the ATFL more effectively than the CFL. Two difficulties may be encountered while performing the Watson-Jones technique: first, it may be difficult to drill a tunnel in the neck of the talus; second, the peroneus brevis tendon may be too short. The Evans technique[71] is performed by directing the transected peroneus brevis tendon through a drill hole in the distal fibula. Then the tendon is sutured back to the musculotendinous junction in an overlapping fashion (Fig. 23–8). The Elmslie procedure[69] involves lateral reconstruction of the ankle using a fascia lata graft.

Details of the operative techniques of an-

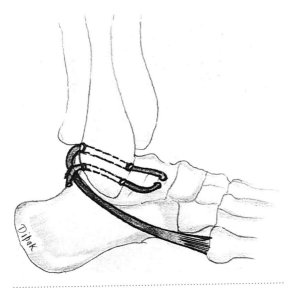

Figure 23–7. The Watson-Jones procedure.

atomic reconstruction and various tenodesis procedures have been reported in standard textbooks of foot and ankle surgery, and their detailed description is beyond the scope of this chapter. Satisfactory clinical results have been obtained using the Watson-Jones, Evans, and Elmslie procedures.

Chrisman and Snook[72] reported a modification of the Elmslie procedure whereby the ATFL and CFL are reconstructed using one half of the peroneus brevis tendon. The tendon is passed either through a subperiosteal tunnel along the neck of the talus or through a drill hole in the talus and then through the distal fibula, down to the os calcis (Fig. 23–9). The purpose is to enhance both lateral ankle and subtalar stability.

Snook and associates[65] reviewed the long-term results of this procedure and found that 45 of 48 ankles had excellent or good results and 3 had fair or poor results. The fair or poor results were caused by persistent lateral instability. These authors have slightly modified the procedure originally described in 1969 by (1) drilling a tunnel in the calcaneum, which is stronger and easier to make than the original "trapdoor" tunnel; (2) suturing the end of the graft in front of the lateral malleolus rather than at the base of the fifth metatarsal, thus providing a stronger repair; and (3) putting the foot and ankle in mild rather than forced eversion while the graft is sutured in place. We

believe that the Chrisman and Snook modification of the Elmslie procedure is useful for patients with chronic, symptomatic ankle and subtalar instability and for those who are engaged in strenuous athletic sports. In our experience with this technique, excellent lateral and anterior stability has been obtained. Some loss of subtalar motion may occur. In addition, the incision is long, and potential wound problems may occur.

St. Pierre and associates[63] reviewed the results of various reconstructive procedures (Evans procedure[71]; two modifications of the Elmslie procedure by Chrisman and Snook[72]; and the Watson-Jones procedure[70]). They found that there was no significant differences in the amount of postoperative pain, swelling, and functional instability among the just-mentioned reconstructive techniques. They concluded that excellent results can be obtained in greater than 90% of cases with any of these procedures provided they are technically correctly performed.

In performing the lateral reconstructions of the ankle, the status of the peroneal tendons should be noted because peroneal tendon instability may be concomitantly present in a patient with lateral instability of the ankle. Sobel and associates[77] reported an association between lateral ankle instability and dislocation of the peroneal tendons in a 29-year-old man. The Chrisman-Snook procedure was used to reconstruct the superior peroneal retinaculum and the lateral ligaments of the ankle. When reviewed at 2-year follow-up, the patient had returned to all athletic activities. His physical examination demonstrated a well-healed scar and stable peroneal tendons and ankle.

Longitudinal rupture of the peroneal tendons in association with lateral ankle sprain has been reported by Bassett and Speer.[78] One should be aware of such combined lesions. If a split in the peroneus brevis tendon is found at operation, it may preclude its use for reconstruction. In such cases, the peroneus brevis tendon should be repaired as part of the procedure. The ankle joint must be carefully explored for the presence of loose bodies from osteochondral injuries.

Functional Instability

The term *functional instability* was first used by Freeman and associates.[48, 79] Func-

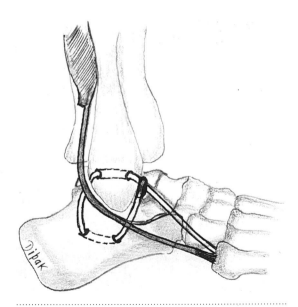

Figure 23–9. The Chrisman-Snook procedure.

tional instability is defined as a subjective feeling of giving way or recurrent sprains of the injured ankle, usually during physical activity. It implies motion beyond voluntary control but not necessarily exceeding the physiologic range of motion.[49] Functional instability is a complex syndrome in which neural (proprioception, reflexes, and muscular reaction time), muscular (strength, power, and endurance), and mechanical (lateral ligamentous laxity) factors are all possibly involved. Functional instability commonly affects physically active individuals and athletes.[34] It can occur with sporting activities or during activities of daily living, such as walking on uneven ground or pivoting to make a sharp turn. Its incidence has been reported to occur in approximately 15 to 60% of patients with injuries to the lateral ligamentous complex of the ankle[14, 15, 40, 49, 51, 56, 73, 79] Functional instability of the ankle seems to be independent of the severity (grade I, II, or III) of the initial injury.[40]

It is well known that, after an acute ankle injury, there is no correlation between the mechanical instability of the ankle and the patients' subjective complaints of functional instability. Freeman and associates[79] reported that functional instability of the ankle is usually due to motor incoordination consequent on capsular deafferentation (disorder of proprioception). Freeman and associates[79] performed a prospective, randomized trial and showed that the incidence of this sequela could be considerably reduced by a treatment program consisting of coordination exercises using an ankle tilt board. Freeman and colleagues' findings have been confirmed by Tropp[49] and Gauffin and associates.[50]

Treatment of Functional Instability

The treatment of functional instability mainly consists of a well-supervised ankle rehabilitation program. Peroneal muscle strengthening, Achilles tendon stretching, and proprioceptive training exercises are important components of ankle rehabilitation. Proprioceptive exercises are performed with the help of a tilt board or ankle disc to return balance and neuromuscular control to the ankle. Tilt board exercises should be continued for at least 10 weeks.

In recent years, external supporting devices (such as ankle taping or a brace) have become increasingly popular in the treatment of mechanical and functional instabilities of the ankle. Various studies have shown that ankle taping is of value in the prevention of ankle injuries.[80, 81] The ankle taping reduces supination and plantar flexion at the ankle. It has been reported that adhesive taping loses up to 50% of its original support after 10 minutes of exercise.[82]

Although patients subjectively often experience a positive effect when using ankle taping or a functional brace, the exact mechanism behind this positive effect is unknown. At the beginning of a performance, they provide a mechanical support. It has also been suggested that these devices provide increased proprioceptive feedback to the ankle.[22] Millar[83] suggested that this results from facilitation of signals from intramuscular and capsular receptors by the skin receptors. The psychologic effect of taping or bracing on the patient's mind should also be considered.

Criteria for Return to Sports

After an ankle sprain, several criteria must be met before allowing the patient to return to sports:

1. A full range of passive and active motion in the ankle should be obtained.
2. The patient should be able to walk and run without limping.
3. The patient should have at least 90% strength in the injured ankle compared with the strength in the normal, noninjured side.
4. The results of physical therapy functional assessment (such as single-leg hop test, high-jump, 30-yard zigzag run, or 40-yard shuttle run) should show greater than 90% performance before allowing the patient to return to normal practice schedule.
5. The patient should be able to reach his or her maximum speed in running and cutting before allowing return to full competition.

Failure to adhere to these guidelines may result in repeated ankle injuries with subsequent functional instability and disability, ultimately delaying a successful return to desired sports.

Chronic Ankle Pain After Inversion or Eversion Sprain

In a patient who presents with a chronic ankle pain after an inversion or eversion sprain, several lesions should be considered.

1. Osteochondral fractures (medial or lateral) of the dome of the talus should be ruled out. MRI or arthroscopy of the ankle, or both, is helpful in this setting. The treatment consists of arthroscopic or open debridement of the lesion and drilling of the base of the crater to promote healing.

2. Lateral impingement of the ankle can result from an overgrowth of the soft tissue along the anterolateral capsule. In a patient who presents with a refractory, symptomatic lateral impingement, arthroscopic debridement of the thick capsule may be necessary.

3. In a patient who presents with chronic ankle pain after an eversion sprain that has not responded to conservative measures, we have found that arthroscopic débridement of the synovium at the distal tibiofibular joint will lead to resolution of symptoms.

4. Sinus tarsi syndrome after an ankle sprain may also occur. This usually results from scar formation in the interosseous ligament area. Occasionally, it can also occur from ganglion formation in the sinus tarsi after ankle sprain.[84] In refractory cases, exploration of the sinus tarsi, with excision of the scar tissue, may be required to alleviate pain and restore ankle function.

5. Subluxation or dislocation of the peroneal tendons should be ruled out in a patient with a chronic lateral ankle pain. Stabilization of the peroneal tendons may be required for a patient presenting with a chronic, symptomatic subluxation or dislocation of the tendons.

6. Peroneal brevis tendon split should also be considered as a cause of chronic pain over the lateral aspect of the ankle. In a patient who has persistent lateral ankle symptoms that have not responded to nonoperative measures, exploration of the tendon and repair of the lesion are required.

SUMMARY AND FUTURE DIRECTIONS

Ankle sprain is one of the most common injuries sustained in both the nonathletic and the athletic patient population. We emphasize the importance of a good history and a detailed physical examination to obtain a correct diagnosis. Early appropriate treatment is required to enable patients to return safely to full function and sports without any residual morbidity.

Standard AP and lateral radiographs should be obtained for patients with a grade II or grade III ankle sprain. In addition, an AP view with the foot in 15 to 20° of internal rotation (mortise view) may be taken if one needs to evaluate the ankle mortise in detail. Some authors prefer to obtain stress radiographs (anterior drawer stress and inversion stress) for evaluation and documentation of the injury to the lateral ligamentous complex. However, we have not found this to be of significant value. In patients who present with a constant, unexplained pain and disability after an ankle sprain, selective use of other investigative modalities such as radioisotope bone scan, tomography, CT scan, and MRI may be of value. Ankle arthroscopy may be required in some cases to obtain a definitive diagnosis.

Patients who present with an acute ankle sprain are mostly treated by nonoperative measures. A functional treatment program consisting of rest, cold, compression, and elevation is begun immediately after an acute injury. Patients with a grade III lateral ankle sprain require a short period of immobilization (1–3 weeks), and then early controlled mobilization of the ankle is commenced. It should be noted that the eversion injuries of the ankle are slow to recover compared with inversion injuries. Early weight bearing is allowed within the limits of pain. After 3 weeks, the rehabilitation program consists of inversion and eversion exercises, stationary biking, proprioceptive tilt board training, and calf muscle–stretching exercises.

In patients who have a chronic mechanical instability of the ankle, a program of intensive rehabilitation is initially tried. If the patient fails to respond to conservative treatment, anatomic reconstruction of the ATFL and CFL (using the Brostrom procedure) is undertaken. If the tissue is insufficient or if the patient has a generalized ligamentous laxity, a Chrisman-Snook type of ankle reconstruction may be necessary. Factors such as patient's occupation, activity level, and sporting demand on the ankle should be considered before planning surgery.

The patient with functional instability of the ankle should initially be treated by a tilt board training program to improve proprioception and neuromuscular control of the injured ankle. Reconstruction of the ankle is required for patients who still have a persistent mechanical and functional disability despite adequate conservative measures. An organized functional rehabilitation program is then commenced to restore full mobility and strength in the ankle. The ultimate goal is to enable the patients to return to full function and sports without any residual symptoms in the ankle. We must ensure that the athletes are safely able to return to their respective sports at top performance level without aggravating or worsening the ankle injury.

REFERENCES

1. Ruth CJ. The surgical treatment of injuries of the fibular collateral ligaments of the ankle. J Bone Joint Surg Am 43:229, 1961.
2. Brooks SC, Potter BT, Rainey JB. Treatment for partial tears of the lateral ligament of the ankle: a prospective trial. BMJ 282:606, 1981.
3. McCulloch PG, Holden P, Robson DJ, et al. The value of mobilization and non-steroidal anti-inflammatory analgesia in the management of inversion injuries of the ankle. Br J Clin Pract 39:69, 1985.
4. Jackson DW, Ashley RL, Powell JW. Ankle sprains in young athletes: relation of severity and disability. Clin Orthop 101:201, 1974.
5. Sandelin J. Acute sports injuries: a clinical and epidemiological study. Thesis. Helsinki, Finland: University of Helsinki, 1988:1–66.
6. Maehlum S, Daljord OA. Acute sports injuries in Oslo: a one-year study. Br J Sports Med 18:181, 1984.
7. Nilsson S. Sprains of the lateral ankle ligaments: part II. Epidemiological and clinical study with special reference to different forms of conservative treatment. J Oslo City Hosp 33:13, 1983.
8. Mack RP. Ankle injuries in athletics. Clin Sports Med 1:71, 1982.
9. Glick JM, Gordon RB, Nishimoto D. The prevention and treatment of ankle injuries. Am J Sports Med 4:136, 1976.
10. Garrick JG. The frequency of injury, mechanism of injury, and epidemiology of ankle sprains. Am J Sports Med 5:241, 1977.
11. Hardaker WT Jr, Margello S, Goldner JL. Foot and ankle injuries in theatrical dancers. Foot Ankle 6:59, 1985.
12. Smith RW, Reischl SF. Treatment of ankle sprains in young athletes. Am J Sports Med 14:465, 1986.
13. Lassiter TE Jr, Malone TR, Garrett WE Jr. Injury to the lateral ligaments of the ankle. Orthop Clin North Am 20:629, 1989.
14. Balduini FC, Tetzlaff J. Historical perspectives on injuries of the ligaments of the ankle. Clin Sports Med 1:3, 1982.
15. Balduini FC, Vegso JJ, Torg JS, Torg E. Management and rehabilitation of ligamentous injuries to the ankle. Sports Med 4:364, 1987.
16. Rasmussen O. Stability of the ankle joint: analysis of the function and traumatology of the ankle ligaments. Acta Orthop Scand (Suppl) 211:1, 1985.
17. Brostrom L. Sprained ankles: I. Anatomic lesions in recent sprains. Acta Chir Scand 128:483, 1964.
18. Brostrom L. Sprained ankles: V. Treatment and prognosis in recent ligament ruptures. Acta Chir Scand 132:537, 1966.
19. Brostrom L. Sprained ankles: VI. Surgical treatment of "chronic" ligament ruptures. Acta Chir Scand 132:551, 1966.
20. Chapman MW. Sprains of the ankle. Instr Course Lect 24:294, 1975.
21. Diamond JE. Rehabilitation of ankle sprains. Clin Sports Med 8:877, 1989.
22. Drez DJ Jr, Kaveney MF. Ankle ligament injuries: practical guidelines for examination and treatment. J Musculoskeletal Med 6:21, 1989.
23. Ryan JB, Hopkinson WJ, Wheeler JH, et al. Office management of the acute ankle sprain. Clin Sports Med 8:477, 1989.
24. Lahde S, Putkonen M, Puranen J, Raatikainen T. Examination of the sprained ankle: anterior drawer test or arthrography. Eur J Radiol 8:255, 1988.
25. Linstrand A. Lateral lesions in sprained ankles: a clinical and roentgenological study with special reference to anterior instability of the talus. Thesis. Lund, Sweden: University of Lund, 1976:1–140.
26. Glasgow M, Jackson A, Jamieson AM. Instability of the ankle after injury to the lateral ligament. J Bone Joint Surg Br 62:196, 1980.
27. Seligson D, Gassman J, Pope M. Ankle instability: evaluation of the lateral ligaments. Am J Sports Med 8:39, 1980.
28. Grace DL. Lateral ankle ligament injuries: inversion and anterior stress radiography. Clin Orthop 183:153, 1984.
29. Korkala O, Rusanen M, Jokipii P, et al. A prospective study of the treatment of severe tears of the lateral ligament of the ankle. Int Orthop 11:13, 1987.
30. Johnson EE, Markolf KL. The contribution of the anterior talofibular ligament to ankle laxity. J Bone Joint Surg Am 65:81, 1983.
31. Renstrom P, Wertz M, Incavo S, et al. Strain in the lateral ligaments of the ankle. Foot Ankle 9:59, 1988.
32. Johannsen A. Radiological diagnosis of lateral ligament lesion of the ankle: a comparison between talar tilt and anterior drawer sign. Acta Orthop Scand 49:295, 1978.
33. Prins JG. Diagnosis and treatment of injury to the lateral ligament of the ankle: a comparative clinical study. Acta Chir Scand (Suppl) 486:3, 1978.
34. Niedermann B, Andersen A, Andersen SB, et al. Rupture of the lateral ligaments of the ankle: operation or plaster cast? A prospective study. Acta Orthop Scand 52:579, 1981.
35. Moller-Larsen F, Wethelund JO, Jurik AG, et al. Comparison of three different treatments for ruptured lateral ankle ligaments. Acta Orthop Scand 59:564, 1988.
36. Sommer HM, Arza D. Functional treatment of recent ruptures of the fibular ligament of the ankle. Int Orthop 13:157, 1989.
37. Black HM, Brand RL, Eichelberger MR. An improved technique for the evaluation of ligamentous injury in severe ankle sprains. Am J Sports Med 6:276, 1978.
38. Derscheid GL, Brown WC. Rehabilitation of the ankle. Clin Sports Med 4: 527, 1985.

39. Hamilton WG. Foot and ankle injuries in dancers. Clin Sports Med 7:143, 1988.
40. Schaap GR, de Keizer G, Marti K. Inversion trauma of the ankle. Arch Orthop Trauma Surg 108:273, 1989.
41. Viljakka T, Rokkanen P. The treatment of ankle sprain by bandaging and antiphlogistic drugs. Ann Chir Gynaecol 72:66, 1983.
42. Dupont M, Beliveau, P, Theriault G. The efficacy of antiinflammatory medication in the treatment of the acutely sprained ankle. Am J Sports Med 15:41, 1987.
43. Williamson JB, George TK, Simpson DC, et al. Ultrasound in the treatment of ankle sprains. Injury 17:176, 1986.
44. Michlovitz S, Smith W, Watkins M. Ice and high voltage pulsed stimulation in treatment of acute lateral ankle sprains. J Orthop Sports Phys Ther 9:301, 1988.
45. Hocutt JE Jr, Jaffe R, Rylander CR, Beebe JK. Cryotherapy in ankle sprains. Am J Sports Med 10:316, 1982.
46. Meeusen R, Lievens P. The use of cryotherapy in sports injuries. Sports Med 3:398, 1986.
47. Cote DJ, Prentice WE Jr, Hooker DN, Shields EW. Comparison of three treatment procedures for minimizing ankle sprain swelling. Phys Ther 68:1072, 1988.
48. Freeman MAR. Treatment of ruptures of the lateral ligament of the ankle. J Bone Joint Surg Br 47:661, 1965.
49. Tropp H. Functional instability of the ankle joint (medical dissertation no. 202. pp 1–92). Linkoping, Sweden: Linkoping University, 1985.
50. Gauffin H, Tropp H, Odenrick P. Effect of ankle disc training on postural control in patients with functional instability of the ankle joint. Int J Sports Med 9:141, 1988.
51. Staples OS. Ruptures of the fibular collateral ligaments of the ankle: result study of immediate surgical treatment. J Bone Joint Surg Am 57:101, 1975.
52. Redler I, Brown GG Jr, Williams JT. Operative treatment of the acutely ruptured lateral ligament of the ankle. Southern Med J 70:1168, 1977.
53. Brand RL, Collins MD, Templeton T. Surgical repair of ruptured lateral ankle ligaments. Am J Sports Med 9:40, 1981.
54. Jaskulka R, Fischer G, Schedl R. Injuries of the lateral ligaments of the ankle joint: operative treatment and long-term results. Arch Orthop Trauma Surg 107:217, 1988.
55. Henning CE, Egge LN. Cast brace treatment of acute unstable lateral ankle sprain: a preliminary report. Am J Sports Med 5:252, 1977.
56. Hansen H, Damholt V, Termansen NB. Clinical and social status following injury to the lateral ligaments of the ankle: follow-up of 144 patients treated conservatively. Acta Orthop Scand 50:699, 1979.
57. Drez D Jr, Young JC, Waldman D, et al. Nonoperative treatment of double lateral ligament tears of the ankle. Am J Sports Med 10:197, 1982.
58. Clark BL, Derby AC, Power GRI. Injuries of the lateral ligament of the ankle: conservative vs. operative repair. Can J Surg 8:358, 1965.
59. Gronmark T, Johnsen O, Kogstad O. Rupture of the lateral ligaments of the ankle: a controlled clinical trial. Injury 11:215, 1980.
60. Evans GA, Hardcastle P, Frenyo AD. Acute rupture of the lateral ligament of the ankle. To suture or not to suture? J Bone Joint Surg Br 66:209, 1984.
61. Kannus P, Renstrom P. Treatment for acute tears of the lateral ligaments of the ankle: operation, cast, or early controlled mobilization? J Bone Joint Surg Am 73:305, 1991.
62. Gould N, Seligson D, Gassman J. Early and late repair of lateral ligament of the ankle. Foot Ankle 1:84, 1980.
63. St. Pierre R, Allman F Jr, Bassett FH III, et al. A review of lateral ankle ligamentous reconstructions. Foot Ankle 3:114, 1982.
64. Cass JR, Morrey BF, Katoh Y, Chao EYS. Ankle instability: comparison of primary repair and delayed reconstruction after long-term follow-up study. Clin Orthop 198:110, 1985.
65. Snook GA, Chrisman OD, Wilson TC. Long-term results of the Chrisman-Snook operation for reconstruction of the lateral ligaments of the ankle. J Bone Joint Surg Am 67:1, 1985.
66. Sammarco GJ, DiRaimondo CV. Surgical treatment of lateral ankle instability syndrome. Am J Sports Med 16:501, 1988.
67. Ahlgren O, Larsson S. Reconstruction for lateral ligament injuries of the ankle. J Bone Joint Surg Br 71:300, 1989.
68. Karlsson J, Bergsten T, Lasinger O, Peterson L. Reconstruction of the lateral ligaments of the ankle for chronic lateral instability. J Bone Joint Surg Am 70:581, 1988.
69. Elmslie RC. Recurrent subluxation of the ankle joint. Ann Surg 100:364, 1934.
70. Watson-Jones R. Recurrent forward dislocation of the ankle joint. J Bone Joint Surg Br 34:519, 1952.
71. Evans DL. Recurrent instability of the ankle—a method of surgical treatment. Proc R Soc Med 46:343, 1953.
72. Chrisman OD, Snook GA. Reconstruction of lateral ligament tears of the ankle: an experimental study and clinical evaluation of seven patients treated by a new modification of the Elmslie procedure. J Bone Joint Surg Am 51:904, 1969.
73. Termansen NB, Hansen H, Damholt V. Radiological and muscular status following injury to the lateral ligaments of the ankle: follow-up of 144 patients treated conservatively. Acta Orthop Scand 50:705, 1979.
74. Gillespie HS, Boucher P. Watson-Jones repair of lateral instability of the ankle. J Bone Joint Surg Am 53:920, 1971.
75. Ottosson L. Lateral instability of the ankle treated by a modified Evans procedure. Acta Orthop Scand 49:302, 1978.
76. Althoff B, Peterson L, Renstrom P. Simple plastic surgery of inveterate ligament damage in the ankle joint. Lakartidningen 78:2857, 1981.
77. Sobel M, Warren RF, Brourman S. Lateral ankle instability associated with dislocation of the peroneal tendons treated by the Chrisman-Snook procedure: a case report and literature review. Am J Sports Med 18:539, 1990.
78. Bassett FH III, Speer KP. Longitudinal rupture of the peroneal tendons. Am J Sports Med 21:354, 1993.
79. Freeman MAR, Dean MRE, Hanham IWF. The etiology and prevention of functional instability of the foot. J Bone Joint Surg Br 47:678, 1965.

80. Garrick JG, Requa RK. Role of external support in the prevention of ankle sprains. Med Sci Sports Exerc 5:200, 1973.

81. Lindenberger U, Reese D, Andreasson G, et al. The effect of prophylactic taping of ankles. Thesis. Gothenburg, Sweden: Chalmers University of Technology, 1985.

82. Rarick GL, Bigley G, Karst R, Malina RM. The measurable support of the ankle joint by conventional methods of taping. J Bone Joint Surg Am 44:1183, 1962.

83. Millar J. Joint afferent fibres responding to muscle stretch, vibration and contraction. Brain Res 63:380, 1973.

84. Warren RF. Ganglion of the sinus tarsi: a case report. Am J Sports Med 8:133, 1980.

24 Lateral Ankle Instability: An Overview

Jan Willem K. Louwerens
Chris J. Snijders

Injury to the ligaments on the lateral side of the ankle and foot, caused by a sudden excessive inversion or torsion of the foot in relation to the leg, is probably the most common everyday injury of the locomotory system. Most of these injuries are sustained during sport, but, with increasing age, activities of daily life become a more dominant cause. It is estimated that one inversion injury of the ankle per 10,000 persons per day occurs. Despite adequate treatment, it is estimated that approximately 40% of the patients suffer from residual symptoms after sustaining this injury. These symptoms include recurrent sprains, "giving way" sensations, pain, swelling, and stiffness. The severity of these complaints is related to the level of demands regarding physical activities, but the great majority of the patients who note these complaints are not incapacitated by them. Presumably, only a small percentage of patients with chronic lateral instability consult a general practitioner or a specialist. On the basis of these percentages, it can be deduced that chronic lateral instability of the foot is a very common problem.

Multiple factors, such as dysfunction of the ligaments, proprioceptive deficit, and decrease of central motor control, are involved in this clinical syndrome. A review of the literature concerning these factors is presented in this chapter. Although assumptions are made in the literature regarding the role of the peroneal muscles, the influence of foot geometry, and the role of subtalar instability, little or no studies have actually quantified these factors or presented a standardized method to examine them. There are no reports regarding the influence of foot positioning or passive stability of the foot on chronic lateral instability.

ACUTE LATERAL LIGAMENT INJURIES

Epidemiology

Injury to the lateral ankle ligaments is a common, everyday injury. Both athletics and activities of daily life cause ankle ligament sprain.[1] Most ankle sprains occur in the 15- to 35-year age group.[2] The incidence is highest for young males. After the age of 40, the incidence becomes higher for women than for men. Most sprains are sustained during sport, but with increasing age other activities become dominant.[3] It has been estimated that there is one inversion injury of the ankle per 10,000 persons per day.[4–6] One third of West Point cadets were found to have sustained ankle sprains within a 4-year time period.[7] Ankle sprains account for 25 to 50% of injuries in sports such as soccer, basketball, volleyball and other sports that include running and jumping activities.[8] In The Netherlands, it is estimated that more than 500,000 persons consult their general practitioner or attend a hospital with ankle injuries every year. In 50% of cases, the injury was the result of a sporting accident.[9]

FUNCTION AND ANATOMY OF THE LATERAL ANKLE LIGAMENTS AND DAMAGE CAUSED BY AN INVERSION INJURY

Classically, the lateral ligament complex of the ankle is described as consisting of the anterior talofibular ligament (ATFL), the calcaneofibular ligament (CFL), and the posterior talofibular ligament (PTFL). The ATFL is a thickening in the anterolateral joint capsule. Its attachment is the anterior aspect of the lateral malleolus, close to the apex, and it proceeds forward and medially to gain insertion on the lateral aspect of the talar neck. The fibers run almost horizontally when the foot is in a neutral standing position. The ATFL primarily limits internal rotation of the talus.[10] Together with forces transmitted to the talus through the contact surfaces of the bones, this ligament plays a crucial role in bringing the talus into an external rotation, which results in inversion of the foot by the tarsal mechanism, as described by Huson.[11, 12] Thus, the function of this ligament is to tune the coupling of longitudinal rotation from the leg to the talus and vice versa by the talocrural joint. This ligament is not built to stabilize the foot or to carry the body weight and cannot resist high forces without active protection of the muscles. The function of the lateral ankle ligament complex is different from that of the medial ligament complex. The ligaments on the medioplantar side of the foot form a magnificent strong, thick structure and are built to stabilize the foot passively and to resist high forces, as during sporting activities.[13] The direction of the ATFL fibers varies according to the degree of dorsal or plantar flexion in the talocrural joint.[10, 14] The ATFL becomes taut and parallel to the tibia when the foot is plantar flexed. With further forced plantar flexion or inversion of the foot, this ligament tears. This finding is probably why so many authors stress the plantar flexion component in describing the trauma mechanism.[15] Broström, however, recorded that rupture of the lateral ankle ligaments was generally caused by internal rotation or adduction of the weight-bearing foot, and it seems logical that rotation is generally the more important component in the trauma mechanism. The ATFL is the most commonly injured lateral ligament.[15–17] Severing of the ATFL with its adjacent capsular structures results, depending on the position of the talocrural joint, in increased anterior talar translation and increased inversion or adduction of the talus within the talocrural mortise (this is usually called talar tilt [TT]). More importantly, the mechanism of talocrural transmission may be damaged,[18] resulting in an increase of tibiotalar delay, particularly in feet of patients with rather lax talocrural ligaments.[19] In clinical studies, this feature is described as anterolateral rotary instability; in this regard, the ATFL must be considered the "key ligament."

The CFL is an extra-articular structure. It extends from the tip of the lateral malleolus to the lateral surface of the calcaneus and is intimately associated with the posteromedial part of the peroneal tendon sheath. This ligament has an oblique orientation ranging from almost vertically downward to almost horizontally backward and is relaxed when the foot is in neutral position.[16] The CFL, being a biarticular structure, thus permits subtalar motion. The fibers are tensed when the foot is dorsiflexed and also during inversion of the foot, when they take in a more vertical orientation perpendicular to the joint.[14] The CFL inhibits inversion first and foremost.[10] It is rarely injured alone but is associated with ATFL tears in more severe injuries.[18] Damage results in further increase of inversion or adduction by 11 to 12°, independent of the position of the ankle.[10] Broström[17] observed that combined rupture of the talofibular and calcaneofibular ligaments occurred in less than 30% of his patients and that the calcaneofibular ligament was never ruptured alone. Rasmussen[10] stated that isolated cutting of the CFL did not influence inversion stability of the talocrural joint; however, Kjaersgaard-Anderson and colleagues[20] found an increased adduction in the talocalcaneal joint to a maximum of 5°, constituting two thirds of total increment in adduction of the hindfoot joint complex. They also found small, but relatively substantial, increments in external and internal rotation in the talocalcaneal joint, and thus concluded that this ligament is an important structure in stabilizing the movements of the hindfoot.[21]

The PTFL is the strongest ligament of the lateral ligament complex. It originates in the fossa of the lateral malleolus and spreads in the shape of a fan, its anterior short fibers inserting laterally on the posterior edge of the talus and its posterior long fibers inserting medially on the lateral tubercle of the posterior process of the talus.[14, 18] This ligament has no independent stabilizing function. The PTFL primarily inhibits external rotation and to some degree dorsiflexion.[10] The PTFL is rarely injured, except in severe ankle lesions.

DIAGNOSIS AND TREATMENT

The diagnosis and treatment of acute tears of the lateral ankle ligaments have received a vast amount of attention in the literature. In The Netherlands, it has been the subject of numerous theses.[9, 22–25] In clinical practice, sprains of the ankle have been classified as grade I (mild), II (moderate), and III (severe). Almost all authors agree that patients with a grade I or grade II injury recover quickly with a conservative treatment program, usually called functional treatment, and that the prognosis is almost without exception excellent or good. The treatment of acute complete (grade III) tears, however, has generated much controversy in the literature. Although the long-term prognosis is excellent or good in most patients, regardless of the treatment, some studies cited one reservation: the young, active athlete for whom primary operative repair should be considered.[26–28] In The Netherlands, Prins[18] and van der Ent[22] recommended operative repair as the basic method of treatment, and until recently 4000 acute ankle ligament ruptures per year were still treated operatively.[29] After a critical review of 12 prospective, randomized studies whose purpose was to identify the proper treatment of complete tears, Kannus and Renström[30] concluded that functional treatment is clearly the treatment of choice. Functional treatment with a bandage is the standard treatment propagated by the Dutch Society of General Practitioners.[31] Consequently, specific radiologic examinations such as arthrography or stress radiography are not indicated. Also the indication for routine radiography can be established on grounds of careful physical examination, and the number of X-ray examinations can be drastically reduced without harm to the patient and with appreciable reductions in workload, radiation levels, and costs.[9, 29]

Functional treatment includes ICE treatment (*ice, compression,* and *elevation*); involves only a short period of protection by tape, bandage, or a brace; and allows early weight bearing. Range of motion (ROM) exercises, as well as motor control training of the ankle and foot, should begin early. This program clearly provides the quickest recovery to a full ROM and return to work and physical activity. It does not compromise the late mechanical stability more or produce more late symptoms than the other treatments. In addition, functional treatment seems to be virtually free from complications, whereas after other methods, especially operation, serious complications sometimes occur.

There are other reasons to consider functional treatment as the treatment of choice. First, for patients who do need secondary operative reconstruction or delayed repair of the lateral ankle ligaments, the results of surgical treatment compare favorably with those of primary acute repair, also when performed years after the injury.[30, 32] Furthermore, in the cost-benefit analysis of functional versus operative treatment, functional treatment achieves excellent results for the majority of patients without the expense of hospitalization, surgery, and treatment of surgical complications. Functional treatment means enormous economic savings compared with operation, especially when one also considers that the great majority of ankle injuries can be treated by the specialist and do not need to be seen in emergency rooms.

In some situations, however, operation should be considered. Such situations include the presence of lesions such as displaced osteochondral fracture or large avulsions of bone. An elective operative procedure may also be appropriate when the injury is severe and combined with a long history of chronic instability and multiple severe sprains, despite adequate previous conservative treatment. Obtaining a complete medical history is important to discover patients at risk for complications, also with functional treatment. One of these risk factors is the presence of neuropathy. Severe deformation as a result of neuropathic disintegration of the foot and ankle can occur after a simple sprain of the ankle.

RESIDUAL COMPLAINTS AFTER ACUTE LATERAL LIGAMENT INJURY

Despite adequate treatment, 10 to 40% of patients suffer from residual symptoms after sustaining an acute lateral ligament injury.[18, 23, 26, 33–38] These symptoms include recurrent sprains, pain, swelling, stiffness and sensations of giving way. In a prospective study comparing four conservative methods of treatment of acute lateral ligament injuries, Zeegers[9] found that 30% of the patients complained of pain, and 44% suffered some degree of instability 5 years after their injury. The incidence of these chronic complaints might be thought to be surprisingly high; however, the great majority of the patients who note these complaints are not incapacitated by them. Linde and associates[37] performed a prospective study following 150 patients after functional treatment of a lateral ligament injury. After 1 month 90% were free from pain and 97% had resumed work. Sport was resumed by 70% of athletes after 1 month and 90% after 3 months. At 1-year follow-up (n = 137), 18% had not fully recovered and experienced pain (14%) or instability (7%) or had not resumed sport at their normal level (7%). Only 8% found the condition inconvenient. Increased risk of residual symptoms was clearly related to athletic activities and symptoms occurred in 32% of top athletes after 1 year. These findings are comparable with those of other studies. Hansen and colleagues[36] found that of 144 patients 20.8% had residual symptoms after a mean follow-up of 4.2 years. Only 4 patients had major complaints. The symptoms influenced work or sport if these activities severely strained the foot. Freeman[35] recorded an incidence of 39%. Almost all his patients were fit, young soldiers with high demands regarding sport and probably their complaints would have passed unnoticed in a sedentary life. As explained by van Dijk,[25] the variation in the percentage of residual symptoms can also be caused by other factors such as the duration of follow-up and the interpretation of the concept "residual symptoms."

CHRONIC LATERAL INSTABILITY

The diagnosis of chronic lateral instability relies primarily on the history. In the majority of cases, the history includes an injury of the lateral ligaments, but not all patients remember a primary injury. Patients complain of "giving way" sensations or the feeling of instability, pain, swelling, and actual reinjuries. These may occur during sports, walking on uneven ground, or activities of daily life.

Clinically, it seems practical to differentiate between patients who predominantly complain of pain, swelling, or stiffness and patients with mainly instability complaints. When patients mainly complain of pain, this can be attributed to several intra-articular lesions, such as chondral lesions, osteochondral lesions, intra-articular adhesions, and

pinching of perisynovial tissue.[39–42] Pain is typically related to activity when walking or running or to a particular sport. Pain located on the medial side of the ankle joint can be caused by injury of the cartilage with or without loose body formation as found arthroscopically by van Dijk[25] in a high percentage of patients after acute rupture of the lateral ligaments. Other diagnoses that should be looked for when rehabilitation does not progress as anticipated include fractures resulting from traction or compression around the "axis" of inversion, ligamentous injury in the lines of Chopart and Lisfranc, peroneal tendon subluxation or dislocation, Achilles tendon rupture, and reflex sympathetic dystrophy.[43]

Another patient group is formed by those who predominantly have instability complaints. They complain of "giving way" sensations and often of recurrent sprains. Typically, the patients say that they already give way or sprain the foot when they misstep on a small stone or walk on an uneven surface. Symptoms like pain and swelling are less prominent and are more related to actual reinjuries. Between injuries these patients generally walk without pain and without limping. Although they might present with synovitis because of recurrent sprains, there are otherwise no signs of intra-articular damage.

CAUSE OF CHRONIC LATERAL INSTABILITY

Mechanical Instability

In 1944 Bonnin[33] described the "hypermobile ankle" as a distinct entity capable of radiologic proof. He found unilaterally increased inversion in 24% of all sprained ankles and bilateral hypermobility in patients with severely sprained ankles in a higher percentage (42%) than in a group of controls (13%). He concluded that hypermobility, being excessive inversion tilt either of the talocrural or of the tarsal joints, was a prime factor in the incidence of sprains and produced a feeling of instability with complaints of "going over." Motion beyond the physiologic ROM will further be referred to as mechanical instability.

Other authors have also reported a significant correlation between mechanical instability and chronic lateral instability complaints.[17, 26, 44, 45] Karlsson[45] performed a radiographic investigation showing that a diagnosis of mechanical instability can be reached in more than 90% of the chronic unstable ankles. A so-called Telos device is used to perform stress radiography in a standardized manner. Two provocation tests are performed, one in the sagittal plane and one in the frontal plane. Thus, the amount of anterior talar translation (ATT) and the amount of inversion tilt of the talus (TT) within the ankle mortise are determined. Karlsson[45] defined the ATT as the shortest distance (in millimeters) between the posterior border of the joint surface of the distal tibia and the talus, as proposed by Landeros and associates.[46] The TT is measured as the angle made by the superior articular trochlear facet of the talus and the inferior tibial joint surface. He concluded that mechanical instability can be defined as an ATT of 10 mm or more and a TT of 9° or more, or a difference in ATT and TT between stable and unstable ankle joints of more than 3 mm and 3°, respectively.

The majority of the available literature on chronic lateral instability consists of reports on operative treatment. More than 50 procedures or modifications have been described.[45] Both nonanatomic and anatomic repairs are used to reconstruct the function of the injured ligaments. Although, most commonly, other indications than the presence of mechanical instability (based on radiographic criteria) are used to proceed to surgery, the fact that the outcome of these procedures is good and excellent in about 90% of the patients seems to indicate that mechanical stability plays an important role.[47]

Subtalar Mechanical Instability

Mechanical instability is most often located at the talocrural level. Since Rubin and Witten for the first time suggested the clinical significance of subtalar instability, this topic has received increasing attention.[48–55] Subtalar instability must be considered as a cause of symptoms after an inversion injury, particularly if other causes of instability have been excluded. Mechanical instability of the subtalar joint must also be considered when patients continue to complain of instability after reconstructive procedures, not taking into account reconstruction of a ruptured calcaneofibular ligament.[50, 54]

In addition to the calcaneofibular ligament, ligaments located in the sinus and canalis tarsi are reported to play a role in hindfoot instability. The sinus and canalis tarsi are located in the region between the neck of the talus and the anterosuperior surface of the calcaneus. The canalis tarsi, which is bordered by a sulcus in both the talus and the calcaneus, contains the interosseous talocalcaneal ligament centrally and extends medially in the canal and the three roots of the inferior extensor retinaculum laterally.[56–57] These roots are described as the intermediate and medial roots derived from a layer deep to the extensor tendons and a lateral root deriving from a superficial layer. In the sinus tarsi, slightly anterior to the intermediate root, is a relatively thick ligament, the cervical ligament, which passes from the neck of the calcaneus to the neck of the talus. Significant variability is described; however, in general, a lateral talocalcaneal ligament can be found crossing the posterior facet of the subtalar joint. This ligament is relatively narrow, thin, and parallel with, but slightly anterior to, the calcaneofibular ligament.

Isolated cutting of the calcaneofibular ligament results in increased inversion and rotation.[20–21] The increments found at the talocalcaneal level are small, but, because they involve a large percentage of total increment found in the tibiotalocalcaneal joint complex, they are considered important. The same arguments account for the situation found after cutting of only the ligaments of the sinus and canalis tarsi, which also results in small increments of inversion and rotation.[58] Zwipp and Tscherne[52] found tilting of the calcaneus of more than 5° and medial shift of more than 5 mm to be indicative of subtalar instability.

Different methods have been proposed for measuring instability of the subtalar joint.[48–52, 59] It seems that, in spite of continuing efforts, methods for documenting or quantifying inversion instability of the foot remain elusive.

Proprioceptive Deficit

Proprioceptive sensory feedback is used by the central nervous system for conscious appreciation of the position and movement of the body and limbs. It is suggested that proprioceptive deficit is caused by ligamentous and capsular trauma, which damages the many articular nerve fibers terminating in mechanoreceptors in the capsule and ligaments of joints.[60] Freeman and Wyke[61] described four types of receptors in feline ankle ligaments. It is thought that type I receptors provide postural sense to the central nervous system, type II receptors convey a sense of the beginning of joint motion, type III receptors provide sensation at the extremes of movement, and type IV receptors are responsible for nociceptive sensation. Michelson and Hutchins showed the presence of type II and III receptors to be abundant in human ankle ligaments.[62] They infrequently found type I receptors and were unable to demonstrate the presence of type IV receptors. Aside from the proprioception, it is suggested that the sensory output from mechanoreceptors in the ligaments assists in controlling muscle stiffness and coordination around a joint, thereby increasing stability. They are thought to have roles in kinesthesia, muscle tone, and articular reflexes.[63] Thus, rupture of ligaments may lead to partial joint deafferentation, and this leads to disturbances of control of locomotion and reflex behavior.

Freeman performed an extensive study of injuries to the lateral ligaments of the ankle.[35, 60, 64, 65] He introduced the term *functional instability* to designate the disability to which patients refer when they say that their foot tends to give way. He found that mechanical instability of the talus in the ankle mortise, in fact, rarely, if ever, was responsible for initiating functional instability. He concluded that (1) ligamentous injuries at the foot and ankle frequently produce a proprioceptive deficit affecting the muscles of the injured leg, (2) such a deficit is responsible for the symptom of giving way of the foot, and (3) the incidence of both the proprioceptive deficit and the symptom of giving way can substantially be reduced by treatment with coordination exercises. The finding of a prolonged peroneus reaction time in unstable legs seems to substantiate this theory. Studies have been performed using a trap door to elicit and simulate ankle sprains. Karlsson[45] used surface electromyography (EMG) to measure the time from tilting of the plate to the first response of the peroneus longus or brevis muscles. Comparing the symptomatic unstable and the asymptomatic stable ankles of patients with unilateral instability, he found that the mean reaction time was 68.8 ms (peroneus longus) and 69.2 ms (peroneus brevis) in the stable ankles compared with 84.5 and 81.6 ms, respectively, in the unstable ankles. Using a biomechanical model, he also suggested that the receptors are stimulated at a common fraction of the statically measured talar tilt angle.

Konradsen and Ravn[66] performed a similar study. However, they also measured EMG activity of the rectus femoris and biceps femoris muscles; in addition, joint movements of the ankle, knee, and hip were recorded, as were alternations of the body center of pressure using a force plate mounted under the trap door. The time from the first muscular response of the peroneus muscles to the first response over one of the upper leg muscles was defined as the central reaction time. Stable and unstable patients showed a similar reaction pattern to sudden inversion; first a peripheral reflex action, namely contraction of the peronei, and then a centrally elicited pattern by which the vertical pressure on the ankle is relieved through flexion of the hip and knee and dorsiflexion of the ankle. The central reaction time did not differ, but a prolonged peroneal reaction time (comparable with the results of Karlsson) was found in the unstable group. These findings suggest that functional instability is not associated with disturbance of the central processing, but substantiate the theory of a proprioceptive deafferentation being responsible for this entity.

To improve the sensitivity of one leg stabilometry, when compared with the method used by Tropp and associates,[67] Fridén and coworkers[68] performed a stabilometry in the frontal plane only. They not only analyzed the distance but also variables such as speed and frequency. Contrary to Tropp and associates,[67] they could well discriminate between the injured and the uninjured leg of patients with unilateral instability. Thus, their results seem to confirm the theory of Freeman.[60]

In a study of seven patients with normal joints, Konradsen and associates[69] tested active and passive position sense of ankle inversion, peroneal reflex reaction time, and postural control during single-leg stance. These tests were performed before and after regional anesthetic blockade of the ankle and foot. Passive position sense was greatly impaired by anesthesia, but active position sense, with the calf muscles activated, was preserved, and the peroneal reaction time was not altered. The stabilometric values were also unchanged by anesthesia. The authors suggested that the afferent input from intact ankle ligaments is important in seeing correct placement of the foot while walking, but that this input can be replaced by afferent information from active calf muscles. This mechanism might also be responsible for dynamic protection against sudden ankle inversion. The authors did not believe that higher centers quickly learned to replace afferent impulses from the ankle ligaments with those from the muscles and tendons, because the results from the last tests were no better than those from the first.

Central Coordination

Postural control is a complex function of cerebral, cerebellar, spinal, and peripheral afferent and efferent signals as well as muscle fiber function all working together to keep the line of gravity within the area of support.[61] Freeman and associates[65] suggested the use of the Romberg test to examine decrease of proprioception of the ankle and to evaluate functional instability. Tropp and colleagues[67, 70, 71] maintained this assumption and used stabilometry to objectify postural control and, following Freeman, assumed this method to evaluate proprioception of the ankle and functional instability. Stabilometry is a quantitative modified Romberg test. Information from a force plate (e.g., mark Kistler) is processed on line in a computer. The coordinates of the center of force of the patient when standing on one leg, in the x-y plane corresponding to the force plate, are calculated; thus, the total body sway in the frontal as well as in the sagittal plane is measured.

Tropp and coworkers[67, 70, 71] observed no difference between the injured and uninjured leg in a group of soccer players after a previous ankle joint injury; thus, they could not demonstrate that an injury itself produces functional instability. On the other hand, players without previous injury but showing abnormal stabilometric values ran a significantly higher risk of sustaining an ankle injury during the following season compared with players with normal values.[67] The stabilometric values of players with functional instability were abnormal but were not associated with a positive anterior drawer sign on clinical examination.[70, 71] Recording movements of different body segments in the frontal plane showed increased movement of upper body segments in patients with functional instability.[72] The results of stabilometry, and subjective giving way feeling, and control of the movement of the body segments could successfully be improved with coordination training on an ankle disk.[70, 73] Improvement reached even supranormal values, however, in the trained as well as the untrained foot. In summary, they found that (1) decreased postural control is associated with functional instability, (2) mechanical instability has no correlation to the degree of functional instability, (3) functional instability is associated with a higher risk for sustaining an ankle lesion, and (4) a deficit of central motor control and not of peripheral proprioception is associated with functional instability.

As reported, Fridén and associates[68] did find a difference between the injured and uninjured leg of patients with unilateral instability; however, they also found impaired postural control of the uninjured leg of these patients compared with the control group. Thus, they also concluded that impaired postural control is predisposing to lateral ligament injuries.

Peroneal Muscles

Bonnin[33] stressed the importance of mechanical instability. However, he also noted that hypermobility may be symptomless in people with developed muscular control. He suggested that exercise of the peroneal muscles was the method to develop muscle control. Peroneal weakness is thought to be a source of symptoms after an inversion injury.[32, 34, 74, 75] Tropp[75] associated peroneal muscle weakness with functional instability. They believed this weakness to be secondary to inadequate rehabilitation and to factors such as pain and immobilization. It is generally assumed that the peroneus muscles are not only involved in positioning the foot in the period about heel contact, but they protect the foot against inversion injuries. A peripheral reflex action with contraction of the peroneus muscles is described to counteract sudden ankle inversion.[66] However, there is controversy as to whether the peroneal muscles are active at all at the time of heel contact.[76–79]

Peroneal Nerve Palsy

Another factor that may be involved in the occurrence of functional instability is the possibility of palsy of the peroneal nerve. Peroneal nerve injuries after ankle sprains have been reported.[80, 81] A prolonged peroneal reaction time, as described previously, can also be caused by a lowered motor conduction velocity. Kleinrensink and associates[82] measured the motor conduction velocity of both the superficial and deep peroneal nerves in 22 patients. Three recordings were made starting 1 week after trauma and ending 5 weeks after trauma. A control group of 28 asymptomatic patients was also included. The conduction velocity of both nerves was found to be lowered directly after the injury, and in the following 5 weeks both nerves recovered to a collection velocity equal to that of the contralateral leg. The conduction velocity found in the patient group and control group proved to be equal with regard to the superficial nerve; however, the conduction velocity of the deep peroneal nerve in both the injured and uninjured leg of the patients was always lowered compared with that of the control group. This seems to indicate that the patients are characterized by a pre-existent low motor nerve conduction velocity of the deep peroneal nerve in both legs, thus predisposing them to inversion injuries.

FOOT BUILD AND FOOT POSITIONING

Functional anatomic studies have demonstrated how the foot in the weight-bearing situation moves from a neutral, more or less pronated position to a cavovarus position during inversion.[11, 12, 83, 84] From a biomechanical point of view, it is acceptable that a foot with a cavovarus configuration is more prone to lateral instability, because a smaller moment of force is needed to enforce further inversion. As soon as the point of calcaneal floor contact is reached medial to the line of body weight transmission and the axis of rotation proximal in the hindfoot, an inversion lever will be produced. The relation between a cavovarus foot build and chronic lateral instability has been supported by numerous reports.[55, 83, 85–89]

Foot build will influence the position of the foot. The position of the foot and the way the foot is placed on the ground during gait, however, is probably also determined by other passive and active factors.

GENERAL JOINT LAXITY

The ROM at a given joint follows a Gaussian distribution throughout the population.[90] At the extreme of range are patients with lax, hypermobile joints. Generalized hypermobility is associated with chronic lateral instability in numerous studies. Bonnin[33] differentiated between patients with bilateral instability and unilateral instability. The hypermobility found in the first group was believed to be congenital and to predispose to sprains. Hypermobility of the symptomatic foot of patients with unilateral instability was found to be the result of ligamentous rupture. Increase of tibiotalar delay, which clinically results in anterolateral instability complaints, is reported particularly to be found in patients with general joint laxity.[19] Karlsson[45] concluded that patients with generalized hypermobility of the joints should be considered poor risks when anatomic reconstructions are planned. In Kato's study,[59] many of the patients with subtalar joint instability had no history of injury, and he suggested that laxity of the interosseous talocalcaneal ligament may occur as one symptom of generalized joint laxity.

General joint laxity is generally associated with mechanical instability, but it was suggested that patients with hypermobility syndrome have poorer proprioceptive feedback than controls.[91]

TIBIOFIBULAR SPRAIN

Tibiofibular sprain has been reported as a cause of chronic lateral instability.[74, 92] Bonnin[92] found persistent pain at the lower tibiofibular joint and increased mobility of the fibula in the tibial groove at the injured side in a group of patients with chronic instability complaints. More recently, Löfvenberg and associates[93] recorded a slight increase of fibular rotations in patients with chronic lateral instability during plantar flexion and dorsiflexion and at adduction (inversion) in some patients with bilateral symptoms. They suggested that this perhaps reflects generalized joint laxity and not a separate pathophysiologic entity.

SINUS TARSI SYNDROME

The subjective manifestations of the sinus tarsi syndrome are diffuse pain on the lateral side of the foot; a feeling of hindfoot instability, especially when walking on uneven ground; and in most patients, a history of a supination trauma to initiate the complaints.[94-96] At examination, pain is provoked by pressure over the sinus tarsi and at attempt of supination. Meyer and Lagier[97] observed arthrographic features corresponding with synovial inflammation and fibrous scarring tissue in the lateral talocalcaneal recess in most of their patients with sinus tarsi syndrome. They found no disease at routine and stress radiographic examination. Zwipp and Tscherne,[52] however, determined talocalcaneal instability in a number of patients with this clinical syndrome. This association was also suggested by Kjaersgaard-Andersen and associates.[95]

TREATMENT OF CHRONIC LATERAL INSTABILITY

Most reports in the literature deal with the operative treatment of ankle instability. Some authors reported that conservative treatment was undertaken before surgery, but little is known regarding the specific type and outcome of this treatment. It is stated that conservative treatment should be tried for all patients with chronic lateral instability and is definitely indicated for less active, low demand, and minimally symptomatic patients.[47] No randomized studies report on the success rate of treating individuals with chronic unstable ankles by conservative means, as reported next.[47]

The common nonoperative treatment consists of physiotherapy modalities and taping and bracing. On the basis of the findings of the just-mentioned studies,[65, 71, 73, 75] muscle strengthening and tilt board or ankle disk training are emphasized. These exercises have shown to give objective and subjective improvement. Theoretically, these exercises address a whole range of the factors that seem to be involved in chronic lateral instability simultaneously. Probably as important as exercises to reestablish motor control is the prevention of reinjury and termination of the vicious circle of recurrent sprains and subsequent peripheral deficits. Both ankle taping and braces are used, and continuation of this treatment for 3 to 6 months is recommended.[32, 98] Taping has shown to decrease the incidence of ankle injury in basketball players.[1] In addition to restricting the extremes of ankle motion, ankle taping positively affects the proprioceptive function[99] and stimulates the peroneus brevis muscle round heel contact during gait.[76] However, the mechanical properties of ankle taping are dubious because it loses 40% of its effectiveness after 10 minutes.[76, 100]

More mechanical support is expected to be provided by an ankle orthosis. It may act by holding the ankle in a neutral position, thus preventing initiation of inversion, and it may also give more mechanical support to ligamentous structure.[101] Ankle orthotics, such as pneumatic ankle braces and lace-up braces, are reported to be more effective than taping in preventing ankle injuries in football players.[102] The use of a brace was found to compensate the decrease of postural control found in the symptomatic legs of patients with chronic lateral instability.[68]

Frequently, patients with significant mechanical instability can still function when these braces are worn in situations such as sports. Patients with chronic lateral instability can improve with functional rehabilitation; thus, conservative treatment should be attempted before surgical intervention.[32, 47] The indications for operative treatment are ill defined. Most authors report that failure of nonoperative management is an indication to proceed to surgery. Generally, positive stress tests (to examine increase of talar translation and increase of inversion at the talocrural and subtalar level) on clinical examination are also included as a criterion. The importance of finding an increase of anterior talar translation or increase of talar tilt using stress radiography to demonstrate instability preoperatively is controversial. Only a few authors found a good correlation between these findings and the subjective complaints of the patients and use radiographic criteria as an indication for surgery.[45] In one review article, it was concluded that surgery is indicated when chronic lateral instability occurs in the normal day-to-day situation in which a brace is not practical.[32] Others might include patients with higher physical demands regarding their work or sport.

More than 50 surgical techniques for reconstruction of the lateral ankle ligaments have been described. They can be divided into two groups: (1) reconstructions in which another structure or material substitutes for the injured ligament and (2) repairs in which the injured ligament is repaired secondarily with or without augmentation (anatomical repair). On the basis of a review of the literature, Peters and associates[47] recommend anatomic repair of the ligaments. They recommended a nonanatomic reconstruction, as described by Chrisman-Snook, based on its ability to reconstruct both the ATFL and the CFL for the treatment of patients with generalized joint laxity, greater than 10 years from time of injury to repair, significant arthritis, and failed anatomic repair.

SUMMARY

Although most authors choose to emphasize the importance of one certain factor, they cannot, however, deny the influence of other elements. For example, hypermobility as a result of general joint laxity found bilaterally is reported to be of importance but also hypermobility found unilaterally in an injured foot.[33] Both are mechanical factors, but in one group of patients this is a predisposing factor, and in other groups this is acquired. In the same study, it is reported that these factors might only result in symptoms in those individuals with less developed muscular control. Thus, not only mechanical factors but also muscle or motor control are involved. The same mix of different factors can be found in practically all studies. Karlsson[45] is one of the few authors to find a strong correlation between mechanical instability and the subjective complaints of the patients. However, he also reported on the finding of a prolonged peroneal reaction time in the symptomatic legs, which is generally explained to be the result of a proprioceptive deficit. Again, both mechanical and so-called functional

factors seem to be involved at the same time. Freeman[65] introduced the term *functional instability*, found no correlation between mechanical instability and the subjective complaints, and suggested proprioceptive deficit to be responsible for the symptoms. However, he also found that persistent varus instability of the talus plays a part in the cause in a small group of patients. Tropp[75] found decreased central postural control to be a predisposing factor correlating with symptoms of functional instability. In addition, he reported on peripheral deficits in the form of peroneal muscle weakness.[75] Friden and associates[68] were able to discriminate between the injured and the uninjured leg and found lesser postural control when patients stood on the injured leg. However, they also found the postural control in the uninjured leg to be impaired compared with the control group. Thus, both central predisposing factors as well as peripheral acquired factors are involved. The same can be concluded with regard to the lowered motor conduction velocity of the deep peroneal nerve found by Kleinrensink and associates.[82] The finding that hypermobility and poorer proprioceptive feedback might be associated would imply that proprioceptive malfunction can be either a predisposing or an acquired factor.[91]

Listing most of the factors that are involved in the cause of chronic lateral instability demonstrates that practically all factors have been reported both as predisposing and as acquired. Generally, two types of instability are described: mechanical and functional instability. One can now try to divide all factors into those that are in-

Table 24–1. Endogenous Passive and Active Factors that Determine Stability of the Foot

Passive	Active
Axes of rotation (determined by the geometry of the bones and articular surfaces)	Muscles Muscle forces are determined by central motor control, which, among others, depends on
Ligaments	Proprioceptive feedback
Soft tissue characteristics (e.g., stiffness)	Motor nerve conduction Muscle strength Concentration Vision

volved in mechanical stability and those that determine functional stability. However, from a biomechanical (and orthopedic) point of view, it is more practical to differentiate between passive and active factors (Table 24–1).

In conclusion, it is obvious from the previous review of the literature that multiple factors are involved in chronic lateral instability of the foot. There seems to be general consensus that numerous factors can play a role at the same time.

REFERENCES

1. Garrick JG, Requa RK. Role of external support in the prevention of ankle sprains. Med Sci Sports Exerc 5:200–203, 1973.
2. Boruta PM, Bishop JO, Braly WG, Tullos HS. Acute lateral ankle ligament injuries: a literature review. Foot Ankle 11: 107–113, 1990.
3. Hölmer P, Sondergaard L, Konradsen L, et al. Epidemiology of sprains in the lateral ankle and foot. Foot Ankle 15:72–74, 1994.
4. Brooks SC, Potter BT, Rainey JB. Treatment for partial tears of the lateral ligaments of the ankle: a prospective trial. BMJ 282: 606–607, 1981.
5. McCullouch PG, Holden P, Robson DJ, et al. The value of mobilization and non-steroidal anti-inflammatory analgesia in the management of inversion injuries of the ankle. Br J Clin Pract 2:69–72, 1985.
6. Ruth CJ. The surgical treatment of injuries of the fibular collateral ligament of the ankle. J Bone Joint Surg Am 43:229–239, 1961.
7. Jackson DW, Ashley RL, Powell JW. Ankle sprains in young athletes. Clin Orthop 101:201–215, 1974.
8. Mack RP. Ankle injuries in athletes. Clin Sports Med 1:71–84, 1982.
9. Zeegers AVCM. Het supinatieletsel van de enkel. Thesis. Utrecht, The Netherlands: University of Utrecht, 1995.
10. Rasmussen O. Stability of the ankle joint: analysis of the function and traumatology of the ankle ligaments. Acta Orthop Scand 56 (Suppl):211, 1985.
11. Huson A. Een ontleedkundig, funktioneel onderzoek van de voetwortel. Thesis. Leiden, The Netherlands: University of Leiden, 1961.
12. Huson A. Functional anatomy of the foot. In Jahss MH, ed. Disorders of the Foot and Ankle, vol 1, ed 2. Philadelphia: W. B. Saunders, 1991:409–432.
13. Bøjsen-Møller F. Physical properties of normal and injured ligaments. In Gotzen L, Baumgaertel F, eds. Hefte zur Unfallheilkunde, Bandverletzungen am Sprunggelenk. Grundlagen, Diagnostiek, Therapie, Hefte 204. Berlin: Springer-Verlag, 1989.
14. Vogel PL de. Enige functionaeel-anatomische aspecten van het bovenste sprongewricht. Thesis. Leiden, The Netherlands: University of Leiden, 1970.
15. Broström L. Sprained ankles: III. Clinical obser-
16. vations in recent ligament ruptures. Acta Chir Scand 130:560–569, 1965.
16. Broström L. Sprained ankles: I. Anatomic lesions in recent sprains. Acta Chir Scand 128:483–495, 1964.
17. Broström L. Sprained ankles: VI. Surgical treatment of "chronic" ligament ruptures. Acta Chir Scand 132:551–565, 1966.
18. Prins JG. Diagnosis and treatment of injury to the lateral ligament of the ankle: a comparative clinical study. Acta Chir Scand 486(Suppl):3–149, 1978.
19. Fievez AWFM, Spoor CW. A kinematical analysis of the ankle joint in relation to lateral ligamentous and capsular injuries. In Op de voet gevolgd (course book of the Boerhaave Committee for Postgraduate Courses of Leiden University). Leiden, The Netherlands: University of Leiden, 1987:101–112.
20. Kjaersgaard-Anderson P, Wethelund JO, Nielsen S. Lateral talocalcaneal instability following section of the calcaneofibular ligament; a kinesiologic study. Foot Ankle 7:355–361, 1987.
21. Kjaersgaard-Anderson P, Wethelund JO, Helmig P, Nielsen S. Effect of the calcaneofibular ligament on hindfoot rotation in amputation specimens. Acta Orthop Scand 58:135–138, 1987.
22. Ent FWC van der. Lateral ankle ligament injury. Thesis. Rotterdam, The Netherlands: University of Rotterdam, 1984.
23. Van Moppes FI, van den Hoogenband CR. Diagnostic and therapeutic aspects of inversion trauma of the ankle joint. Utrecht, The Netherlands: Bohn, Scheltema and Holkema, 1982.
24. Bleichrodt RP. Diagnostiek van letsels van het laterale enkelbandapparaat. Thesis. Groningen, The Netherlands: University of Groningen, 1987.
25. Van Dijk CN. On diagnostic strategies in patients with severe ankle sprain. Thesis. Amsterdam, The Netherlands: University of Amsterdam, 1994.
26. Broström L. Sprained ankles: V. Treatment and prognosis in recent ligament ruptures. Acta Chir Scand 132:537–550, 1966.
27. Gørnmark T, Johnsen O, Kogstad O. Rupture of the lateral ligaments of the ankle: a controlled clinical trial. Injury 11:215–218, 1980.
28. Korkala O, Rusanen M, Jokipii P, et al. A prospective study of the treatment of severe tears of the lateral ligament of the ankle. Int Orthop 11:13–17, 1987.
29. Van Linge B. De verstuikte enkel. Ned Tijdschr Geneeskd 132: 660–662, 1988.
30. Kannus P, Renström P. Current concept review: treatment for acute tears of the lateral ligaments of the ankle. J Bone Joint Surg Am 73:305–312, 1991.
31. Nederlands Huisarten Genootschap. Enkeldistorsie. Standaard MO4, Huisarts en Wetenschap 32:182–185, 1989.
32. Trevino SG, Davis O, Hecht PJ. Management of acute and chronic lateral ligament injuries of the ankle. Orthop Clin North Am 25:1–16, 1994.
33. Bonnin JG. The hypermobile ankle. Proc R Soc Med 37:282–286, 1944.
34. Bosien WR, Staples OS, Russel SW. Residual disability following acute ankle sprains J Bone Joint Surg Am 37:1237–1243, 1955.
35. Freeman MAR. Instability of the foot after injur-

ies to the lateral ligament of the ankle. J Bone Joint Surg 47:669–677, 1965.

36. Hansen H, Damholt V, Termansen NB. Clinical and social status following injury to the ligaments of the ankle joint. Acta Orthop Scand 50:669–704, 1979.

37. Linde F, Hvass I, Jurgensen U, Madsen F. Early mobilizing treatment in lateral ankle sprains: course and risk factors for chronic painful or function-limiting ankle. Scand J Rehabil Med 18:17–21, 1986.

38. Zwipp H, Hoffman F, Thermann H, Wippermann BW. Rupture of the ankle ligaments. Int Orthop 15:245–249, 1991.

39. Hutton PAN. Ankle lesions. In Jenkins DHR, ed. Ligament Injuries and Their Treatment. London: Chapman and Hall, 1985:95–112.

40. Biedert R. Anterior ankle pain in sports medicine: aetiology and indications for arthroscopy. Arch Orthop Trauma Surg 110:293–297, 1991.

41. Borelli AH. Osteochrondral fracture of the talofibular joint. J Am Podiatr Med Assoc 79:151–153, 1989.

42. Stone JW, Guhl JF. Meniscoid lesions of the ankle. Clin Sports Med 10:661–676, 1991.

43. DeMaio M, Paine R, Drez D Jr. Chronic lateral ankle instability-inversion sprains: part I. Orthopaedics 15:87–96, 1992.

44. Anderson KJ, Lecocq JF. Operative treatment of injury to the fibular collateral ligament of the ankle. J Bone Joint Surg Am 36:825–832, 1954.

45. Karlsson J. Chronic lateral instability of the ankle joint; a clinical, radiological and experimental study. Thesis. Goteborg, Sweden: University of Goteborg, 1989.

46. Landeros O, Frost HM, Higgins CC. Post-traumatic anterior ankle instability. Clin Orthop 56:169–178, 1968.

47. Peters JW, Trevino SG, Renstrom PA. Current topic review: chronic lateral ankle instability. Foot Ankle 12:182–191, 1991.

48. Rubin G, Witten M. The subtalar joint and the symptom of turning over on the ankle: a new method of evaluation utilizing tomography. Am J Orthop 4:16–19, 1962.

49. Laurin CA, Oellet R, St. Jacques R. Talar and subtalar tilt: an experimental investigation. Can J Surg 11:270–279, 1968.

50. Brantigan JW, Pedegana LR, Lippert FG. Instability of the subtalar joint: diagnosis by stress tomography in three cases. J Bone Joint Surg Am 59:321–324, 1977.

51. Zollinger H, Meier CH, Waldis M. Diagnostik der unteren Sprunggelenks-instabilitat mittels Stress-tomographie. In Hefte Unfallheilkd, Heft 165. Heidelberg: Springer-Verlag, 1983:175–177.

52. Zwipp H, Tscherne H. Die radiologische Diagnostik der Rotationsinstabilitat im hinteren unteren Sprunggelenk. Unfallheilkunde 85:494–498, 1982.

53. Zell BK, Shereff MJ, Greenspan A, Liebowitz S. Combined ankle and subtalar instability. Bull Hosp Joint Dis Orthop Inst 46:37–46, 1986.

54. Clanton TO. Instability of the subtalar joint. Orthop Clin North Am 20:583–592, 1989.

55. Vidal J, Fassio B, Buscayret Ch, et al. Instabilite externe de la cheville. Importance de l'articulation sous-astragalienne; nouvelle technique de reparation. Rev Chir Orthop 60:635–642, 1974.

56. Cahill DR. The anatomy and function of the contents of the human tarsal sinus and canal. Anat Rec 153:1–17, 1965.

57. Schmidt HM. Shape and fixation of band systems in human sinus and canalis tarsi. Acta Anat 102:184–194, 1978.

58. Kjaersgaard-Anderson P, Wethelund JO, Helmig P, Søballe K. The stabilizing effect of the ligamentous structures in the sinus and canalis tarsi on movements in the hindfoot: an experimental study. Am J Sports Med 16:512–517, 1988.

59. Kato T. The diagnosis and treatment of instability of the subtalar joint. J Bone Joint Surg Br 77:400–406, 1995.

60. Freeman MAR. Ligamentous injury: a study of injuries to the lateral ligament of the ankle. Thesis. Cambridge, England: Cambridge University, 1964.

61. Freeman MAR, Wyke B. The innervation of the knee joint: an anatomical and histological study in the cat. J Anat 101:505–532, 1967.

62. Michelson JD, Hutchins C. Mechanoreception in human ankle ligaments. J Bone Joint Surg Br 77:219–224, 1995.

63. Freeman MAR, Wyke B, Hanham IWF. Articular reflexes at the ankle joint: an electromyographic study of normal and abnormal influences of ankle-joint mechanoreceptors upon reflex activity in the leg muscles. Br J Surg 54:990–1001, 1967.

64. Freeman MAR. Treatment of ruptures of the lateral ligament of the ankle. J Bone Joint Surg Br 47:661–668, 1965.

65. Freeman MAR, Dean MRE, Habham IWF. The etiology and prevention of functional instability of the foot. J Bone Joint Surg 47:678–685, 1965.

66. Konradsen L, Ravn JB. Ankle instability caused by prolonged peroneal reaction time. Acta Orthop Scand 61:388–390, 1990.

67. Tropp H, Ekstrand J, Gillquist J. Stabilometry recordings in functional and mechanical instability of the ankle joint. Int J Sports Med 6:180–182, 1985.

68. Fridén T, Zatterstrom R, Lindstrand A, Moritz U. A stabilometric technique for evaluation of lower limb instabilities. Am J Sports Med 17:118–122, 1989.

69. Konradsen L, Ravn JB, Sørenson AL. Proprioception at the ankle: the effect of anaesthetic blockade of ligament receptors. J Bone Jont Surg 75:433–436, 1993.

70. Tropp H, Askling C, Gillquist J. Factors affecting stabilometry recordings of single limb stance. Am J Sports Med 12:185–188, 1984.

71. Tropp H. Functional instability of the ankle joint. Thesis. Linköping, Sweden: University of Linkoping, 1985.

72. Tropp H, Odenrick P. Postural control in single-limb stance. J Orthop Res 6:833–839, 1988.

73. Gauffin H, Tropp H, Odenrick P. Effect of ankle disk training on postural control in patients with functional instability of the ankle joint. Int J Sports Med 9:141–144, 1988.

74. Staples OS. Ruptures of the fibular collateral ligaments of the ankle. Result study of immediate surgical treatment. J Bone Joint Surg 57:101–107, 1975.

75. Tropp H. Pronator muscle weakness in functional instability of the ankle joint. Int J Sports Med 7:291–294, 1986.

76. Glick JM, Gordon RB, Nishimoto D. The prevention and treatment of ankle injuries. Am J Sports Med 4:136–141, 1976.
77. Shiavi R. Electromyographic patterns in adult locomotion: a comprehensive review. J Rehabil Res Dev 22:85–98, 1985.
78. Mann RA, Moran GT, Dougherty SE. Comparative electromyography of the lower extremity in jogging, running and sprinting. Am J Sports Med 14:501–510, 1986.
79. Van Linge B. Activity of the peroneal muscles, the maintenance of balance, and prevention of inversion injury of the ankle: an electromyographic and kinematic study. Acta Orthop Scand 59(Suppl 227):67–68, 1988.
80. Hyslop GH. Injuries to the deep and superficial peroneal nerves complicating ankle sprain. Am J Surg 51:436–438, 1941.
81. Nitz AJ, Dobner JJ, Kersey D. Nerve injury and grades II and III ankle sprains. Am J Sports Med 13:177–182, 1985.
82. Kleinrensink GJ, Stoeckart R, Meulstee J, et al. Lowered motor conduction velocity of the peroneal nerve after inversion trauma. Med Sci Sports Exerc 26:877–883, 1994.
83. Benink RJ. The constraint-mechanism of the human tarsus: a radiological experimental study. Acta Orthop Scand (Suppl)215:1–135, 1985.
84. van Langelaan EJ. A kinematical analysis of the tarsal joints: an x-ray photogrammetric study. Acta Orthop Scand (Suppl)204:1–269, 1983.
85. Ayres MJ, Bakst RH, Baskwill DF, Pupp GP. Dwyer osteotomy: a retrospective study. J Foot Surg 26:322–328, 1987.
86. Bremer SW. The unstable ankle mortise-functional ankle varus. J Foot Surg 24:313–317, 1985.
87. Lassiter TE, Malone TR, Garrett WE. Injury to the lateral ligaments of the ankle. Orthop Clin North Am 20:629–639, 1989.
88. Subotnick SI. The biomechanics of running: implications for the prevention of foot injuries. Sports Med 2:144–153, 1985.
89. Larsen E, Angermann P. Association of ankle instability and foot deformity. Acta Orthop Scand 61:136–139, 1990.
90. Wood PHN. Is hypermobility a discrete entity? Proc R Soc Med 64:690–692, 1971.
91. Hall MG, Ferrel WK, Sturrock RD, et al. The effect of the hypermobility syndrome on knee joint proprioception. Br J Rheumatol 34:121–125, 1995.
92. Bonnin JG. Editorials and annotations. Injury to the ligaments of the ankle. J Bone Joint Surg Br 47:609–611, 1965.
93. Löfvenberg R, Karrholm J, Selvik G. Fibular mobility in chronic lateral instability of the ankle. Foot Ankle 11:22–29, 1990.
94. O'Connor D. Sinus tarsi syndrome: a clinical entity. J Bone Joint Surg Am 40:720, 1958.
95. Kjaersgaard-Andersen P, Soballe K, Pilgaard S. Sinus tarsi syndrome: presentation of seven cases and review of the literature. J Foot Surg 28:3-6, 1989.
96. Taillard W, Meyer JM, Garcia J, Blanc Y. The sinus tarsi syndrome. Int Orthop 5:117–130, 1981.
97. Meyer JM, Lagier R. Post-traumatic sinus tarsi syndrome: an anatomical and radiological study. Acta Orthop Scand 48:121–128, 1977.
98. Drez D, Young JC, Wladman D. Nonoperative treatment of double lateral ligament tear of the ankle. Am J Sports Med 10:197–200, 1982.
99. Karlsson J, Andreasson GO. The effect of external ankle support in chronic lateral ankle joint instability: an electromyographic study. Am J Sports Med 20:257–261, 1992.
100. Laughmann RK, Carr TA, Chao EY. Three dimensional kinematics of the taped ankle before and after exercise. Am J Sports Med 8:425–431, 1984.
101. Tropp H, Askling C, Gillquist J. Prevention of ankle sprains. Am J Sports Med 13:259–262, 1985.
102. Rovere GD, Clarke TJ, Yates CS. Retrospective comparison of taping and ankle stabilizers in preventing ankle injuries. Am J Sports Med 15:228–233, 1988.

25

The Chronically Unstable Ankle: Anatomic, Biomechanical, and Neurologic Considerations

Gerrit J. Kleinrensink
Chris J. Snijders
Rob Stoeckart

Injuries of the locomotor system are generally self-limiting, because the human body has a tremendous capacity of self-healing. Exclusively in serious cases, assistance of an expert is needed: a general practitioner, a physiotherapist, a podiatrist or orthopedic surgeon, or another specialist. In discussing dysfunction of the locomotor system, two different approaches must be discerned: clinical-practical and scientific-theoretical. In both views, anatomy plays an important role, although the questions asked in these disciplines are different.

First, we examine the clinical-practical point of view. In treating patients with pain or dysfunction of the locomotor system, attention is generally focused on localizing the structure causing the pain. For this, knowledge of topographic anatomy is essential. For localization of the injured structure and subsequent (surgical) treatment, knowledge of the topographic anatomy is relevant. However, in many cases, no structural disease can be found while the patient is complaining of pain and dysfunction, sometimes for a very long period. Often structural damage is found and treated, but complaints recur and become chronic. In these cases, one must address the questions of "Why is this structure injured?" and "How can reinjury be prevented?" Then, a more scientific-theoretical approach is needed. Functional anatomy and the closely related biomechanics play an important role.

In the clinical-practical line of thought, posture and motion are often "translated" into two closely related aspects: joint stability and joint mobility. These aspects are illustrated by discussing cause and effects of inversion trauma. Ankle stability is generally thought to be based on intact joint capsule and ligaments. After inversion trauma, stretched or torn ligaments are supposed to

be the cause of the instability. Treatments, varying from tape bandages to reconstructive surgery of ligaments, focus on the healing of anatomic structures. Generally, these treatments are effective, but about 30% of patients keep complaining about instability of the ankle, reinjury, fear of giving way, and fear of reinjury.[1-3] Because the collagen of the ligaments is structurally healed and restored to its original strength within 6 to 12 weeks, "something else" must be responsible for the chronicity of the injury. Here we have to focus on the discrepancy between load and capacity. In normal gait, the loading of the ankle joint is estimated to be about three times body weight (about 200 kg/cm² for a 70-kg person). Strength tests of the anterior talofibular ligament have shown that the tensile strength of this ligament at failure is about 70 kg/cm². To compensate for forces arising during normal walking, and more so during running and jumping, ligaments are not sufficient; leg muscles are needed in addition. To fulfill this task, muscles have to be recruited in time. This implicates the introduction of the central and peripheral part of the nervous system. Here the concept of the arthrokinetic reflexes,[4] also called joint protecting reflexes, offers a useful model. In addition to capsule and ligaments, now seen as "structures containing receptors," several other elements come into the picture: joint and muscle receptors (proprioceptors), the afferent and efferent nerves of the ankle joint (the peroneal nerves), the spinal cord, and higher parts of the central nervous system (e.g., cerebellum, cerebral cortex).

In fact, the situation is rather complex because even a minor trauma like inversion trauma has widespread effects. For instance, alterations in the electromyogram (EMG) of the gluteal muscles[5] and in the

354

motor nerve conduction velocity (MNCV) of the contralateral deep peroneal nerve[6] show that also other regions of the ipsi- and contralateral extremity have to be taken into account. It is not unusual that the affected structures are separately seen as a specific cause of pain and dysfunction. However, their interaction or, better, the lack of interaction is probably more important.

Before trauma, all structures can be assumed to function in a more or less harmonious and coordinated way, creating joint stability. At a certain moment, this obviously changes; as a result, the ligaments are damaged: inversion trauma. So the question should be transformed from "*Why* are the ligaments injured?" to "Why are *the ligaments* injured?" In inversion trauma, the ligaments are the "victims" of abnormal loading or of a system (temporarily) out of order. The ligaments should not be seen as the structural cause of trauma but merely as the weakest link in a set of structures involved in a chain of events leading to inversion trauma. Each link of the chain must be analyzed on its specific qualitative and quantitative contribution; otherwise, there is the risk of underestimating the role of an essential link. For instance, adequate treatment of the ligamentous injury can nevertheless result in chronic complaints of pain and instability if treatment is restricted to the ligaments.

RELATIONSHIP BETWEEN INVERSION TRAUMA AND LOWERED MOTOR NERVE CONDUCTION VELOCITY OF THE PERONEAL NERVES

Since Cohen proposed the "arthrokinetic reflex" as the mechanism for stabilizing joints,[4] several authors accepted ankle stability to be dependent on an intact reflex mechanism.[7-10] They suggested that functional instability is predominantly caused by injured joint receptors (disturbed propriocepsis). The possibility of lowered MNCV as a possible cause is not mentioned, but in our view this can be an additional factor. For instance, it could explain the prolonged peroneal muscle reaction time in patients suffering from chronic instability of the ankle, found by Konradsen and Ravn.[10]

To analyze the possibility of peroneal nerve lesion after inversion trauma, we as-

sessed the MNCV of the superficial and deep peroneal nerves. The MNCV of both nerves turned out to be lowered after inversion trauma, and we hypothesized that this was due to a traction lesion. In discussing a traction lesion, it is relevant to know whether the nerve is stretched beyond its critical limit (Fig. 25-1).

Stretch of the Peroneal Nerves: Normal Range of Motion Versus Inversion Trauma

Because of a variety of compensating mechanisms, normally damage to the peroneal nerves will not occur from normal range-of-motion (ROM) inversion.[11-14] However, during inversion trauma, extensive displacement can take place. Stretching a peripheral nerve beyond a certain percentage of in vivo length leads to acute and long-term deficiencies in intraneural circulation and thus to alterations in the conduction properties.[12, 15, 16] In rabbit tibial nerve irreversible functional deficit has been shown after strain of more than 12%.[17]

In determining whether inversion stretches the superficial and deep peroneal nerves beyond critical values, four factors should be considered. First, the length of the nerve segment over which the elongation has to be compensated for. Assuming the total length of the peroneal nerve to be 100 cm from radix to the end of the intermediate cutaneous nerve, a 3-cm displacement of the nerve at the lateral side of the foot results in an elongation of 3%. However, the peroneal nerve has an awkward position just distal to the caput fibulae. Here the nerve enters a musculotendinous arch in the peroneus longus muscle. In about 40% of anatomic preparations, we found a strongly diminished gliding mechanism, and in 20% this mechanism was not present at all (unpublished data). In the latter cases, the total length over which the elongation has to be compensated for is about 50 cm, enlarging the elongation to 6% in normal inversion. Furthermore, where the nerve pierces the crural fascia, an analogous entrapment can be expected.[18] With a fixation of the nerve at this site, a 3-cm elongation has to be compensated over about 20 cm, whereas an elongation of 15% is probably already in the critical area.

Second, the total amount of displacement

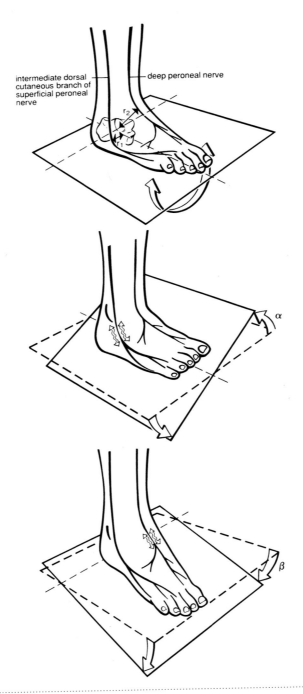

Figure 25–1. Because of its relative lateral position on the dorsum of the foot, displacement of the superficial peroneal nerve at the level of the ankle occurs especially through the supination component of inversion. Displacement of the deep peroneal nerve is mainly due to the plantar flexion component of inversion. The displacement of both nerves is mainly due to the plantar flexion component of inversion. The displacement of both nerves can be seen as a part of a circle. According to the equation $S = \alpha \times r$, with $\alpha = 45°$ (0.8 rad) and $r_1 = 4$ cm in *normal* inversion, a 3-cm displacement of the intermediate dorsal cutaneus branch of the superficial peroneal nerve has to be compensated for. For the branches of the deep peroneal nerve, $\beta = 45°$ and $r_2 = 5$ cm, a 4-cm displacement has to be compensated for.

in the foot is of importance. When the entire body weight is exerted to the inverted ankle, a larger inversion angle and, consequently, a larger nerve displacement can be expected.

A third factor is the velocity of the traction forces. In daily life, marked dysfunction is not likely to occur because the traction force will be exerted gradually and slowly. In inversion trauma an abrupt, fast traction will be exerted on the nerve. Such an accelerated force is much more damaging to the nerve.[19, 20]

The last factor that has to be taken into account is the simultaneity of traction and compression forces. In moving the foot medially (adduction component of inversion), the fibular head becomes a pulley to the peroneal nerve. In rounding this pulley, an additional transverse force is exerted, resulting in compression of the nerve. Actually the nerve is double crushed.

Considering these four facts, it is obvious that a lesion of the peroneal nerves can occur as a result of inversion trauma.

Whether there is a clinically relevant relationship between inversion trauma and lowered MNCV was the object of a series of studies.

LOWERED MOTOR NERVE CONDUCTION VELOCITY OF THE PERONEAL NERVES *AFTER* INVERSION TRAUMA

It must be stated that MNCV values of both the superficial and deep peroneal nerves after trauma did not correlate with the clinical (mechanical) grading of the inversion trauma. Patients with grade I inversion trauma (i.e., little or no pain, swelling, or mechanical instability) could have a large (up to 30%) decrease of MNCV compared with control group values and vice versa. This might indicate the necessity of adding functional testing to mechanical grading.

Superficial Peroneal Nerve

Four to 8 days after trauma, the MNCV of the superficial peroneal nerve in the injured leg was significantly reduced compared with both the contralateral leg and the control group values (Table 25–1, Recording I). Recordings II and III (18–22 and 32–36 days after trauma) do not show significant differences (see Table 25–1). Apparently recovery occurred within 3 weeks after trauma.

Deep Peroneal Nerve

For the deep peroneal nerve 4 to 8 days after trauma, significant differences in MNCV were found only between injured leg and control group values (Table 25–2). Within the 5-week follow-up period, this difference did not disappear, showing that for this nerve recovery did not occur in this period. Whether recovery did occur at all could not be ascertained.

When compared with the contralateral leg, 4 to 8 days after trauma, the MNCV of the injured leg was not lowered. This unexpected finding can be explained by the fact that MNCV values of the contralateral (uninjured) leg were also lower when compared with control group values. Lowered MNCV in the uninjured leg could mean either of the following:

1. The inversion trauma also affects the deep peroneal nerve of the contralateral leg.

Table 25–1. Mean ($\pm$ SD) Motor Nerve Conduction Velocities of Superficial Peroneal Nerve Between the Knee and Caput Fibulae

Group	Recording I* (4–8 days post trauma)	Recording II† (18–22 days post trauma)	Recording III‡ (32–36 days post trauma)	Linear Trend in Recordings I, II, III
Injured leg	52.0 ± 6.3	55.0 ± 10.2	58.3 ± 8.9†	Yes ($P < 0.05$)
Contralateral leg	60.8 ± 8.8*	58.0 ± 10.3	60.8 ± 9.8	No
Control group	60.5 ± 7.0*	63.0 ± 10.3‡	61.0 ± 9.7	No

* Compared with injured leg: $P < 0.01$.
† Compared with Recording I: $P < 0.05$.
‡ Compared with injured leg: $P < 0.05$.

Table 25–2. Mean (±SD) Motor Nerve Conduction Velocities of Deep Peroneal Nerve

Group	Recording I	Recording II	Recording III	Linear Trend
Caput fibulae-ankle				
Injured leg	44.6 ± 3.0	45.7 ± 3.4	46.6 ± 0.0††	Yes ($P < 0.05$)
Contralateral leg	45.5 ± 3.3	45.5 ± 3.6	46.3 ± 3.5	No
Control group	48.0 ± 2.5*†	49.6 ± 3.6*†	49.1 ± 4.0*†	No
Knee-ankle				
Injured	44.5 ± 2.4	46.0 ± 3.0**	46.4 ± 2.9†	Yes ($P < 0.05$)
Contralateral leg	45.7 ± 3.1	45.7 ± 3.6	46.4 ± 2.6	No
Control group	49.0 ± 2.8*†	50.0 ± 4.3*†	49.29 ± 4.2*¶	No
Knee-caput fibulae				
Injured	50.1 ± 9.2	52.5 ± 10.5	55.1 ± 10.0	No
Contralateral leg	55.5 ± 8.5	55.3 ± 9.9	56.5 ± 8.2	No
Control group	57.0 ± 11.8‖	60.4 ± 12.0‖	55.3 ± 9.2	No

* Compared with injured leg: $P < 0.01$.
† Compared with contralateral leg: $P < 0.01$.
‡ Compared with injured leg: $P < 0.02$.
§ Compared with contralateral leg: $P < 0.02$.
‖ Compared with injured leg: $P < 0.05$.
¶ Compared with contralateral leg: $P < 0.05$.
** Compared with Recording I: $P < 0.01$.
†† Compared with Recording I: $P < 0.05$.

This possibility is supported by both the findings of Gauffin[21] and the tendency of MNCV values of the contralateral leg to increase during the 5-week period of this study (see Table 25–2).

2. The patients are characterized by a pre-existent low MNCV of the deep peroneal nerve in both legs, predisposing them for inversion trauma. To investigate this possibility, a prospective study in volunteer soldiers of the Royal Dutch Infantry was performed.

LOWERED MOTOR NERVE CONDUCTION VELOCITY OF THE PERONEAL NERVES *CAUSED BY* INVERSION TRAUMA

From the first study, it can be concluded that after inversion trauma patients showed a relatively low MNCV of the peroneal nerve. Because preinjury values of MNCV were not available, it could not be established whether the low MNCV was pre-existent or whether it was actually caused by inversion trauma. To study this causal relationship, we assessed the MNCV of the peroneal nerve before and after trauma.

In this study, preinjury MNCV values (Recording I) were obtained from a group very homogenous in age, length, gender, activities, and even footwear. MNCV of the deep and superficial peroneal nerves was measured in both legs of 120 healthy male recruits of the Dutch Royal Army (age range, 18–26 years; mean age, 20.4 ± 2.0 years). Measurements were performed within the first 3 weeks after entering military service. During the following 3-month training period, 9 recruits suffered an inversion trauma. Two of them were lost for posttrauma follow-up because of detachment in another army camp. Seven recruits (age range, 19–23 years; mean age, 20.8 ± 1.7 years) were available for all posttrauma measurements. Four to 8 days after trauma, the MNCV in the Caput-Ankle and Knee-Ankle segments of the deep peroneal nerve of the injured leg was significantly lowered compared with preinjury values. This proves a causal relationship between inversion trauma and lowered MNCV of the deep peroneal nerve. Although in the superficial peroneal nerve values statistical significance was not reached, a tendency in lowering of the MNCV values was observed.

Eighteen to 22 days after trauma, MNCV values in the just-mentioned two segments of the deep peroneal nerve of the injured leg tended to be higher compared with both preinjury and control values. This is not in line with the results of our previous study, in which MNCV was still significantly lower 32 to 36 days posttrauma compared with control values. Probably this discrepancy is related to a difference in treatment. In the previous study, the patients were immobilized rather rigidly (semirigid bandage for 4 or 6 weeks) compared with the patients in this trial (tape bandage for 10 days followed by remobilization). We assume that the fast recovery of MNCV in the second study is due to the beneficial effects of early remobilization and exercise.[22, 23] Besides these findings, some other interesting observations have to be discussed.

RISK OF USING NORMAL OR REFERENCE VALUES

Four to 8 days after trauma, MNCV values in all four segments of the contralateral leg tended to be lower than MNCV values of the control group. This is consistent with our previous findings. However, compared with their own baseline (preinjury) values, the MNCV of the contralateral leg tended to increase. This discrepancy needs attention because normally clinicians do not have the opportunity to compare a patient's post-trauma and pretrauma values. They have to rely on "normal" values. The necessity to be cautious in comparing patient data with "normal" data becomes even more poignant when realizing that in this study the reference ("normal") values are obtained from a group perfectly comparable with the patients and exceptionally homogenous. The increase in the MNCV of the contralateral leg seen after trauma compared with baseline values is remarkable but not unexpected. We assume that as a result of trauma the contralateral legs were used more intensively. Also, in this case, we attribute this increase in MNCV in the contralateral legs to the effect of exercise.[22, 23] In fact, during the trial period, not only did MNCV values of the contralateral leg tend to rise but those of the controls did as well. This could reflect a general increase of peroneal activity as a result of the (military) training.

CONCLUSIONS

The results of both studies support the hypothesis of an injury to the peroneal nerve caused by inversion trauma. In the concept of the joint stabilizing "arthrokinetic" reflexes, such a deficiency can jeopardize the functional stability of the ankle joint in two ways. First, normally the relevant muscles function as a spring, absorbing and storing energy. In this way, large forces can be neutralized by muscle action. Second, there is an important relation between muscle action and the bony and articular configuration of the foot. In this regard, it is helpful to recall the work of Bojsen-Møller.[24] In his considerations about stability of the foot, he emphasizes that pronation is the most stable position of the foot, especially needed in running; in pronation the foot is in its close-packed position. To establish these positions, it is essential to recruit the pronating muscles, especially the peroneal muscles. When there is a lengthened reaction time of these muscles because of a lowered MNCV of the peroneal nerves, stability of the foot is seriously endangered. When no adequate measures are taken, normal loading patterns (e.g., walking, jumping) can already be hazardous to the joint, leading to secondary inversion trauma and eventually to chronic instability of the ankle joint.

Finally, MNCV measurements performed with surface electrodes mean practically no extra inconvenience to the patient and do not take much time. In contrast to, for instance, depolarization potential measurements, MNCV measurements can be performed within 4 to 8 days after trauma. These advantages can make MNCV measurements (in addition to mechanical testing) a useful tool in the early assessment and therapy of functional instability of the ankle joint.

REFERENCES

1. Van de Ent FWC. Lateral ankle ligament injury. Doctoral thesis. Rotterdam, The Netherlands: Erasmus University, 1984.
2. Homminga GN, Kluft O. Long-term inversion stability of the ankle after rupture of the lateral ligaments. Neth J Surg 38:103, 1986.
3. Schaap GR, De Keizer G, Marti K. Inversion trauma of the ankle. Arch Orthop Trauma Surg 108:273, 1989.
4. Cohen LA, Cohen ML. Arthrokinetic reflex of the knee. Am J Physiol 184:433, 1956.
5. Bullock Saxton JE, Janda V, Bullock MI. The influence of ankle sprain injury on muscle activation during hip extension. Int J Sports Med 15:330, 1994.
6. Kleinrensink GJ, Stoeckart R, Meulstee J, et al. Lowered motor conduction velocity of the peroneal nerve after inversion trauma. Med Sci Sports Exerc 26:877, 1994.
7. Freeman MAR, Wyke BD. Articular contributions to limb muscle reflexes (1). J Physiol 171:20P, 1964.

8. Freeman MAR. Instability of the foot after injuries to the lateral ligaments of the ankle. J Bone Joint Surg Br 47:669, 1965.

9. Freeman MAR, Dean MRE, Hanham IWF. The etiology and prevention of functional instability of the foot. J Bone Joint Surg Br 47:678, 1965.

10. Konradsen L, Ravn B. Ankle instability caused by prolonged peroneal reaction time. Acta Orthop Scand 61:388, 1990.

11. Sunderland S, Bradley KC. Stress strain phenomena in denervated peripheral nerve trunks. Brain 84:125, 1961.

12. Sunderland S. Traumatized nerves, roots and ganglia: musculoskeletal factors and neuropathological consequences. In Korr IM, ed. The Neurobiologic Mechanisms in Manipulative Therapy. New York: Plenum Press, 1977:137.

13. Lundborg G. Nerve Injury and Repair. Edinburgh: Churchill Livingstone, 1988:91.

14. Millesi H, Zöch G, Rath TH. The gliding apparatus of peripheral nerves and its clinical significance. Ann Hand Surg 9:87, 1990.

15. Lundborg G, Rydevik B. Effects of stretching the tibial nerve of the rabbit: a preliminary study of the intraneural circulation and the barrier function of the perineurium. J Bone Joint Surg Br 55:390, 1973.

16. Lundborg G. Structure and function of the intraneural microvessels as related to trauma, edema formation and nerve function. J Bone Joint Surg Am 57:938, 1975.

17. Kwan MK, Wall EJ, Massie J, Garfin SR. Strain, stress and stretch of peripheral nerve: rabbit experiments in vitro and in vivo. Acta Orthop Scand 63:267, 1992.

18. Kopell HP, Thompson WAL. Peripheral entrapment neuropathies. New York: Robert E. Krieger, 1976:36.

19. Mumenthaler M, Schliack H. Läsionen peripherer Nerven. Diagnostik und Therapie, ed 4. Stuttgart: Thieme Verlag, 1982:23.

20. Rydevik BL, Kwan MK, Myers RR, et al. An in vitro mechanical and histological study of acute stretching on rabbit tibial nerve. J Orthop Res 8:694, 1990.

21. Gauffin H. Knee and ankle kinesiology and joint instability. Doctoral thesis. Linköping, Sweden: University of Linköping, 1991.

22. Sale DG, Upton ARM, McComas AJ, MacDougall JD. Neuromuscular function in weight-trainers. Exp Neurol 82:521, 1983.

23. Kamen G, Taylor P, Beehler PJ. Ulnar and posterior tibial nerve conduction velocity in athletes. Int J Sports Med 5:26, 1984.

24. Bojsen-Møller F. Calcaneocuboid joint and stability of the longitudinal arch of the foot at high and low gear push off. J Anat 129:165, 1979.

26 Fractures of the Ankle

Craig S. Bartlett III
David L. Helfet
Ely L. Steinberg

HISTORY

Ankle fractures are among the most common injuries seen by the orthopedic surgeon. Reports of their treatment date back to the time of Hippocrates in the fifth century B.C.[1] when he recommended traction for closed fractures. For open fractures, he delayed reduction for at least 7 days, believing that if performed earlier the patient would die from "inflammation and gangrene." Until the 18th century, diagnosis was based on clinical findings without the benefit of radiography or surgical observation, and most of the cases reported were sporadic. However, for the first time, physicians tried to explain the mechanism of the injury. In 1775, Pott noted the importance of the fibula in the treatment of ankle fracture.[2] By the beginning of the 19th century, other studies focused on the mechanism of the injury in cadavers.[2] Since then, more and more experiments have been performed and reported with regards to the structure and function of the ankle joint and the mechanisms of the injury. These have led to a better understanding of the stabilizing function of the surrounding ligaments and the mechanism of pure abduction or rotation of the syndesmosis.

The introduction of radiology at the beginning of this century made fracture assessment and diagnosis both easier and more accurate.[3] This allowed clinical reports and treatment to be objectively based on x-ray imaging.[4, 5] Closed treatment and immobilization in a plaster cast could be assessed by the x-ray film.

However, the unsatisfactory results of closed treatment, combined with advances in technology, better design of surgical instruments, and improvements in anesthesia, encouraged many surgeons to try operative treatment.[3, 6] At first, open reduction was limited to failed closed reduction, fractures of the medial or lateral malleolus, and dislocation of the joint.[7–9] With increased improvement of implant technology and introduction of antibiotics to prevent infection, more surgeons tried to achieve an anatomic reduction by surgery.

Even today, as experience continues to be gained, the indications for open reduction and fixation of fractures are constantly being extended. Still, good results are reported with closed treatment as well, and treatment decisions must be made based on the personality of the fracture.[6, 10–13] Certainly, accurate anatomic reduction and early ankle mobilization provide the best outcomes, a goal achieved mainly by open reduction and internal fixation (ORIF).[14–17]

ANATOMY

The ankle is a synovial joint surrounded by a thin capsule. Although primarily functioning as a hinge, there is a component of rotation and widening during flexion and extension.[2, 13]

OSSEOUS. The ankle joint consists of three bones: tibia, fibula, and talus. The tibial articular surface is composed of the tibial plafond (pilon) and the medial malleolus (Fig. 26–1A–C). The lateral malleolus on the most distal part of the fibula stabilizes the ankle from the lateral side. Body weight is transferred through the tibial plafond to the talus. The plafond is mildly concave and continuous with the medial malleolus, a bony prominence on the medial aspect of the distal tibia. On the posterior part of the medial malleolus, a groove exists for the tibialis posterior tendon. The lateral side of the tibial plafond articulates with the fibula. Posterolaterally lies the posterior malleolus, a slight prominence, and, medial to this, a groove for flexor hallucis longus tendon.

The lateral malleolus is a bony promi-

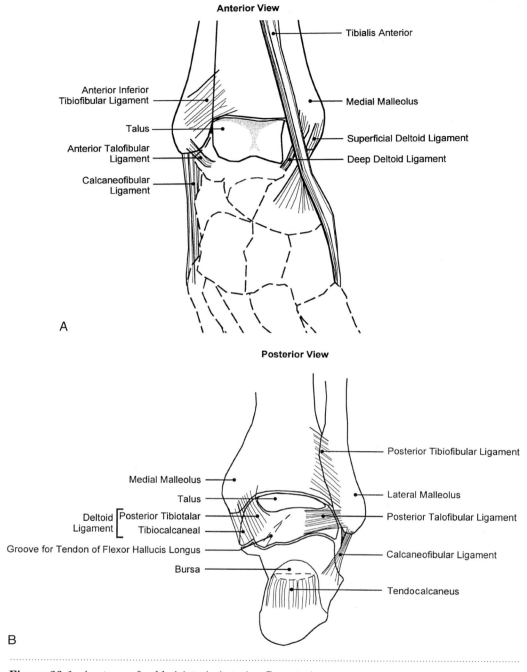

Anterior View

Tibialis Anterior

Anterior Inferior Tibiofibular Ligament

Talus

Anterior Talofibular Ligament

Calcaneofibular Ligament

Medial Malleolus

Superficial Deltoid Ligament

Deep Deltoid Ligament

A

Posterior View

Medial Malleolus

Talus

Deltoid Ligament — Posterior Tibiotalar / Tibiocalcaneal

Groove for Tendon of Flexor Hallucis Longus

Bursa

Posterior Tibiofibular Ligament

Lateral Malleolus

Posterior Talofibular Ligament

Calcaneofibular Ligament

Tendocalcaneus

B

Figure 26–1. Anatomy of ankle joint: *A,* Anterior; *B,* posterior.

nence on the lateral aspect of the distal fibula. It is more posterior and projects further distally than the medial malleolus. Medially, its triangular surface is covered by cartilage and articulates with the talus. A groove on the posterolateral aspect of the lateral malleolus is for the peroneus brevis tendon.

The talus transfers body weight from the tibia to the calcaneus. Its convex superior surface is covered by cartilage and articulates with the tibial plafond. This surface is

Lateral View

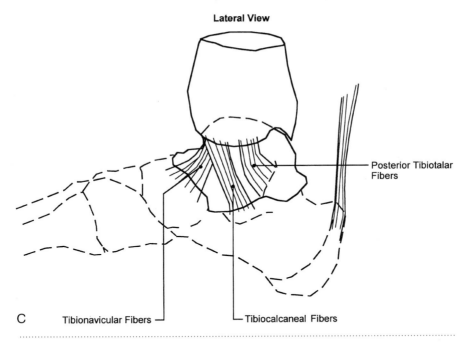

Posterior Tibiotalar Fibers

C   Tibionavicular Fibers —   — Tibiocalcaneal Fibers

Figure 26–1 *Continued. C,* Lateral.

continuous medially and laterally, covering the talar body and articulating on both sides with the medial and lateral malleoli.

LIGAMENTS. Ankle stability is provided by the periarticular ligaments. On the medial aspect of the ankle is a double-laminar ligament known as the deltoid ligament. It is a triangular ligament originating from the medial malleolus and inserting posteriorly on the talus and calcaneus and anteriorly to the ligaments of the talonavicular joint. On the plantar aspect of the foot, the deltoid ligament blends into the plantar fascia, which extends from the calcaneus to provide support for the longitudinal arch. Its superficial layer prevents valgus displacement and the deeper layer, lateral translation.

On the posterior aspect of the ankle is a complex consisting of two main ligaments: posterior tibiotalar and posterior talofibular. This complex is strengthened by the posterior tibiofibular ligament.

The lateral (fibular) collateral ligaments are divided into three groups: posterior talofibular, calcaneofibular, and anterior talofibular.

One of the most important structures that maintains ankle stability is the syndesmotic ligament complex. It is made up of the anterior tibiofibular, posterior tibiotalar, transverse tibiofibular, and interosseous ligaments. Some stability between the distal tibia and fibular is also provided by the interosseous membrane.

CAPSULE AND SYNOVIAL MEMBRANE. The ankle is covered by a thin hyaline capsule. This capsule is attached to the articulating surfaces of the joint and, to some degree, the intracapsular portion of the talar neck.

TENDONS. On the medial side of the ankle lie the tendons of the main muscles for inversion: tibialis posterior, flexor hallucis longus, and flexor digitorum longus. Posteriorly lie the tendons of the triceps surae (tendocalcaneus, Achilles tendon) and the plantaris. The former is the main plantar flexor of the foot. Laterally are the tendons of the main evertors of the foot: peroneus longus and peroneus brevis. Anteriorly are the tendons of the dorsiflexors: tibialis anterior, extensor digitorum longus, extensor hallucis longus, and peroneus tertius.

NEUROVASCULAR STRUCTURES. The anterior neurovascular bundle is composed of the anterior tibial artery and deep peroneal nerve. It crosses the joint between the tibialis anterior and the extensor hallucis longus. On the medial aspect of the ankle, a neurovascular bundle consisting of the posterior tibial artery and tibial nerve passes behind the posterior part of the medial malleolus. Anteriorly to the medial malleolus, the saphenous nerve and vein pass the joint. The superficial peroneal nerve crosses the lateral side of the joint anteriorly and the sural nerve posteriorly to the lateral malleolus.

Applied Anatomy

ANTERIOR ASPECT. Keeping the ankle in neutral position (90° to the tibial shaft), the tibialis anterior tendon can be observed in the anteromedial aspect on the ankle. On both sides of the ankle are the two prominences, the medial and lateral malleoli. Between them and lateral to tendon of the tibialis anterior, the pulsation of the anterior tibial artery can be felt.

MEDIAL ASPECT. The most prominent structure is the medial malleolus. The pulsation of the posterior tibial artery can be felt behind the posterior cortex of the medial malleolus.

POSTERIOR ASPECT OF THE ANKLE. The lateral malleolus is more posterior than the medial malleolus. The most posterior structure is the Achilles tendon.

LATERAL ASPECT. The lateral malleolus is anterior to the Achilles tendon. Adjacent and posterior to this are the peroneus longus and brevis tendons.

BIOMECHANICS AND MECHANISM OF INJURY

Biomechanics

The ankle joint absorbs the load from the limb. This load is centered on the midline of the ankle and divided in two vectors. The first is oriented posteriorly toward the heel and calcaneus, and the second anteriorly toward the foot. The latter passes through the neck of the talus, navicular, cuneiforms, and metatarsals.

Normal range of motion of the ankle joint is between 20° of dorsiflexion and 20 to 30° of plantar flexion. Some authors have described different values. This includes a total range of motion of 62° by Hicks,[18] 30 to 50° dorsiflexion and 20 to 30° plantar flexion by Kapandji,[19] and 32.5° for dorsiflexion and 44.7° for plantar flexion by Lindsjö.[20] Ten degrees of dorsiflexion is required for normal activities, whereas 20 to 30° is necessary for most sporting endeavors.[20]

Inman[21] showed that the talus is not a perfect hinge joint, with the body of the talus closely resembling a section of a frustum (a shape cut from a cone with the apex oriented medially). During motion, the lateral malleolus translates laterally as much as 2.0 mm.[21, 22]

Four groups of muscles cross and affect the ankle joint:

1. Dorsiflexors, adductors, and supinators: tibialis anterior and extensor hallucis longus

2. Dorsiflexors, abductors, and pronators: peroneus tertius and extensor digitorum longus

3. Plantar flexors, abductors, and pronators: peroneus brevis and peroneus longus

4. Plantar flexors, adductors, and supinators: tibialis posterior, flexor digitorum longus, flexor hallucis longus, and triceps surae (gastrocnemius and soleus)

During ankle motion the subtalar joint is also affected by these muscles. The resulting maximal contraction of triceps surae muscle in plantar flexion is associated with adduction and supination.[19] In normal walking, two phases are recognized: stance and swing. The stance phase is typically described in terms of five segments: initial contact, loading response, midstance, terminal stance, and preswing. Swing phase has been described in terms of initial swing, midswing, and terminal swing.

At initial contact, the ankle is slightly plantar flexed. As the limb moves into the next segment, the ankle joint dorsiflexes. At midstance phase, the ankle remains in a dorsiflexed position. In the terminal stance, the ankle plantar flexes. In the next phase of initial swing, the ankle moves toward dorsiflexion position. In terminal swing, the knee extends for heel strike, and the ankle plantar flexes.

Mechanism of Injury

The pattern of ankle injury is affected by many factors, especially patient age, bone quality, and direction and magnitude of the force. More than 40 years ago, Lauge-Hansen contributed significantly to our present understanding of the ankle fracture mechanism.[52, 53] He emphasized the influence of foot position and the forces acting on the ankle at the time of the injury. These forces include adduction, abduction, dorsal and plantar flexion, and rotation. Pronation and supination forces are generated around the axis of the subtalar joint. Adduction and abduction forces result from rotation of the talus around the long axis. Internal and external rotational movements are around the long axis of the tibia.

Lauge-Hansen also created a two-word classification system, later duplicated by Pankovich. The first word refers to the position of the foot at the time of the trauma, and the second indicates the direction of the force that causes the injury.[23, 24] There are four main fracture patterns (Fig. 26–2) discussed next. A fifth pattern, vertical shear, leads to fractures of the tibial plafond. Lauge-Hansen described the four stages as the injury progresses.[26–28]

SUPINATION-ADDUCTION (SAD) INJURY. The foot is in supination, and an adduction force inwardly rotates the lateral side of the ankle, stressing the lateral ligament complex and resulting in either rupture of the ligaments or avulsion of the lateral malleolus. Next, the talus is forced medially, creating a fracture of the medial malleolus.

SUPINATION-EXTERNAL ROTATION (SER) INJURY. The foot is in supination, and the force rotates it externally. The anterior syndesmosis of the ankle tightens and tears or avulses a fragment of bone from the tibia (Tillaux-Chaput) or fibula (Wagstaffe-Lefort). The force then externally rotates the lateral malleolus, producing a spiral fracture, mainly up to the level of the syndesmosis. The third stage involves posterior tibiofibular ligament tearing or avulsion from the posterior malleolus (Volkmann's triangle). The fourth and final stage involves tearing of the deltoid ligament or avulsion of medial malleolus.

PRONATION-ABDUCTION (PAB) INJURY. The foot is in pronation, and the force is directed externally. This results in an avulsion fracture of the medial malleolus. The force drives the talus into the lateral malleolus, resulting in rupture of the syndesmosis and oblique fracture of the lateral malleolus above the syndesmosis.

PRONATION-EXTERNAL ROTATION (PER) INJURY. The pronated ankle is forced into external rotation. This higher energy injury involves an avulsion of the malleolus or deltoid ligament tear. The rotation moment will next tear the syndesmosis and the interosseous membrane. The third stage results in a high spiral fibular fracture at or above the syndesmosis. In some cases, this fracture is very high, in the proximal fibula (Maisonneuve fracture).[2, 25]

PHYSICAL EXAMINATION

A complete history of the event should be recorded. Age, previous injuries, general health condition, drugs, and activity level are all important for making a definitive treatment decision. One must first observe any deviation of normal ankle joint con-

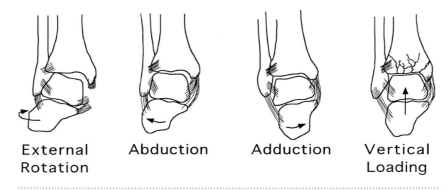

External
Rotation   Abduction   Adduction   Vertical
Loading

Figure 26–2. Biomechanics of the ankle fracture.

tours. Unless rapid radiographic evaluation is available, any ankle dislocation should be reduced immediately and immobilized in a padded splint. A careful evaluation of the skin is vital to identify lacerations, blisters, swelling, and discoloration. It is important to palpate all bony landmarks and localize any pain, crepitus, and bone tenderness. Pathologic motion of the ankle or the subtalar joint should be recorded. The joints should be stressed to rule out ligamentous rupture with instability. The presence or absence of medial (deltoid) injury/tenderness is a very important finding; it is used in selecting the conservative versus operative reduction.[7]

The anterior drawer maneuver evaluates the anterior talofibular ligaments. The knee is flexed in 90°, and the ankle is in neutral position. The foot is held in place, and a backward force is applied to the tibia. Posterior translation of the tibia with respect to the talus compared with the contralateral joint implies ankle instability. Inversion stress to the foot tests the lateral calcaneofibular ligament. Eversion stress in neutral position is to assess the deltoid ligament.

To complete the examination, a neurovascular evaluation is mandatory, especially after a crush injury. If there is any suspicion of impending compartment syndrome, it is imperative to measure the intracompartmental pressures of the lower extremity.

RADIOGRAPHIC EVALUATION

The standard trauma radiographs to be taken include the anteroposterior (AP), lateral, and mortise views (Fig. 26–3A–C).

ANTEROPOSTERIOR VIEW. This view is taken with the foot in neutral in line with the long axis of the leg. It images the malleoli and the distance between them, the tibial plafond, and the talar dome.

LATERAL VIEW. The foot is in neutral, and the x-ray beam is perpendicular to the long axis of the leg. The congruency of the talus on the tibia is best visualized with this view. Posterior and anterior dislocation of the talus and foot and fracture of the anterior or posterior margins are best diagnosed using this view.

MORTISE VIEW. This view is an anteroposterior view obtained with the leg internally rotated approximately 15 to 20° It visualizes the distance between the malleoli and talar congruity and shift.

Radiographic Measurements

Radiographic measurements are as follows (Fig. 26–4A, B).[4]

TIBIOFIBULAR LINE. This is a continuous line of the tibia and fibula in relation to the talar dome and is best evaluated on the mortise view.

TALOCRURAL ANGLE. On the mortise view, this angle is determined by the intersection of a line parallel to the tibial plafond or the talar dome and a line between the tips of both malleoli. This normally ranges from 8 to 15°.

TALAR TILT. This is determined on the AP view by two parallel lines, one along the distal tibial surface and the second along the talar dome. Up to 1.5° is accepted as normal. With an inversion stress, up to 5° is considered acceptable.

MEDIAL CLEAR SPACE. On the mortise view, this is the distance between the medial malleolus and the medial talar surface. This space should be the same size as the distance between the tibial plafond and the talar dome.

TIBIOFIBULAR OVERLAP. On AP view, the distal tibia is anterior and medial to the fibula. Thus, the anterolateral border of the tibia normally overlaps the fibula by 10 mm. A smaller overlap is indicative of syndesmotic injury.

Stress Tests

Stress roentgenograms should be performed if there is suspicion of a ligamentous injury. Any stress views of the injured ankle should be compared with those of the uninjured side. For lateral ligament evaluation, an AP view and a mortise view are taken with the ankle in inversion and the foot in plantar flexion. More than 5° of talar tilt indicates ligament injury. For anterior tibiotalar ligaments, a lateral view is taken with the foot in neutral, and the force is applied to the

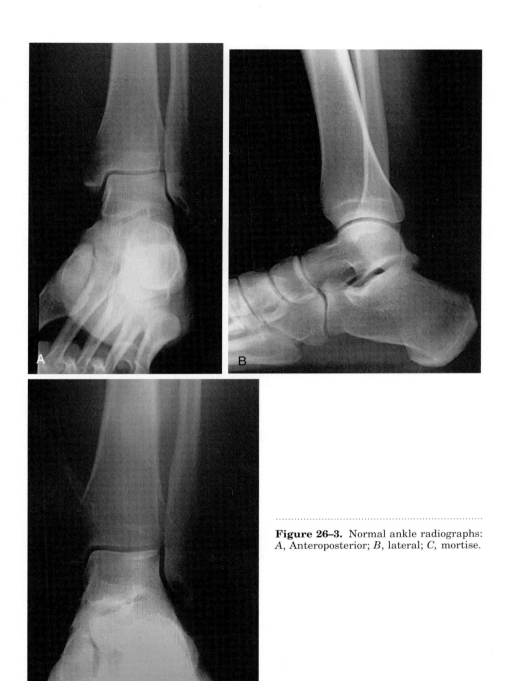

Figure 26–3. Normal ankle radiographs:
A, Anteroposterior; *B,* lateral; *C,* mortise.

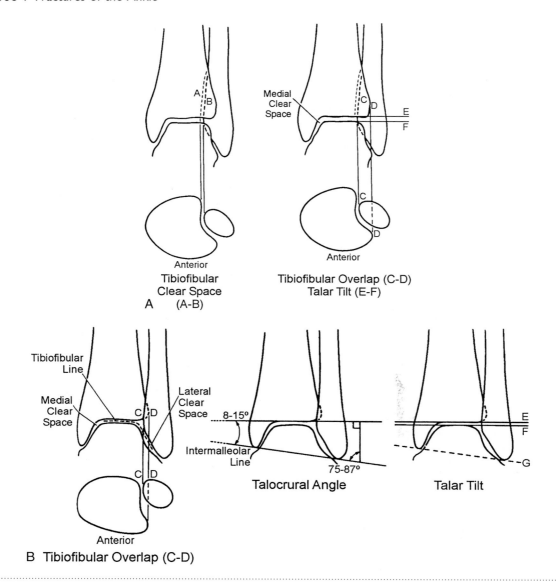

Figure 26–4. Radiographic measurements: *A*, Parameters measured in the anteroposterior view; *B*, parameters measured in the mortise view. Adapted from Müller ME, et al. Manual of Internal Fixation, ed 3. New York: Springer-Verlag, 1990. Used with permission.

ankle as the drawer test. More than 5° of talar tilt and anterior subluxation of the talus on the tibial surface indicate ligament injury. These tests may be affected by generalized ligament laxity, muscular spasm or pain, and the amount of force. To avoid some of these pitfalls, a special measuring device (Telos equipment) has been developed for quantitative assessment of ankle instability.[21]

Arthrography

This involves the use of radiopaque dye injected into the joint. Although this examination is rarely performed because of its high cost and technical difficulty, it can be useful to assess capsular integrity in some cases. Extravasation of the dye outside of the capsular limits is diagnostic of ligament injury. More recently, the use of magnetic resonance imaging (MRI) arthrography has gained increased interest because of its superior imaging capabilities.[27]

Tomography

Anteroposterior and lateral roentgenographic views of the ankle are taken at different focal distances, allowing for a three-dimensional reconstruction of the area. Although this technique has been used for distal tibia fractures or triplane fractures in adolescents,[28] it has been virtually replaced by the advent of computed tomography (CT).

COMPUTED TOMOGRAPHY

CT includes two- and three-dimensional (2- and 3-D) reconstruction capability. The addition of orthogonal planar sections and 3-D reconstruction to routine axial imaging enhances the visualization of structures. Such capabilities are readily applied to ankle trauma and pilon fractures as well as other bone fractures. Rotation of the 3-D image allows inspection of the bone from all angles. In addition, 3-D reformation allows for surgical simulation. One of the significant disadvantages of CT scanning is the radiation exposure to the patient.

MAGNETIC RESONANCE IMAGING

MRI is based on the use of magnetic fields, radiofrequency (RF) waves, and complex image reconstruction techniques. MRI allows multiplanar imaging without radiation. It is the newest and most sophisticated of the imaging technologies. MRI easily depicts the normal anatomy and disorders not only of osseous structures but of all the soft tissue and cartilage as well. It is especially helpful in evaluating large joints, such as the knee, shoulder, and ankle.

In imaging of the ankle, MRI has been an accurate modality to detect osteochondral lesions and soft tissue disorders such as tendon and ligament injuries. A 1994 report comparing the use of three techniques for obtaining images in the same patients with ligamentous injuries of the ankle and chronic instability indicates that the addition of intra-articular contrast improves the sensitivity of MRI in detecting ligamentous tears.[27]

ARTHROSCOPY

Arthroscopy of the ankle is used mainly to evaluate osteochondral lesions of the talus and intra-articular disorders. There is, at present, inadequate experience with arthroscopy-assisted reduction of ankle fractures, and further evaluation is needed.[29]

CLASSIFICATION

In 1948 Lauge-Hansen[2] stated that "the classification of the malleolar fractures in the literature is almost chaotic." There was no specific and accepted classification, and most surgeons used terms such as malleolar fractures, marginal fractures, ligament rupture, or directional dislocation.[2, 7] There have been many different classification systems based on etiology or biomechanics, anatomy, clinical evaluation, and radiographic feature of the fracture. The two main classifications in use today are that of Lauge-Hansen and Danis-Weber.[13, 17, 23]

Lauge-Hansen Classification

As discussed earlier (see Biomechanics), Lauge-Hansen's experimental, clinical, and radiographic studies resulted in the classification system that bears his name. More than 95% of ankle fractures can be classified into the four groups of this system. A fifth group, pronation-dorsiflexion, was added later for fractures caused by axial load, such as a fall from a height.[14] In the Lauge-Hansen classification, the first word is the position of the foot at time of the injury, and the second word is the direction of the force. Each group has several stages, up to four.

Supination-Adduction (SA)

1. Transverse fracture of the fibula below the level of the joint, or rupture of the lateral collateral ligaments

2. Vertical fracture of the medial malleolus

Supination-Eversion (External Rotation) (SER)

1. Rupture of the anterior tibiofibular ligament
2. Spiral or oblique fracture of the distal fibula
3. Rupture of the posterior tibiofibular ligament or fracture of posterior malleolus
4. Rupture of deltoid ligament or fracture of the medial malleolus

Pronation-Abduction (PA)

1. Fracture of the medial malleolus or rupture of deltoid ligament
2. Rupture of the syndesmotic (anterior and posterior tibiofibular) ligaments or avulsion fracture of their osseous attachments
3. Short, oblique fracture of the fibula above the level of the joint

Pronation-External Rotation (PER)

1. Rupture of the deltoid ligament or avulsion fracture of the medial malleolus
2. Rupture of the anterior tibiofibular and interosseous ligament
3. Short spiral fracture of the fibula above the level of the joint
4. Rupture of the posterior tibiofibular ligaments or avulsion fracture of posterior tibial margin

Pronation-Dorsiflexion (PD)

1. Fracture of the medial malleolus
2. Fracture of the anterior margin of the tibia
3. Supramalleolar fracture of the fibula
4. Transverse fracture of the posterior tibial surface

Danis-Weber Classification

In 1949, Danis[54] described an anatomic classification that was later modified by Weber and is now known as the Danis-Weber, or AO-ASIF group classification (Fig. 26–5). In this system, the ankle fracture is divided into three classes (A, B, or C) according to the relationship of the fibular fracture to the syndesmosis and interosseous ligaments.

Müller,[55] in the *Comprehensive Classification of Fractures,* further classified these three types into groups and subgroups, to qualify the spectrum of the injury according to the morphologic complexity of the fracture.

AO-ASIF Classification

Type A fractures are distal to both the interosseous ligament and syndesmosis (infrasyndesmoidal)

A1: isolated
A2: with fracture of the medial malleolus
A3: with posteromedial fracture

Type B fractures, which occur obliquely through the fibula, involve part or all of the syndesmosis and have an unstable syndesmosis approximately 50% of the time. They are typically at the level of the syndesmosis (transsyndesmotic).

B1: isolated
B2: medial lesion (ligament or malleolus)
B3: with medial lesion and fracture of the posterolateral margin

Type C fractures include fractures of the fibula proximal to the distal tibiofibular ligament and syndesmosis. These high fractures above the level of the syndesmosis (suprasyndesmotic) are considered unstable.

C1: simple diaphyseal fracture
C2: complex fracture of the diaphysis
C3: proximal fracture of the fibula

Classification systems are intended to provide therapeutic guidelines and to allow accurate comparison of results of different modalities of treatment. In an interobserver study, both systems were noted to have acceptable reliability. However, there was poor precision of staging within the categories of the Lauge-Hansen system, and the author recommended that the system's usefulness diminishes for daily practice.[30] The Lauge-Hansen system has also been criticized as too comprehensive without a significant contribution to the prognosis of the injury.[20, 22, 31]

TREATMENT

The goal of the treatment of any articular fracture is to reduce the joint and the frac-

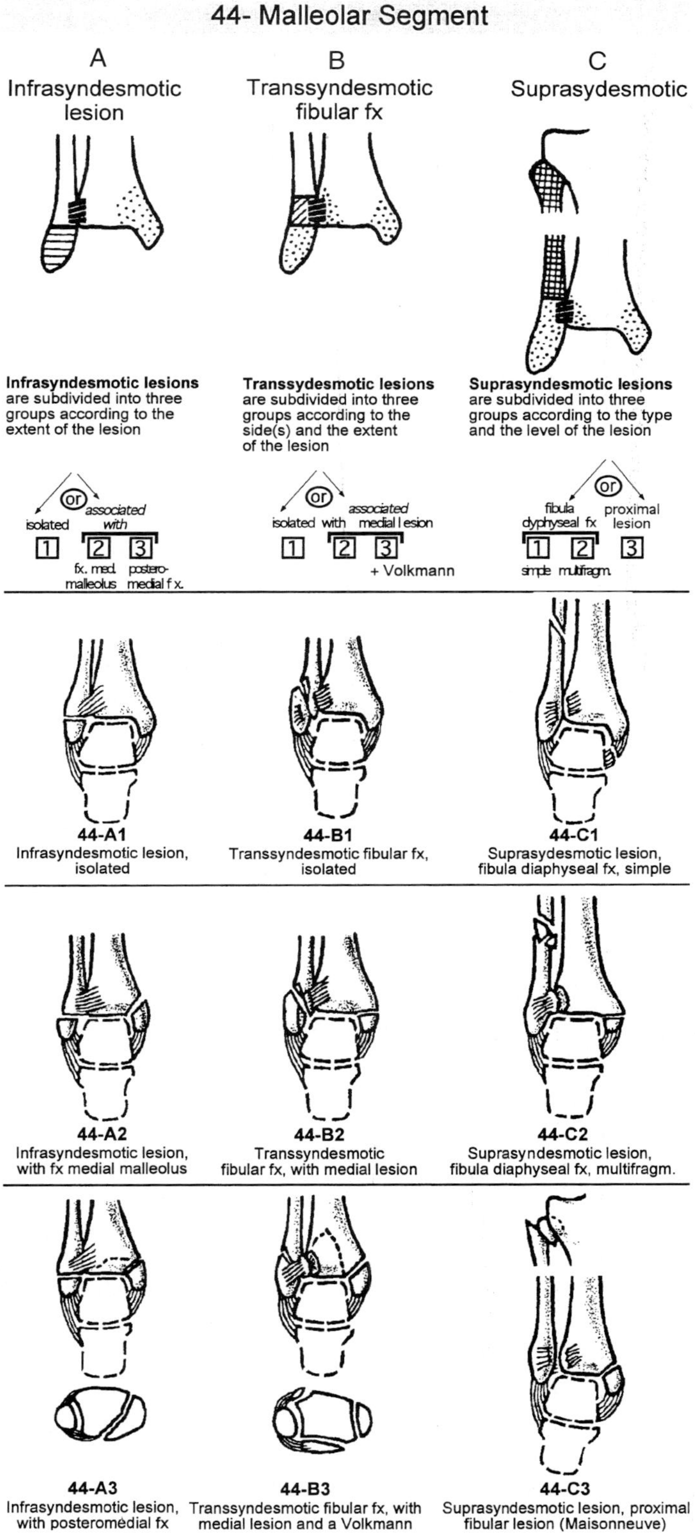
44- Malleolar Segment
A
Infrasyndesmotic lesion
B
Transsyndesmotic fibular fx
C
Suprasydesmotic
Infrasyndesmotic lesions are subdivided into three groups according to the extent of the lesion
Transsydesmotic lesions are subdivided into three groups according to the side(s) and the extent of the lesion
Suprasyndesmotic lesions are subdivided into three groups according to the type and the level of the lesion
or
isolated
associated with
1
2
3
fx. med. malleolus
postero-medial fx
isolated
with medial lesion
+ Volkmann
fibula dyphyseal fx
proximal lesion
simple
multifragm.
44-A1
Infrasyndesmotic lesion, isolated
44-B1
Transsyndesmotic fibular fx, isolated
44-C1
Suprasydesmotic lesion, fibula diaphyseal fx, simple
44-A2
Infrasyndesmotic lesion, with fx medial malleolus
44-B2
Transsyndesmotic fibular fx, with medial lesion
44-C2
Suprasyndesmotic lesion, fibula diaphyseal fx, multifragm.
44-A3
Infrasyndesmotic lesion, with posteromedial fx
44-B3
Transsyndesmotic fibular fx, with medial lesion and a Volkmann
44-C3
Suprasyndesmotic lesion, proximal fibular lesion (Maisonneuve)

Figure 26–5. Maurice E. Müller comprehensive classification of fractures of the ankle. Adapted from Griend RAV, Savoie FH, Hughes JL. Fractures of the ankle. In Rockwood CA, Green DP, Bucholz RW, eds. Fractures in Adults. Philadelphia: J. B. Lippincott, 1990, pp. 1983–2039.

ture, maintain the reduction until union, and return the patient to the previous level of activity.

Many factors affect the selection of the proper treatment regimen. Each fracture has a unique personality. Some fractures are best treated conservatively in plaster, and others mandate ORIF. Many studies have attempted to compare closed and open treatment.[10, 14, 16, 32–38] However, the criteria for selecting patients for each of these are often biased as well as imprecise. Still, outcomes in ankle fractures usually correlate with the adequacy of the reduction, and better overall results have been achieved by ORIF.[6, 16, 24, 32, 39] Thus, the inability to obtain or maintain a reduction of the joint or the fracture is often the prime indication for surgery. Other factors that affect the indications for surgery include patient age and activity level, past illness, drug use, and condition of the leg.

Conservative Treatment

Closed reduction is indicated in cases of undisplaced fractures, stable fractures, or displaced fractures that can be reduced and maintained in a plaster cast without many manipulations. When surgery is delayed, temporary closed reduction is used to keep the ankle in an acceptable position and immobilized. Good reduction is achieved by understanding the mechanism of the fracture and the stability of the joint. The stability of the reduction is then assessed with sequential postreduction x-ray films. Depending on the amount of swelling, a bulky dressing may be needed for several days after injury. After resolution of the swelling, the fracture may then be reduced and reinforced in a long leg cast (above the knee).

Fractures of the lateral or medial malleolus below the syndesmosis type A (Weber) or supination-adduction (Lauge-Hansen) are usually stable and can be treated in plaster cast with good results.[16, 36, 38] An associated oblique fracture of the medial malleolus makes closed reduction difficult and unstable and may require open reduction. Eversion relaxes the lateral ligaments, facilitating reduction of the lateral malleolus.

Fractures at the level of the syndesmosis, Weber type B or supination-external rotation, associated with a fracture of the medial malleolus are difficult to treat closed and are best treated by ORIF. The fracture is reduced by distraction, internal rotation, and varus stress.

Fractures above the syndesmosis with syndesmotic ligament disruption, Weber type C or pronation-external rotation, are usually unstable, and most often require ORIF. Closed reduction is achieved by gentle traction, inversion, and adduction of the foot. The reduction is maintained in a long leg cast (above the knee) for 4 to 6 weeks, followed by a short ankle brace. Weight bearing is permitted with early evidence of fracture healing.

Operative Treatment

ORIF is indicated for displaced and unstable fractures, failed closed reduction, widening of the mortise greater than 2 mm, and open fractures[16, 17, 20, 22, 31, 40] (Fig. 26–6A–F). Surgery should be performed as soon as possible. However, it is important first to evaluate properly the patient, ascertaining general health, and ensuring that soft tissue status will allow safe surgical exposure. In the presence of significant swelling, edema, or fracture blisters, surgery should be delayed, usually only a few days but sometimes as long as 2 weeks, until soft tissue swelling begins to decrease and the skin wrinkles (wrinkle test). In certain cases involving displacement or ankle instability, closed reduction, traction, or even temporary external fixation is required to maintain reduction.

Lateral Approach for Fractures of the Lateral Malleolus

The patient is placed in the supine position with a tourniquet. Exposure is improved by internally rotating the leg, placing a sandbag under the ipsilateral buttock, and rotating the table away from the surgeon. Either an anterolateral or posterolateral incision may be used, depending on the fracture. However, the incision should be centered over the fracture site and should be long enough to provide good exposure without soft tissue tension. Careful and gentle dissection of the subcutaneous tissue exposes the lateral cortex of the fibula. For more proximal (higher) fractures of the lateral malleolus, the superficial peroneal nerve may be at risk for injury.

Only 1 to 2 mm of periosteum needs to be elevated proximal and distal to the fracture site to enable and visualize an accurate reduction. The fracture site is opened to remove hematoma, interposed soft tissue, and bone chips using irrigation or a small probe. If possible, the articular surface is also inspected through the fracture site and is irrigated, and any small, loose fragments are removed. The remaining fragments are reduced and provisionally stabilized with a reduction clamp or Kirschner wires (K-wires).

The selection of the proper form of fixation depends on the fracture pattern of the fibula. Avulsion fractures associated with medial malleolus fractures require ORIF by a tension band or lag screw construct. For large fragments, a lateral plate and screws are used.

Tension band wiring involves the placement of two parallel K-wires inserted from the distal fragment into the medial cortex of the proximal fragment above the fracture line. A 1.6-mm stainless steel wire is then passed under the K-wires and through a transverse drill hole proximal to the fracture in a figure-eight fashion. Finally, the K-wires are bent and cut to the desired length to avoid penetration of the skin or irritation of the peroneal tendons.

Oblique or spiral fractures above the joint (Weber type B) should be fixed by one or two lag screws and a one-third tubular plate used as a neutralization plate. First, the distal part of the plate is contoured to accommodate the bowing of the lateral malleolus, and then 3.5-mm screws are placed. Fluoroscopy should be used to assess the fracture reduction and placement of hardware.

Weber type C fractures usually involve disruption of the syndesmosis. The fibula is reduced and fixed with a one-third tubular plate. Anatomic reduction and restoration of fibular length are important for this type of fracture to avoid talar tilt. Proximal one-third fibular fractures (Maisonneuve type) usually do not require fixation, but, if associated with a syndesmotic ligament tear, the syndesmosis should be reduced and stabilized with one or two syndesmotic screws.

The syndesmotic screw is placed from the fibula anteromedially into the tibia at the proximal level of the tibiofibular ligament. The foot must be in dorsiflexion during the placement of any syndesmotic screws. This action rotates the widest part of the talus into the mortise, thereby avoiding overcompression by the screw and resultant narrowing of the ankle joint. Two cortices of the fibula and the lateral cortex of the tibia are drilled and taped, and a 3.5- or 4.5-mm nonlag screw is placed.

Other methods of fibular fixation that have been used include the Steinmann or Rush pins. These provide poor rotational control at the fracture site and should only be considered in unusual circumstances.

Before wound closure, radiographic examination of the ankle is required to confirm mortise reduction, ligamentous stability, and proper extraarticular placement of screws outside the joint and syndesmosis. Finally, the wound is closed in layers, and the leg is placed in a bulky Jones-type dressing.

Medial Approach for Fractures of the Medial Malleolus

In unstable fractures of the medial malleolus with displacement of more than 2-mm open reduction is usually required. In stable fractures, open reduction is necessary when there is failure of closed reduction. This is often due to interposition of soft tissues such as the torn deltoid ligament or tibialis tendon. Either an anterior approach or a posterior approach may be used. The *anteromedial* approach offers an excellent view of the medial malleolus and the anteromedial part of the joint. The incision is curved over the anterior aspect of the medial malleolus and centered over the ankle joint. The *posteromedial* approach offers good visualization of the posterior aspect of the tibia. The incision is curved posterior to the medial malleolus and centered over the ankle joint. Subcutaneous dissection is performed, taking into consideration the saphenous nerve and vein anterior to the malleolus; the tibialis posterior, flexor digitorum, and flexor hallucis longus tendons; and the posterior tibial neurovascular bundle posteriorly.

As with the lateral malleolus, the periosteum is elevated only 1 to 2 mm proximally and distally to expose the fracture surfaces. Articular inspection, irrigation, and removal of debris are then completed before reduction is performed. Any associated osteochondral injuries to the talus should be noted.

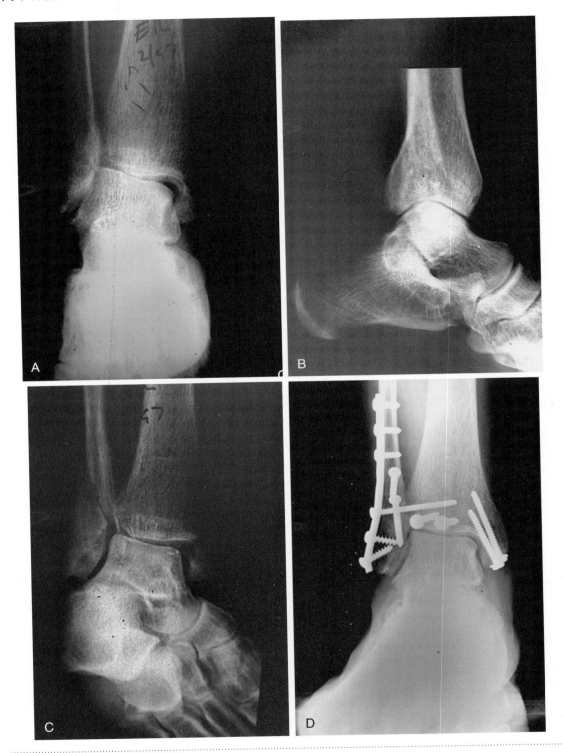

Figure 26–6. Radiographs of open reduction and internal fixation of the three malleoli: *A*, Preoperative anteroposterior; *B*, preoperative lateral; *C*, preoperative mortise; *D*, postoperative anteroposterior.

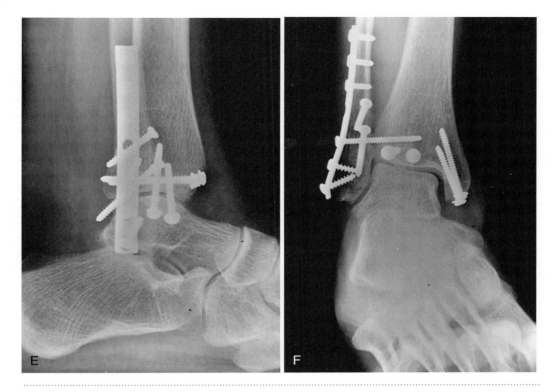

Figure 26–6 *Continued. E*, Postoperative lateral; *F*, postoperative mortise.

Avulsion fractures of the medial malleolus are treated by a figure-eight tension band wiring construct. Fractures above the deltoid may be reduced and fixed with two 4.0-mm cancellous screws or two cannulated cancellous screws (3.5 mm). An additional buttress is required in the presence of oblique or vertical fractures of the malleolus, in which shear forces may lead to proximal translation and loss of fixation. This may be in the form of a small one-third plate with one or two screws proximal to the fracture.

Posterior Malleolus Fixation

Internal fixation of the posterior malleolus is required when more than 25% of its surface is involved or more than 2 mm of displacement is present. Two techniques for reduction and fixation exist: direct and indirect.

Using a posterior surgical approach, the fragment may be reduced and fixed under direct vision. The approach involves a plane between the peroneal tendons and flexor hallucis longus, which is developed to ex-pose the posterior tibia. The posterior fracture fragment is overdrilled with a 3.5-mm gliding hole, reduced temporarily with K-wires, and then stabilized by one or two 3.5-mm cortical lag screws placed into the anterior part of the tibia.

Indirect reduction is achieved using the technique of ligamentotaxis (i.e., ligamentous and capsular). Relying on the soft tissue attachments between the fragment and the lateral malleolus, reduction and fixation of the lateral malleolus will often reduce the posterior malleolus. After reduction, the posterior malleolus may be fixed by placing the screws from anterior to posterior under fluoroscopic guidance.

Anterior Margin of the Tibia (Anterior Malleolus) Fixation

Isolated fractures of the anterior margin of the tibia are very uncommon. Occasionally, avulsion of a large fragment (more than 25% of the surface) of bone may necessitate ORIF. An anterior approach to the ankle joint is needed to reduce the fragment, which is usually fixed with two lag screws.

Postoperative Management

The postoperative care of the patient is as controversial as the initial management of the fracture. The main goals of rigid stabilization are to achieve early mobilization and restoration of function. However, although early active motion appears critical in most intra-articular fractures, there is some evidence that this is not so for ankle fractures. Many different protocols with and without early motion have been used without any difference in the outcome.[41-43] Some surgeons prefer protected weight bearing in a cast until there is evidence of fracture healing. Others prefer non-weight bearing with a cast or brace for 6 weeks. Implant removal should be performed in symptomatic patients. However, routine removal is controversial, and the decision left to both the physician and the patient.

OPEN FRACTURES OF THE ANKLE

For open ankle injuries, the same principles apply as to other open fractures. Antibiotics—depending on the type of injury—early irrigation, debridement, and stabilization are required at the time of injury.[11] The ankle joint should not be left open, and early soft tissue coverage with a free flap is occasionally necessary because of the paucity of local tissue available for transfer. Re-evaluation and multiple debridement of soft tissue and bone should be performed, usually at 2- or 3-day intervals, until the wound is clean of necrotic tissue.

Bone fixation is carried out with a minimum number of implants. Hardware and bone should be covered with soft tissue. In cases of extensive comminution or contamination, the use of internal fixation is not advisable, and external fixation becomes a valuable alternative. In severe cases of open fractures with high-energy injury to the soft tissue and bone loss, a combined treatment of debridement, temporary placement of antibiotic beads, soft tissue coverage, intravenous antibiotic treatment, fusion of the ankle, and bone grafting may be required.[44]

COMPLICATIONS AND PROGNOSIS

The incidence and severity of complications and the prognosis for the patient depend on many factors, including energy of the injury, bone quality, soft tissue involvement, general health of the patient, presence of open fracture and its degree of contamination, accuracy of reduction, rigidity and quality of stabilization, soft tissue handling at time of the operation, and postoperative management. Complications may be classified as early, intermediate, and late.

Compartment Syndrome

Compartment syndrome of the foot is uncommon in ankle fractures, but may occur in the presence of severe crush or contusion or with an unreduced dislocation of the ankle. Early recognition, evaluation with compartment pressure measurement, and fasciotomy when indicated, are critical.[45-47]

Wound Complications

Marginal skin necrosis after surgery occurs in approximately 3 to 5% of cases and can be minimized by delaying surgery until swelling decreases, with careful surgical handling of the soft tissues and by wound closure without tension.

Infection

The reported incidence of infection is approximately 2% and can be further reduced by minimizing soft tissue trauma, performing adequate debridement and irrigation, and achieving wound closure without tension.[16, 48] Treatment depends on the extent of the infection. Superficial wound infections usually respond to systemic antibiotics and local care. Deep infection requires a more aggressive approach.

Nonunion

Soft tissue interposition, ankle instability, malreduction, and infection are common causes of ankle nonunion. These occur more commonly on the medial side, especially after cast treatment. Treatment of nonunion of the medial malleolus is operative with lag screw fixation or of figure-eight tension band wiring with bone graft. Very distal ununited avulsion fractures of both malleoli are rarely symptomatic, but if so can be excused.

Malunion

Malunion is usually related to a lack of reduction, as seen with a poor closed reduction, improper ORIF, an unrecognized loss of reduction, or an underreduced depressed fracture (most commonly of the tibial plafond). The deformity most often seen with malunion of the lateral malleolus is shortening external rotation. The lateral talar tilt and the shortened rotated fibula should be corrected with a lengthening osteotomy.[9] Malunion of the medial malleolus, at or above the level of the mortise, must be corrected to restore the anatomy of the joint.

Osteoarthritis

The incidence of posttraumatic arthritis is approximately 10 to 20%.[22, 32, 48, 49] Improper reduction of the fracture is the most commonly associated factor, although anatomic reduction does not necessarily prevent degenerative changes. The incidence of arthritic changes are increased with the severity of the injury. For posttraumatic symptomatic arthritis, ankle fusion is the treatment of choice.

Reflex Sympathetic Dystrophy

Reflex sympathetic dystrophy (RSD) may be seen in all types of ankle injuries. Physical findings include vasomotor changes and dysfunction, skin temperature changes, joint stiffness, bone osteopenia, swelling, and pain.[50] Treatment is directed toward reducing pain and restoring function by energetic physiotherapy. Regional or intravenous sympathetic blockades are used to release the pain.

Heterotopic Bone Formation

Synostosis or heterotopic bone formation between the distal fibula and tibia may occur in severe injuries of the ankle with syndesmosis disruption. A synostosis may interfere with normal joint motion. However, in the presence of good motion, there is usually no need for active treatment of the synostosis.

Osteochondral Fractures of the Talus

Osteochondral fractures of the talus may be present either medially or laterally and may occur with ligament sprains as well as with fractures of the ankle.

In their classic 1959 study, Berndt and Harty[51] demonstrated that those lesions are transchondral and caused by a trauma. They classified the lesion into four stages: stage I, small area of indentation in the talar margin: stage II, an osteochondral chip that is partially detached; stage III, completely detached osteochondral fragment undisplaced; stage IV, completely detached and displaced into the joint.[51]

The mechanism of injury on the medial border is plantar flexion with inversion of the foot and talar rotation on the tibia. Medial injuries typically heal with conservative treatment and rarely require surgical treatment.

The mechanism for lateral border transchondral fracture is inversion and compression of the talar dome against the face of the lateral malleolus. In contrast to the medial side, lateral osteochondral fractures are more likely not to heal and may need operative intervention.

Open (arthrotomy) or arthroscopic excision or fixation of these osteochondral fragments is needed in cases that do not respond to conservative treatment with immobilization in a plaster cast or brace.[29]

REFERENCES

1. Hippocrates. On Joints: (ET. Withington, trans.) Cambridge, MA: Loeb Classical Library, Harvard University Press, 1984.
2. Lauge-Hansen N. Fractures of the ankle: analytic historic survey as the basis of new experimental roentgenologic and clinical investigations. Arch Surg 56:259–317, 1948.
3. Scudder CL. The classic: the open or operative treatment of fresh fractures: is it ever justifiable? With an analysis of the results of the present methods of treatment in one hundred and fifty-three fractures of the lower extremity (1900). Clin Orthop 199:3–11, 1985.
4. Joy G, Patzakis MJ, and Harvey JP, Jr. Precise evaluation of the reduction of severe ankle fractures. J Bone Joint Surg Am 56:979–993, 1974.
5. Lauge-Hansen N. Fractures of the ankle: III. Ge-

netic roentgenologic diagnosis of fractures of the ankle. AJR Am J Roentgenol 71:456–471, 1954.

6. Yde J. Ankle fractures: primary and late results of operative and non-operative treatment. Acta Orthop Scand 51:981–990, 1980.

7. Lewin P. The Foot & Ankle. Philadelphia: Lea & Febiger, 1947.

8. Weber BG. Lengthening osteotomy of the fibula to correct a widened mortice of the ankle after fracture. Int Orthop 4:289–293, 1981.

9. Weber BG, Simpson LA. Corrective lengthening osteotomy of the fibula. Clin Orthop 199:61–67, 1985.

10. Bauer M, Jonsson K, Nilsson B. Thirty-year follow-up of ankle fractures. Acta Orthop Scand 56:103–106, 1985.

11. Chapman MW, Mahoney M. The role of early internal fixation in the management of open fractures. Clin Orthop 138:120–131, 1979.

12. Kristensen KD, Hansen T. Closed treatment of ankle fractures: stage II supination-eversion fractures followed for 20 years. Acta Orthop Scand 56:107–109, 1985.

13. Last RJ. Anatomy, Regional and Applied. London: Churchill Livingstone, 1973.

14. Burwell HN, Charnley AD. The treatment of displaced fractures at the ankle by rigid fixation and early joint movement. J Bone Joint Surg Br 47:634–660, 1965.

15. Desouza LJ, Gustilo RB, Meyer TJ. Results of operative treatment of displaced external rotation-abduction fractures of the ankle. J Bone Joint Surg Am 67:1066–1074, 1985.

16. Hughes JL, Weber H, Willenegger H, Kuner EH. Evaluation of ankle fractures: non-operative and operative treatment. Clin Orthop 138:111–119, 1979.

17. Muller ME, Allgower M, Schneider R, Wilenegger H. Manual of Internal Fixation Techniques Recommended by the AO Group. New York: Springer-Verlag, 1979.

18. Hicks JH. The mechanism of the foot. J Anat 87:345–357, 1953.

19. Kapandji IA. The Physiology of Joints. New York: Churchill Livingstone, 1970.

20. Lindsjö U, Danckwardt-Lilliestrom G, Sahlstedt B. Measurement of the motion range in the loaded ankle. Clin Orthop 199:68–71, 1985.

21. Inman VT. The joints of the ankle. Baltimore: Williams & Wilkins, 1976.

22. Lindsjö U. Operative treatment of ankle fractures. Acta Orthop Scand Suppl 189:1–131, 1981.

23. Lauge-Hansen N. "Ligamentous" ankle fractures: diagnosis and treatment. Acta Chir Scand 97:544–550, 1949.

24. Wagner UA, Sangeorzan BJ, Harrington RM, Tencer AF. Contact characteristics of the subtalar joint: load distribution between the anterior and posterior facets. J Orthop Res 10:535–543, 1992.

25. Pankovich AM. Maisonneuve fracture of the fibula. J Bone Joint Surg Am 58:337–342, 1976.

26. Karlsson J, Bergsten T, Lansinger O, Peterson L. Lateral instability of the ankle treated by the Evans procedure: a long-term clinical and radiological follow-up. J Bone Joint Surg Br 70:476–480, 1988.

27. Chandnani VP, Harper MT, Ficke JR, et al. Chronic ankle instability: evaluation with MR arthrography, MR imaging, and stress radiography. Radiology 192:189–194, 1994.

28. Ertl JP, Barrack RL, Alexander AH, Van Buecken K. Triplane fracture of the distal tibial epiphysis: long-term follow-up. J Bone Joint Surg Am 70:967–976, 1988.

29. Pritsch M, Horoshovski H, Farine I. Arthroscopic treatment of osteochondral lesions of the talus. J Bone Joint Surg Am 68:862–865, 1986.

30. Thomsen NO, Overgaard S, Olsen LH, et al. Observer variation in the radiographic classification of ankle fractures. J Bone Joint Surg Br 73:676–678, 1991.

31. Yablon IG, Heller FG, Shouse L. The key role of the lateral malleolus in displaced fractures of the ankle. J Bone Joint Surg Am 59:169–173, 1977.

32. Bauer M, Bergstrom B, Hemborg A, Sandegard J. Malleolar fractures: nonoperative versus operative treatment. A controlled study. Clin Orthop 199:17–27, 1985.

33. Eventov I, Salama R, Goodwin DR, Weissman SL. An evaluation of surgical and conservative treatment of fractures of the ankle in 200 patients. J Trauma 18:271–274, 1978.

34. Leeds HC, Ehrlich MG. Instability of the distal tibiofibular syndesmosis after bimalleolar and trimalleolar ankle fractures. J Bone Joint Surg Am 66:490–503, 1984.

35. Phillips WA, Schwartz HS, Keller CS, et al. A prospective, randomized study of the management of severe ankle fractures. J Bone Joint Surg Am 67:67–78, 1985.

36. Rowley DI, Norris SH, Duckworth T. A prospective trial comparing operative and manipulative treatment of ankle fractures. J Bone Joint Surg Br 68:610–613, 1986.

37. Sangeorzan BJ, Wagner UA, Harrington RM, Tencer AF. Contact characteristics of the subtalar joint: the effect of talar neck misalignment. J Orthop Res 10:544–551, 1992.

38. Yde J, Kristensen KD. Ankle fractures: supination-eversion fractures stage II. Primary and late results of operative and non-operative treatment. Acta Orthop Scand 51:695–702, 1980.

39. Yde J. The Lauge-Hansen classification of malleolar fractures. Acta Orthop Scand 51:181–192, 1980.

40. Griend RAV, Savoie FH, Hughes JL. Fractures of the ankle. In Rockwood CA, Green DP, Bucholz RW, Fractures in adults. eds New York: J. B. Lippincott, 1991: 1983–2039.

41. Finsen V, Benum P. Osteopenia after ankle fractures: the influence of early weight bearing and muscle activity. Clin Orthop 245:261–268, 1989.

42. Finsen V, Saetermo R, Kibsgaard L, et al. Early postoperative weight-bearing and muscle activity in patients who have a fracture of the ankle (see comments). J Bone Joint Surg Am 71:23–27, 1989.

43. Segal D, Wiss DA, Whitelaw GP. Functional bracing and rehabilitation of ankle fractures. Clin Orthop 199:39–45, 1985.

44. Sanders R, Pappas J, Mast J, Helfet D. The salvage of open grade IIIB ankle and talus fractures. J Orthop Trauma 6:201–208, 1992.

45. Fakhouri AJ, Manoli A II. Acute foot compartment syndromes. J Orthop Trauma 6:223–228, 1992.

46. Manoli A II. Compartment syndromes of the foot: current concepts. Foot Ankle 10:340–344, 1990.

47. Manoli A II, Weber TG. Fasciotomy of the foot: an anatomical study with special reference to release of the calcaneal compartment. Foot Ankle 10:267–275, 1990.

48. Lindsjö U. Operative treatment of ankle fracture-dislocations: a follow-up study of 306/321 consecutive cases. Clin Orthop 199:28–38, 1985.
49. Mont MA, Sedlin ED, Weiner LS, Miller AR. Postoperative radiographs as predictors of clinical outcome in unstable ankle fractures. J Orthop Trauma 6:352–357, 1992.
50. Amadio PC. Pain dysfunction syndromes. J Bone Joint Surg Am 70:944–949, 1988.
51. Berndt AL, Harty M. Transchondral fractures (osteochondritis dissecans) of the talus. J Bone Joint Surg Am 41:988–1020, 1959.
52. Lauge-Hansen N. Fractures of the ankle: II. Combined experimental surgical and experimental roentgenologic investigations. Arch Surg 60:957–985, 1950.
53. Lauge-Hansen N. Fractures of the ankle: IV. Clinical use of genetic roentgen diagnosis and genetic reduction. Arch Surg 64:488–500, 1952.
54. Danis R. Theorie et pratique de l'osteosynthese. Edited by Masson, Paris: 1949.
55. Müller ME, Nazarian S, Koch P, Schatzker J. The Comprehensive Classification of Fractures of Long Bones. Berlin: Springer-Verlag, 1990.

27

Pilon Fractures: Classification, Diagnosis, and Treatment

Craig S. Bartlett III
David L. Helfet

Fractures of the distal tibia that involve a significant portion of the weight bearing articular surface and overlying metaphysis are notoriously difficult to treat.[1–6] In 1905, Albin Lambotte[7] was perhaps the first to perform an open reduction and internal fixation (ORIF) of this type of fracture, calling it a "fracture de l'epiphyse." The term *pilon tibial* ("hammer" or "pestle") was later introduced by the French radiologist Destot[1] in 1911. In 1950, Bonin[8] added the term *plafond* ("ceiling") to emphasize the region of injury where there is impaction superiorly of the articular surface and overlying metaphyseal bone. This is caused by the talus as it is driven up into the tibial articular surface like a hammer striking a nail.

Disturbingly, 10 to 30% of these are open fractures, and one third to one half are associated with other injuries.[9–11] The most common associated fractures involve the calcaneus and tibial shaft.[9] Fractures of the talus, tibial plateau, proximal fibula, femur, pelvis, acetabulum, and spine are also seen.[2, 9–12] Additionally, degloving and crushing of the skin frequently lead to necrosis.[4, 9, 12–15] Treatment is fraught with complications, including infection, soft tissue damage, nonunion or malunion, and post-traumatic arthrosis. Fortunately, these devastating fractures account for only 3 to 10% of all fractures of the tibia and less than 1% of all fractures of the lower extremity.[3, 16–20]

MECHANISM OF INJURY

The injury is most commonly sustained after a fall from a height, a motor vehicle accident with a sudden stop, or a fall forward with a trapped foot.[2, 4, 19–22] Both axial compression and rotation (shear) forces produce variable degrees of fracture separation.[3, 5, 11, 17–20, 23] Furthermore, the amount of energy involved directly affects the fracture severity and its prognosis.[2, 18–20]

High-energy injuries tend to be associated with greater degrees of articular and metaphyseal comminution with more severe soft tissue trauma. In contrast, torsional injuries tend to be lower energy injuries occurring most commonly during sporting activities, usually skiing accidents (the "boot-top" fracture).

An associated fibula fracture occurs in approximately 75 to 85% of cases.[11, 19] Its presence implicates valgus shear forces, which usually result in damage to the lateral articular surface and valgus deformity or a rotational mechanism. Open injuries are more commonly associated with the valgus displacement type,[9] resulting primarily from tearing of the thin medial soft tissues.

CLASSIFICATION

The system proposed by Ruedi and Allgower[19, 20] makes a distinction between non-displaced, low-energy injuries and severely comminuted and impacted fractures.[5, 16]

A Ruedi type I fracture is a cleavage fracture of the distal tibia without significant displacement of the articular surface. A type II fracture has significant displacement of articular surface cleavage lines. However, the joint surface is neither crushed nor grossly comminuted. The more severe type III fracture involves both comminution and impaction of the distal tibial articular surface and its overlying metaphysis. Maale and Seligson[3] modified this scheme by identifying a spiral fracture of the distal tibial diaphysis with intra-articular extension as a separate injury. Although involving the tibial plafond, this is a low-energy rotational fracture with a relatively good prognosis.

The Comprehensive Classification System (Fig. 27–1)[24] is the most descriptive and possibly prognostic system in the literature. The same system applies to all periarticular

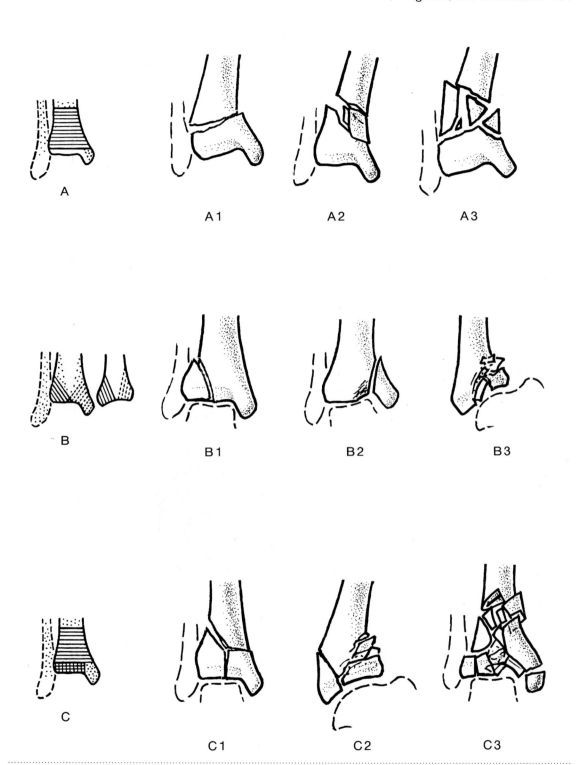

Figure 27–1. The Comprehensive Classification System for pilon fractures. (From Müller ME, et al. Manual of Internal Fixation, ed. 3. New York: Springer-Verlag, 1991, p. 147.)

fractures; type A is extra-articular and type B partial articular. The most severe pilon fractures are type C, which are complete articular with metaphyseal-diaphyseal dissociation.

Each type is further subdivided into three groups: a simple pattern (no comminution or impaction) in both the articular and metaphyseal areas makes up the C1 fracture group. Impaction involving only the supra-articular metaphysis comprises those fractures in group C2. In addition to meta-physeal impaction, group C3 fractures involve comminution and impaction of the articular surface and are a "worst-case scenario" (Figs. 27–2 and 27–3).

DIAGNOSIS AND EVALUATION

Examination of the ankle should primarily include a careful evaluation of the soft tissues, especially amount of swelling, skin integrity (Fig. 27–2C, D), neurologic status,

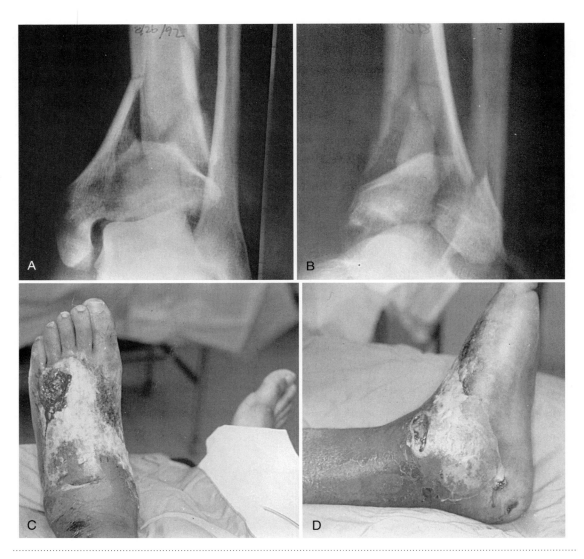

Figure 27–2. *A,* Anteroposterior and *(B)* lateral roentgenograms, left tibia and fibula, of a 35-year-old man with an AO type C3 (Ruedi type III) pilon fracture after a fall at a construction site. On the basis of these films, most surgeons would recommend a formal open approach. *C,* Anteroposterior and lateral *(D)* clinical appearance of left foot. Not appreciable on the plain films is the severe soft tissue compromise evident in this patient, precluding any open procedure. It cannot be overemphasized that, in the case of the pilon fracture, the soft tissues are often more likely to dictate treatment than the fracture itself!

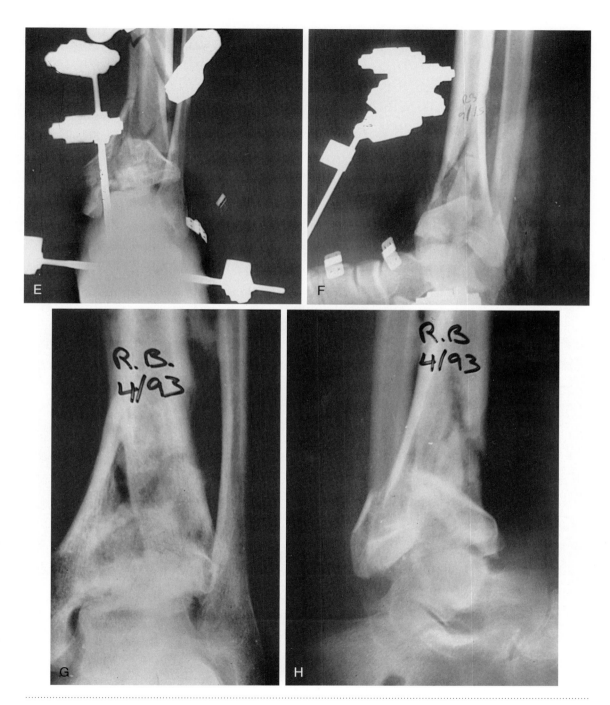

Figure 27–2 *Continued. E,* Anteroposterior and lateral *(F)* roentgenograms after spanning external fixation was used to provide ligamentotaxis, realignment, and stabilization of the foot and distal tibia. Note the inability to obtain an articular reduction indirectly with external fixation. *G,* Anteroposterior and lateral *(H)* roentgenograms, 8 months later with residual articular step-off and gapping but an "autofusion" of the ankle (without infection).

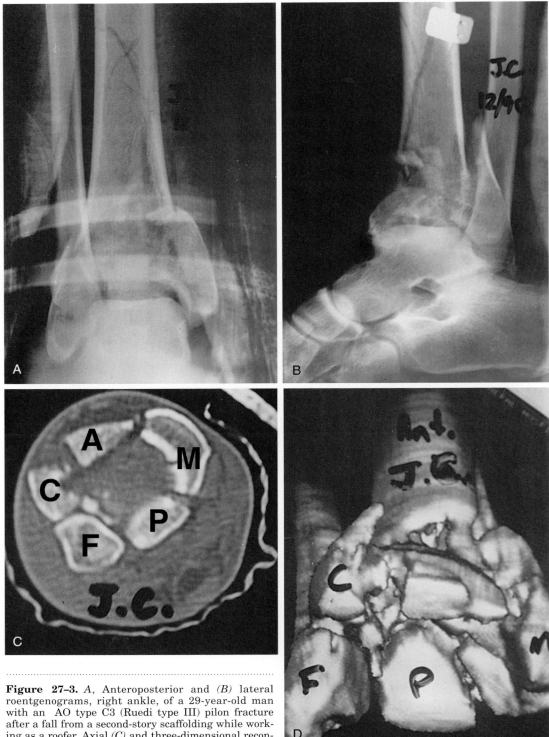

Figure 27–3. *A,* Anteroposterior and *(B)* lateral roentgenograms, right ankle, of a 29-year-old man with an AO type C3 (Ruedi type III) pilon fracture after a fall from a second-story scaffolding while working as a roofer. Axial *(C)* and three-dimensional reconstruction *(D)* computed tomography images delineate the multiple fracture fragments. Note the presence of a central defect on the axial CT, heralding a "die punch" fracture fragment, and its corresponding location on the plain films. (C = Chaput fragment; F = distal fibula; P = posterior malleolus; M = medial malleolus; A = anterior plafond.)

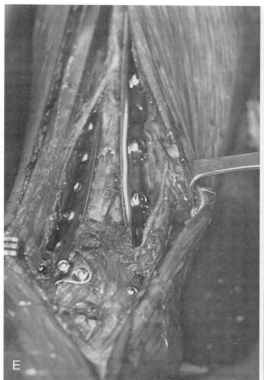

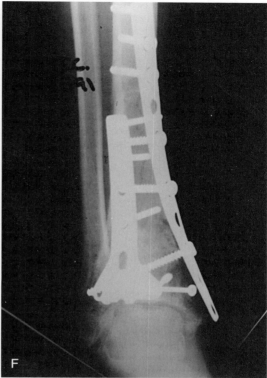

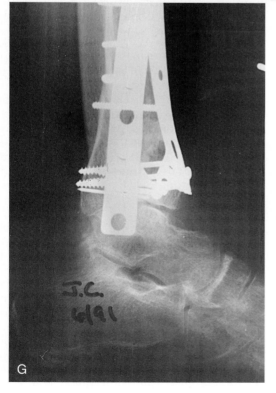

Figure 27–3 *Continued. E,* Intraoperative clinical picture of formal open reduction and internal fixation of pilon fracture with two buttress plates (anterior and medial). Such extensive incisions are becoming less frequent with the development of more modern techniques of indirect reduction and limited internal fixation. Anteroposterior *(F)* and lateral *(G)* roentgenograms 6 months later, showing healing but some early joint space narrowing.

and status of the peripheral pulses. Of particular importance is the identification of an open injury or any early signs or symptoms of compartment syndrome.

Anteroposterior, lateral, mortis, and 45° external rotation roentgenograms should be obtained to delineate the anteromedial and posterolateral surfaces of the tibia.

Additional radiographs of the contralateral ankle are also helpful, providing a model for templating and reduction. Computed tomography (CT) can also provide valuable information with regards to fracture pattern, comminution, and displacement (see Fig. 27–3C and D). The addition of sagittal and coronal CT cuts will complete the three-dimensional representation of the fracture. This will allow the surgeon to visualize and understand the fracture quite well and hence allow adequate preoperative planning for approach, reduction, and fixation of the fracture.

HISTORY AND RESULTS OF TREATMENT

Early surgical results of severely comminuted and impacted fractures of the distal tibial articular surface were dismal. Good results were achieved in only 43 to 50% of cases.[2, 20] This led to an initial emphasis on nonoperative treatment, which, unfortunately, also produced consistently poor results.[2, 16, 20, 23, 25, 26]

In 1963, the AO group (Arbeitsgemeinschaft fur Osteosynthesefragen) introduced the principles of ORIF,[27] which restimulated a wave of enthusiasm for ORIF of these joint fractures. As a result, in 1969, Ruedi and Allgower[19] reported good to excellent results in 74% of 84 pilon fractures monitored for 4.2 years. Ninety percent of patients returned to their previous occupation and, by 9 years, 85% had a good to excellent outcome.[18] Heim[9] reported similar results, noting 90% good function and only a 1.4% infection rate. However, 75% and 90% of patients, respectively, in each study sustained lower energy skiing-type injuries.

Other authors have been less optimistic, reporting dismal complication rates and frequently suboptimal end results using AO techniques to treat high-energy pilon fractures.[2–6, 12, 16, 17, 20] In 1986, Ovadia and Beals[4] reviewed 145 pilon fractures, the majority of which were high energy. When comparing

the 80 treated with ORIF versus all other methods, good to excellent results were obtained in 74% and 54%, respectively. However, with ORIF, good or better results were obtained in only 38% of their most severe fractures. Grades II and III open injuries had significantly higher complication rates, which are consistent with other reports.[14, 28]

Teeny and Wiss[6] reported even more dismal results of ORIF in a series of 60 pilon fractures. Unacceptable results were found in 75% of their patients, with a 37% rate of skin slough and dehiscence in 30 Ruedi type III fractures. The presence of these wound problems increased the incidence of deep infection sixfold from 7 to 43%! Arthrodesis was ultimately required in 26% of cases. Not surprisingly, the fracture severity and inadequate reduction were key factors correlating with their poor results.

In an effort to improve on the previous poor results associated with open reduction and plate and screw fixation, Tornetta and colleagues[22] treated 26 pilon fractures with limited internal and hybrid external fixation. Thirteen were Ruedi type III, of which 69% had good to excellent results. These authors concluded that this method yielded anatomic and functional results comparable with ORIF but without the related soft tissue complications.

More recently, Wyrsch and coworkers[29] performed a prospective study comparing the results of ORIF of pilon fractures versus external fixation with or without limited internal fixation. Although ankle scores for the two groups were equivalent, complications were more frequent and severe in those patients treated with ORIF. There were 15 complications in 7 of 18 patients treated with ORIF, including amputation in 3. In contrast, only 4 complications occurred in 4 of 20 patients treated with external fixation.

Other investigators have also endorsed the concept of limited surgery for severe pilon injuries.[2, 22, 23, 30, 31] From this desire to produce minimal insult have evolved modern biologic principles, which emphasize meticulous soft tissue dissection, limited stripping of fracture fragments, indirect reduction techniques, and stable fixation.[11] Helfet and associates[32] expanded these concepts to include percutaneous plate fixation of the reconstructed articular surface to the diaphysis with resultant fewer complications in their initial series of 20 patients.

Unfortunately, most studies to date are too small, retrospective, not controlled, and without consistent grading or classification systems. This makes comparisons very difficult. However, few argue that the treatment of pilon fractures remains a dilemma. Although nonsurgical methods, ORIF, and external fixation have all met with varying degrees of success, it is apparent that no one method is ideal for all pilon fractures. Thus, it is up to the surgeon to determine individually the most appropriate form of treatment in each case, dependent not only on the fracture type but also the status of the soft tissues and the patient (i.e., the personality of the patient and injury).

INITIAL TREATMENT

Care should begin the moment the patient is examined in the emergency room. Some form of lower leg immobilization is imperative before moving the patient to prevent any further soft tissue damage. Once radiographs are obtained and the severity of the fracture is documented, preliminary reduction and more rigid cast or splint immobilization should be applied as necessary.

While awaiting definitive treatment, four basic principles must be adhered to: the fracture must be reduced, length and rotational alignment of the extremity must be restored, the ankle must be stabilized, and the limb must be elevated on a Böhler frame.[11, 21]

TREATMENT OPTIONS

Most surgeons agree that, in the absence of other problems, anatomic reduction of the articular surface and early joint motion lead to a lower incidence of posttraumatic arthrosis and subsequently a better functional result.[2, 5, 8, 10, 11, 14, 17–21, 23, 25, 26, 33, 34] However, the ability to achieve these goals is also directly related to the severity of the initial injury, primarily the soft tissues. The most important factor and determinant of outcome is the soft tissues (see Fig. 27–2C and D); hence, their integrity and involvement determine the treatment option available, timing of definitive surgery, approaches, and so on. Any treatment plan should also be based on the presence of tibial shaft fracture extension, amount of displacement or comminution, quality of bone stock, and presence of an open fracture.

Methods of conservative management include closed reduction with immobilization in plaster[2, 4, 12, 17, 23] or traction with early range of motion,[2, 11] generally by way of calcaneal pin placement. Common to these measures is the reliance on ligamentotaxis to reduce and maintain the alignment of the fracture fragments. This, however, will have no effect on displaced intra-articular "die punch" fracture fragments (see Fig. 27–2E–H). In addition, plaster generally fails to maintain alignment, and late displacement is common because of the presence of associated comminution and metaphyseal bone loss.[9, 28] Prolonged immobilization also prevents joint motion, which is important in promoting cartilage nutrition and healing. The end result of such conservative treatment is often joint incongruity, stiffness, and osteodystrophy.[9] Thus, the use of closed treatment is recommended only for minimally displaced fractures, debilitated patients, or temporary measure to allow for soft tissue healing before definitive surgical management.[3, 10]

There are several options for ORIF of the fracture. Internal fixation can be formal ORIF (see Fig. 27–3), using a variety of plates and screws,[2, 5, 10, 12, 16, 18–21, 27] or it can be performed on a limited basis[2, 3, 5, 12] with minimal soft tissue stripping (Fig. 27–4).

A third option, external fixation,[4, 14, 21] may be combined with limited internal fixation of the fibula[12] or tibial articular surface.[2, 14, 22, 31] A number of external fixator designs are available from which to choose. They fall into three basic categories: joint spanning-rigid,[14, 16] joint spanning-articulated,[30, 31] and nonjoint spanning.[2, 22] The benefit of the latter two is the presence of ankle motion. Regardless of design, the fixator is often best supplemented with some form of reduction and limited internal fixation of the distal tibial articular surface. Arthrodesis[4, 5, 26, 28] and amputation[4, 5, 9, 28, 36, 37] are salvage procedures and have limited indications in primary fracture treatment.

Open fractures are treated emergently using accepted surgical principles.[38–40] These include tetanus prophylaxis, initiation of appropriate antibiotics, early and repeated surgical debridement, rigid fixation, and delayed wound closure. The more severe open injuries and closed injuries associ-

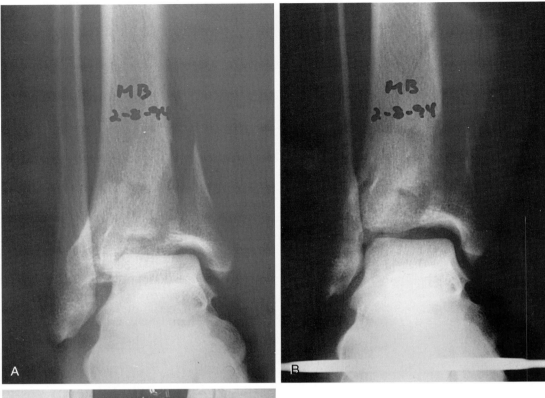

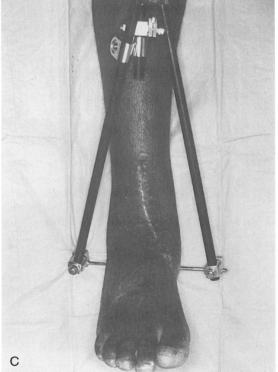

Figure 27–4. *A,* Anteroposterior roentgenogram, right ankle, of 26-year-old man with an AO type C2 (Ruedi type II) pilon fracture after fall from one-story window. In addition to his clinical shortening, this patient had severe swelling. *B,* Intraoperative anteroposterior roentgenogram after placement of a spanning external fixator to stabilize the fracture and provide length. This allowed open reduction–internal fixation to be delayed until 10 days later, when the severe swelling of the soft tissues had subsided. *C,* Anteroposterior clinical appearance 6 weeks later, just before removal of external fixator, demonstrating the healing of the soft tissues and good clinical alignment.

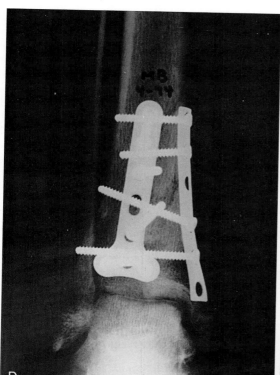
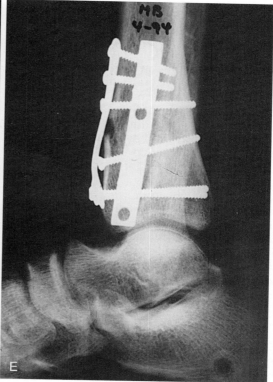

Figure 27–4 *Continued. D,* Anteroposterior and lateral *(E)* roentgenograms at 8 weeks showing healing. Union was complete by 3 months. Note the presence of lower profile implants, which have been used in concert with limited soft tissue stripping.

ated with extensive soft tissue compromise are candidates for joint spanning external fixation, which provides stability until definitive treatment can be performed (Fig. 27–4). Unfortunately, poor soft tissue healing often leaves this technique as the only alternative for definitive care (see Fig. 27–2).

Because soft tissue healing around the distal tibia is notoriously poor,[4–6] timing of surgical intervention is critical. After 8 to 12 hours, swelling is primarily due to intradermal edema, which increases the likelihood of postoperative wound problems.[10, 11] Marked edema, skin blistering, deep abrasions, and contusions of skin, subcutaneous fat, and muscle are significant indicators of soft tissue compromise, which will require a period of soft tissue management before definitive fracture fixation. Maximal soft tissue compromise generally occurs over the first 3 to 6 days.[9, 41, 42]

If surgery is performed during this high-risk period, outcomes can be disastrous.[3, 43]

Thus, operative intervention should often be deferred for a period of 7 to 10 days.[3, 10, 19, 21, 26] An important sign that heralds improvement of the tissues is the reappearance of skin creases. With delay beyond 3 weeks, onset of granulation tissue, organization of hematoma, and development of disuse osteoporosis make the operation more technically difficult.[9]

SURGICAL APPROACH

Fractures of the fibula are typically approached posterolaterally.[19] By placing the incision anterior to the peroneal tendons but near the posterior border of the fibula, a delayed wound closure may be performed, if necessary, without risking exposure of either the implants or the tendons.[21] This approach will also provide an adequate anterior soft tissue bridge for an anteromedial tibial incision. For an uncompromised skin bridge, a minimum width of 7 to 8 cm should prevent skin slough.[10, 11, 21, 35, 41]

The anteromedial incision begins proximally, 1 cm lateral to the anterior tibial crest, and curves distally, following the medial border of the tibialis anterior tendon. Full-thickness flaps must be maintained and retracted with minimal trauma to the skin edges. The paratenon of the tibialis anterior should not be violated, because this, unlike the tendon itself, will except any skin grafting should soft tissue problems develop later.[11]

A limited open approach is most appropriate for nondisplaced fractures or a joint surface that has major fragments that reduce after application of distraction. An additional advantage of the limited approach is that the incision can be positioned over a major fracture line as seen on CT scan. This allows the surgeon to obtain optimal exposure.[2, 31]

TECHNIQUES OF OPEN REDUCTION AND INTERNAL FIXATION

Four sequential steps are required for successful surgical reconstruction of a pilon fracture[19]: (1) restoration of the fibula or extremity length, (2) reconstruction of the articular surface, (3) bone grafting, and (4) neutralization of the metaphysis to the diaphysis with the use of buttress plating or external fixation.

The value of the first step is reconstruction of the lateral column and reduction of anterolateral and posterolateral fragments.[2, 11, 16, 18–21, 27, 34, 43] Furthermore, in some cases of soft tissue compromise, early fixation of the fibula will preserve length and allow the definitive ORIF of the pilon to be delayed until the soft tissue status has improved.[21] However, fibular reduction may not always be beneficial.[22, 31, 44] An inability to achieve anatomic reduction of a comminuted fibula may interfere with each subsequent stage of the pilon reconstruction.[19, 43] Additionally, a second incision increases the risk of wound complications and potentially delays healing.[44]

Reconstruction of the articular surface should be performed with a minimum of soft tissue stripping. Provisional fixation is obtained with Kirshner wires. Before definitive fixation with screws or plates, this provisional construct should be evaluated using the image intensifier or plain films. In some cases, the application of tibialcalcaneal or tibiotalar distraction with either the AO femoral distractor[11] or an external fixator may facilitate reduction. These devices provide restoration of extremity length and alignment by increasing tension on the soft tissue sleeve (ligamentotaxis).[2, 11, 34] If enough soft tissue attachments to comminuted fragments still exist, then peripheral joint anatomy may also be restored. Finally, distraction can open the joint space to allow inspection of the reduction.[10, 34]

Because of the presence of joint impaction into the soft metaphyseal bone, autologous bone grafting should be performed at the time of the open reduction.[43] However, when significant metaphyseal-diaphyseal comminution is present, delayed bone grafting at 4 to 6 weeks may improve the chance for union and decrease the likelihood of malunion.

The final step of reconstruction is the neutralization of the metaphysis to the diaphysis using a medial buttress to prevent varus deformity. This can be accomplished by plating techniques, external fixation, or a combination of internal and external fixation. Determination of the correct technique is multifactorial. The technique of reconstruction of the joint and neutralization with a plate is ideal for fractures confined to the metaphysis and fractures in which neutralization of "key" fragments has stabilized the medial column. When soft tissue injury or severe comminution will not permit ORIF, external fixation must be considered.

CLOSURE AND COVERAGE

Meticulous soft tissue handling can help reduce the incidence of complications. Dead space and fluid collections are avoided by closing atraumatically over small suction drains. The anterior tibial wound is closed meticulously in layers with 4-0 nylon Allgower-Donati skin sutures.[11] Skin staples should be avoided because tension at the wound edge may lead to necrosis.[42]

The absence of skin wrinkles, presence of fracture blisters, and loss of palpable bony landmarks are considered relative contraindications for primary closure.[21, 35] Open wounds, poor capillary refill, and blanching of skin flaps on attempted approximation are absolute contraindications.[35, 42] In these cases, a primary skin graft or delayed primary closure can be performed after repeat debridement in 3 to 5 days.[35, 43]

Any significant skin slough should prompt consideration of a soft tissue transfer procedure such as a free muscle flap. When flaps become necessary, more likely with open fracture, they should be performed within 5 to 10 days of the injury and only if there is no evidence of infection.[38, 45]

POSTOPERATIVE CARE

Postoperative care varies to some extent depending on the type of treatment. Patients are generally placed in a well-padded, nonconstricting, removable U splint or brace, which is used to maintain the ankle at 90° to avoid equinus deformity. Strict elevation of the extremity for at least 2 to 3 days is mandatory. Prophylaxis against thromboembolism should be performed.

Antibiotic coverage is best continued for 24 to 72 hours postoperatively depending on the condition of wounds. If an external fixator has been used, pin care is performed at least two to three times daily with half-strength hydrogen peroxide solution.

Although desirable, early and active range of motion of the ankle should not begin until the soft tissues appear healthier and the surgical wounds have sealed, usually in 48 hours. When the tissues are healthy and postoperative swelling is diminished, toe-touch weight bearing with crutches is instituted. Initially, elastic stockings are helpful because they counteract the hemostatic pressure of the dependent leg.[9, 11] Once good ankle control has been obtained, a cooperative patient may discard his or her splint and begin more aggressive active range of motion, usually by 10 to 14 days.[11]

Because union usually requires 10 to 16 weeks,[21] patients should remain toe-touch weight bearing for approximately 3 months and then advanced based on their clinical examination and the roentgenograms. For severely comminuted fractures and those with significant chondral damage, a longer period of protected weight bearing, up to 14 to 20 weeks, has been suggested.[2, 9, 19–22]

COMPLICATIONS AND PROGNOSIS

Complications after operative treatment of pilon fractures, especially the high-energy injuries, are frequent and often severe.[2, 4, 5, 9, 12, 15, 17, 18, 29, 42, 49] Soft tissue disorders, including hematoma formation, wound dehiscence, skin slough problems (see Fig. 27–2C, D), chronic edema, stasis ulceration, and infection, have reportedly ranged from 0 to 37%, correlating closely with injury severity.[4, 9, 12, 15, 17, 21, 29, 35, 41, 42, 45] This may be attributed to the poor vascularity of the skin over the anteromedial surface of the tibia[42] and compounded by poor surgical techniques, incisions, and timing.

The development of chronic osteomyelitis can be devastating with an unpredictable outcome. The basic principles of treatment are aggressive debridement of all infected and necrotic bone and surrounding soft tissues, removal of any hardware present, immobilization, appropriate antibiotic therapy, including the use of antibiotic-impregnated polymethylmethacrylate beads, and management of the resulting dead space.[37, 47]

Placement of external fixation wires or pins through tendons, vessels, and nerves damages these structures and increases the risk of infection. Pin tract infections are among the most common complications of external fixation.[2, 22] However, these tend to clear with the administration of antibiotics. Skinny wires or metaphyseal screws placed too close to the joint are prone to deep infection.

Delayed and nonunion rates as high as 36%[2, 4, 6, 9, 12, 16, 17] and, depending on the treatment used, malunion rates as high as 58% have been reported.[4, 6, 12, 16–18] Joint stiffness is also common because of a combination of articular damage, immobilization, and soft tissue scarring.

Ruedi and Allgower[18, 19] and others[6, 9, 16, 17, 25] directly correlated the adequacy of the articular reduction and the presence of stable fixation with functional and radiographic results at long-term follow-up. However, regardless of the reduction, the presence of avascular necrosis,[2, 4, 9, 13] plafond chondral damage,[4, 33] and associated talar chondral damage,[17, 18, 22, 25] increase the likelihood of posttraumatic arthritis. This complication has been reported to occur in anywhere from 13 to 54% of cases.[2, 4, 9, 12, 16–18]

Importantly, Ruedi[18] noted that the lack

of joint arthrosis at 1 to 2 years indicates a more favorable prognosis. Subjective results also tend to improve over time in spite of persistent restriction of motion.[20]

THE UNRECONSTRUCTABLE FRACTURE

When severe comminution, articular damage, or loss of bone stock precludes satisfactory reduction, arthrodesis becomes a viable alternative.[4, 5, 26, 28] However, primary arthrodesis should rarely be performed because of high rates of infection and nonunion and the difficulty of the procedure acutely.[9, 25, 47] Furthermore, some patients regain a considerable degree of painless motion despite residual deformity and arthrosis.[2, 20]

Ultimately, despite the best planning and use of modern technique, a few patients will require amputation.[4, 5, 28, 36, 37] Even when limb salvage is successful, functional results are often poor.[28, 37] In contrast, the use of modern prostheses allows for early and nearly normal return to function after below-knee amputations. Thus, consideration of primary amputation must be entertained in the most severe injuries.

SUMMARY

As techniques of biologic reduction and stabilization are refined, they are playing an increasingly crucial role in the management of these severe fractures. Adhering to the principles of restoration of length, alignment, and rotation, with anatomic articular reduction and fixation stable enough to allow early functional rehabilitation but without further soft tissue compromise, appears to improve results with fewer complications.

One fact is clear: a pilon fracture is not an injury to be taken lightly or treated by the inexperienced surgeon. Dillin and Slabaugh[46] noted disastrous results (a 55% incidence of osteomyelitis and 36% incidence of delayed wound healing or superficial infection) when such hands were involved. Thus, only those familiar with the anatomy, pathophysiology, and modern principles and techniques of pilon fracture care should tackle this challenging and often frustrating injury.

REFERENCES

1. Destot E. Traumatismes du pied et rayons x malleoles. Astragale, Calcaneum, Avant-pied. Paris: Masson, 1911.
2. Kellam JF, Waddell JP. Fractures of the distal tibial metaphysis with intra-articular extension: the distal tibial explosion fracture. J Trauma 19:593–601, 1979.
3. Maale G, Seligson D. Fractures through the distal weight-bearing surface of the tibia. Orthopaedics 3:517–521, 1980.
4. Ovadia DN, Beals RK. Fractures of the tibial plafond. J Bone Joint Surg Am 68:543–551, 1986.
5. Pierce FO, Heinrich JH. Comminuted intra-articular fractures of the distal tibia. J Trauma 19:828–832, 1979.
6. Teeny SM, Wiss DA. Open reduction and internal fixation of tibial plafond fractures: variables contributing to poor results and complications. Clin Orthop 292:108–117, 1993.
7. Lambotte A. Chirurgie operatoire des fractures. Paris: Masson, 1913.
8. Bonin JG. Injuries to the Ankle. London: William Heinemann, 1950, pp. 248–260.
9. Heim U. The Pilon Tibial Fracture: Classification, Surgical Techniques, Results. Philadelphia: W. B. Saunders, 1995.
10. Helfet DL, Koval K, Pappas J, et al. Intra-articular "pilon" fractures of the tibia. Clin Orthop 298:221–228, 1994.
11. Mast JW, Spiegal PG, Pappas JN. Fractures of the tibial pilon. Clin Orthop 230:68–82, 1988.
12. McFerran MA, Smith SW, Boulas HJ, Schwartz HS. Complications encountered in the treatment of pilon fractures. J Orthop Trauma 6:195–200, 1992.
13. Beck E. Results of operative treatment of pilon fractures. In Tscherne H, Schatzker J, eds. Major Fractures of the Pilon, the Talus, and the Calcaneus. Heidelberg: Springer, 1993, pp. 49–51.
14. Bone L, Stegeman P, McNamara K, Seibel R. External fixation of severely comminuted and open tibial pilon fractures. Clin Orthop 292:101–107, 1993.
15. Muhr G, Breitfuss H. Complications after pilon fractures. In Tscherne H, Schatzker J, eds. Major Fractures of the Pilon, the Talus, and the Calcaneus. Heidelberg: Springer, 1993, pp. 65–67.
16. Bourne RB. Pylon fractures of the distal tibia. Clin Orthop 240:42–46, 1989.
17. Moller BN, Krebs B. Intra-articular fractures of the distal tibia. Acta Orthop Scand 53:991–996, 1982.
18. Ruedi T: Fractures of the lower end of the tibia into the ankle joint: results nine years after open reduction and internal fixation. Injury 5:130–134, 1973.
19. Ruedi T, Allgower M. Fractures of the lower end of the tibia into the ankle joint. Injury 1:92–99, 1969.
20. Ruedi TP, Allgower M. The operative treatment of intra-articular fractures of the lower end of the tibia. Clin Orthop 138:105–110, 1979.
21. Tile M. Fractures of the distal tibial metaphysis involving the ankle joint: the pilon fracture. In Schatzker J, Tile M, eds. The Rationale of Operative Fracture Care. Berlin: Springer-Verlag, 1987, pp. 343–369.
22. Tornetta P, Weiner L, Bergman M, et al. Pilon fractures: treatment with combined internal and

external fixation. J Orthop Trauma 7:489–496, 1993.

23. Ruoff AC, Snider RK. Explosion fractures of the distal tibia with major articular involvement. J Trauma 11:866–873, 1971.

24. Muller ME, Nazarian S, Koch P, Schatzker J. The Comprehensive Classification of Fractures of Long Bones. New York: Springer-Verlag, 1987, pp. 170–179.

25. Etter C, Ganz R. Long-term results of tibial plafond fractures treated with open reduction and internal fixation. Arch Orthop Trauma Surg 110:277–283, 1991.

26. Jergesen F. Open reduction of fractures and dislocations of the ankle. Am J Surg 98:136, 1959.

27. Allgower M, Muller ME, Willenegger H. Technik der operativen Frakturbehandlung. New York: Springer-Verlag, 1963.

28. Sanders R, Pappas J, Mast J, Helfet D. The salvage of open grade IIIB ankle and talus fractures. J Orthop Trauma 6:201–208, 1992.

29. Wyrsch B, McFerran MA, McAndrew M, et al. Operative treatment of fractures of the tibial plafond: a randomized prospective study. J Bone Joint Surg Am 78:1646–1657, 1996.

30. Fitzpatrick DC, Marsh JL, Brown TD. Articulated external fixation of pilon fractures: the effects on ankle joint kinematics. J Orthop Trauma 9:76–82, 1995.

31. Marsh JL, Bonar S, Nepola JV, et al. Use of an articulated external fixator for fractures of the tibial plafond. J Bone Joint Surg Am 77:1498–1509, 1995.

32. Helfet DL, Borrelli J, Shonnard P, Levine DB. Minimally invasive plate osteosynthesis of distal tibia fractures. Injury 28:A42–A48, 1997.

33. Leach RE. Fractures of the tibial plafond. In Yablon IG, Segal D, Leach R, eds. Ankle Injuries. New York: Churchill Livingstone, 1983.

34. Mast JW. Reduction techniques in fractures of the distal tibial articular surface. Tech Orthop 2:29–36, 1987.

35. Leone VJ, Ruland R, Meinhard B. The management of soft tissue in pilon fractures. Clin Orthop 292:315–320, 1993.

36. Helfet CK, Howey T, Sanders R, Johansen K. Limb salvage versus amputation: preliminary results of the mangled extremity severity score. Clin Orthop 256:80–86, 1990.

37. Stasikelis PJ, Calhoun JH, Ledbetter BR, et al. Treatment of infected pilon nonunions with small pin fixators. Foot Ankle 14:373–379, 1993.

38. Collins DN, Temple SD. Open joint injuries. Clin Orthop 243:48–56, 1989.

39. Franklin JL, Johnson KD, Hansen ST. Immediate internal fixation of open ankle fractures: report of thirty-eight cases treated with a standard protocol. J Bone Joint Surg Am 66:1349–1356, 1984.

40. Gustilo RB, Anderson JT. Prevention of infection in the treatment of one thousand and twenty-five open fractures of the long bones: retrospective and prospective analysis. J Bone Joint Surg Am 58:453–458, 1976.

41. Trentz O, Friedl HP. Critical soft tissue conditions and pilon fractures. In Tscherne H, Schatzker J, eds. Major Fractures of the Pilon, the Talus, and the Calcaneus. Heidelberg: Springer, 1993, pp. 59–64.

42. Trumble TE, Benirschke SK, Vedder NB. Use of radial forearm flaps to treat complications of closed pilon fractures. J Trauma 6:358–365, 1992.

43. Mast J. Pilon fractures of the distal tibia. In Tscherne H, Schatzker J, eds. Major Fractures of the Pilon, the Talus, and the Calcaneus. Heidelberg: Springer, 1993, pp. 7–27.

44. Marsh JL, DeCoster TA, Hurwitz SR, et al. Tibial plafond fractures: is routine plating of the fibula necessary? Paper presented at the 11th annual meeting of the Orthopaedic Trauma Association. Tampa, FL, September 1995.

45. Cierny G, Byrd HS, Jones RE. Primary versus delayed soft tissue coverage for severe open tibial fractures. Clin Orthop 178:54–63, 1983.

46. Dillin L, Slabaugh P. Delayed wound healing, infection, and nonunion following open reduction and internal fixation of tibial plafond fractures. J Trauma 26:1116–1119, 1986.

47. Green SA, Roesler S. Salvage of the infected pilon fracture. Tech Orthop 2:37–41, 1987.

28

Chronic Compartment Syndrome and Shin Splints

David S. Levine
Stephen J. O'Brien

Since the 1970s, the number of athletic participants, either at the recreational or world-class level, has skyrocketed. Concomitantly, the development of advanced technology, the understanding and implementation of improved nutrition concepts, and increased access to recreational facilities have all contributed to this increased participation. As a result, there has been an increase in the absolute numbers of musculoskeletal injuries. Acute injuries to the lower extremity such as fractures and dislocations frequently present little difficulty in establishing a diagnosis. However, lower extremity injuries that develop insidiously, often presenting as a vague leg pain, can challenge the physician's clinical acumen.

The clinician who maintains a practice in sports medicine or foot and ankle surgery will encounter leg pain in approximately 4 to 30% of their practice.[1] Three of the most common clinical entities presenting as chronic leg pain include "shin splints, "chronic exertional compartment syndrome, and stress fractures. The diagnosis and management of stress fractures are discussed in Chapter 20. Although much has been learned in recent years about the causes and management of these chronic leg syndromes, much remains to be understood. In addition, other entities in the differential diagnosis of chronic leg pain, including peripheral vascular disorders (such as the popliteal artery entrapment syndrome), nerve entrapment syndromes, inflammatory and infectious processes, as well as central neurological disorders (i.e., radiculopathies), need to be ruled out.

CHRONIC COMPARTMENT SYNDROME

Davey and colleagues defined compartment syndrome as a condition of neurovascular compromise of soft tissues within a nondistensible space resulting from elevated tissue pressures.[2] Acute compartment syndromes of the leg can result from a direct injury to the lower extremity, such as a tibial fracture. Additional causes include, for example, crush injuries, burns, reperfusion injury after vascular repairs, and constrictive circumferential dressings or casts. An untreated acute compartment syndrome can result in significant permanent disability and even limb loss. Fortunately, the diagnosis and management of acute compartment syndrome have been extensively studied, and such clinical sequelae can usually be avoided with timely intervention (i.e., fasciotomy). Chronic or exertional compartment syndrome represents a transient and reversible interruption of adequate blood flow to the lower extremity. Through the work of multiple investigators, the diagnosis and management of this condition have been refined and have subsequently brought relief of chronic leg pain to many of those so affected.

Anatomic Considerations

The leg has been classically described as containing four compartments: anterior, lateral, superficial, and deep posterior (Fig. 28–1). Chronic exertional compartment syndrome occurs most commonly in the anterior compartment, followed in frequency by the deep posterior compartment.[3] Each compartment contains skeletal muscle and neurovascular elements surrounded by a relatively nondistensible fascial envelope. It has been estimated that during exercise muscle can experience a 20% increase in its volume.[4] Within the noncompliant osseofascial compartments, the increase in muscular volume as a result of exercise is reflected as a concomitant rise in compartmental pressures. When such pressures exceed the capillary perfusion pressures, the result is the

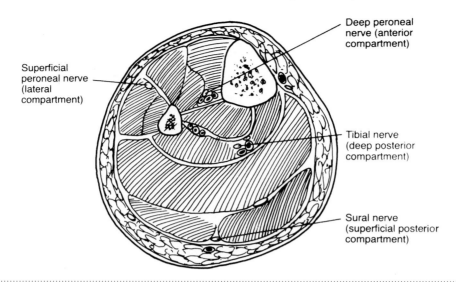

Figure 28–1. Cross-section demonstrating the four osseofascial compartments of the leg. From Andrish JT. The leg. In DeLee JC, Drez D Jr, eds. Orthopaedic Sports Medicine: Principles and Practice. Philadelphia: WB Saunders, 1994, p 1603.

lack of blood supply to the contents of the compartment, including the neural elements.

Investigations combining contrast injection techniques, in vivo and cadaveric dissections, have suggested that a fifth compartment exists in the leg that contributes to chronic exertional compartment syndrome. According to Davey and associates[2] and Rorabeck,[5] the tibialis posterior muscle exists in its own osseofascial compartment, distinct from the deep posterior muscle compartment. Radiopaque contrast injected into the substance of the muscle was noted to remain within its fascial boundaries without extravasating into the remainder of the deep posterior compartment. These investigators demonstrated that traditional four-compartment fasciotomies failed to release the fascia of the tibialis posterior muscle in cadaveric compartment syndrome models. In addition, compartmental pressure measurements of athletes with clinical presentations of posterior compartment syndrome demonstrate elevated pressures within the tibialis posterior muscle, whereas those of the deep posterior compartment were within normal limits. The authors concluded that during fasciotomy for deep posterior compartment syndrome the surgeon should include the release of the thick investing fascia overlying the tibialis posterior muscle.

Clinical Presentation

The most common presenting complaint of a patient suspected of having a chronic exertional compartment syndrome is pain in the leg. The pain typically occurs during an activity (e.g., running) typically involving repetitive muscular contraction. Often noted in the history is a change in training habits of an athlete such as a recent increase in mileage or a change in equipment (e.g., running shoes, terrain). The symptoms begin at some predictable time after the activity is begun and promptly subside with the cessation of the activity. The pain is often dull in character at its onset, but with continued activity the intensity can be disabling, precluding the activity altogether. A sense of fullness in the involved compartment is a consistent symptom, again promptly relieved with rest. The pain may be localized to the involved muscle masses themselves. Alternatively, the patient may present with radicular pain or weakness involving the peripheral nerve traversing that particular compartment. Most commonly, the anterior compartment is involved followed by the deep posterior compartment (together these two compartments make up 80% of the cases of exertional compartment syndrome).[1] Often no history of trauma can be elicited. Neurologic symptoms may include paresthesias, dysesthesias, or burning in the distribution of the cutaneous nerve within the involved compartment. History of stress fracture of the involved lower extremity may be present in up to 17% of patients with chronic exertional compartment syndrome.[6]

Physical Examination

Recall that chronic compartment syndromes are exertional. That is, the patient may be pain free during a routine office visit. To elicit positive signs on examination, it is often necessary to exercise the patient. Exercise similar to the activity that causes the symptoms is most appropriate. Typically, the patient will experience a tenseness present in the involved compartment not present in unaffected compartments. Tenderness is noted in the muscle bellies within the affected compartment with continued exercise. The bony structures of the affected lower extremity are not usually tender. Tenderness of the osseous structures should make the examiner question the diagnosis of chronic exertional compartment syndrome. Stress fractures and periostitis are much more likely to result in bony tenderness. Pedal pulses are routinely intact and symmetric. Pulses should be checked with maximal ankle dorsiflexion and maximal plantar flexion. Loss of pulses in either of these extremes, particularly plantar flexion, may represent a popliteal artery entrapment syndrome. Arteriography should be performed to identify the site of entrapment in such patients. The loss of two-point discrimination and the presence of paresthesias may be noted over the distribution of a cutaneous nerve affected by an exertional compartment syndrome.

The presence of fascial hernias in the leg has been noted in many studies involving chronic exertional compartment syndrome. This association has been reported in up to 60% of patients with exertional compartment syndromes.[7] Paresthesias are more common in the presence of muscle hernias, because nerve entrapment can occur along the sharp edge of the fascial defect. The presence of these fascial hernias has implications for the placement of skin and fascial incisions and is discussed under Treatment.

Diagnostic Testing

Anteroposterior and lateral plain radiographs typically are unremarkable. The presence of a stress fracture would routinely be observed on plain radiographs. Patients with early stress fractures will have normal radiographs; however, the average duration of symptoms in a patient with chronic compartment syndrome before presenting to a clinician is 22 months.[1] At this time, radiologic stigmas of a stress fracture would be readily apparent.

The patient who presents with an objective neurologic abnormality should undergo nerve conduction velocities and electromyographic studies. These investigations can identify the nerve entrapment neuropathies commonly seen with muscle herniations through fascial defects. The lateral branch of the superficial peroneal nerve is the most commonly involved nerve.

A 1990 investigation evaluated the usefulness of magnetic resonance imaging (MRI) in the diagnosis of chronic exertional compartment syndrome.[8] Amendola and colleagues used methoxy isobutyl isonitrile, a radiotracer compound known to be "taken up by muscle in direct proportion to its blood flow" along with both pre- and postexercise MRI to determine the pathophysiology of chronic exertional compartment syndrome.[8] Blood flow studies were normal in all symptomatic patients studied irrespective of normal or elevated compartment pressures. However, in a small subset of patients with a history consistent with exertional compartment syndrome, postexercise MRI demonstrated significant signal alterations on T1 signal sequences, with failure to return to baseline levels with activity cessation. These signal alterations paralleled abnormally elevated postexercise pressure measurements, and with further study may provide a reliable noninvasive alternative to compartmental pressure measurements.

A patient who presents with a clinical picture consistent with a stress fracture or periostitis, who has normal radiographs, should undergo a labeled technetium bone scan. Either of these entities has a characteristic nuclear medicine pattern that readily distinguishes one from the other. The patient with chronic exertional compartment syndrome does not demonstrate increased uptake on the delayed (osseous) phase of a bone scan.

Clinical evaluation with a detailed history and physical examination is often sufficient to establish the diagnosis of a chronic exertional compartment syndrome. To add objective verification of a chronic compartment syndrome, measurement of intracompartmental pressure has become an integral part of the work-up. Although the use of intracompartmental pressure measurements is widely accepted by those who treat such disorders, the method of measurement and the temporal relationship to exercise are often matters of debate.

Various techniques used to measure compartment pressures have been described in the literature, including the wick catheter,[9] slit catheter,[10] Strykes Intra-Compartmental (STIC) method,[11] constant infusion method,[12] and fiber optics.[13] The STIC and slit-catheter methods are the two most commonly used. As mentioned, chronic exertional compartment syndrome is a dynamic condition. Its manifestations are often absent at rest and occur with exercise. It is not difficult to measure intracompartmental pressures at rest before exercise. Nor is it difficult to measure pressures after exercise completion. Some authors, however, have attempted to measure pressures during exercise. Such dynamic pressure measurements, especially if accompanied by a patient's characteristic symptoms, may offer a more prognostic measurement. These dynamic techniques are often more difficult to perform and are significantly more difficult to standardize.

Mubarak and colleagues[14] used the wick and slit-catheter methods to measure intracompartmental pressures before, during, and after exercise in athletes who complained of exercise-induced pain along the posteromedial border of the leg. These patients, according to Mubarak and coworkers, had medial tibial stress syndrome but provided them with the normal values for pressure measurements. They described the mean resting pressure in the anterior compartment of the leg while supine as 4 ± 4 mm Hg. During exercise, the pressures rose to more than 50 mm Hg. After exercise, the mean pressures decreased to below 30 mm Hg almost immediately and at 5 minutes after exercise were at the pre-exercise resting level in most cases. They described another group of patients with chronic anterior compartment syndrome. The resting intramuscular pressures were usually greater than 15 mm Hg. During exercise, pressures often rose greater than 75 mm Hg and on occasion over 100 mm Hg. Postexer-

cise pressures remained greater than 30 mm Hg at 5 minutes or longer.[14]

Other investigators have noted similar elevated dynamic pressures as well as a failure of postexercise pressures to return to normal. Mannarino and Sexson[7] compared the differences in compartment pressures between patients with clinical anterior and posterior chronic compartment syndromes with asymptomatic controls. Using the wick catheter method, resting pressures in the symptomatic cases averaged 13.7 mm Hg compared with 9.9 mm Hg for the controls. The average exercise pressures in the symptomatic cases was 81.5 mm Hg; peak pressures were consistently above 100 mm Hg, often reaching 120 to 130 mm Hg. Those patients whose exercise pressures did not reach 60 mm Hg could not complete the exercise protocol as a result of intense pain in the affected muscle compartment. The average exercise pressures in the control group was 62.5 mm Hg. The postexercise pressures did not return to normal levels in the majority of symptomatic patients, whereas 70% of the asymptomatic patients did return to resting levels within 5 minutes after activity cessation. None of the asymptomatic control patients exhibited pain during the exercise protocols. The authors concluded that resting pressures are suggestive of, but not diagnostic for, chronic exertional compartment syndrome, whereas peak exercise pressures above 100 mm Hg are more predictive. The authors stressed that the clinical evaluation and reproduction of symptoms during exercise testing are most predictive.[7]

Puranen and Alavaikko[3] similarly measured compartment pressures at rest and during running in patients who had the clinical presentation of chronic compartment syndrome. Compared with a group of asymptomatic controls, the symptomatic patients had a significantly higher exercise pressure increase. There were no differences in the pressures at rest between the two groups.[3] Once again, the postexercise pressures did not return to pre-exercise levels for many minutes.

Pedowitz and colleagues[15] developed criteria to be used for the diagnosis of chronic compartment syndrome of the leg based on their evaluation of 159 patients with chronic exertional leg pain. All patients underwent compartment pressure measurements. The only difference between those with elevated pressures and those with normal pressures was a 46% incidence of muscle hernias in the patients with chronic compartment syndrome compared with 13% in those without the syndrome. Through the comparison of the two groups, modified criteria for the objective diagnosis of chronic exertional compartment syndrome were developed. One or more of the following pressure criteria must be present for the diagnosis to be established: (1) a pre-exercise pressure of 15 mm Hg or greater, (2) a 1-minute postexercise pressure of 30 mm Hg or greater; (3) a 5-minute postexercise pressure of 20 mm Hg or greater.[15]

Treatment
Nonoperative

Avoidance of the activity that causes and incites the symptoms is a very effective treatment for chronic exertional compartment syndrome. However, most of the people who seek a professional opinion for the treatment of activity-related leg pain are interested in continuing the activity. A trial of activity modification (e.g., cross-training, intensity reduction) is warranted in most patients. A controlled, staged reintroduction of the patient's exercise program, often with the use of an anti-inflammatory agent and other adjunctive treatment modality, may then be attempted. However, the majority of patients will experience a return of their symptoms as they approach their prior levels of training.

Operative

The treatment of choice for a documented chronic exertional compartment syndrome of the leg is fasciotomy. Unlike the management of an acute compartment syndrome, which routinely requires a four-compartment fasciotomy, selective compartment release may be appropriate in the chronic syndrome in which only certain compartments demonstrate elevated pressures.

Several techniques have been proposed for performing fasciotomy of the leg: fibulectomy,[16] perifibular four-compartment fasciotomy,[12] and two-incision four-compartment fasciotomy.[17]

Technique for Anterior / Lateral Compartment release (Fig. 28–2)

1. An incision is made longitudinally over the anterolateral aspect of the leg approximating the position of the anterolateral intermuscular septum. The incision ex-

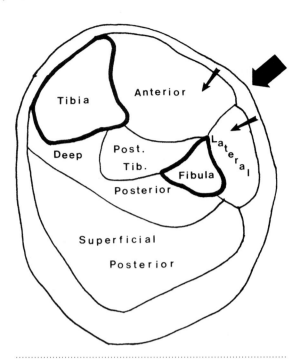

Figure 28–2. Cross-section demonstrating placement of skin and fascial incisions for anterior and lateral compartmental release. From Eisele SA, Sammarco J. Chronic exertional compartment syndrome. In Heckman JD, ed. Instructional Course Lectures, Vol 42. Rosemont, IL: American Academy of Orthopaedic Surgeons, 1993, p 213.

tends for approximately 10 cm from just below the level of the tibial tubercle.

2. A transverse incision is made in the fascia to identify the lateral intermuscular septum.

3. The anterior compartment fascia is released longitudinally approximately 1 cm anterior to the intermuscular septum.

4. The lateral compartment is released longitudinally approximately 1 cm posterior to the intermuscular septum.

5. The superficial peroneal nerve pierces the fascia just lateral to the intermuscular septum approximately 10 to 12 cm above the tip of the lateral malleolus. The surgeon should exercise caution because the nerve lies subcutaneously distal to this point.

6. After hemostasis has been achieved, the skin is closed.

Technique for Superficial / Deep Posterior Compartment Release (Fig. 28–3)

1. A longitudinal skin incision is made approximately 2 cm posterior to the postero-

medial border of the tibia. Care should be taken to avoid injury to the saphenous vein and nerve in the subcutaneous tissues.

2. The fascia overlying the superficial compartment is released longitudinally. In the middle and distal thirds of the leg, the fascia of the soleus muscle inserts directly on the posteromedial border of the tibia. It must be released, providing complete exposure of the deep posterior compartment.

3. The fascia of the deep posterior compartment may then be released. Of note, a separate release of the fascia overlying the tibialis posterior muscle should be performed. Exposure of the fascia overlying the tibialis posterior muscle can be difficult, however. The tibialis posterior can be exposed through a perifibular approach posterior to the fibula as described by Davey and others.[2] Alternatively, it can be approached through the interosseous membrane from the anterolateral incision as described by Nghiem and Boland.[18] Finally, the tibialis posterior muscle can be approached through the posteromedial incision posterior to the tibia.[19]

4. The skin is closed after hemostasis is achieved.

Postoperative Care

A gentle compressive bandage is placed in the operating room. Elevation of the postoperative extremity is recommended for 48 to 72 hours to minimize swelling. Progressive weight bearing with crutches for comfort is begun immediately. Motion exercises and isometrics are begun as soon as the acute operative pain subsides. At 3 to 4 weeks, light running is usually tolerated with a return to full, unlimited activity by 4 to 6 weeks in most cases.

Conclusions

Chronic exertional compartment syndrome presents with a characteristic history and physical examination. Examination after a period of exercise is often the key to establishing the diagnosis. Compartment pressure testing is helpful in confirming the diagnosis and directing treatment. Nonoperative treatment measures are largely ineffective in this population of patients, who generally desire to maintain their active lifestyles. Fasciotomy of the involved compartments provides predictable relief of the

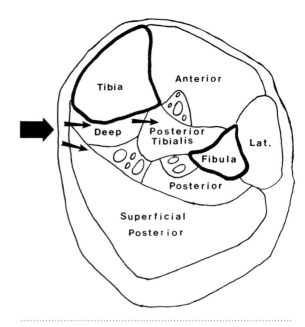

Figure 28–3. Cross-section demonstrating placement of skin and fascial incisions for superficial and deep posterior compartmental release. From Eisele SA, Sammarco J. Chronic exertional compartment syndrome. In Heckman JD, ed. Instructional Course Lectures, Vol 42. Rosemont, IL: American Academy of Orthopaedic Surgeons, 1993, p 213.

signs and symptoms of compartment syndrome when performed on the carefully selected patient, with little risk of complications.

SHIN SPLINTS

The term *shin splints* is vague, often used as a catch-all phrase by the recreational athlete to refer to pain over the lower end of the leg that prevents further athletic activity. It probably should be abandoned because its causes are varied, including chronic exertional compartment syndrome, stress fractures of the tibia and fibula, fascial herniations, tears of the interosseous membrane, periostitis, tendinitis, and muscle strains. As investigation into chronic leg pain syndromes continues, the distinction between the different syndromes widens. Drez proposed the term *medial tibial stress syndrome*.[14] Detmer[20] subclassified this syndrome, as follows: type I represents posteromedial stress fracture; type II is a lesser degree of periosteal reaction from the overpull of the soleus fascia on the posteromedial border of the tibia; type III is a deep posterior or tibialis posterior compartment syndrome.

The most recent consensus in the literature indicates that medial tibial stress syndrome is a condition of periostitis.[14, 21–25] This implies that cases of stress fracture and chronic exertional compartment syndromes are excluded. We concur with this definition, and the presentation, evaluation, and management of periostitis, therefore, comprise the remainder of this discussion.

Clinical Presentation

The main complaint among patients with medial tibial stress syndrome is pain along the posteromedial border of the middle and distal thirds of the tibia. Similar to those afflicted with chronic compartment syndromes, the pain is intermittent and associated with a strenuous physical activity. Initially, the pain may be dull and occur toward the end of the activity. However, with continuation of the training, the character and intensity of the pain increase predictably and often occur with less exertion. The pain, which was relieved with rest initially, now may persist for some time even over the ensuing days after the activity. Symptoms are often exacerbated by running on banked surfaces. As with most other overuse conditions, medial tibial stress syndrome often occurs after a change in athletic activity, such as an increase in running mileage. The literature is not in agreement about the protective nature of preconditioning in the prevention of medial tibial stress syndrome. Andrish and colleagues found that Navy midshipmen who had no prior physical training before entering the Naval Academy were twice as likely to experience medial tibial stress syndrome as those who had prior training.[26] However, Milgrom and colleagues[27] found no association between prior aerobic fitness and sports participation and the development of medial tibial stress syndrome in military recruits.

Physical Examination

Tenderness along the posteromedial border of the tibia is the most reproducible finding on examination. It is often located over the middle and distal thirds of the tibia, typically between 4 and 12 cm from the medial malleolus. Swelling and induration may be noted locally. Bony tenderness is unusual and should raise the clinician's suspicions for a stress fracture. Percussion of the tibia proximally should not elicit tenderness. Active resisted flexion of the ankle may elicit pain. Neurologic examination is normal, and pedal pulses should be present at rest and with active ankle dorsi- and plantar flexion. Limb alignment should be carefully evaluated. Sommer and Vallentyne noted the association of either hindfoot or forefoot varus with the incidence of medial tibial stress syndrome.[28]

Diagnostic Evaluation

Routine evaluation of the anteroposterior and lateral radiographs are often normal. However, certain subtle signs may be present, including posterior tibial cortical hypertrophy and periosteal new bone formation. Evidence of a healed stress fracture may be noted.

The most useful diagnostic tool in the evaluation of the patient with symptoms consistent with medial tibial stress syndrome is the bone scan. Technetium-99 bone scans demonstrate a characteristic pattern of increased radiotracer signal uptake. In medial tibial stress syndrome, there is increase signal noted along the posteromedial border of the tibia on the delayed phase of the scan. The character of the uptake as described by Rupani and colleagues distinguishes medial tibial stress syndrome from tibial stress fracture.[29] In medial tibial stress syndrome, the signal uptake is moderate and extends for about one-third the length of the tibia itself. The ratio of the length of the lesion and the length of the tibia is 1:3 to 3:4. Bone scan abnormalities in tibial stress fractures, on the other hand, are typically more intense and focal. The uptake has been described as fusiform, although it is often transverse. The ratio of the lesion on the scan and the length of the tibia is closer to 1:5.

If some doubt remains in distinguishing a medial tibial stress syndrome from a chronic exertional compartment syndrome in a particular patient, compartment pressures should be measured. They are normal in medial tibial stress syndrome. Finally, diagnostic local injection of a short-acting anesthetic such as lidocaine into the periosteum on the posteromedial border of the tibial should be helpful. In medial tibial stress syndrome, the symptoms should transiently be relieved.[30]

Anatomic Considerations

Multiple causes of medial tibial stress syndrome have been offered by various authors. As mentioned, compartment syndromes can be ruled out by pressure measurement studies; tibial stress fractures can be ruled out by radiographs and characteristic bone scan appearance. The anatomic cause of medial tibial stress syndrome is still debated. Many investigators consider the tibialis posterior muscle to be the cause of the syndrome.[31, 32] Detmer[20] and Michael and Holder[33] proposed that the medial fibers of the soleus muscle and fascia caused the syndrome. Finally, Garth and Miller have implicated the flexor digitorum longus muscle as the causative agent in medial tibial stress syndrome.[34]

Beck and Osternig performed an anatomic study to identify the tibial origins of various structures thought to cause medial tibial stress syndrome. The purpose was to determine whether each structure has the potential to cause a traction periostitis at the site of the symptoms of medial tibial stress syndrome. The investigators found in 50 cadavers that the soleus, the flexor digitorum longus, and the deep crural fascia were found to attach to the tibia at the site where medial tibial stress syndrome symptoms occur. In no specimen was the tibialis posterior muscle found to attach to this site.[35]

Treatment

Nonoperative

In the study of Naval midshipmen mentioned previously, patients were treated with one of a number of nonoperative therapies, including rest, anti-inflammatory medications, heel cord stretching, orthoses, and casting. No treatments alone or in combination were superior to rest alone.[26] As in all overuse syndromes, modification of activities or avoidance altogether may prove effective for the patient willing to do so.

Recall that certain limb alignment abnormalities such as forefoot and hindfoot varus as well as tibial varus are associated with an increased incidence of medial tibial stress syndrome. Properly fitted orthoses may prove beneficial in such circumstances.

Recurrence of symptoms is the most common outcome of nonoperative treatment of medial tibial stress syndrome. The most common error leading to the recurrence of symptoms is the premature return to the preinjury level of activity. At least 6 weeks of a graduated program of activity reintroduction should be followed to ensure the greatest possibility of nonoperative success.

Operative

The individual who suffers from the signs and symptoms of medial tibial stress syndrome who fails repeated attempts at activity reduction or modification is a candidate for operative intervention. Recall that the most agreed-on theory regarding the cause of medial tibial stress syndrome is the chronic periostitis of the posteromedial tibia caused by the pull of the soleus muscle and its fascia. Operative treatment, therefore, is directed at the medial insertion of the soleus muscle into the tibia.

Technique

1. A longitudinal incision is made parallel to the posteromedial border of the tibia in its middle third. The saphenous vein and nerve should be carefully preserved.

2. The soleus muscle and its investing fascia should be released from the medial border of the tibia. This is best accomplished from distal to proximal.

3. The skin is closed after hemostasis is achieved.

Postoperative Care

A gentle compressive bandage is applied in the operating room. Progressive weight bearing with crutches is begun at 2 to 4 days. Range-of-motion exercises are begun immediately. Light running is begun at 2 weeks when incisional pain subsides with a full return to sport expected at 4 to 6 weeks.

Conclusions

The incidence of activity-related leg pain is increasing as the population assumes a more active lifestyle. The clinician whose practice concentrates in sports medicine and foot and ankle disorders will certainly encounter chronic exertional compartment syndromes and medial tibial stress syndromes. If the clinician takes a careful history and performs a complete physical examination, the diagnosis will not be missed. When the diagnosis is less obvious, various diagnostic modalities offer the practitioner further insight into the cause of the condition. Nonoperative treatment of chronic exertional compartment syndrome and medial tibial stress syndrome is often ineffective, and surgical treatment provides long-lasting relief in the majority of patients.

REFERENCES

1. Andrish JT. The leg. In Delee JC, Drez D Jr, eds. Orthopaedic Sports Medicine. Principles and Practice. Philadelphia, W. B. Saunders, 1994, p. 1603.
2. Davey JR, Rorabeck CH, Fowler PJ. The tibialis posterior muscle compartment: an unrecognized cause of exertional compartment syndrome. Am J Sports Med 12:391, 1984.
3. Puranen J, Alavaikko A. Intracompartmental pressure increase on exertion in patients with chronic compartment syndrome in the leg. J Bone Joint Surg Am 63:1304, 1981.
4. Jones DC, James SL. Overuse injuries of the lower extremity: shin splints, iliotibial band friction syndrome, and exertional compartment syndromes. Clin Sports Med 6:273, 1987.
5. Rorabeck CH. Exertional tibialis posterior compartment syndrome. Clin Orthop 208:61, 1986.
6. Detmer DE, Sharpe K, Sufit RL, Girdley FM. Chronic compartment syndrome: diagnosis, management and outcomes. Am J Sports Med 13:162, 1985.
7. Mannarino F, Sexson S. The significance of intracompartmental pressures in the diagnosis of chronic exertional compartment syndrome. Orthopedics 12:1415, 1989.
8. Amendola A, Rorabeck CH, Vellett D, et al. The use of magnetic resonance imaging in exertional compartment syndromes. Am J Sports Med 18:29, 1990.
9. Mubarak SJ, Hargens AR, Owen CA, et al. The wick catheter technique for measurement of intramuscular pressure: a new research and clinical tool. J Bone Joint Surg Am 58: 1016, 1976.
10. Rorabeck CH, Castle GSP, Hardie R, et al. Compartmental pressure measurements: an experimental investigation using the slit catheter. J Trauma 21:446, 1981.
11. McDermott AGP, Marble AE, Yabslev RH, et al. Monitoring dynamic anterior compartment pressures during exercise: a new technique using the STIC catheter. Am J Sports Med 10:83, 1982.
12. Matsen FA, Winquist RA, Krugmire RB. Diagnosis and management of compartment syndromes. J Bone Joint Surg Am 62:286, 1980.
13. Crenshaw AG, Hargens AR, Mubarak SJ. A new fiber optic "transducer tipped" catheter for measuring intramuscular pressures. Orthop Trans 13:173, 1988.
14. Mubarak SJ, Gould RN, Lee YF, et al. The medial tibial stress syndrome: a cause of shin splints. Am J Sports Med 10:201, 1982.
15. Pedowitz RA, Hargens AR, Mubarak SJ, Gershuni DH. Modified criteria for the objective diagnosis of chronic compartment syndrome of the leg. Am J Sports Med 18:35, 1990.
16. Whitesides T, Haney T, Morimoto K, Harada H. Tissue pressure measurements as a determinant for the need of fasciotomy. Clin Orthop 135:45, 1975.
17. Mubarak SJ, Owen C. Double-incision fasciotomy of the leg for decompression in compartment syndromes. J Bone Joint Surg Am 59:184, 1977.
18. Nghiem D, Boland J: Four compartment fasciotomy of the lower extremity without fibulectomy: a new approach. Am Surg 46:414, 1980.
19. Eisele SA, Sammarco GJ. Chronic exertional compartment syndrome. In Heckman JD, ed. Instructional Course Lectures, vol 42. Park Ridge, IL: American Academy of Orthopaedic Surgeons, 1993:213.
20. Detmer DE. Chronic shin splints: classification and management of medial tibial stress syndrome. Sports Med 3: 436, 1986.
21. Andrish JT, Work JA. How I manage shin splints. Phys Sports Med 18:113, 1990.
22. Holder LE, Michael RH. The specific scintigraphic pattern of "shin splints in the lower leg": concise communication. J Nucl Med 25: 865, 1984.
23. Johnell O, Rausing A, Wendeberg B, Westlin N. Morphological bone changes in shin splints. Clin Orthop 167:180, 1982.
24. Mattalino AJ, Deese JM, Campbell ED. Office evaluation and treatment of lower extremity injuries in the runner. Clin Sports Med 8:461, 1989.
25. Styf J. Diagnosis of exercise-induced pain in the anterior aspect of the lower leg. Am J Sports Med 16:165, 1988.
26. Andrish JT, Bergfeld JA, Walheim J. A prospective study on the management of shin splints. J Bone Joint Surg Am 56:1697, 1974.
27. Milgrom C, Giladi M, Stein M, et al. Medial tibial pain: a prospective study of its cause among military recruits. Clin Orthop 213:167, 1986.
28. Sommer HM, Vallentyne SW. Effect of foot posture on the incidence of medial tibial stress syndrome. Med Sci Sports Exerc 27:800, 1995.
29. Rupani H, Holder L, Espinola D, Engin S. Three-phase radionuclide bone imaging in sports medicine. Radiology 156:187, 1985.
30. Allen JM, Barnes MR. Exercise pain in the lower leg. J Bone Joint Surg Br 68: 818, 1986.
31. D'Ambrosia RD, Zelis RF, Chuinard RG, Wilmore J. Interstitial pressure measurements in the anterior and posterior compartments in athletes with shin splints. Am J Sports Med 5: 127, 1977.
32. Slocum DB. The shin splint syndrome: medical aspects and differential diagnosis. Am J Surg 114:875, 1967.
33. Michael RH, Holder LE. The soleus syndrome: cause of medial tibia stress (shin splints). Am J Sports Med 13:87, 1985.
34. Garth WP, Miller ST. Evaluation of claw toe deformity, weakness of the foot intrinsics, and posteromedial shin pain. Am J Sports Med 17:821, 1989.
35. Beck BR, Osternig LR. Medial tibial stress syndrome: the location of muscles in the leg in relation to symptoms. J Bone Joint Surg Am 76: 1057, 1994.

29 Peroneal Tendon Disorders

Stuart D. Katchis
Eric J. Lindberg

Peroneal tendon injuries present with lateral ankle pain, swelling, or ankle instability. They are often underdiagnosed as simple ankle sprains. These disorders may occur in isolation or, frequently, in concert with other disease of the lateral ankle. In this section, we review the anatomy of the peroneal tendons, their function, pathology, and treatment options.

ANATOMY AND FUNCTION

The peronei include the peroneus longus, brevis, tertius, and quartus muscles. The peroneus longus and brevis are most often involved with lateral ankle disease and are contained in the lateral leg compartment. This distinct fascial compartment also contains the superficial peroneal nerve and, if present, the peroneus quartus muscle. The peroneus tertius is located in the anterior compartment of the leg; because it is not involved with lateral foot and ankle pathology, it is not discussed in this section. The blood supply to the lateral compartment is via perforating branches of the peroneal artery, which originates from the posterior tibial artery traveling in the posterior compartment of the leg.

The peroneus longus and peroneal brevis muscles each take origin from two thirds of the fibula: the longus from the proximal two thirds of the fibula and the brevis from the distal two thirds. From knee to ankle, the lateral aspect of the fibula spirals to a posterior position in the retromalleolar position; the respective origins of the muscles follow this spiral. In the central third of the fibula, the brevis origin is anterior to the longus origin, and the muscles and tendons retain this relationship throughout their course.[1] The muscle belly of the peroneus brevis extends distal to that of the longus. It usually ends superior to the superior peroneal retinaculum but occasionally lies below this level. The brevis tendon then curves around the tip of the lateral malleolus to travel just superior to the peroneal trochlea on the lateral aspect of the calcaneus. It continues distal, inferiorly, and laterally to insert on the base of the fifth metatarsal. The longus tendon remains posterior and inferior to the brevis tendon and passes inferior to the peroneal trochlea. The tendon then curves around the cuboid to travel distal medially across the sole of the foot to insert on the base of the first metatarsal and medial cuneiform. There are variable additional slips of tendinous insertion along the plantar aspect of the foot, of which those to the base of the second metatarsal and the first dorsal interosseous muscle are the most common.[2]

The anomalous peroneus quartus muscle is present in 13 to 21.7% of the population.[3, 4] The origin, insertion, and size of this muscle vary considerably. It originates from the muscular portion of the peroneus brevis 63% of the time.[5] The most common insertion is on the peroneal tubercle, but it may insert into the tuberosity of the cuboid or into the tendon of the peroneus longus. When the tendon inserts into the peroneal tubercle, the tubercle is often enlarged.

Anatomic constraints, including the synovial sheaths, the superior and inferior peroneal retinacula, and the retromalleolar groove, are important in maintaining the tendons along their course. The peroneal tendons are contained in separate synovial sheaths proximal to the lateral malleolus; these sheaths combine to form a common sheath in the retromalleolar region but split again at the level of the peroneal tubercle. The brevis sheath ends proximal to its insertion into the base of the fifth metatarsal, and the longus sheath ends before its turn around the cuboid. A second synovial sheath then forms around the longus tendon to enclose the tendon across the sole of the foot.

Two retinacula stabilize the tendons in their anatomic positions.[2] The superior peroneal retinaculum (SPR) is a Y-shaped fascial band that arises from the lateral border of the retromalleolar groove on the distal fibula. One limb inserts on the aponeurosis of the Achilles tendon, and the other on the posterolateral calcaneal surface paralleling that of the calcaneofibular ligament (Fig. 29–1). This, along with the strong aponeurotic tunnel on the posterior aspect of the fibula, retains the tendons in their retromalleolar position. The inferior peroneal retinaculum (IPR) is in continuity with the inferior extensor retinaculum on the dorsum of the foot. It originates on the lateral rim of the sinus tarsi and inserts on the lateral aspect of the calcaneus near the peroneal trochlea. The IPR forms two separate fibrous tunnels enclosing each tendon in its own synovial sheath at the level of the trochlea.

The retromalleolar groove is located in the posterior distal aspect of the fibula. It is variable in size and shape. Edwards[6] dissected 178 fibulas and found that in 145 (81%) a definite sulcus was present. In 19 (11%) the groove was a flat, transverse surface, and in 13 (7%) the groove was convex in shape. The average width of the sulcus was 6 mm and usually shallow, only occasionally exceeding 3 mm in depth. A dense lateral fibrocartilaginous ridge is present on the posterolateral surface of the fibula, which physiologically deepens this groove (Fig. 29–2).

The os peroneum, a sesamoid bone, is usually present in the longus tendon at the level of the cuboid.

The peroneal tendons are prime movers and dynamic stabilizers of the ankle joint.[7] They act to strongly evert the foot, but they also pronate and abduct the forefoot, thereby stabilizing the supinating triceps surae to produce straight plantar flexion.[8] The peroneus longus is also a plantar flexor of the first ray. If the peroneus longus loses this function, a dorsal bunion can result because of the unopposed action of the tibialis anterior. Although most actions of the peroneus longus tendon can be substituted by the primary movers of the foot, this function is unique.[9]

SPECIFIC DISORDERS

Several specific disorders of the peroneal tendons are described. They may represent, in part, a continuum of pathologic processes involving the peroneal tendons, and thus they may occur in concert with one another.

Tendinitis

Peritendinitis is a common overuse injury of the peroneal tendons resulting from mechanical stress on the tendons in and around the retromalleolar groove.[10] The patient complains of pain in the posterolateral ankle, which increases with activity. Clinical signs include focal tenderness, swelling, and reproduction of pain in the retromalleolar region with active eversion against resistance.[7] The pathophysiology involves both micro- and macroruptures of the tendons and may be associated with the deposition of calcium salts. Radiographs are not diagnostic for tendinitis, but are important to

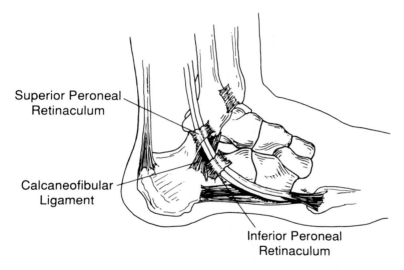

Superior Peroneal Retinaculum

Calcaneofibular Ligament

Inferior Peroneal Retinaculum

Figure 29–1. Superior and inferior peroneal retinacula. Main stabilizers of the peroneal tendons at the ankle. (From Clanton TO, Schon LS. Athletic injuries to the soft tissues of the foot and ankle. In Mann RA, Coughlin HJ, eds. Surgery of the Foot and Ankle, ed 6. St. Louis: C.V. Mosby, 1993, p. 1169.)

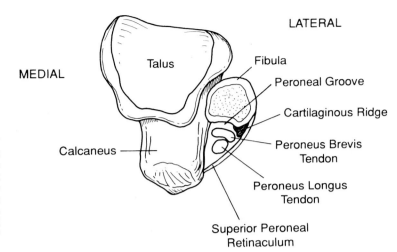

LATERAL

MEDIAL

Talus

Fibula

Peroneal Groove

Cartilaginous Ridge

Peroneus Brevis Tendon

Calcaneus

Peroneus Longus Tendon

Superior Peroneal Retinaculum

Figure 29–2. The cartilaginous ridge serves to deepen the retromalleolar peroneal groove. (From Clanton TO, Schon LS. Athletic injuries to the soft tissues of the foot and ankle. In Mann RA, Coughlin HJ, eds. Surgery of the Foot and Ankle, ed 6. St. Louis: C.V. Mosby 1993, p. 1169.)

rule out peroneus longus rupture (see later discussion).

Treatment

The initial treatment of peroneal tendinitis includes measures to decrease inflammation, among them nonsteroidal anti-inflammatory drugs (NSAIDs), rest, ice, compression splinting, and elevation. Splinting should be tailored to the severity of the symptoms, and may include simple lateral heel wedges, fixed walker boots, or a trial of casting to ensure decreased motion and activity.[7] Certainly, activity modification such as avoidance of ladder work should be encouraged.[8] If conservative measures fail to resolve symptoms, a more advanced pathologic condition should be sought and treated accordingly.

Longitudinal Ruptures

Longitudinal ruptures or splits of the peroneal tendons are a common cause of lateral ankle pain, occurring in 11.3% of cadaveric specimens in one study.[11] These splits may be caused by an acute inversion injury, but are often associated with chronic lateral laxity of the ankle.[12] Longitudinal rupture must be considered before performing a lateral ankle ligament reconstruction because procedures relying on the integrity of the peroneus brevis tendon may have to be aborted.[11] Degenerative splits in the peroneus tendons have also been reported in patients with calcaneal fractures and can be

a cause of residual lateral ankle pain in patients with healed calcaneus fractures.

Etiology

Peroneal tendon splits are most likely the result of mechanical wear and tear of the tendon in and around the retromalleolar groove.[13, 14] During contraction, the peroneus longus tendon is forced anteriorly against the brevis tendon. This pressure can splay the brevis tendon along the posterior border of the fibula. If laxity of the SPR is present and it cannot hold the tendons in the retromalleolar position, partial subluxation of the peroneus brevis (PB) tendon over the sharp posterior border of the fibula will cause further tearing. After calcaneal fractures, splits in the tendon occur secondary to impingement of the peroneal tendons between the fibula and the displaced lateral calcaneal wall.[15]

Clinical Presentation

The patient usually presents months after an acute lateral ankle sprain with persistent lateral ankle pain and swelling. Often there is a mechanical snapping or popping sensation that can be aggravated by walking or running on uneven ground.[12] This sensation can mimic lateral ankle instability but may be present in stable ankles.

Physical examination demonstrates focal swelling in the retromalleolar region with tenderness proximal to the fibular tip. Popping may be noted with active foot rotation. Sobel and colleagues[13] described the peroneal tunnel compression test to attempt to reproduce these symptoms on physical exam. The patient sits at the end of the examining table with the knee flexed 90° and the foot relaxed. While palpating the posterior border of the fibula at the origin of the superior peroneal retinaculum, the patient dorsiflexes and everts the involved ankle against resistance. If a split is present, snapping, popping, or partial tendon subluxation may occur. Lidocaine injections into the peroneal sheath are useful diagnostically and should temporarily eliminate the patient's pain if the pain is originating from within the synovial sheath.

Radiology

Plain radiographs are not diagnostic for degenerative tendon splits, but are important to rule out other causes of lateral ankle pain. Peroneal tenography has been used to evaluate peroneal tendon disease but is being replaced by magnetic resonance imaging (MRI). An MRI study can demonstrate morphologic changes in the brevis tendon. Images may show "three" peroneal tendons in the retromalleolar region as the longus tendon essentially bisects the split brevis tendon[16] (Fig. 29–3). An MRI may also demonstrate anatomic anomalies, including a low-lying peroneus brevis muscle belly or the presence of a peroneus quartus muscle, which can assist preoperative planning.

Pathology

Pathologic findings intraoperatively and in cadaveric specimens usually demonstrate a longitudinal split in the brevis tendon, although splits in the longus tendon have also been described. They are 1 to 3 cm in length and are almost always located in the inferior portion of the retromalleolar groove.[12] A variable amount of tendon degeneration with granulation tissue is present. A partial subluxation of the anterior portion of the split brevis tendon can often be demonstrated at surgery (see Fig. 29–3).

Treatment

Symptomatic peroneal tendon splits are usually refractory to conservative care. Most have had significant conservative treatment for presumed uncomplicated tendinitis. A short course of rest, NSAIDs, immobilization, and rehabilitation should be tried if prior rehabilitation efforts were inadequate to decrease the tenosynovitis associated with peroneus brevis splits.

Surgical treatment options include tenolysis, tenosynovectomy, debridement of hypertrophic tissue, primary tendon repair, and tenodesis of the longus and brevis tendons.[12] Exploration of the peroneal tunnel in the retromalleolar region is performed through a curvilinear posterolateral incision. The SPR is split, and the tendons are identified. If the tear is minimal, tenolysis or tenosynovectomy is all that is necessary to return the retromalleolar anatomy to normal. With chronic tears, the splits are often associated with abundant hypertrophic granulation tissue. This tissue should be débrided to narrow the tendon before repair

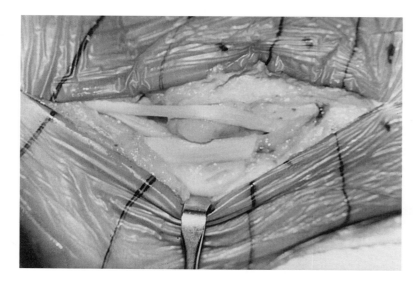

Figure 29–3. Dislocation of the anterior portion of the torn brevis tendon at surgery. Note that the posterior portion of the brevis tendon and the longus tendon remain in the retromalleolar groove.

of the tendon (tubulization). If fraying is extensive, tenodesis of the brevis tendon to the longus tendon may be necessary because primary repair becomes impossible. A low-lying peroneus brevis or peroneus quartus, if present, should be excised to recreate more normal anatomy in the retromalleolar region[17] (Fig. 29–4). Laxity of the SPR should be addressed by débridement of the sharp posterior border of the fibula to cancellous bone. The SPR is then repaired or reefed onto the exposed cancellous surface of the fibula to tighten the peroneal constraints and prevent further brevis subluxation and degeneration. Additionally, if chronic lateral ankle instability exists, the lateral ligamentous complex should also be reconstructed to prevent recurrent injury to the peroneal tendons. A modified Chrisman-

Snook procedure with the graft position over the tendons before insertion into the calcaneus has been reported to give good results.[18] The postoperative course includes 3 to 4 weeks in a short leg walking cast followed by peroneal strengthening and gradual return to activities.

Transverse Ruptures of the Peroneus Tendons

Transverse ruptures of the peroneal tendons may also rarely occur. Ruptures most often involve the peroneus longus tendon, but acute traumatic rupture of the brevis tendon has been reported.[19, 20] They are usually secondary to an acute traumatic event but are most commonly associated with an un-

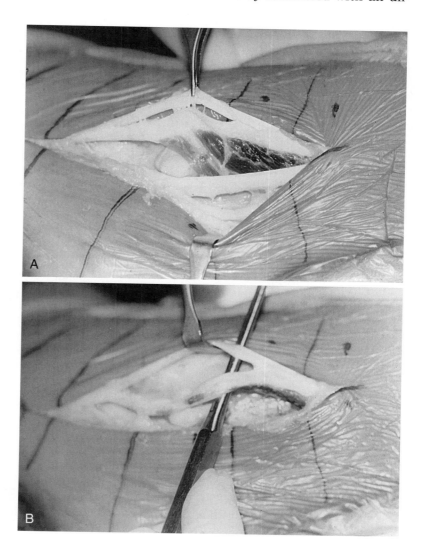

Figure 29–4. *A,* Low-lying muscle belly of the peroneal brevis, which caused overcrowding of the retromalleolar space and subsequent tear of the brevis tendon. *B,* The muscle has been débrided. The brevis tendon is now ready for repair.

derlying tendinitis or earlier less traumatic injury. Varus alignment of the hindfoot may predispose the patient to a peroneus longus rupture.[21]

Etiology

McMaster demonstrated that normal tendons do not rupture in midsubstance without underlying anatomic, traumatic, inflammatory, or degenerative conditions.[22] When predisposing factors are present, peroneus longus ruptures can occur and are usually associated with three general situations: (1) rupture associated with significant tendinitis; (2) direct blow injury to the lateral aspect of the foot; (3) failure in tension secondary to attempted eversion of the supinating foot.[23] Chronic inflammation, when present, can weaken the tensile strength of the tendon, predisposing to rupture.

A direct blow to the lateral aspect of the foot can cause direct injury to the tendon or, more likely, the os peroneum. It is hypothesized that this direct trauma causes an undisplaced fracture of the os peroneum, which then subsequently fails in tension during the secondary acute injury.[24]

Forced eversion in an attempt to counter a sudden inversion or supinating force on the foot has been reported to occur in both sporting events and after a misstep into a hole or off a curb.[21, 23] This provides a significant tension force across the tendon. If the tendon is previously damaged from chronic or acute tendinitis, the tendon may fail in the midsubstance of the tendon.

Clinical Presentation

The patient presents with pain and swelling over the lateral aspect of the foot and ankle. Tenderness extends from the posterior lateral malleolus to the base of the fifth metatarsal. Range of motion of the ankle may be limited secondary to pain, but active eversion of the ankle is both painful and weak.

Radiology

X-ray films demonstrate lateral foot and ankle soft tissue swelling and may show a fracture of the os peroneum. If the rupture occurs proximal or distal to the os peroneum, a change in position of the entire sesamoid bone with serial radiographs may be noted.[25] This diagnosis is often made ret-rospectively, with longitudinal re-review of the x-ray films. Only with increased awareness of this diagnosis will subtle changes be noted in initial x-ray films.

Treatment

Because of the rarity of this injury, treatment has been reported infrequently and is based on anecdotal personal experience rather than well-conducted prospective studies. Both surgical and conservative treatments are advocated and reported to give satisfactory results. Thompson and Patterson[25] and Evans[26] reported four cases of peroneal tendon ruptures that were treated surgically with débridement of the chronic inflammatory tissue and tenodesis of the distal aspect of the longus stump to the peroneus brevis tendon. Three patients had a history of chronic tendinitis, and one had an acute injury 8 months previously. Postoperatively, all patients were treated with protected weight bearing for 4 to 6 weeks followed by range-of-motion exercises. Thompson and Patterson additionally used a functional ankle brace for an additional month. The results were excellent in all four patients.

Bianchi and coworkers reported the results of three patients also diagnosed with peroneal tendon ruptures.[24] All patients were treated conservatively because they each refused surgery. A short leg cast was used for 6 weeks, followed by range-of-motion therapy. Two of the three had satisfactory results; the third had some residual pain and weakness.

Peacock and associates[23] reported one case associated with an os peroneum fracture. This was repaired through drill holes to allow bone to bone healing. The patient had satisfactory results with healing of the fracture and only occasional pain.

Peroneus brevis ruptures are more infrequently reported. One case of brevis rupture in association with a bimalleolar ankle fracture and a base of the fifth metatarsal fracture has been reported.[20] This patient did well with repair of the peroneus brevis back to its insertion to the base of the fifth metatarsal. Direct repair and tenodesis to the peroneus longus tendon are additional surgical options.

Peroneal Tendon Dislocations

Traumatic dislocations of the peroneal tendons are considered uncommon injuries, but should be a consideration in evaluating a patient with a lateral ankle sprain. Often when this diagnosis is made, it is done in a delayed manner.[27] This delay allows the transition from an acute injury to a neglected chronic one and has treatment and prognostic implications.

Etiology

As discussed, the peroneal muscles usually terminate into their respective tendons proximal to the ankle joint. As they course posteriorly to the lateral malleolus, they are held in place by local anatomic constraints. These constraints include the retromalleolar groove, the fibrocartilaginous ridge, and the SPR complex (see Fig. 29–2). The bony constraints, even with the augmentation of the fibrous ridge, are often not sufficient to contain the peroneal tendons in their anatomic position. Peroneal tendon dislocation is usually secondary to an acute traumatic event compromising the integrity of the SPR complex. Predisposing factors to peroneal tendon dislocation include a shallow retromalleolar groove and an absence or laxity of the superior peroneal retinaculum.[28] Causes of SPR laxity include recurrent ankle sprains, prior dislocation of the peroneal tendons, and overcrowding of the peroneal tunnel by a low-lying peroneus brevis muscle belly or the presence of a peroneus quartus tendon.[20] The inciting mechanism in the dislocation of the peroneal tendons involves reflex contraction of the peroneal tendons with the ankle in the dorsiflexed position in response to further violent dorsiflexion of the ankle. The injury has been reported with a plantar-flexed position of the ankle as well.[27, 28] This contraction overpowers the limited bony and soft tissue restraints, leading to anterior and lateral dislocation. Peroneal tendon dislocation occurs often during downhill skiing, where the relatively dorsiflexed ankle is often further stressed into more dorsiflexion. Injuries while participating in other sporting events, including football, water-skiing, running, dancing, baseball, and mountain climbing have also been reported.[29]

Peroneal tendon subluxation or dislocation may also occur with other acute traumatic events about the foot and ankle, including calcaneal fractures and ankle dislocations.[30, 31] Ebraheim and others[32] examined 21 calcaneal fractures with computed tomographic (CT) scans and found that 8 (38%) had dislocated or subluxated tendons. Of note, in these patients, this was not suspected or determined clinically. Residual widening of the calcaneal tuberosity causes impingement of the tendons between the lateral calcaneal wall and the fibula. The CT scan with soft tissue windows should be routinely examined for the possibility of peroneal tendon involvement with acute calcaneal fractures. In their series, three additional patients were found to have avulsion fractures from the posterior aspect of the fibula. This is pathognomonic for peroneal tendon dislocation.

Some patients with dislocations of the peroneal tendons do not report an acute traumatic event and are found to have chronic laxity of the SPR as a result of ankle instability.[33] Numerous inversion injuries in an unstable ankle stress the calcaneal band of the SPR, causing retinacular incompetence and leading to subluxation or dislocation of the peroneal tendons in association with sprains of the lateral ankle ligaments.

Clinical Presentation

Patients present with acute onset of severe pain on the lateral side of the ankle and can often recall hearing or feeling a "snap" during the traumatic event. Patients are unable to continue with their current activity, and are often prevented from ambulating after an acute, first-time injury.[28] On examination, there is soft tissue swelling. In those patients who present within the first few hours, there is focal swelling in the retromalleolar region.[34] Those who present later will have diffuse soft tissue swelling of the lateral ankle, making it more difficult to localize the precise zone of injury. Palpation reveals tenderness in the retromalleolar region and may reveal anterior displacement of the tendons if presentation is acute and swelling is minimal. Active eversion against resistance is painful. DeHaven and colleagues reported that 50% of patients who have experienced spontaneous relocation will do so again with forced eversion against resistance; this is difficult to produce clinically because of pain at presentation.[35]

Radiology

Plain radiographs will usually demonstrate only soft tissue swelling but should be carefully evaluated for fibular fracture. In one series, 16% of cases demonstrated an avulsion of the posterior lateral aspect of the fibula best seen on the internal rotation view (mortise view) of the ankle.[28] This small avulsion "flake" of bone is pathognomonic for a dislocation of the peroneal tendons. Magnetic resonance imaging (MRI) can also aid in the diagnosis of peroneal retinacular rupture and tendon dislocation when clinical diagnosis is uncertain. Zeiss and colleagues report the MRI findings in 15 ankles in 10 volunteers, 2 patients suspected of having a peroneal retinacular injury, and 3 cadaveric specimens.[36] They found that the peroneal tendon location could be identified with certainty, and all but the thinnest retinacula were visualized with enough clarity to determine its integrity.

Pathology

Eckert and Davis examined 73 patients with an acute ankle injury and dislocation of the peroneal tendons.[34] They described three grades of injury (Fig. 29–5). A grade I injury involves a separation of the retinaculum from the fibrocollagenous lip and lateral malleolus; the peroneal tendons lie between the periosteum and the bare bone surface (Fig. 29–5A). In a grade II injury, the distal 1 to 2 cm of the dense fibrous lip on the posterior aspect of the malleolus was elevated with the retinaculum (Fig. 29–5B). A grade III injury involves an avulsion of a thin fragment of bone along with the fibrocollagenous lip and attached to the deep surface of the retinaculum (Fig. 29–5C). These injury grades occurred in 51%, 33%, and 16%, respectively. Importantly, none of the cases demonstrated a tear in the retinaculum itself.

Treatment

Conservative treatment for acute peroneal tendon dislocations is controversial. Several authors advocate an initial trial of conservative treatment by either casting or with a soft dressing, but the results are difficult to interpret.[29] Results were generally positive, and some patients did well clinically despite recurrent dislocations. Grade I injuries are stable once reduced and could be appropriately treated in a short leg walking cast. It is difficult, however, to determine a grade I injury clinically, so most authors advocate

surgical exploration of all acute peroneal dislocations to prevent the attritional changes in the tendons associated with recurrent dislocations.[27, 28]

Reconstruction of the SPR can be performed using a variety of procedures to stabilize the tendons in the retromalleolar groove. The procedures can be divided into four general categories: (1) anatomic repair of the retinacular complex; (2) retromalleolar groove–deepening procedures; (3) soft tissue reconstruction and augmentation of the SPR complex; and (4) tendon-rerouting procedures.[37–39] Most acute injuries can be treated with direct repair of the retinacular complex. Chronically dislocated tendons, or recurrent subluxators, however, usually require more extensive reconstruction procedures. Elements of these different procedures can be combined for maximum benefit, in cases of anatomic abnormalities. Examples of each category follow.

Anatomic repair of the damaged SPR complex is commonly used to treat acute dislocations of the peroneal tendons. The specific repair procedure depends on the pathoanatomy of the individual injury. If a grade I injury is present, it can be repaired by suturing the anterior edge of the fascia to the intact fibrocollagenous lip. Grade II injuries require accurate reduction of the avulsed fibrocartilaginous lip and retinaculum and firm suture fixation of the fibrous retinaculum through bone. For grade III injuries, two Kirschner wires directed from posterolateral to anteromedial through the fragment provide adequate fixation. This procedure can be supplemented by soft tissue repair as done for grades I and II. The postoperative course involves 3 weeks in a short leg non-weight-bearing cast, followed by 2 to 3 weeks in a weight-bearing cast.

Results of surgical treatment of acute peroneal tendon dislocations are excellent. Eckert and Davis reported only three recurrent dislocations of 73 patients.[34] Twelve patients experienced mild pain with vigorous activities, but in none was it severe enough to alter activities or require further treatment. Alm and colleagues performed direct repair of the retinacular complex through drill holes in the posterior aspect of the fibula.[40] A short leg walking cast was applied for 3 to 4 weeks and weight bearing was encouraged. Nine of 10 patients were able to return to their previous sporting events, and only 1 experienced a redislocation but had an excellent result after reoperation.

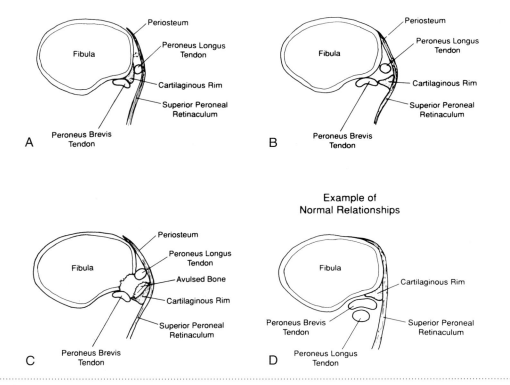

Figure 29–5. Eckert classification of pathology in peroneal tendon dislocations. *A:* Grade I; *B:* Grade II; *C:* Grade III; *D:* Normal anatomy. See text for discussion. (From Mann RA, Coughlin MJ. Surgery of the Foot and Ankle, ed 6, vol 2. St Louis, CV Mosby, 1993, p. 1170. Adapted from Eckert WR, Davis EA Jr. Acute rupture of the peroneal retinaculum. J Bone Joint Surg 58:670–672, 1976.)

Marti reported uniformly excellent results in acute peroneal dislocations.[27] He advocated an acute repair of the torn retinaculum complex with early protected motion. Once motion is attained, the patients are protected in a short leg walking cast for 5 additional weeks.

Retromalleolar groove–deepening procedures can be done by methods that either deepen the retromalleolar groove directly or functionally increase the depth and stability of the groove by adding an additional bony block to prevent tendon dislocation. Kelly described a veneer graft procedure for deepening the groove by incising the subcutaneus portion of the distal fibula and displacing this distally and posteriorly.[41] This was then internally fixed with two screws. A short leg cast was then applied for 5 months. Marti reported the results of 12 patients with recurrent subluxation of the peroneal tendons treated with a slightly modified Kelly procedure.[27]* All patients

were able to return to their previous level of vocational and avocational activities. A similar procedure involving sliding a portion of the lateral fibula distally to contain the peroneal tendons has also been reported with good results.[42]

An alternative groove-deepening procedure involves removing a portion of the cancellous bone from the posterior and inferior aspects of the distal fibula. To deepen the groove, an incision 5 to 7 mm posterior to the lateral malleolus along the peroneal tendons is made. The tendons are then freed from their sheaths and retracted anteriorly. A cortical osteoperiosteal flap measuring 3 × 1 cm is raised along the posterolateral aspect of distal fibula, leaving the posteromedial border intact to act as a hinge. The flap is then hinged posteriorly, and cancellous bone is removed from the posterior aspect of the fibula. This deepens the groove 6 to 9 mm (Fig. 29–6). The flap is then tamped back into position, which replaces the smooth gliding surface of the fibula. The repair is then augmented by a reefing of the SPR or by creation of a periosteal sling. A

*The original procedure described by Kelly was modified by leaving a periosteal and cortical hinge posteriorly.

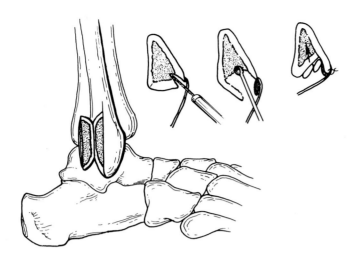

Figure 29–6. Deepening of the retromalleolar groove using a posterior fibular osteoperiosteal flap. See text. (From Arrowsmith SR, Fleming LL, Allman FL. Traumatic dislocations of the peroneal tendons. Am J Sports Med 11:142–146, 1983.)

short leg cast is used for 3 weeks, followed by a hinged short leg cast for 3 more weeks. Progressive range-of-motion exercises and strengthening are then begun. Zoellner and Clancy reported the results of nine patients treated in this manner.[43] At 2-year follow-up, all patients had excellent results without limitations in their activities.

Soft tissue reconstruction of the SPR complex may be done with reefing of the remaining retinacular tissue, or it may be augmented with the use of periosteum.[44, 45] Several different tendons have been used to reconstruct the SPR, including the Achilles tendon,[46] the plantaris tendon,[47] the peroneus brevis tendon,[48] and the peroneus quartus tendon when present.[5] Jones described a procedure in which a sling of Achilles tendon is used to recreate the SPR.[26] A slip of the lateral aspect of the Achilles tendon ¼ inch wide and 2½ inches long is detached proximally and left attached to the calcaneus distally. It is then passed transversely through a hole drilled in the fibula 1 inch proximal to the tip. The tendon is then looped posteriorly and sutured to itself and to the fibular periosteum. Two weeks in a short leg cast follow, with protected weight bearing for an additional 4 weeks. Escalas and colleagues reported on 28 patients treated with the Jones technique.[49] The patients were injured skiing and failed initial conservative care with a compressive dressing. All patients except one were asymptomatic and unlimited in their activities on follow-up.

Tendon-rerouting procedures are used to place the tendons in a position where additional soft tissue or bony restraints prevent further subluxation or dislocation. Poll and Duijfjes described a procedure for rerouting the tendons under the calcaneofibular ligament.[50] The tendons are exposed in the retromalleolar and inframalleolar positions by incising the peroneal sheath. The calcaneofibular ligament is identified, and a cancellous bone block with the calcaneal insertion of the ligament is mobilized and raised. The tendons are then placed under the ligament, and the bone block is replaced and secured with a cancellous screw. A groove-deepening procedure can be added, if necessary. A short leg cast is used for 6 weeks, the last 4 of which are weight bearing. Nine of 10 patients treated in this manner returned to their previous levels of activities, although 2 had slight pain and 4 complained of scar sensitivity.[50] Rerouting of the peroneal tendons under the calcaneofibular ligament by temporarily removing the fibular insertion of the ligament has also been described, as has dividing the tendons proximal to the SPR and reanastomosing them.[51, 52]

Chronic, unrecognized dislocations or recurrent subluxations are treated with a number of procedures to increase soft tissue or bony restraints of the retromalleolar peroneal groove. Because of the presence of attritional changes in the tendons associated with these disorders, early operative intervention is warranted.[28]

REFERENCES

1. Last RJ. Anatomy, Regional and Applied. New York: Churchill Livingstone, 1984.
2. Sarrafian SK. Anatomy of the Foot and Ankle:

Descriptive, Topographic, Functional. Philadelphia: J. B. Lippincott, 1993.

3. Hecker P. Study on the peroneus of the tarsus. Anat Rec 26:79–82, 1923.

4. Sobel M, Levy ME, Bonhe WHO. Congenital variations of the peroneus quartus muscle: an anatomic study. Foot Ankle 11:81–89, 1990.

5. Mick CA, Lynch F. Reconstruction of the peroneal retinaculum using the peroneus quartus. J Bone Joint Surg 69:296–297, 1987.

6. Edwards ME. The relations of the peroneal tendons to the fibula, calcaneus, and cuboideum. Am J Anat 42:213–253, 1928.

7. Frey CC, Shereff MJ. Tendon injuries about the ankle in athletes. Clin Sports Med 7:103–118, 1988.

8. Roggatz J, Urban A. The calcaneous peritendinitis of the long peroneal tendon. Arch Orthop Trauma Surg 96:161–164, 1980.

9. Bowker JH, Olin FH. Complete replacement of the peroneus longus muscle by a ganglion with compression of the peroneal nerve: a case report. Clin Orthop Rel Res 140:172–174, 1979.

10. Cox D, Paterson FWN. Acute calcific tendinitis of peroneus longs. J Bone Joint Surg Br 73:342, 1991.

11. Sobel M, Bohne WHO, Levy ME. Longitudinal attrition of the peroneus brevis tendon in the fibular groove: an anatomic study. Foot Ankle 11:124–128, 1990.

12. Bassett FH III, Speer KP. Longitudinal rupture of the peroneal tendons. Am J Sports Med 21:354–357, 1993.

13. Sobel M, Geppert MJ, Olson EJ, et al. The dynamics of peroneus brevis tendon splits: a proposed mechanism, technique of diagnosis, and classification of injury. Foot Ankle 13:413–422, 1992.

14. Sobel M, Geppert MJ, Warren RF. Chronic ankle instability as a cause of peroneal tendon injury. Clin Orthop Rel Res 296:187–191, 1993.

15. Schweitzer ME, Karasick D. MRI of the ankle and hindfoot. Semin Ultrasound CT MR 15:410–422, 1994.

16. Schweitzer ME. Magnetic resonance imaging of the foot and ankle. Magn Reson Q 9:214–234, 1993.

17. Sobel M, Mizel MS. Peroneal tendon injury. In Pfeffer GB, Frey CC, eds. Current Practice in Foot and Ankle Surgery. New York: McGraw-Hill, 1993, p. 38.

18. Sobel M, Warren RF, Brourman S. Lateral ankle instability associated with dislocation of the peroneal tendons treated by the Chrisman-Snook procedure: a case report and literature review. Am J of Sports Med 18:539–543, 1990.

19. Springer KR. Isolated transverse rupture of the peroneus brevis tendon treated with a free split-thickness tendon graft. Foot Surg 31:595–598, 1992.

20. Stiehl JB. Concomitant rupture of the peroneus brevis tendon and bimalleolar fracture: a case report. J Bone Joint Surg 70:936–937, 1988.

21. Burman M. Subcutaneous tear of the tendon of the peroneus longus: its relation to the giant peroneal tubercle. Arch Surg 67:686–698, 1953.

22. McMaster PE. Tendon and muscle ruptures: clinical and experimental studies on the causes and location of subcutaneous ruptures. J Bone Joint Surg 15:705–722, 1933.

23. Peacock KC, Resnick EJ, Thoder JJ. Fracture of the os peroneum with rupture of the peroneus longus tendon: a case report and review of the literature. Clin Orthop Rel Res 202:223–226, 1986.

24. Bianchi S, Abdelwahab IF, Tegaldo G. Fracture and posterior dislocation of the os peroneum associated with rupture of the peroneus longus tendon. Can Assoc Radiol J 42:340–344, 1991.

25. Thompson FM, Patterson AH. Rupture of the peroneus longus tendon: report of three cases. J Bone Joint Surg Am 71:293–295, 1989.

26. Evans JD. Subcutaneous rupture of the tendon of peroneus longus: report of a case. J Bone Joint Surg Br 48:507–509, 1966.

27. Marti R: Dislocation of the peroneal tendons. Am J Sports Med 51:19–22, 1977.

28. Arrowsmith SR, Fleming LL, Allman FL. Traumatic dislocations of the peroneal tendons. Am J Sports Med 11:142–146, 1983.

29. McLennan JG. Treatment of acute and chronic luxations of the peroneal tendons. Am J Sports Med 8:432–436, 1980.

30. Bradley SA, Davies AM. Computed tomographic assessment of soft tissue abnormalities following calcaneal fractures. Br J Radiol 65:105–111, 1992.

31. Segal LS, Lynch CJ, Stauffer ES. Anterior ankle dislocation with associated trigonal process fracture: a case report and literature review. Clin Orthop Rel Res 278:171–176, 1992.

32. Ebraheim NA, Zeiss J, Skie MC, Jackson WT. Radiological evaluation of peroneal tendon pathology associated with calcaneal fractures. J Orthop Trauma 5:365–369, 1991.

33. Geppert MJ, Sobel M, Bohne WH. Lateral ankle instability as a cause of superior peroneal retinacular laxity: an anatomic and biomechanical study of cadaveric feet. Foot Ankle 14:330–334, 1993.

34. Eckert WR, Davis EA Jr. Acute rupture of the peroneal retinaculum. J Bone Joint Surg Am 58:670–672, 1976.

35. DeHaven KE, Allman FL, Cox JS, et al. Symposium: ankle sprains in athletes. Contemp Orthop 1:56–78, 1979.

36. Zeiss J, Saddemi SR, Ebraheim NA. MR imaging of the peroneal tunnel. J Comput Assist Tomogr 13:840–844, 1989.

37. Brage ME, Hansen ST Jr. Traumatic subluxation/dislocation of the peroneal tendons. Foot Ankle 13:423–431, 1992.

38. DasDe S, Balasubramaniam P. A repair operation for recurrent dislocation of peroneal tendons. J Bone Joint Surg Br 67:585–587, 1985.

39. Duvries HL. Surgery of the Foot, ed 2. St Louis: C. V. Mosby, 1978, pp. 540–541.

40. Alm A, Lamke LO, Liljedhl SO. Surgical treatment of dislocation of the peroneal tendons. Injury 7:14–19, 1975.

41. Kelly RE. An operation for the chronic dislocation of the peroneal tendons. Br J Surg 7:502–504, 1920.

42. Micheli LJ, Waters PM, Sanders DP. Sliding fibular graft repair for chronic dislocation of the peroneal tendons. Am J Sports Med 17:68–71, 1989.

43. Zoellner G, Clancy W Jr. Recurrent dislocation of the Peroneal tendon. J Bone Joint Surg Am 61:292–294, 1979.

44. Gould N. Repair of dislocating peroneal tendons. Foot Ankle 6:208–213, 1986.

45. Scheller AD, Kasser JR, Quigley TB. Tendon injur-

ies about the ankle. Orthop Clin North Am 11:806–809, 1980.

46. Jones E. Operative treatment of chronic dislocation of the peroneal tendons. J Bone Joint Surg 14:574–576, 1932.

47. Miller JW. Dislocation of the peroneal tendons: a new operative procedure. Am J Orthop 9:136–137, 1967.

48. Stein RE. Reconstruction of the superior peroneal retinaculum using a portion of the peroneus brevis tendon: a case report. J Bone Joint Surg 69:298–299, 1987.

49. Escalas F, Figueras JM, Merino JA. Dislocation of the peroneal tendons, long-term results of surgical treatment. J Bone Joint Surg 62:451–453, 1980.

50. Poll RG, Duijfjes F. The treatment of recurrent dislocation of the peroneal tendons. J Bone Joint Surg Br 66:98–100, 1984.

51. Pozo JL, Jackson AM. A rerouting operation for dislocation of peroneal tendons: operative technique and case report. Foot Ankle 5:42–44, 1984.

52. Sarmiento A, Wolf M. Subluxation of peroneal tendons case treated by rerouting tendons under calcaneofibular ligament. J Bone Joint Surg 57:115–116, 1975.

30 Posterior Tibial Tendon Dysfunction

Stuart D. Katchis

Posterior tibial tendon dysfunction (PTTD) is the most common cause of acquired flatfoot in the adult. Since the initial report of this condition by Kettelkamp and Alexander[1] in 1969, many reports have appeared in the literature concerning diagnosis and treatment. Despite this, PTTD often remains an elusive and overlooked diagnosis. Indeed, PTTD should probably be considered a spectrum of disorders involving not only the posterior tibial tendon (PTT) itself but also the capsule and ligamentous structures of the hindfoot and midfoot. The clinical presentation may vary from as little as isolated medial ankle pain and swelling to as much as severe rigid and painful foot deformities. In this section, the anatomy and function of the posterior tibial tendon and the pathophysiology, clinical presentation, and treatment of PTTD are presented.

ANATOMY AND FUNCTION

The posterior tibial muscle is the most deeply situated muscle in the deep posterior compartment of the leg. It takes its origin from nearly the entire interosseous membrane, the posterolateral surface of the upper two thirds of the tibia, and the posterolateral surface of the upper two thirds of the fibula. The tendon emerges from the medial side of muscle at about the middle of the leg, but continues to receive muscle fibers nearly to the level of the medial malleolus.[2] The tendon lies just behind the medial malleolus and passes under the flexor retinaculum in its own synovial sheath. It passes to the plantar surface of the foot to have an extensive insertion primarily into the tuberosity of the navicular bone, but also into the plantar surfaces of the three cuneiforms, the cuboid, and the second, third, and fourth metatarsal bases.[3]

The posterior tibial tendon lies medial to the axis of rotation of the subtalar joint. By virtue of its long lever arm to the subtalar joint, the PTT is the main dynamic stabilizer of the hindfoot against valgus (ever-sion) deformity.[4] It also lies posterior to the axis of rotation of the ankle joint and is a secondary plantar flexor of the hindfoot. The main function of the PTT is inversion of the subtalar joint and adduction of the forefoot.[5] Its main antagonist is the peroneus brevis muscle, which everts the subtalar joint and abducts the forefoot. By stabilizing the hindfoot, the PTT helps to create a lever arm for the gastrocnemius-soleus complex during ankle plantar flexion. During a single-leg heel rise, for example, the initial contraction of the PTT inverts and stabilizes the subtalar joint, allowing the gastrocnemius-soleus complex to work across the ankle to effect plantar flexion. In addition, the inversion of the subtalar joint moves the insertion of the Achilles tendon medially and allows the gastrocnemius-soleus complex to function as an invertor of the hindfoot as well as a plantar flexor of the ankle.

In the normal gait cycle, from heel strike to foot flat, the tibia undergoes internal rotation, the hindfoot undergoes eversion, and the transverse tarsal joints (calcaneocuboid and talonavicular) unlock. This progressive foot pronation allows for the gradual deceleration of the foot and the absorption of the ground reaction force. Although it has been stated often that the PTT functions in an eccentric manner to control this hindfoot eversion, it is more likely that static ligament restraints on the medial side of the hindfoot are responsible.[6, 7] As the body's center of gravity passes over the foot, the tibia externally rotates, and the hindfoot undergoes active inversion via the pull of the PTT. This hindfoot inversion causes a locking of the transverse tarsal joint and allows the foot to become a rigid lever for push-off. Total excursion of the PTT is only approximately 2 cm.

The structural integrity of the longitudinal arch of the foot is probably not dependent on the function of the PTT, but rather on bone shape and conformity and the integrity of the ligamentous structures such as the spring ligament. With posterior tibial tendon dysfunction, however, there is chronic unopposed pull of the peroneus brevis muscle, the ligaments fail, and a flatfoot deformity develops. A more detailed discussion of the biomechanics of the gait cycle is beyond the scope of this chapter, and the reader is referred to Mann's[8] excellent review.

ETIOLOGY

The most frequent site of posterior tibial tendon disease is between the medial malleolus and the insertion into the navicular. Frey and associates[9] demonstrated a critical zone of hypovascularity in the PTT posterior and distal to the medial malleolus in all 28 cadaver specimens injected with India ink. The authors speculated that the decreased blood supply may be related to the anatomic course of the posterior tibial tendon as it turns sharply around the medial malleolus. This may cause a "wringing out" of the tendon and render it more susceptible to degeneration. Jhass[10] suggested that midsubstance tears are caused by tendon constriction beneath the flexor retinaculum. Holmes and Mann[11] found that PTTD was associated with a significantly higher incidence of diabetes, hypertension, and obesity than in the general population. Dyal and colleagues[12] studied the contralateral foot in patients with PTTD and found that preexisting flexible pes planus may also be an etiologic factor. Trauma may also cause PTTD. In these cases, the tendon may become entrapped within fracture callus or occasionally lacerated. Johnson believed that PTTD was secondary to a combination of traumatic and degenerative processes.[4] Finally, the multiple insertions of the PTT may predispose it to degeneration because of an increase in intratendinous shear forces as different segments of the tendon become taut at different times.

PATHOLOGY

The most common finding on exploration of the PTT in the adult with acquired flatfoot is varying degrees of degenerative changes within the tendon itself. The degeneration may be central, which appears as a swelling of the tendon and where the diseased tissue is seen only after the tendon is split open longitudinally. Alternatively, there may be a more generalized degeneration or an avulsion from the navicular bone.[13] Funk and coworkers[14] reviewed 19 patients undergoing surgical exploration for PTTD and found four distinct types of lesions. Group I patients had a complete avulsion of the PTT from the navicular bone. Group II patients had a complete midsubstance rupture just distal to the medial malleolus. Group III patients had a longitudinal tear without complete rupture of the tendon, and Group IV patients had synovitis around the tendon without any signs of tendon disruption or frank tears. Group I patients were treated by reinsertion of the PTT to the navicular, Group II by flexor digitorum longus (FDL) tendon transfer, and Groups III and IV by tenosynovectomy. At minimum 2-year follow-up, group I patients demonstrated no improvement, whereas group II, III, and IV patients all showed objective and subjective improvement.

The presence of synovial reaction is variable. Often there is abundant synovial reaction about the tendon, whereas at other times there is significant tendon degeneration without any evidence of tenosynovitis. Occasionally, the disease will be seen to be most significant around the spring ligament and the plantar medial aspect of the talonavicular joint. Gazkag and Cracchiolo[15] examined the spring ligament complex in 22 patients undergoing surgery for acquired flatfoot. They found varying degrees of injury to the ligament complex in 18 of the 22 patients. The authors stated that a damaged spring ligament complex should be repaired, if possible, to strengthen static support to the hindfoot.

CLINICAL PRESENTATION

Most patients with PTTD will give a history of a gradual onset of pain and swelling on the medial side of the affected ankle. A few may relate a specific traumatic incident, but most cannot. They do, however, notice a gradual loss of the longitudinal arch on the affected foot and increased wear on the medial side of the shoe. Very often, patients complain of increased fatigue with walking distances or having to give up sports activities such as tennis or golf.

Findings on physical examination are classic and often conclusive. The patient is first observed standing and walking. Flattening of the longitudinal arch is seen with weight bearing, as is increased hindfoot valgus. Depending on the severity of the disease, the forefoot may demonstrate increased abduction (Fig. 30–1). When viewed from behind, the medial malleolus and the talar head sag medially and the "too many toes" sign may be present (Fig. 30–2). This sign is positive when the combination of forefoot abduction and hindfoot valgus causes more of the lateral toes to be seen on the affected foot when viewing the loaded foot from behind.[4]

Tendon function is evaluated by asking the patient to perform a single-leg heel rise. Although some patients may be able to do a heel rise, careful observation demonstrates that they are unable to invert the calcaneus (a function of the PTT). Fatigue is easily tested by having the patient do multiple heel rises. Most patients with PTTD will be unable to complete a set of 10 single-leg heel rises without significant pain.

With the patient sitting, swelling, tenderness, muscle strength, and range of motion are evaluated. Swelling is seen over the PTT, especially if there is significant tenosynovitis. Tenderness is most commonly elicited directly over the tendon distal to the medial malleolus. In the later stages of the disease process, with hindfoot collapse, there is often lateral impingement of the fibular tip or the lateral talar process with the anterior process of the calcaneus. This

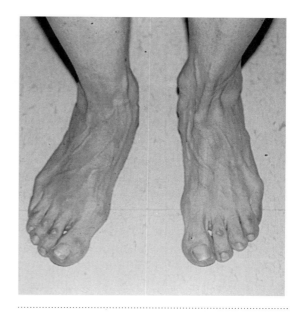

Figure 30–1. Posterior tibial tendon dysfunction. Note increased forefoot abduction on the patient's right foot.

causes lateral tenderness in the sinus tarsi region. Muscle strength is tested manually. Often, the patient will attempt to substitute tibialis anterior function to make up for PTT weakness. To avoid this and test only PTT function, the foot is placed in maximum equinus and hindfoot eversion, and the patient is asked to invert the foot against resistance.

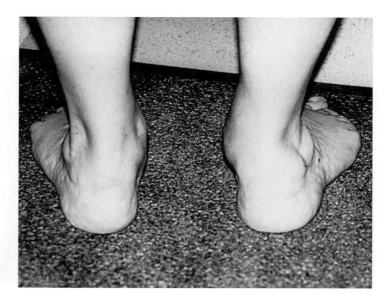

Figure 30–2. "Too many toes" sign. Note increased hindfoot valgus and forefoot abduction.

Ankle joint motion is usually not affected, but subtalar motion is often restricted. Depending on the severity and stage of the disease, subtalar motion may be normal, restricted, or ankylosed (see later discussion). Hindfoot inversion is affected first and most severely. Motion through the transverse tarsal joint (talonavicular and calcaneocuboid joints) is measured as forefoot abduction and adduction. With long-standing PTTD, forefoot adduction may be lost. Finally, the relationship of the forefoot to the hindfoot is evaluated. In the patient with PTTD and hindfoot valgus, the forefoot naturally assumes a varus position (supination). This is necessary to keep all metatarsal heads on the floor. With long-standing PTTD, this forefoot varus can become fixed. Determining the flexibility or rigidity of the various joints in PTTD is critical to planning treatment because tendon transfers are ineffective in the absence of normal passive range of joint motion. With fixed joint contractures present, arthrodeses may be necessary.

CLASSIFICATION

Patients with posterior tibial tendon dysfunction are classified according to the system first described by Johnson and Strom.[16] This classification system takes into account the length of the posterior tibial tendon and the mobility of the joints of the hindfoot. In stage I PTTD, the tendon is of normal length, and the hindfoot has normal motion and alignment. The patient has medial ankle swelling, inversion weakness, and fo-

cal tenderness to palpation. In stage II disease, the tendon is elongated. The hindfoot has normal passive motion, but with stance the foot adopts a pes planovalgus position. The pain is more severe and continues after cessation of weight bearing. Weakness is also more severe. In stage III disease, the tendon is elongated and the deformity fixed. The hindfoot is in valgus, and the forefoot is in abduction and supination. There is marked weakness or complete absence of PTT function. The patient has pain medially and often laterally in the sinus tarsi because of impingement of the fibular tip or the lateral talar process with the anterior process of the calcaneus.

ROENTGENOGRAPHIC EVALUATION

Routine lateral and anteroposterior (AP) roentgenograms of the foot and ankle should always be taken while weight bearing. Bordelon[17] used the talus–first metatarsal angle on the lateral x-ray film to classify pes planus. Normal was said to be 0° (i.e., a straight line), mild deformity between 1° and 15°, moderate deformity between 16° and 30°, and severe deformity greater than 30° (Fig. 30–3). The sag in the longitudinal arch may take place at the talonavicular joint, the naviculocuneiform joint, or a combination of both.

The talonavicular coverage angle is used to measure forefoot abduction.[18] The angle is that between the long axis of the navicular and the long axis of the talus, as meas-

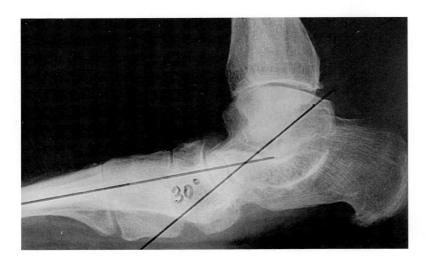

Figure 30–3. Method of measuring pes planus using the lateral talus–first metatarsal angle.

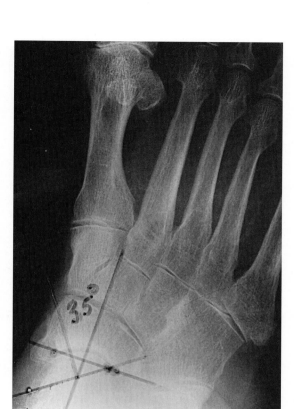

Figure 30–4. The talonavicular coverage angle. See text.

ured on the weight-bearing AP x-ray film (Fig. 30–4).

Magnetic resonance imaging (MRI) is the imaging modality of choice for evaluation of PTTD.[19] The fluid in the tendon sheaths that accompanies tenosynovitis will appear as bright signal on T2-weighted images (Fig. 30–5). In cases of acute tenosynovitis, the tendon itself will appear normal, whereas in chronic tenosynovitis, there will be tendon enlargement (Fig. 30–6). Tendon tears seen on MRI are classified as type I (partial ruptures associated with increased tendon girth and focal areas of fiber rupture and degeneration), type II (more severe rupture with attenuation of the remaining tendon), or type III (complete rupture with a gap in the tendon and retraction of the free edges).

TREATMENT

The treatment of PTTD depends on the Johnson stage of the disease at presentation.

Stage I

The treatment of stage I PTTD is largely conservative. The patient is placed in a walking cast or a fracture brace to put the tendon at rest and is given nonsteroidal anti-inflammatory medications. The patient is re-evaluated monthly. The immobilization may last 2 or 3 months. When the pain and swelling subside, physical therapy is begun for muscle strengthening and range of motion. Shoe modifications to limit hindfoot hyperpronation are helpful. These include a long medial counter, Thomas heel, or a medial heel and sole wedge. Custom-molded orthotic devices such as University of California Berkeley shoe inserts with arch support and medial heel and sole posting are also useful. Chao and associates[20] reported that 67% of patients achieved good or excellent results with nonoperative treatment.

If the symptoms of swelling and pain do not subside despite immobilization, early surgical intervention is indicated. Early synovectomy is important to prevent active synovitis from destroying the posterior tibial tendon and allowing a progression from stage I to stage II disease.[13] According to Teasdall and Johnson,[21] 84% of their stage I PTTD patients subjectively reported being "much better" after surgical synovectomy and tendon debridement. These authors recommended surgical treatment for stage I PTT dysfunction.

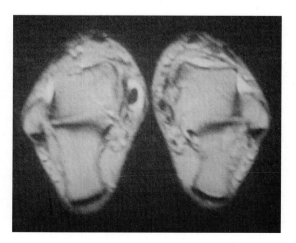

Figure 30–5. T2-weighted magnetic resonance image demonstrating marked tenosynovitis around the posterior tibial tendon. Note the bright signal around the tendon on the left image.

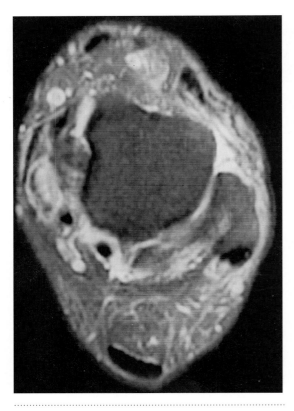

Figure 30–6. Magnetic resonance image demonstrating chronic tenosynovitis and probable rupture of the posterior tibial tendon. Note the normal signal of the flexor hallucis longus and flexor digitorum longus tendons and the enlarged and abnormal PTT signal.

Stage II

The treatment for stage II PTTD is surgical. By definition, in stage II disease, the PTT is enlarged, elongated, and functionally incompetent. The foot is in a position of pes planovalgus, but the deformity is flexible. Tendon transfer to compensate for the diseased PTT is the hallmark of treatment. In order for any tendon transfer to succeed, however, no fixed joint deformity can be present. In patients with PTTD, care should be taken to ensure preoperatively that there is full inversion of the subtalar joint and no more than 5° to 7° of fixed forefoot varus before tendon transfer is undertaken.[13] The best candidates for tendon transfer are of medium build, younger than 60 years, active, and athletic.[22] Patients older than 60 years are probably better served with an arthrodesis, which will predictably provide a stable foot. In patients with hypermobility

of the joints, even if young and active, tendon transfer should not be performed because the hyperelasticity of the tissues will lead to failure of the transfer.[13]

The goal of surgery is to maintain foot motion and function. Many different procedures have been described; currently, the best treatment is controversial. Mann and Thompson[23] reported on PTT reconstruction by transferring the flexor digitorum longus to the navicular bone. Results were initially good, especially with relief of pain. Long-term follow-up, however, demonstrated that results deteriorated with time. Myerson and associates[24] added a medial displacement osteotomy of the calcaneus to the tendon transfer to reduce the antagonistic deforming force of heel valgus (Fig. 30–7). This is essentially a "double" tendon transfer. The calcaneal osteotomy serves to shift the Achilles attachment medially. This improves the mechanical advantage of the FDL transfer while also decreasing the hindfoot valgus force of the Achilles tendon itself. They reported an overall improvement in the radiographic parameters studied. Long-term functional results are not yet available. Pomeroy and Manoli[25] reported preliminary results with an FDL tendon transfer, calcaneal osteotomy, lateral column lengthening, and Achilles tendon lengthening. Again, preliminary results are encouraging, but long-term results are pending.

Stage III

PTT dysfunction associated with fixed deformity of the hindfoot and forefoot is best managed with arthrodesis. In stage III disease, there is usually collapse of the medial longitudinal arch, fixed hindfoot valgus and subtalar eversion, and forefoot abduction and supination through the talonavicular joint.[25] The goal of treatment is realignment of the foot followed by arthrodesis. The surgical choices include talonavicular arthrodesis, double arthrodesis (talonavicular and calcaneocuboid joints), subtalar arthrodesis, or triple arthrodesis. Cadaver studies by Astion and others[26] demonstrated that the talonavicular joint is the key joint of the triple joint complex, and that any fusion that involves this joint will limit motion of the other joints in the complex to less than 2% of normal. After isolated subtalar joint

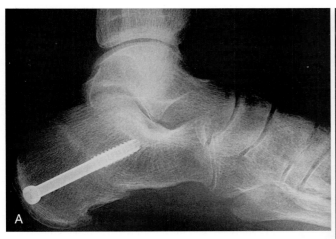

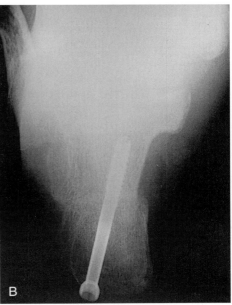

Figure 30–7. Lateral *(A)* and axial *(B)* views after medial displacement calcaneal osteotomy performed in conjunction with flexor digitorum longus transfer for posterior tibial tendon dysfunction.

arthrodesis, 26% of talonavicular joint motion and 56% of calcaneal cuboid joint motion were preserved.

The ability of selected arthrodeses to correct the deformities of the acquired flatfoot have also been studied in the cadaver model.[27] Isolated talonavicular arthrodesis

and double arthrodesis were each able to correct fully the flatfoot deformity, whereas subtalar arthrodesis and isolated calcaneocuboid arthrodesis were not.

The choice of the proper arthrodesis procedure for the patient with stage III disease is controversial. Isolated talonavicular fu-

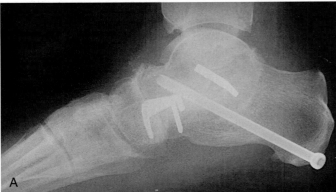

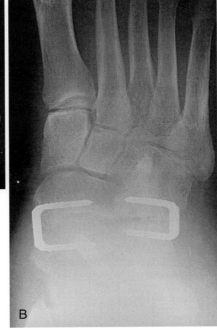

Figure 30–8. Lateral *(A)* and AP *(B)* views after triple arthrodesis performed for posterior tibial tendon dysfunction. Note the correction of the pes planus and the forefoot abduction.

sion is indicated in the face of isolated talo-navicular joint instability when the rest of the foot is supple. It is best reserved for the older less active patient. In younger patients, the double arthrodesis is an excellent choice as long as the subtalar joint is stable. The stability achieved is similar to that of a triple arthrodesis, but the morbidity is less without the subtalar fusion.[28] A triple arthrodesis is indicated in the presence of fixed deformities of the subtalar joint and the transverse tarsal joints. Hindfoot valgus should be corrected to a maximum of 5°, and forefoot abduction and supination should be corrected to neutral (Fig. 30–8).

Regardless of arthrodesis performed, postoperative care involves 6 to 8 weeks of immobilization and non-weight bearing followed by 4 to 6 weeks protected weight bearing and physical therapy. Appropriately selected and successfully performed hindfoot arthrodeses will provide long-term stability and pain relief for the patient with stage III PTT dysfunction.[28, 29]

REFERENCES

1. Kettelkamp DB, Alexander HH. Spontaneous rupture of the posterior tibial tendon. J Bone Joint Surg Am 51:759, 1969.
2. Netter FH. The Ciba Collection of Medical Illustrations: Volume 8, The Musculoskeletal System. Summit, NJ: Ciba-Geigy, 1987.
3. Hollingshead WH. Textbook of Anatomy, ed 3. New York: Harper & Row, 1974.
4. Johnson KA: Tibialis posterior tendon rupture. Clin Orthop 177:140–147, 1983.
5. Duchenne GBA. Physiology of Motion (Kaplan EB, ed and trans). Philadelphia: W. B. Saunders, 1949.
6. Keenan MAE, Peabody TD, Gronley JK, Perry J. Valgus deformities of the feet and characteristics of gait in patients who have rheumatoid arthritis. J Bone Joint Surg Am 73:237–247, 1991.
7. Perry J. Anatomy and biomechanics of the hindfoot. Clin Orthop 177:9–15, 1983.
8. Mann RA. Biomechanics of the foot and ankle. In Mann RA, Coughlin MJ, eds. Surgery of the Foot and Ankle, ed 6. St. Louis: C. V. Mosby, 1993, p. 3.
9. Frey C, Shereff M, Greenidge N. Vascularity of the posterior tibial tendon. J Bone Joint Surg Am 72:884–888, 1990.
10. Jhass MH. Spontaneous rupture of the posterior tibial tendon: clinical findings, tenographic studies, and a new technique of repair. Foot Ankle 3:158–166, 1982.
11. Holmes GB, Mann RA. Possible etiological factors associated with rupture of the posterior tibial tendon. Foot Ankle Int 13:70–79, 1992.
12. Dyal CM, Feder J, Deland JT, Thompson FM. Pes planus in patients with posterior tibial tendon insufficiency: asymptomatic versus symptomatic foot. Foot Ankle Int 18:85–88, 1997.
13. Mann RA. Flatfoot in adults. In Mann RA, Coughlin MJ, eds. Surgery of the Foot and Ankle, ed 6. St. Louis: C. V. Mosby, 1993, p. 757.
14. Funk DA, Cass JR, Johnson KA. Acquired adult flat foot secondary to posterior tibial tendon pathology. J Bone Joint Surg Am 68:95–102, 1986.
15. Gazkag AR, Cracchiolo A III. Rupture of the posterior tibial tendon: evaluation of injury of the spring ligament and clinical assessment of tendon transfer and ligament repair. J Bone Joint Surg Am 79:675–681, 1997.
16. Johnson KA, Strom DE. Tibialis posterior tendon dysfunction. Clin Orthop 239:196–206, 1989.
17. Bordelon RL. Correction of hypermobile flatfoot in children by molded insert. Foot Ankle 1:143–150, 1980.
18. Sangeorzan BJ, Mosca V, Hansen ST. Effect of calcaneal lengthening on relationships among the hindfoot, midfoot and forefoot. Foot Ankle Int 14:136–141, 1993.
19. Rosenberg ZS, Cheung Y, Jhass MH, et al. Rupture of the posterior tibial tendon: CT and MR imaging with surgical correlation. Radiology 169:229–235, 1988.
20. Chao W, Wapner KL, Lee TH, et al. Nonoperative management of posterior tibial tendon dysfunction. Foot Ankle Int 17:736–741, 1996.
21. Teasdall RD and Johnson KA. Surgical treatment of stage I posterior tibial tendon dysfunction. Foot Ankle Int 15:646–648, 1994.
22. Pedowitz WJ, Kovatis P. Flatfoot in the adult. J Am Acad Orthop Surg 3:293–302, 1995.
23. Mann RA, Thompson FM. Rupture of the posterior tibial tendon causing flatfoot: surgical treatment. J Bone Joint Surg Am 67:556–561, 1985.
24. Myerson MS, Corrigan J, Thompson F, Schon LC. Tendon transfer combined with calcaneal osteotomy for treatment of posterior tibial tendon insufficiency: a radiological investigation. Foot Ankle Int 16:712–718, 1995.
25. Pomeroy GC, Manoli A II. A new operative approach for flatfoot secondary to posterior tibial tendon insufficiency: a preliminary report. Foot Ankle Int 18:206–212, 1997.
26. Astion DJ, Deland JT, Otis JC, Kenneally SL. Motion of the hindfoot after simulated arthrodesis. J Bone Joint Surg Am 79:241–246, 1997.
27. O'Malley MJ, Deland JT, Kyung-Tai L. Selective hindfoot arthrodesis for the treatment of adult acquired flatfoot deformity: an in vitro study. Foot Ankle Int 16:411–417, 1995.
28. Clain MR, Baxter DE. Simultaneous calcaneocuboid and talonavicular fusion: long-term follow-up study. J Bone Joint Surg Br 76:133–136, 1994.
29. Harper MC, Tisdel CL. Talonavicular arthrodesis for the painful adult acquired flatfoot. Foot Ankle Int 17:658–661, 1996.

31 Achilles Tendinitis

Raymond D. Reiter
Vijay B. Vad

Achilles tendinitis has been reported as the most common overuse injury seen in the sports medicine setting.[1–6] In runners, the incidence of Achilles tendinitis has ranged from 6.5 to 18%.[7, 8] Also athletes participating in soccer, dance, tennis, and basketball as well as middle-aged men lacking gastrocnemius-soleus flexibility are at risk for this disorder.[7–12] Seronegative spondyloarthropathies and gout can also predispose an individual to this disorder.[13, 14]

Achilles tendinitis is the result of accumulative impact loading and repetitive microtrauma.[1, 2, 11, 12, 15–17] There are, however, intrinsic and extrinsic factors that can place an individual at greater risk for Achilles tendinitis. Intrinsic factors include areas of decreased vascularity within the tendon,[18] tendon degeneration,[15, 19] anatomic factors such as overpronation of the foot,[1, 2, 15, 20, 21] and poor gastrocnemius-soleus flexibility.[1, 4, 6]

Extrinsic factors include sudden increase in training intensity, running surface change, and worn-out or inappropriate footwear.[1, 5] Clain and Baxter[22] separated Achilles tendinitis into two categories: insertional and noninsertional. The insertional type of Achilles tendinitis involves the adjacent bursa along with attritional tendon changes usually in conjunction with Haglund deformity, whereas the noninsertional type affects the hypovascular zone 2 to 6 cm proximal to the insertion of Achilles tendon into the calcaneus.[23, 24]

CLINICALLY RELEVANT ANATOMY

The triceps surae comprises two heads of the gastrocnemius and the soleus and combines to form the Achilles tendon. It is the thickest and strongest tendon in the body, able to withstand up to 7000 N of force.[22] However, the stresses placed on the Achilles tendon are equally large, equaling up to 10 times the body weight during vigorous activities.[25] Furthermore, because of the presence of talocalcaneal motion, there are uneven stresses placed on the Achilles tendon. Overpronation of the foot is another factor implicated in placing greater stresses on the Achilles tendon.[26] These biomechanical factors make the Achilles tendon susceptible to injury.

The tendinous fibers from the gastrocnemius insert posterolaterally, and those from the soleus insert posteromedially on the calcaneus. Proximal to the insertion site lies the retrocalcaneal bursa. The narrowest part of the tendon is approximately 4 cm proximal to the insertion. An area 2 to 6 cm proximal to the insertion site has been shown to be hypovascular,[24] making it susceptible to injury. This area of hypovascularity has been shown to be the most common site of peritendinitis, tendinosis, and tendon rupture.[1, 5, 6, 11, 27] Moreover, the Achilles tendon has a deterioration in nutrition with aging as a result of decreased vascularity, further predisposing it to injury.[18]

The pathologic changes seen in Achilles tendinitis is a continuum of abnormalities separated into three stages by Puddu and colleagues.[28] The tendon in stage I is normal, but there is inflammation in the peritendinous tissue and is described as paratendinitis. Stage II is associated with paratendinitis combined with tendinosis. Tendinosis is defined as degenerative changes within the tendon. Macroscopic examination reveals calcification, nodular thickening, and lack of normal luster. Microscopic examination reveals mucoid degeneration, fibrinoid necrosis, and tendon fiber tearing. Stage III is characterized by macroscopically visible tendon fiber disruption occurring peripherally and centrally.

CLINICAL EVALUATION

Pain localized to 2 to 6 cm above the Achilles insertion is the predominant symptom of Achilles tendinitis.[5] Clement and associates[1] have reported overtraining, functional overpronation, and poor gastrocnemius-soleus flexibility as the three most common etiologic factors of Achilles tendinitis. In the early stages of tendinitis, there is pain with prolonged running. With advanced disease, there is pain at the start of a run. In advanced stages, there is morning stiffness with pain at rest.[5] History should be thorough, including miles run per outing, activity in which the patient is involved, shoe condition, running surface, character and quality of pain, review of systems, and previous treatments, including use of local or systemic corticosteroids.

The physical examination should involve both extremities. The physical findings in Achilles tendinitis include soft tissue swelling, local tenderness, and crepitus.[5, 28] In the acute stages, crepitus can be accentuated by active dorsiflexion and plantar flexion of the foot. Clancy and colleagues[9] defined Achilles tendinitis as acute (< 2 weeks), subacute (3–6 weeks), and chronic (> 6 weeks). Any gaps or nodularity in the tendon should be critically inspected. Leg and foot posture should be recorded (i.e., valgus or varus, cavus or pronated, rigid or flexible). Ankle range of motion is recorded with the forefoot supinated in both knee-flexed and knee-extended positions. Thompson test, in which the patient lies prone and the calf is squeezed to check for the integrity of the Achilles tendon, should be performed. Thompson's test is negative in Achilles tendinitis, even with the presence of partial rupture. Factors such as overpronation of foot, tight heel cords (especially limitation of passive ankle dorsiflexion), tight hamstrings, and abnormal anatomy such as tibia varum should be identified.

All these data are gathered to make as specific a diagnosis as possible (e.g., insertional or noninsertional Achilles tendinitis). Other differential diagnoses should be considered, including retrocalcaneal or superficial bursitis, calcaneus or posterior talar process stress fracture, plantaris muscle rupture, os trigonum fracture, and enthesopathy associated with Reiter disease. A tuning fork vibration test or manual percussion will usually elicit pain if there is a stress fracture. Other differential diagnoses include plantaris muscle rupture, in which pain is more proximal and occasionally a

pop is heard. Reiter disease is associated with other systemic symptoms.

ENDOCRINE/NUTRITION

Stress, increased catecholamine release, and glucocorticoids decrease cross-linking of collagen fibers. Collagen synthesis and cross-linking are reliant on adequate amino acid intake as well as cofactors (vitamins A and C, copper) supplied by a normal healthy diet. Calcium-deficient diets have been shown to decrease tensile strength of the myotendinous junction,[29] which may lead to junctional injuries, and an iron-deficient diet can negatively influence healing.[30]

ANTIBIOTICS

Fluoroquinolones, such as norfloxacin, pefloxacin, ciprofloxacin, and ofloxacin, have been associated with tendon disorders since 1992. Arthralgias and myalgias are classic adverse effects of quinolones, but tendinous involvement should be realized to prevent risk of tendon rupture. The rupture may occur on the first day of treatment or after withdrawal of the antibiotic. It has been postulated that the histopathology results form ischemic necrosis. Predisposing risk factors to tendon rupture include age greater than 6 years, renal failure, and prior corticosteroid treatment.[31]

RADIOGRAPHIC INVESTIGATIONS

Plain radiographs should be obtained to evaluate for bony calcaneus contour and os trigonum fracture, presence of Haglund deformity, tendon calcification, and soft tissue swelling. Technetium bone scan can be obtained if a stress fracture is suspected.

Should the patient not respond to conservative measures, a magnetic resonance imaging (MRI) scan should be obtained for further evaluation. Advantage of MRI is that it can define areas of thickening and degree of tendon degeneration (Figs. 31–1 to 31–3) as well as monitor healing response after surgery. Ultrasonography is also used in diagnosing and evaluating Achilles tendinitis, with 0.94 sensitivity and 1.0 specificity[32];

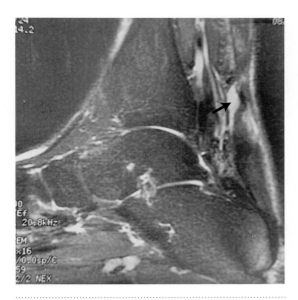

Figure 31–1. Sagittal magnetic resonance image demonstrating partial Achilles tendon disruption.

however, its drawback is that it is operator dependent.

NONOPERATIVE TREATMENT

The nonoperative treatment for insertional and noninsertional Achilles tendinitis is similar. The vast majority of Achilles tendinitis cases are successfully managed nonoperatively. Nonoperative treatment includes rest, protected mobilization, use of ¼- to

⅜-inch heel lift, arch supports if overpronation of the foot is present, oral nonsteroidal anti-inflammatory drugs (NSAIDs), the modality of ultrasound to the tendon, and gastrocnemius-soleus stretching and strengthening.[1]

The athlete should start out with modified rest, which includes swimming and bicycling with curtailment of running activities for 10 days after the patient is asymptomatic.[1] Running should be gradually resumed and increased. Electrical stimulation coupled with ice therapy is useful for pain control.[33] Iontophoresis and phonophoresis can be used for decreasing inflammation.[34–36] Patients tend to find phonophoresis more comfortable. In the meantime, proper stretching and strengthening are of paramount importance. Applying ultrasound to the tendon before stretching is also important for healing of the lesion.[37] Ultrasound has been shown to increase the rate of collagen synthesis, thus aiding in healing of the tendon. After ultrasound treatment, slow and sustained 20- to 30-second stretches should be performed, emphasizing heel cord and hamstring flexibility. Gaining passive ankle dorsiflexion is essential. Tendon-strengthening exercises should slowly be added. Running should gradually begin after the patient is asymptomatic for at least 10 days.

In severe cases with acute symptoms, a period of 7 days of immobilization may be needed.[4] Steroid injections into the retrocalcaneal bursa can be helpful if there is evidence of retrocalcaneal bursitis. However,

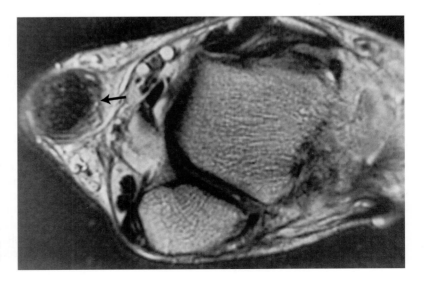

Figure 31–2. Axial magnetic resonance image demonstrating thickened Achilles tendon.

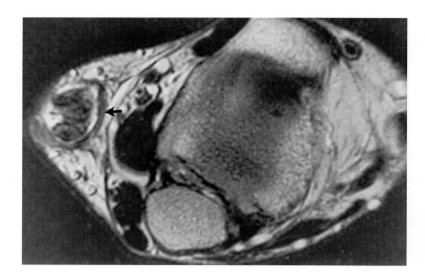

Figure 31–3. Axial magnetic resonance image demonstrating partial Achilles tendon disruption along with evidence of paratendinitis.

steroid injections into the Achilles tendon should be avoided because they may increase the risk of tendon rupture and retard healing.[25, 26, 37, 38] Athletes should be advised to modify extrinsic factors such as overtraining and use of improper shoes so they can remain symptom free. Preventive measures should be taught, such as proper warm-up before running, application of ice for 15 minutes to the tendon after running, maintaining hamstring and heel cord flexibility, and monitoring footwear.[1, 4]

Medications

Initial treatment of the inflamed Achilles tendon is to reduce inflammation. NSAIDs are widely used and are more appropriate for acute rather than chronic injuries. As cyclooxygenase inhibitors, they inhibit prostaglandin synthesis and, therefore, interrupt the inflammatory process. Corticosteroids are the most potent anti-inflammatory medications, and they are commonly used in the treatment of many tendinitis problems. Injection into the Achilles tendon substance is considered taboo because the cortisone preparations used decrease collagen synthesis and may lead to mechanical disruption of the tendon. The NSAIDs differ from the corticosteroids in that they do not inhibit fibroblast or macrophage activity.[39]

Physical Therapy

It has not been determined whether lack of flexibility is a significant cause of tendinitis. It is known that stretching the muscle-tendon unit improves athletic performance. Nevertheless, an aggressive stretching program is a mainstay of any physical therapy program instituted. The period of postinjury immobilization is variable and should be minimized as per pain symptoms with ambulation. The Achilles tendon is to be loaded to augment collagen synthesis, alignment, and maturation via cross-linking.[40] Because there is little tensile force with passive movements of the ankle and knee, passive range of motion is safe and beneficial immediately after injury. Stretching of the tendon to decrease fibrosis is used next, followed by an aggressive exercise regimen.

Physical therapy modalities are used to decrease inflammation and promote healing. Ultrasound has been shown to increase collagen synthesis by fibroblasts. For acute injuries, pulsed ultrasound may be used because it avoids unwanted thermal effects. In and of itself, ultrasound has no effect on inflammation. When used with hydrocortisone cream topically, called phonophoresis, there is an anti-inflammatory effect. Phonophoresis used at the time of maximal synthetic activity of the fibroblasts (the proliferative phase of healing) would maximize its benefit. Electrical stimulation is used to augment tendon healing. Because of the thickness of the Achilles tendon, this may be a more important modality than ultrasound. It prevents soft tissue swelling by decreasing the activity of inflammatory mediators and decreasing the overall metabolic rate of injured tissue.[41] When dexamethasone is applied topically, called ionto-phoresis, the anti-inflammatory effect is greatly increased. Transverse friction massage is used by many therapists, a technique brought forth by Cyriax for a treatment for chronic tendinitis.[42] This form of massage may release adhesions that formed between the Achilles tendon and surrounding soft tissue, causing continuous tissue irritation. Increased blood flow may also occur from the hyperemic response of digital pressure.

OPERATIVE TREATMENT

Resistant cases of Achilles tendinitis after a minimum of 12 weeks of conservative treatment should be considered for operative intervention if the patient wishes to return to previous athletic activities. The surgical approach for insertional and noninsertional Achilles tendinitis differs, as outlined by Clain and Baxter.[22]

In recalcitrant cases of insertional Achilles tendinitis, it is often necessary to eliminate bony deformities and inspect and debulk the thickened tendon anterior to posterior. Bursae should be removed around the insertion site. It may be necessary to remove a small amount of bone at the insertion site. In the case of critical compromise of insertion or vascularity, tendon transfer is warranted.

For noninsertional Achilles tendinitis, the following protocol applies. For paratendinitis, surgical débridement of the paratenon should be performed with immediate motion. For tendinosis, débridement of the tendon defect and paratenon release should be performed. If 20% or less of tendon width is excised, then side-to-side repair is performed. For greater than 20% of tendon width excised, a turn-down flap may be required.[17]

POSTOPERATIVE MANAGEMENT

A functional orthosis rather than cast immobilization, along with progressive active plantar flexion and immediate toe-touch weight bearing for 8 weeks, should be implemented after débridement and tendon repair.[43] This approach reduces the incidence of cast disease with no increased risk of rupture. A plantar flexion splint for the first 3 weeks should be used. By week 3, the patient can initiate swimming. Progressive exercises are begun from weeks 4 to 6. By weeks 6 to 8, stair climbing can begin. Gradual return to running and sports is allowed when the patient has no pain, full range of motion, and sufficient strength in the calf musculature.

CONCLUSION

Achilles tendinitis has multifactorial causes as a result of accumulative impact loading and repetitive microtrauma. Clinical features include pain localized to 2 to 6 cm above the Achilles insertion. Overtraining, functional overpronation, and poor gastrocnemius-soleus flexibility are the common etiologic factors. Conservative treatment, including the use of ultrasonography, stretching, orthotics as needed, modification of training techniques, proper footwear, and gradual return to activities, is successful in the vast majority of patients. Surgical intervention is needed if a minimum of 12 weeks of conservative treatment fails and the patient desires to return to competitive or recreational sports activities.

Acknowledgment

We thank Hollis Potter, MD, for providing the MRI scans.

REFERENCES

1. Clement DB, Taunton JE, Smart GW. Achilles tendinitis and peritendinitis: etiology and treatment. Am J Sports Med 12:179–184, 1984.
2. James SL, Bates BT, Ostering LR. Injuries to runners. Am J Sports Med 6:40–50, 1978.
3. Kvist MH, Lehto MUK, Jozsa L, et al. Chronic Achilles paratendinitis: an immunohistologic study of fibronectin and fibrinogen. Am J Sports Med 16:616–623, 1988.
4. Leach RE, James S, Wasilewski S. Achilles tendinitis. Am J Sports Med 9:93–98, 1981.
5. Nelen G, Martens M, Burssens A. Surgical treatment of chronic Achilles tendinitis. Am J Sports Med 17:754–759, 1989.
6. Schepsis AA, Leach RE. Surgical management of Achilles tendinitis. Am J Sports Med 15:308–315, 1987.
7. Jacobs D, Martens M, Van Andekerce R, et al. Comparison of conservative and operative management of Achilles tendon rupture. Am J Sports Med 6:107–111, 1978.
8. Kirssoff WB, Ferris W. Runners injuries. Physician Sports Med 7:55–64, 1979.

9. Clancy WG, Neidhart D, Brand RL. Achilles tendinitis in runners. Am J Sports Med 4:46–57, 1992.
10. Clement DB, Founton JE, Smart GW, et al. A survey of overuse running injuries. Physician Sports Med 9:47–58, 1981.
11. Fox JM, Blazina ME, Jobe FW, et al. Degeneration and rupture of Achilles tendon. Clin Orthop 107:221–224, 1975.
12. Gould N, Korson R. Stenosing tenosynovitis of the pseudosheath of the tendo Achilles. Foot Ankle 1:179–187, 1980.
13. Scioli M. Other arthritides. In Sammarco GJ, ed. AOFAS Foot and Ankle Manual. Philadelphia: Lea & Febiger, 1991, pp. 186–194.
14. Beskin J, Sanders RA, Hunter SC, et al. Surgical repair of Achilles tendon ruptures. Am J Sports Med 15:81–84, 1987.
15. Inglis AE, Scott WN, Sculco TP, et al. Ruptures of the tendo Achilles. J Bone Joint Surg Am 58:990–993, 1976.
16. Scioli M. Achilles tendinitis. Orthop Clin North Am 25:177–182, 1994.
17. Keene JS. Tendon Injuries of the Foot and Ankle in Orthopaedic Sports Medicine. Philadelphia: W. B. Saunders, 1994.
18. Hastad K, Larsson LG, Lindholm A. Clearance of radiosodium after local deposit in the Achilles tendon. Acta Chir Scand 116:251–255, 1959.
19. Arner O, Lindholm A. Histologic changes in subcutaneous rupture of Achilles tendon. Acta Chir Scand 116:484–490, 1959.
20. Lagergen C, Lindholm A. Vascular distribution in the Achilles tendon. Acta Chir Scand 116:491–495, 1959.
21. Snook GA. Achilles tendon tenosynovitis in long distance runners. Med Sci Sports Exerc 4:155–158, 1972.
22. Clain MR, Baxter DE. Achilles tendinitis. Foot Ankle 13:482–487, 1992.
23. Carr AJ, Norris SH. The blood supply of the calcaneal tendon. J Bone Joint Surg Br 71:10–101, 1989.
24. Lagergren C, Lindholm A. Vascular distribution in the Achilles tendon. Acta Chir Scand 116:491–495, 1958.
25. Scott SH, Winter DA. Internal forces at chronic running injury sites. Med Sci Sports Exerc 22:357–369, 1990.
26. Kleinman M, Gross AE. Achilles tendon rupture following steroid injection. J Bone Joint Surg Am 65:1345–1347, 1983.
27. Gillies H, Chalmers J. The management of fresh ruptures of the tendo Achilles. J Bone Joint Surg Am 52:337–343, 1970.
28. Puddu G, Ippolito E, Postachini F. A classification of Achilles tendon release. Am J Sports Med 4:145–150, 1976.
29. Law DJ, Lightner VA. Divalent cation-dependent adhesion at the myotendinous junction: ultrastructure and mechanics of failure. J Muscle Res Cell Motil 14:173–185, 1993.
30. Andrews FJ, Morris CJ, Lewis EJ, et al. Effect of nutritional iron deficiency on acute and chronic inflammation. Ann Rheum Dis 46:859–865, 1987.
31. Pierfitte C, Gillet P, Royer RJ. Tendinitis and tendon rupture: a side effect of fluoroquinolones. More on fluoroquinolone antibiotics and tendon rupture. N Engl J Med 332:193, 1994.
32. Kalebo P, Allenmark C, Peterson L, et al. Diagnostic value of ultrasonography in partial ruptures of the Achilles tendon. Am J Sports Med 20:378–381, 1992.
33. Lampe GN, Mannheimer JS. Clinical Transcutaneous Electrical Nerve Stimulation. Philadelphia: F. A. Davis, 1984.
34. Gangarosa LP, Park N. Increased penetration of nonelectrolytes into mouse skin during iontophoretic water transport. J Pharmacol Exp Ther 14:377–381, 1980.
35. Glass JM, Stephen RL. The quality and distribution of radiolabeled dexamethasone delivered to tissue by iontophoresis. Int Soc Tropical Dermatol 19:519–525, 1980.
36. Griffin JE, Touchstone JC. Ultrasonic movement of cortisol into pig tissue. Am J Phys Med 42:77–84, 1963.
37. Jackson BA, Schwane JA. Effect of ultrasound therapy on repair of Achilles tendon injuries in rats. Med Sci Sports Exerc 23:171–176, 1991.
38. Balasubramaniam P, Prathap K. The effect of injection of hydrocortisone into rabbit calcaneal tendons. J Bone Joint Surg Br 54:729–734, 1972.
39. Abramson SB. Nonsteroidal anti-inflammatory drugs: mechanisms of action and therapeutic considerations. In Leadbetter WB, Buckwalter JA, Gordon SL, eds. Sports-Induced Inflammation. Park Ridge, IL: American Academy of Orthopaedic Surgeons, 1990, pp. 421–430.
40. Enwemeka CS. Inflammation, cellularity and fibrillogenesis in regenerating tendon: implications for tendon rehabilitation. Phys Ther 69:816–825, 1989.
41. Knight KL. Cold as a modifier of sports-induced inflammation. In Leadbetter WB, Buckwalter JA, Gordon SL, eds. Sports-Induced Inflammation. Park Ridge, IL: American Academy of Orthopaedic Surgeons, 1990, pp. 463–477.
42. Cyriax J. Textbook of Orthopaedic Medicine, Volume II: Treatment by Manipulation, Massage and Injection, ed 11. London: Bailliere Tindall, 1984.
43. Carter TR, Fowler PJ, Blokker C, et al. Functional postoperative treatment of Achilles tendon repair. Am J Sports Med 2:459–462, 1992.

32 Achilles Tendon Injuries

John M. Wright
Heber C. Crockett
Andrew J. Weiland

Injuries to the Achilles tendon are quite common, particularly among recreational athletes. Achilles disease spans a broad spectrum ranging from paratenonitis (inflammation of the encompassing tissue) to complete tendon rupture. Between these two extremes are the phenomena of tendinosis (degenerative change within the tendon structure itself) and partial tendon rupture.

After reviewing the relevant anatomy and pathophysiology, we then describe the clinical manifestations, evaluation, and treatment options for the various forms of Achilles disease.

ANATOMY

The Achilles is the largest and strongest tendon in the body. Linking the gastrocnemius and soleus muscles to the calcaneal tuberosity, it is the chief effector of ankle plantar flexion. The tendon insertion is slightly medial to the midline of the calcaneus such that it imparts a mild inversion movement to the calcaneus as well. A superficial layer of fibers arises from the two heads of the gastrocnemius and joins a deeper layer from the soleus in the distal calf. As these fibers descend, they form an ovoid tendon and spiral approximately 90° around one another before inserting on the posterior surface of the calcaneus. The left Achilles spirals clockwise, and the right Achilles spirals counterclockwise. Thus, the gastrocnemius fibers insert lateral to the soleus fibers. The spiral orientation of the tendon fibers serves as a theoretical source of dynamic ischemia. Tensioning the twisted fibers creates a "wringing" effect, thereby compromising blood flow and promoting ischemic degeneration of the central fibers. Hyperpronation exacerbates this wringing effect by imparting further torsion on the fibers.[1, 2]

The Achilles has no investing synovium. Rather, it is enveloped by paratenon, which provides a mucopolysaccharide-rich surface to facilitate gliding between the tendon and the surrounding pseudosheath (epitenon) (Fig. 32–1). The majority of the tendon's blood supply stems from the ventral paratenon, although it also receives vascular contributions from its muscular origin and osseous insertion.[3] Lagergen and Lindholm have demonstrated a vascular watershed region 2–6 cm proximal to the calcaneal insertion. This region is theoretically susceptible to ischemic breakdown and corresponds to the characteristic site of clinical degeneration and rupture.[3–5] However, despite the long-standing acceptance of Lagergen and Lindholm's hypothesis, their work has been called into question by contradictory data from Schmidt-Rohlfing and colleagues.[6]

PATHOPHYSIOLOGY

The cause of Achilles disease is multifactorial. However, many of the same factors contribute to both Achilles inflammation and Achilles rupture.

BIOMECHANICAL FACTORS

The Achilles transmits forces of two to three times body weight with walking and six to eight times body weight with running and jumping. These forces are highest during midstance and push-off.[7] Given the huge forces to which the Achilles is subjected, it comes as no surprise that it is prone to an overuse mechanism of inflammation and injury.

Microtearing arises when the tendon is unable to resist repetitively applied loads. This initiates a cycle of inflammation and attempted repair. Early scar tissue is poorly organized, and has suboptimal tensile strength to resist recurrent microtrauma when sufficient healing time is not permitted. Chronic inflammation, in turn, stimu-

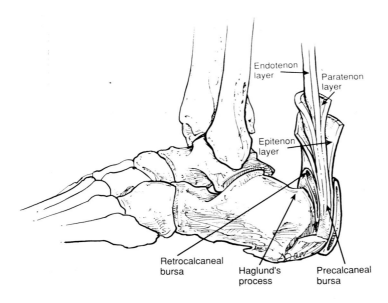

Figure 32–1. Anatomy of the Achilles tendon and adjacent tissues. (From Baker CL. The Hughston Clinic Sports Medicine Book. Baltimore, MD: Williams and Wilkins, 1995.)

lates degeneration with resultant partial rupture.[8]

Extrinsic (Training-Related) Factors

Many training errors promote microtrauma and inflammation. These include insufficient warm-up, inadequate stretching, too abrupt an increase in the amount or duration of activity, rapid return to sport after a period of inactivity, excessive hill running, and excessive running on hard surfaces. A poor-fitting heel counter in running shoes or "ribbon burn" in dancers can lead to friction on the paratenon with resultant inflammation.[9] Excessively stiff running shoe soles impede metatarsophalangeal flexion and, thus, increase Achilles strain by lengthening the lever arm acting on the tendon during late stance and toe-off.[10] Improved running shoe design over the past two decades has significantly reduced the incidence of Achilles tendinitis among runners, but shoes still need to be replaced periodically to maintain adequate shock absorption capacity.

Intrinsic Factors

Multiple intrinsic factors can render the Achilles more vulnerable to inflammation. Poor flexibility in the musculotendinous unit places increased demand on the tendon. Insufficient flexibility and tensile strength can be seen with poor warm-up and improper conditioning, but they are also the result of advancing age.[11] Vascular compromise can promote ischemic degeneration and retard healing. Evidence of ischemic damage has been documented in ruptured specimen.[12] Potential sources of decreased perfusion include the anatomic watershed region described by Lagergen and the dynamic "wringing" effect of pronation[1–3, 10] (Fig. 32–2). Pronation not only in-

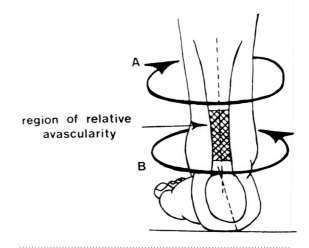

region of relative avascularity

Figure 32–2. Anatomic watershed region, as described by Lagergen (shaded area). The relative avascularity of this region is dynamically exacerbated by pronation. (From Clement DB, Taunton JE, Smart GW. Achilles tendinitis and peritendinitis: etiology and treatment. Am J Sports Med 12:179–184, 1984.)

creases the "wringing" effect, but it also causes medial to lateral Achilles excursion, which in turn creates shear on the paratenon.[10] During normal gait, the calcaneus pronates from heel strike to midstance. Because of the Achilles' roles as a plantarflexor and an accessory hindfoot invertor, this phase of gait eccentrically loads the musculotendinous unit and focuses particular tensile demand at the tendon's medial side (Fig. 32–3). The effects of pronation are exacerbated in individuals who hyperpronate.

A cavus foot has decreased shock absorptive capacity and, thus, causes increased loads to be transmitted to the heel cord. Furthermore, increased dorsal calcaneal pitch in a cavus foot renders the posterosuperior aspect of the os calcis more prominent, which can induce retrocalcaneal bursitis and insertional tendinitis.[9]

Trauma

The mechanism of complete Achilles rupture is typically indirect trauma. This is a secondary phenomenon, with underlying tendon degeneration serving as the diathesis. Most commonly, rupture is caused by a forceful eccentric contraction of the triceps surae such as when a plantar-flexed ankle is abruptly forced into dorsiflexion on landing from a jump. Disruption can also be caused

by excessive concentric gastrocnemius-soleus contracture such as pushing off to initiate a sprint. Concomitant knee extension increases stress on the musculotendinous unit because the gastrocnemius originates above the knee. Under these circumstances, not only gastrocnemius and soleus contraction but also quadriceps forces are transmitted to the Achilles.[13] It has also been proposed that extremely forceful, uncoordinated muscle contraction can contribute to tendon rupture via a mechanism of failed normal protective inhibitory feedback.[10, 14, 15]

Most authorities agree that "normal" Achilles tendons do not spontaneously rupture. Multiple pathologic analyses have confirmed the presence of antecedent chronic inflammation and degeneration in ruptured specimen.[4, 8, 12, 16–21] Despite pre-existing inflammation, the vast majority of these patients are asymptomatic before spontaneous rupture.[9, 19, 20, 22] Patients who lead sedentary lifestyles with intermittent bursts of recreational athletics seem to be at particular risk for Achilles disruption. The combination of poorly conditioned tissues and intermittent extreme forces creates a predisposition for microtrauma and degeneration.[20] Collagen type, remodeling, and regional vascularity are hypothesized to be deleteriously affected by poor conditioning.

Direct trauma from contusion or laceration accounts for a distinct minority of Achilles disruptions and is not predicated on pre-existing tendon degeneration.

Extrinsic (Systemic) Factors

Many systemic factors have been associated with Achilles tendon inflammation and rupture, including the seronegative spondyloarthropathies, hypercholesterolemia (with xanthoma formation), systemic corticosteroids, and fluoroquinolone antibiotic therapy.[23, 24]

PATHOLOGY

Puddu[21] described a useful classification scheme for Achilles disease (Table 32–1). His system consists of three categories of disease: (1) pure peritendinitis (paratenonitis), (2) peritendinitis with tendinosis, and (3) pure tendinosis.[21] In peritendinitis, the tendon itself is macroscopically and histo-

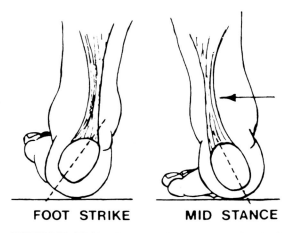

FOOT STRIKE   **MID STANCE**

Figure 32–3. Relative increase in tension of medial side of Achilles with transition from foot strike to midstance. (From Clement DB, Taunton JE, Smart GW. Achilles tendinitis and peritendinitis: etiology and treatment. Am J Sports Med 12:179–184, 1984.)

Table 32–1. Puddu's[21] Pathologic Classification of Achilles Tendinitis

1. Pure peritendinitis (paratenonitis)
2. Peritendinitis with tendinosis
3. Pure tendinosis

From Puddu G. A classification of Achilles tendon disease. Am J Sports Med 4:145–150, 1976.

logically normal. The paratenon displays thickening with an inflammatory cell infiltrate. Adhesions are present between the tendon and paratenon. During acute inflammatory phases, a fibrinous exudate is sometimes encountered within the potential space between the tendon and paratenon. In cases of tendinosis, degeneration (focal or multifocal) exists within the tendon proper. Histologic analysis of these chronic reactive changes has demonstrated myxomatous degeneration, fibrinoid degeneration, fatty degeneration, and metaplastic calcification.[4, 13, 20]

In all spontaneous ruptures without prior symptomatology, Puddu found pure *tendinosis* and no histologic evidence of inflammation in the surrounding tissues.[21] Specimens from patients who had experienced regional discomfort before rupture manifested tendinosis with peritendinitis.[21] In other words, all cases of rupture manifested underlying tendinosis, and all patients with antecedent Achilles discomfort had peritendinitis in addition to tendinosis.

When indicated, surgical intervention should be targeted at the specific disease. For instance, tenolysis should be reserved for cases of recalcitrant pure paratenonitis. Tenolysis accomplishes nothing for tendinosis. Tendinosis requires débridement of the degenerative tissue to promote neovascularization and healing.[25, 26]

It should be noted that Puddu did not recognize "tendinitis" (inflammation of the tendon proper) as a true pathologic entity in the Achilles.[21] However, the term *Achilles tendinitis* is commonly used nonspecifically to refer to all symptomatic inflammatory conditions of the tendon and its adjacent tissues.

ACHILLES TENDINITIS

Manifestations Evaluation

Achilles tendinitis encompasses two principal pathologic conditions: (1) paratenonitis and (2) paratenonitis with coexistent tendinosis. The two conditions present with identical symptoms. Those patients with longer standing symptoms are more likely to have tendinosis in addition to paratenonitis. Many affected individuals are competitive athletes in their 20s and 30s, although older, recreational athletes are also commonly affected.[1, 25] This is in contrast to Achilles ruptures, which occur almost exclusively in middle-aged athletes.

The principal presenting complaint is pain at the Achilles tendon of insidious onset, which is exacerbated by plantar flexion activities and relieved by rest. Other entities that can give rise to pain in the region should be considered and systematically excluded (Table 32–2). These include precalcaneal bursitis ("pump bump"), retrocalcaneal bursitis (with or without Haglund's deformity), calcaneal or distal tibial stress fracture, flexor hallucis longus or tibialis posterior tendinitis, deep posterior exertional compartment syndrome, and posterior shin splints.

Physical examination will reveal varying degrees of focal tenderness and fusiform swelling of the Achilles. Crepitus is sometimes present during episodes of acute inflammation. Ankle dorsiflexion is characteristically limited. This may represent both a cause as well as a consequence of the Achilles disease.

The painful arc sign has been described as a means of clinically differentiating inflammation of the paratenon from involvement of the tendon itself. With paratenonitis, the region of tenderness and swelling does not move as the ankle is plantiflexed and dorsiflexed. With involvement of the tendon itself, the region of tenderness and swelling moves up and down in association with tendon excursion.[75] Distinguishing these two entities from one another is important because it affects prognosis. Conser-

Table 32–2. Differential Diagnosis for Achilles Tendinitis

Precalcaneal bursitis ("pump bump")
Retrocalcaneal bursitis
Stress fracture (calcaneus or distal tibia)
Flexor hallucis longus tendinitis
Tibialis posterior tendinitis
Deep posterior exertional compartment syndrome
Posterior shin splints (symptomatic os trigonum)

vative treatment of the two processes is identical. However, isolated paratenonitis is more likely to respond favorably to conservative treatment. Tendinosis, on the other hand, is less likely to resolve because degenerative tendon has limited healing potential.

Conservative Treatment

The management of Achilles tendinitis is predicated on a two-stage approach. The goal of the first stage is to control and eliminate pain and inflammation. This is accomplished by relative rest, nonsteroidal anti-inflammatory drugs, and ice. Relative rest may simply entail decreasing the mileage that the jogger runs, but for some it may require cessation of the precipitating activity altogether and substitution of a low-impact cross-training activity such as swimming or bicycling. Biking with the ipsilateral heel on the pedal will subject the Achilles to less strain and excursion. The patient should be instructed that continuing the precipitating activity at an intensity or duration that causes pain will increase tissue injury and delay recovery. Heel lifts help to alleviate symptoms in many individuals. Absolute rest is generally not necessary, but in certain acute or recalcitrant cases, brief periods of immobilization in a cast or walking boot may be indicated. Relative rest should be continued for at least 1 week after symptoms have completely resolved.

The goal of the second phase of management is to prevent recurrence. All predisposing biomechanical factors should be eliminated. Weakness and stiffness of the gastrocnemius-soleus musculotendinous unit are both causes as well as sequelae of Achilles tendinitis. Strength and flexibility must be restored. A regimen of heel rise exercises and heel cord stretching should be prescribed (Fig. 32–4). Proper warm-up permits maximal creep and stress relaxation during stretching, which in turn decreases tendon strain. Athletic footwear should be inspected and replaced with appropriate footwear when necessary. Hyperpronation should be addressed with well-molded orthotic inserts (Fig. 32–5). A gradual return to premorbid activity level over several weeks is then permissible.

Operative Treatment for Chronic Tendinitis

The vast majority of patients with pure paratenonitis will respond to conservative therapy. However, surgical intervention may be warranted for the rare individual who fails an appropriate duration of nonoperative management (4–6 months) and who has a strong desire to return to his or her premorbid activity level. At surgery, the crural fascia and paratenon are longitudinally released through a posteromedial incision. Inflamed paratenon is excised, and adhesions between the paratenon and tendon are released. The anterior side of the tendon is not disturbed to avoid compromising its vascular supply from the ventral paratenon. For this procedure, 88 to 97% good to excellent results have been reported.[26, 27]

For patients with recalcitrant tendinitis symptoms who are found to have tendinosis (in addition to paratenonitis), the procedure differs. The diseased tendon is split longitudinally to expose and excise the foci of tendinosis (Fig. 32–6). Foci of tendinosis are identified intraoperatively as regions of macroscopic nodularity, softening, or discoloration (Fig. 32–7). Preoperative magnetic resonance imaging (MRI) can also be used to localize affected areas. The tendon is then closed side to side over the defect with resorbable suture[25, 26] (Fig. 32–8). Good to excellent results have been reported in 73% of patients under these circumstances.[26] If extensive débridement is required, Nelan[26] recommends reinforcement with turn-down tendon flaps with good to excellent results reported in 88% of patients. Reinforcement by other means (such as a plantaris weave or bypass with flexor hallucis longus or flexor digitorum longus tendon) is also acceptable.

Patients with recalcitrant insertional tendinopathy often manifest associated retrocalcaneal bursitis and/or a Haglund deformity.[9, 25] This subset of patients should be treated by excision of the bursa and posterosuperior calcaneal prominence (in addition to debridement of any associated tendinosis).

Glucocorticoid injections have no role in the management of Achilles tendon overuse syndromes because they can further weaken an already compromised tendon and predispose to complete rupture.[28, 29]

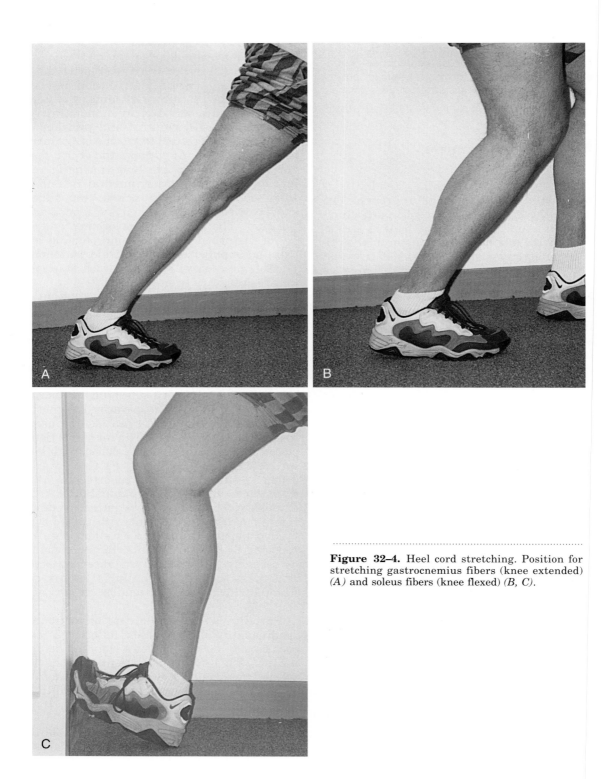

Figure 32–4. Heel cord stretching. Position for stretching gastrocnemius fibers (knee extended) *(A)* and soleus fibers (knee flexed) *(B, C)*.

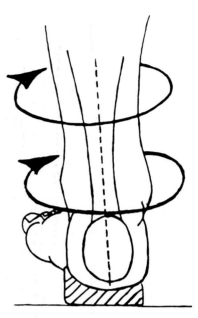

Figure 32–5. Use of an orthosis to neutralize pronation. (From Clement DB, Taunton JE, Smart GW. Achilles tendinitis and peritendinitis: etiology and treatment. Am J Sports Med 12:179–184, 1984.)

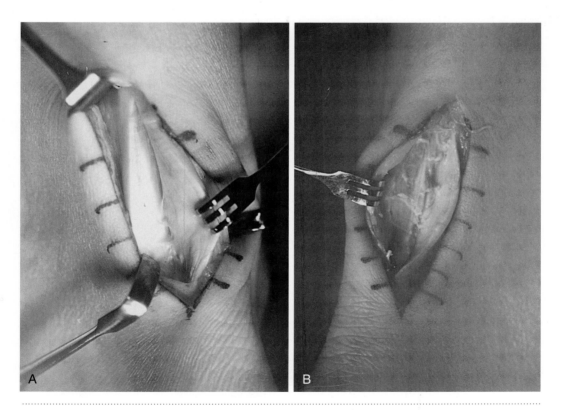

Figure 32–6. *A,* Exposed, split Achilles tendon. *B,* Split Achilles tendon revealing focus of tendinosis.

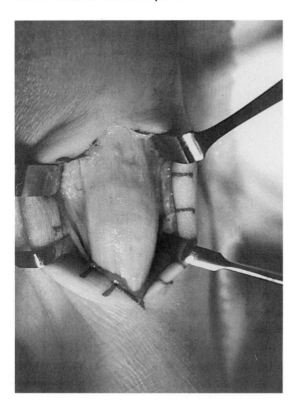

Figure 32–7. Exposure of Achilles tendon with macroscopic region of softening and nodularity.

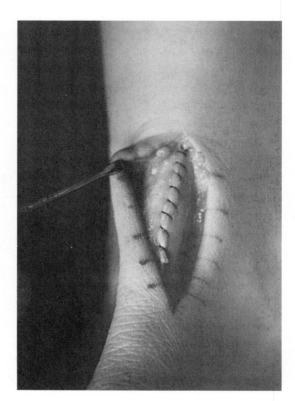

Figure 32–8. Closure of longitudinal split in Achilles tendon after débridement.

COMPLETE ACHILLES RUPTURE

Manifestations and Evaluation

Most Achilles ruptures occur in recreational athletes in their fourth and fifth decades. Men are affected more commonly than women, and the left side ruptures more frequently than the right.[13, 8, 20, 30–33] Patients typically present with a complaint of having experienced sudden posterior ankle pain while lunging or jumping. They often liken the incident to being kicked or struck in the posterior ankle by an object such as an opponent's racket. Patients may also describe having experienced an audible or palpable "snap." Affected individuals will note an inability to run or jump and difficulty with gait because of weakness plantar flexing the affected extremity. Historically, the diagnosis is frequently missed by the primary physician, which may lead to a delay in treatment.[8, 13, 14, 20, 22, 34–36] This is often attributed to the fact that pain and swelling are typically minimal at the time of initial evaluation. Common misdiagnoses include ankle sprain, partial Achilles tear, plantaris tendon rupture, and gastrocnemius strain.[9, 22]

Physical exam will reveal tenderness and ecchymosis at the Achilles with weak plantar flexion. Trace active plantar flexion may be preserved via the deep posterior compartment muscles, but the patient will be unable to perform a single-limb toe rise. Stride length will be shortened. The Thompson squeeze test will produce no plantar flexion[37] (Fig. 32–9). A palpable gap may be appreciated at the point of discontinuity, but this defect may be obscured by organized hematoma. The diagnosis of a complete rupture is made clinically. MRI is rarely necessary as a confirmatory modality, but it may be useful in preoperative planning for cases of recalcitrant tendinosis, or partial rupture, as a means of assessing the extent of disease.

Treatment

The optimal treatment for complete Achilles disruption is highly controversial.[78] The literature pertaining to this topic is contradictory. Multiple reports have advocated nonoperative management,[8, 33, 38–45] but an equally abundant amount of support exists for surgical intervention.[13–16, 19, 22, 30, 34, 46–52] Only nine comparative studies exist, and only those of Nistor and Cetti were randomized[14, 19, 30, 33, 39, 46] (Table 32–3). Comparison and assimilation of the plethora of studies are problematic given the fact that they involve multiple different conservative and surgical techniques used by an assortment of surgeons with different periods of time elapsed between injury and intervention, varied durations of immobilization, multiple different rehabilitation protocols, and evaluations by a wide variety of rating criteria with inconsistent follow-up periods.

Proponents of nonoperative care suggest

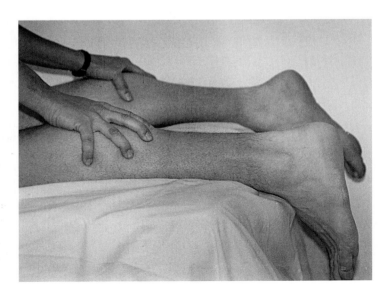

Figure 32–9. Thompson test. Compression of calf should produce plantar flexion (background). With a ruptured Achilles tendon, this compression produces no plantar flexion (foreground).

Table 32–3. Surgical Versus Nonsurgical Treatment of Achilles Rupture (Comparative Studies)

Study	No. Patients	Function	No. Reruptures
Quenu and Stoianovitch (1929)[51]			
Nonoperative	29	6 (21%) good results	
Operative	29	28 (97%) good results	
Christensen (1953)[13]			
Nonoperative	16	12 (75%) patients "normal" function	N/A
Operative	33	30 (90%) patients "normal" function	2 (6%)
Arner (1959)[16]			
Nonoperative	6	5 (83%) poor results*	0
Operative	86	96% good† or excellent‡	4 (5%)
Gillies and Chalmers[39]			
Nonoperative	7	80% strength of normal side	1 (14%)
Operative	6	84% strength of normal side	0
Inglis et al. (1976)[14]			
Nonoperative	23	73% strength of normal side 62% power of normal side 64% endurance of normal side	9 (39%)
Operative	44	101% strength of normal side 88% power of normal side 91% endurance of normal side	0
Jacobs (1978)[19]			
Nonoperative	32	65% strength of normal side	7 (22%)
Operative	26	75% strength of normal side	0
Edna (1980)[46]			
Nonoperative	10	89% power of normal side	3 (30%)
Operative	24	No difference in power vs. nonoperative group	N/A
Nistor (1981)[33]			
Nonoperative	60	Average 9-week absence from work 79% strength of normal side	5 (8%)
Operative	44	Average 13-week absence from work 83% strength of normal side	2 (5%)
Cetti et al. (1993)[30]			
Nonoperative	55	29% returned to sport at same level 35% returned to sport at diminished level 7% stopped sports 47% had abnormal ankle motion 64% had calf atrophy	7 (13%)
Operative	56	57% returned to sport at same level 21% returned to sport at diminished level 14% stopped sports 18% had abnormal ankle motion 39% had calf atrophy	3 (5%)

N/A = not applicable.
* "Poor" indicates gait and strength were markedly affected.
† "Good" indicates gait and strength were slightly hampered.
‡ "Excellent" indicates gait and strength were normal.

that satisfactory functional results can be obtained with cast immobilization alone and that the incidence of operative complications is unacceptably high (Tables 32–4 and 32–5). Advocates of operative treatment cite the lower rate of rerupture and a superior restoration of strength and function after surgical repair[9, 14, 16, 19, 22, 30, 47, 48, 52] (Table 32–6). Nonoperative enthusiasts suggest that many of the reported cases of reruptures and poor functional results after conservative treatment can be attributed to insufficient duration of immobilization.[8, 41, 45] The operative camp argues that open management is the only predictable means to confidently re-establish the appropriate resting length and, thus, optimal function of the musculotendinous unit.

The controversy between surgical and conservative treatment remains unresolved, although there is a general trend in the literature toward surgical management of

Table 32–4. Nonoperative Treatment Outcomes

Study	No. Patients	Function	Rerupture Rate
Christensen (1953)[13]	16	12 (75%) normal function	N/A
Arner (1959)[16]	6	5 (83%) poor results	0
Lea (1970)[41]	55	52 (95%) satisfactory (comfortable and able to return to preinjury activity level)	7 (13%)
Gillies and Chalmers (1970)[39]	7	80% strength of normal side	1 (14%)
Inglis et al. (1976)[14]	23	73% strength of normal side 62% power of normal side 64% endurance of normal side	9 (39%)
Lildholdt and Munch-Jorgensen (1976)[42]	14	N/A	2 (14%)
Jacobs (1978)[19]	32	65% strength of normal side	7 (22%)
Persson and Wedmark (1979)[49]	20	84% strength of normal side	7 (35%)
Edna (1980)[46]	10	89% power of normal side	3 (30%)
Nistor (1981)[33]	60	Average 9-week absence from work 79% strength of normal	5 (8%)
Keller and Bremholm (1984)[40]	37	16 excellent and 18 good (by Arner criteria); all walked normally	2 (5%)
Fruensgaard et al. (1992)[38]	66	Tegner score improved to 0.27, less than preinjury rate	4 (6%)
Mann and Coughlin (1993)[9]	N/A	75–85% normal fixation	25–30%
Cetti et al. (1993)[30]	55	29% returned to sport at same level 35% returned to sport at diminished level 7% stopped sports 47% had abnormal ankle motion 64% had calf atrophy	7 (13%)

N/A = not applicable.

younger individuals who have higher functional demands and expectations.[8, 9, 30, 46–48, 50]

Surgical Treatment

The first step in the operative management of Achilles ruptures is to optimize soft tissue conditions. Swelling is not always extensive enough to warrant postponing surgery. However, when it is significant, elevation and immobilization should be prescribed until swelling has subsided. There is no justification for premature surgical intervention through an area that is recognized for its susceptibility to infection and skin breakdown. Surgical outcomes have not been demonstrated to be altered even by delaying repair up to 4 weeks.[13, 14, 19, 22] On the other hand, conservative measures have been shown to be less effective if initiated after 48 hours post injury.[53]

Patient selection is also crucial. Under most circumstances, patients at greater risk for wound healing difficulties (such as those with diabetes mellitus or peripheral vascular disease) should be treated nonoperatively because the risks of surgery outweigh the potential operative benefits in this patient population.

The principal goal of surgical intervention is to restore the normal resting length of the musculotendinous unit by directly reopposing the torn ends of tendon. With the patient prone, both legs are prepared and draped to allow direct comparison of the Achilles tendon length, after reapproximation, to the contralateral extremity (Fig. 32–10). Exposure should be performed through a posteromedial longitudinal parasagittal incision centered over the level of tendon discontinuity (Fig. 32–11). Medialization keeps the incision away from the sural nerve and minimizes friction on the incision by the heel counter.

The paratenon should be longitudinally incised in line with the overlying skin incision and conscientiously preserved for later repair. The tendon should be exposed with full-thickness flaps to minimize chances of

Table 32–5. Operative Complications

Study	No. Patients	Major (excluding reruptures)	Minor
Arner (1959)[16]	86	2 (2%) DVT (1 fatal PE) 3 (3%) skin slough requiring grafting 4 (5%) fistulas	3 (3%) superficial infection 8 (9%) superficial skin slough
Gillies and Chalmers (1970)[39]	6	1 (16%) deep infection	N/A
Lea and Smith (1972)[41] (literature review)	255	105 (41%) patients had complications 17 (7%) infection 11 (4%) draining fistulas 2 (1%) MI (1 death)	22 (9%) sensory loss 39 (15%) adhesions
Inglis et al. (1976)[14]	44	2 (5%) deep infection	N/A
Ma and Griffith (1977)[57] (percutaneous repair)	18	No skin necrosis No infection No delayed wound healing	1 skin retraction dimple 1 tender nodule at surgical knot No nerve injuries
Jacobs (1978)[19]	26	2 (8%) skin slough 3 (12%) infection	N/A
Shields (1978)[52]	33		1 (3%) wound hematoma No sural nerve injuries
Percy (1978)[50]	75	23% of patients had complications 4 (5%) deep infection 2 (3%) major skin slough 1 (1%) keloid requiring excision 2 (3%) pulmonary emboli 1 (1%) lax repair requiring revision	5 (7%) superficial infection 5 (7%) minor skin slough 6 (8%) inconsequential adhesions
Quigley and Scheller (1980)[34]	40	No skin necrosis	2 (5%) suture granulomas 2 (5%) superficial infection
Lennox et al. (1980)[76]	4 12 4	Laceration group: no complications Acute rupture group: 3 (25%) skin necrosis Subacute rupture group: 2 (50%) skin slough	2 (50%) superficial wound infections
Nistor (1981)[33]	44	2 (5%) deep wound infections	9 (20%) sural nerve injuries 20 (45%) adhesions (skin to tendon)
Nistor (1981)[33] (literature review)	2647	24 (1%) deep infections 76 (3%) fistulas 52 (2%) necrosis of skin and/or tendon	5% total (hematoma, granuloma, adhesions, superficial infection)
Kellam et al. (1985)[48]	68	9 (13%) of patients had complications 1 (1.5%) infection 3 fistulas	1 transient sural dysesthesia 2 delayed wound healing 2 "unsightly" scars
Beskin and Sanders (1987)[22]	42	0	3 (7%) superficial infections
Turco and Spinella (1987)[36]	40	2 (5%) delayed wound healing	
Bradley and Tibone (1990)[58]	15 12	*Open surgery group* No infections No delayed wound healing No skin necrosis *Percutaneous repair group* No infections No delayed wound healing No skin necrosis	No sural nerve problems No sural nerve problems
Cetti et al. (1993)[30]	56	2 (4%) deep infection No skin necrosis	6 (11%) adhesions No superficial infections 7 (13%) sensory disturbances 1 (2%) suture granuloma 1 (2%) delayed wound healing
Fitzgibbons et al. (1993)[59] (percutaneous repair)	14	No infections No delayed wound healing	1 (7%) sural nerve injury

DVT = deep venous thrombosis; PE = pulmonary embolism; N/A = not applicable; MI = myocardial infarction.

Table 32–6. Operative Treatment Outcomes

Study	No. Patients	Function	Rerupture Rate
Christensen (1953)[13]	33	30 (90%) patients "normal" function	2 (6%)
Arner (1959)[16]	86	96% good or excellent	4 (5%)
Gillies and Chalmers (1970)[39]	6	84% strength of normal side	0
Ralston (1971)[35]	49	All returned to comparable level of preoperative activity 11 (22%) had some weakness vs. uninjured side	1 (2%)
Lea and Smith (1972)[41] (literature review)	255		4 (1.6%)
Nistor (1976)[44]	12	No subjective decreased motion strength 70–100% of normal side	1 (8%)
Inglis et al. (1976)[14]	44	101% strength of normal side 88% power of normal side 91% endurance of normal side	0
Ma and Griffith (1977)[57]	18	86% power restoration in 1 year 75% had normal gait at 1 year	0
Percy (1978)[50]	75	56% full function and no weakness 38% full function and slightly questionable weakness 7% some limitation of activities and definite weakness	0
Jacobs (1978)[19]	26	75% strength of normal side	0
Shields et al. (1978)[52]	33	83.5% strength of normal side 82.5% power or normal side 27 (82%) returned to former level of sports activity	0
Lennox et al. (1980)[76]	4	Laceration group: no activity limitation	0
	12	Acute rupture group: full return to preinjury activities; 5 (42%) had weakness or decreased endurance	0
	4	Subacute rupture group: all had some residual weakness; 2 limped; 3 unable to resume preinjury activity level	0
Quigley and Scheller (1980)[34]	40	42% excellent 36% good 15% fair 6% poor	2 (5%)
Nistor (1981)[33]	44	Average 13-week absence from work 83% strength of normal side	2 (5%)
Kellam et al. (1985)[48]	68	92% returned to preinjury activity levels; 13% of patients had residual postoperative weakness	2 (3%)
Beskin and Sanders (1987)[22]	42	88% return of power (if operated <30 days from injury)	0
Turco and Spinella (1987)[36]	40	All patients were able to resume prior level of activity	0
Bradley and Tibone (1990)[58]	15	*Open surgery group:* 84% strength of normal leg *Percutaneous repair group:* 82% strength of normal leg	0
	12		2 (12%)
Cetti et al. (1993)[30]	56	57% returned to sport at same level 21% returned to sport at diminished level 14% stopped sports 18% had abnormal ankle motion 39% had calf atrophy	3 (5%)
Fitzgibbons et al. (1993)[59] (percutaneous repair)	14	13% loss of power vs. normal side @ 180°/sec Cybex (no significant power loss at 60 or 120°/sec)	0

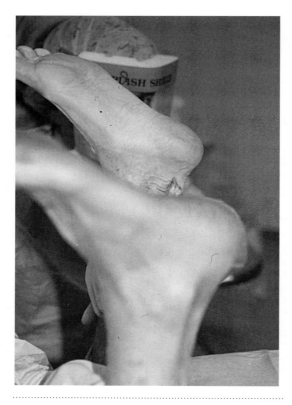

Figure 32–10. Preparation of both lower extremities to allow for intraoperative comparison of resting Achilles tendon length.

skin slough. The tendon ends will manifest varying degrees of "horse tail" or "torn hemp" fraying (Fig. 32–12). These tattered ends should be incorporated into the repair rather than excised unless preserving them creates too much bulk at the repair site.[22] Grossly degenerative tendon should be excised. However, overzealous tendon debridement can excessively shorten the resting length of the repaired musculotendinous unit, with resultant difficulty regaining dorsiflexion. Débrided ends should be brought into direct opposition with one another and held with modified Kessler or Bunnell stitches of no. 5 nonresorbable suture. Beskin and Sanders have reported a "three-bundle" method for preserving and incorporating frayed ends with Bunnell sutures[22] (Fig. 32–13).

Knots should be buried within the tendon substance to avoid friction and minimize the bulk of the repair. An excessively bulky repair creates tension in the overlying skin, which can contribute to wound healing dif-

ficulty. Double-loaded sutures should be used to prevent suture damage during crossing needle passes. Augmentation with fascial turn-down flaps, the plantaris tendon, or the peroneus brevis tendon has been proposed as a means of strengthening the repair, decreasing the chance of rerupture, and permitting earlier weight bearing and functional rehabilitation[36, 54] (Fig. 32–14). Despite these theoretical advantages, the healing response is usually quite vigorous, and these types of reinforcement are not typically necessary in the acute setting unless excessive debridement has produced a gap large enough to require bridging (rather than end-to-end suture). On the other hand, peroneus brevis transfer provides the theoretical advantage of adding an active motor to the repair and has excellent reported results. The peroneus brevis transfer is a particularly valuable adjunct in treating the rare instances when the Achilles tendon has avulsed from the calcaneus.[36]

The wound should be closed in layers with meticulous, atraumatic soft tissue handling and repair of the paratenon whenever

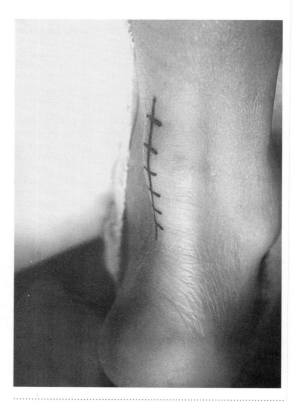

Figure 32–11. Posteromedial parasagittal incision.

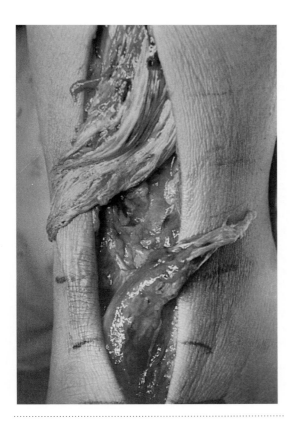

Figure 32–12. Acutely ruptured Achilles tendon with significant fraying.

possible. Certain circumstances (such as chronic pre-existing paratenonitis with adhesions, a bulky tendon repair, or instances when the paratenon was severely damaged in association with the Achilles tear) may preclude paratenon closure. The theoretical benefits of restoring continuity of the paratenon are that (1) it serves as a barrier for adhesion formation between the healing tendon and overlying skin and (2) it is a rich source of fibrocytes for extrinsic tendon healing.

Postoperative immobilization should be as close to neutral flexion as possible without putting undue tension across the repair site. Some tension across the repair is believed to minimize muscle atrophy and promote collagen deposition and remodeling.[36] Standard postoperative immobilization lasts for 6 to 8 weeks. Weight bearing is typically initiated at 3 to 4 weeks, although some authorities permit earlier protected weight bearing. Other authorities still advocate non-weight bearing for the full dura-

tion of immobilization. This variable has not been studied in a randomized, prospective manner. A program of active motion and gentle passive stretching is commenced at the time of cast removal. During this period, partial protection is provided with a heel lift or elevated-heel shoe (i.e., cowboy boot or clog). Strengthening exercises are gradually increased over the next 2 months, and return to sport is typically permitted at 6 months (depending on satisfactory achievement of functional motion and plantar flexion strength).

Carter and Fowler[55] advocated a more aggressive, functional postoperative protocol emphasizing early mobilization with a more rapid return to sporting activities. This is appealing for the athletic-oriented patient compared with the several months of rehabilitation that may be required to regain strength and a functional range of motion after 6 to 8 weeks of casting in relative equinus. Excellent results have been reported in 88% of patients with immediate postoperative free ankle motion in a patellar tendon-bearing cast with a protective frame under the foot for immediate full weight bearing.[56]

The incidence of wound complications remains a drawback to operative management of Achilles ruptures. The literature suggests that wound problems can be minimized via careful soft tissue handling and increased operative experience.[14] Furthermore, the high incidence of fistula formation reported in some of the older literature has been significantly reduced by the use of absorbable suture material.[48]

A technique of percutaneous repair has been described by Ma[57] as a means of averting wound complications encountered with open repair. Excellent results and very few complications have been reported with this technique.[57–59] Some authorities fear that sural nerve injuries may be more likely with this method, particularly if the surgeon has limited experience with the technique.[60] A single comparative study reported a higher rate of rerupture versus open repair.[58]

Nonoperative Treatment

The challenge imposed by conservative management is to bring the tendon ends back into opposition with one another without exposing them. Scar tissue readily forms

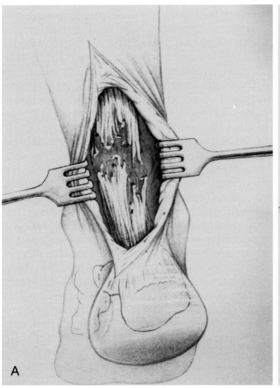

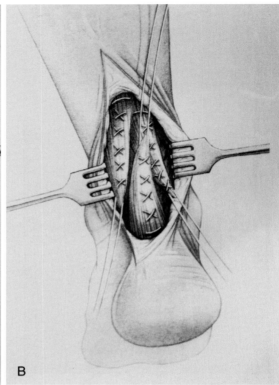

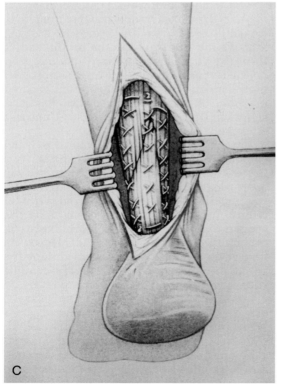

Figure 32–13. *A,* Ruptured Achilles tendon. *B,* Triple-bundle reconstitution of frayed ends. *C,* Reapproximation of reconstituted ends. (From Beskin JL, Sanders RA, Hunter SC, Hughton JC. Surgical repair of Achilles tendon ruptures. Am J Sports Med 15:1–8, 1987.)

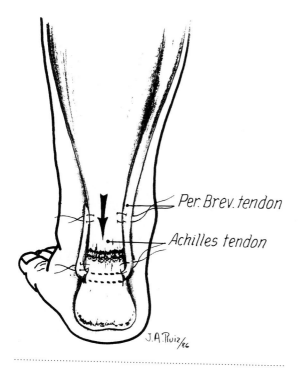

Figure 32–14. Achilles repair augmentation with peroneus brevis tendon transfer. (From Turco VJ, Spinella AJ. Achilles tendon ruptures—peroneus brevis transfer. Foot Ankle 7:253–259, 1987.)

in the region and will bridge virtually any gap.[61, 62] Tendon ends must be reapproximated to avoid healing of the musculotendinous unit in an elongated position. In some centers, ultrasonography is used to assess reapproximation, but the quality and reliability of this modality are technician dependent. MRI can also be used to assess the success of gap reduction.[63]

Nonoperative care typically consists of 6 to 8 weeks of immobilization in the gravity equinus position. Long leg casting has been advocated by some to prevent gapping between the tendon ends via pull from the gastrocnemius origin, but no benefit over a short leg cast has ever been demonstrated. Unlike surgically managed cases, the ankle should not be brought to neutral until the immobilization phase is complete because of concern over the risk for tendon healing in a lengthened position. The postcasting rehabilitation regimen is identical to that for operative cases, although slower return of motion and strength are likely.

The option of no treatment whatsoever (judicious neglect) may be appropriate for very old, sick, or low-demand patients in whom a compromised functional result is acceptable.[9] An ankle-foot orthosis can be useful in this patient population.

PARTIAL ACHILLES RUPTURE

Partial Achilles ruptures represent a diagnostic conundrum. These injuries present with essentially identical signs and symptoms as Achilles tendinitis. Sometimes a history of sudden sharp pain during activity can be elicited, but this is neither sensitive nor specific. Plantar flexion strength is preserved. A classic pain cycle has been described, with discomfort on commencing activity that subsides with further activity but recurs when activity is ceased. This history should raise the clinician's index of suspicion for a partial rupture, but it also lacks sensitivity and specificity. In short, history and physical examination cannot reliably distinguish partial rupture from tendinitis. The diagnosis of a partial tear can be made by a skilled ultrasonographer, but the gold standard is MRI, which can precisely localize and quantify the extent of injury.[63]

Conservative Treatment

Nonoperative management of partial Achilles ruptures uses all of the techniques described for Achilles tendinitis. However, partial tears respond less well to conservative measures than other causes of Achilles pain. In fact, this diagnosis should also come to mind whenever a compliant patient with presumed tendinitis fails conservative treatment. Rest and immobilization mollify the symptoms of partial rupture but rarely provide an enduring curative effect.[64, 65]

Surgical Treatment

Surgery consists of excision of the partial rupture with debridement of associated adjacent degenerative tissue. This procedure eliminates painful, immature scar and promotes healing by encouraging local neovascularization. Thus, the surgeon eliminates unhealthy tissue as well as the local hypoxia, which presumably contributes to the degenerative milieu in which partial rupture typically occurs. Postoperatively, the ankle is immobilized in slight plantar flexion for 6 weeks with subsequent initiation of physical therapy. Full recovery to premorbid activity level usually requires approximately 6 months.

Allenmark[64] compared 35 patients treated surgically for partial Achilles tears with a control group of 26 patients treated conservatively. At 5-year follow-up, only 15% of conservatively treated patients were able to return to premorbid activity level and intensity in comparison to 77% of surgically treated patients. At 10-year follow-up, these numbers were 27% and 88%, respectively. It is apparent that partial Achilles ruptures do not respond favorably to conservative management.[64, 65] Thus, when the diagnosis is objectively established (by ultrasonography or MRI), surgical treatment should be recommended to patients who wish to optimize their chances of returning to their premorbid level of activity.

CHRONIC RUPTURE

The term *chronic* is typically applied to Achilles tears that are not treated for the

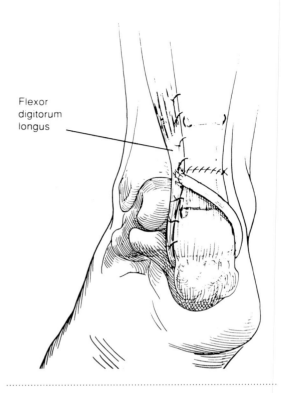

Figure 32–16. Augmentation of Achilles tendon repair with flexor digitorum longus tendon transfer. (From Mann RA, Holmes GB, et al. Chronic rupture of the Achilles tendon: a new technique of repair. J Bone Joint Surg Am 73:214–218, 1991.)

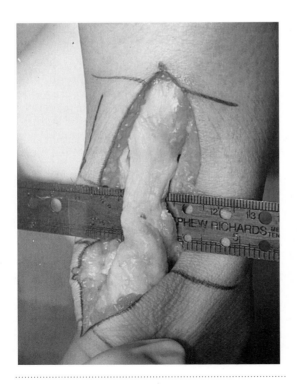

Figure 32–15. Neglected chronic Achilles tendon rupture which healed in an elongated fashion.

initial 4 to 6 weeks. Management of chronic Achilles insufficiency is a challenge because of the gap that arises between the ruptured ends when the injury is initially neglected.

In patients with neglected ruptures, bridging scar does form between the torn tendon ends.[61] Thus, the Thompson test may produce plantar flexion. However, with bridging of the gap by scar, the tendon heals in an elongated fashion, and the gap scar is often fixed to surrounding tissues (Fig. 32–15). The proximal stump is retracted, and there is frequently considerable disuse atrophy of the gastrocnemius and soleus. Thus, these patients present with marked subjective and objective plantar flexion weakness.

Unlike the dispute between operative and nonoperative management for acute Achilles disruptions, there is little disagreement over the fact that operative intervention is the only efficacious means to address the significant functional compromise that stems from a chronic neglected Achilles

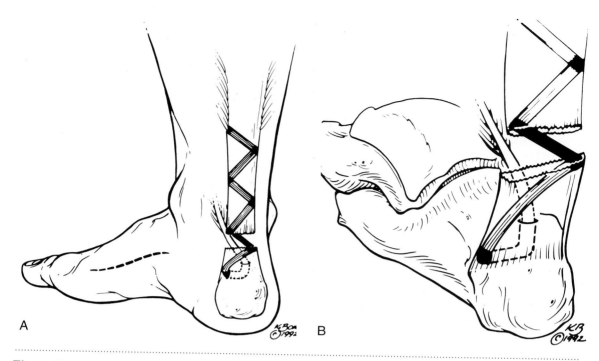

Figure 32–17. *A, B,* Achilles tendon repair with flexor hallucis longus tendon transfer. (From Wapner KL, Pavlock GS, Hecht PJ, et al. Repair of chronic Achilles tendon rupture with flexor hallucis longus tendon transfer. Foot Ankle 14:443–449, 1993.)

tear.[13, 14, 53, 77] However, considerable controversy does exist over what is the ideal material with which to bridge the gap. Proposed intercalary augmentation materials have included aponeurotic turndown flaps,[14, 16] peroneus brevis tendon[36, 66] (see Fig. 32–14), plantaris tendon,[54] flexor digitorum longus tendon[67] (Fig. 32–16), flexor hallucis longus tendon[68] (Fig. 32–17), fascia lata transplantation,[69] V-Y advancement,[70, 71] carbon fiber implants,[72, 73] and Marlex mesh.[74]

Allograft Achilles has also been used under isolated circumstances and is particularly valuable when potential local donor tissues are compromised by systemic disease (T. Wickiewicz, personal communication, 1997).

The potential operative complications are no different than with surgery for acute ruptures. These patients are at slightly greater risk for wound healing difficulties and sural nerve problems because more extensive exposure is generally required in this setting.

REFERENCES

1. Galloway MT, Jokl P, Dayton W. Achilles tendon overuse syndromes. Clin Sports Med 11:773–782, 1992.
2. Schepsis AA, Leach RJ. Surgical management of Achilles tendinitis. Am J Sports Med 15:308, 1987.
3. Carr AJ, Norris SH. The blood supply of the calcaneal tendon. J Bone Joint Surg Br 71:100–101, 1989.
4. Fox JM, Blazina ME, Jobe FW, et al. Degeneration and rupture of the Achilles tendon. Clin Orthop 107:221–224, 1975.
5. Lagergen C Lindholm A. Vascular distribution in Achilles tendon. Acta Chir Scand 116:491–495, 1958.
6. Schmidt-Rohlfing B, Graf J, Schneider U, Niethard F. The blood supply of the Achilles tendon. Int Orthop 16:29–31, 1992.
7. Scott S, Winter D. Internal forces at chronic running injury sites. Med Sci Sports Exerc 22:357–369, 1990.
8. Hattrup SJ, Johnson KA. A review of ruptures of the Achilles tendon. Foot Ankle 6:34–38, 1985.
9. Mann RA, Coughlin MJ. Surgery of the Foot and Ankle, ed 6. St. Louis: C. V. Mosby, 1993.
10. Clement DB. Achilles tendinitis and peritendinitis. Am J Sports Med 12:179–184, 1984.
11. Teitz CC. Scientific Foundations of Sports Medicine. Philadelphia: B.C. Decker, 1989.
12. Kvist M, Jozsa L, Jarvinen M. Vascular changes in the ruptured Achilles tendon and paratenon. Int Orthop 16:377–382, 1992.
13. Christensen I. Rupture of the Achilles tendon: analysis of 57 cases. Acta Chir Scand 106:50–60, 1953.
14. Inglis A, Scott W, Sculco T. Ruptures of the tendo Achillis: an objective assessment of surgical and non-surgical treatment. J Bone Joint Surg Am 58:990–993, 1976.

15. Inglis A, Sculco T. Surgical repair of ruptures of the tendo Achilles. Clin Orthop 156:160–169, 1981.

16. Arner O. Subcutaneus rupture of the Achilles: a study of 92 cases. Acta Chir Scand 239:1–51, 1959.

17. Clancy W. Achilles tendinitis in runners: a report of 5 cases. Am J Sports Med 4:46–57, 1976.

18. Davidsson L. Pathogenesis of subcutaneus tendon rupture. Act Chir Scand 135:209–212, 1969.

19. Jacobs D. Comparison of conservative and operative treatment of Achilles tendon ruptures. Am J Sports Med 6:107–111, 1978.

20. Jozsa L, Kvist, M, et al. The role of recreational sporting activity in Achilles tendon rupture: a clinical, pathoanatomical, and sociological study of 292 cases. Am J Sports Med 17:338–343, 1989.

21. Puddu G. A classification of Achilles tendon disease. Am J Sports Med 4:145–150, 1976.

22. Beskin JL, Sanders RA. Surgical repair of Achilles tendon rupture. Am J Sports Med 15:1–8, 1987.

23. Ribard P, Audisio F. Seven Achilles tendinitis including three complicated by rupture during fluoroquinolone therapy. J Rheumatol 19:1479–1481, 1992.

24. Saraf S, Sharma S. Reconstruction for xanthoma of the Achilles tendon. Int Orthop 16:37–38, 1992.

25. Leach RE, Schepsis A. Long term results of surgical management of Achilles tendinitis in runners. Clin Orthop 282:208–212, 1992.

26. Nelan G, Martens M. A surgical treatment of chronic Achilles tendinitis. Am J Sports Med 17:754–759, 1989.

27. Kvist H, Kvist M. The operative treatment of chronic calcaneal paratenonitis. J Bone Joint Surg Br 62:353–357, 1980.

28. Kleinman M, Gross A. Achilles tendon rupture following steroid injection. J Bone Joint Surg Am 65:1345, 1983.

29. Mahler F, Fritschy D. Partial and complete ruptures of the Achilles tendon and local corticosteroid injections. Br J Sports Med 26:7 1992.

30. Cetti R, Christensen S, Ejsted R, et al. Operative versus nonoperative treatment of Achilles tendon rupture. Am J Sports Med 21:791–799, 1993.

31. Gillespie H. Results of surgical repair of spontaneous rupture of the Achilles tendon. J Trauma 9:247–249, 1969.

32. Goldman S. Disruptions of the tendo Achillis: a review of 33 cases. Mayo Clin Proc 44:28–35, 1969.

33. Nistor L. Surgical and non-surgical treatment of Achilles tendon rupture. J Bone Joint Surg Am 63:394–398, 1981.

34. Quigley T Scheller A. Surgical repair of the ruptured Achilles tendon. Am J Sports Med 8:244–250, 1980.

35. Ralston E. Repair of the ruptured Achilles tendon. J Trauma 11:15–21, 1971.

36. Turco VJ, Spinella AJ. Achilles tendon ruptures: peroneus brevis transfer. Foot Ankle 7:253–259, 1987.

37. Thompson T, Doherty J. Spontaneous rupture of the Achilles: a new clinical diagnostic test. J Trauma 2:126–129, 1962.

38. Fruensgaard S, Helmig P, Riis J, Stovring J. Conservative treatment for acute rupture of the Achilles tendon. Int Orthop 16:33–35, 1992.

39. Gillies H, Chalmers J. Management of fresh ruptures of the teno Achilles. J Bone Joint Surg Am 52:337–343, 1970.

40. Keller J, Bremholm T. Closed treatment of Achilles tendon rupture. Acta Orthop Scand 55:548–550, 1984.

41. Lea RB, Smith L. Non-surgical treatment of tendo Achilles rupture. J Bone Joint Surg Am 54:1398–1407, 1972.

42. Lildholdt T, Munch-Jorgensen T. Conservative treatment of Achilles tendon rupture. Acta Orthop Scand 47:454–458, 1976.

43. Murrell G, Lilly E, Collins A, et al. Achilles tendon injuries: a comparison of surgical versus no repair in a rat model. Foot Ankle 14:400–406, 1993.

44. Nistor L. Conservative treatment of fresh subcutaneous rupture of the Achilles tendon. Acta Orthop Scand 47:459–462, 1976.

45. Stein S, Leukens C. Methods and rationale for closed treatment of Achilles tendon rupture. Am J Sports Med 4:162–169, 1976.

46. Edna T. Nonoperative treatment of Achilles tendon ruptures. Acta Orthop Scand 51:991–993, 1980.

47. Haggmark T, Liedberg H, Eriksson E, Wredmark T. Calf muscle atrophy and muscle function after non-operative vs operative treatment of Achilles tendon ruptures. Orthopedics 9:160–164, 1986.

48. Kellam JF, Hunter GA, McElwain JP. Review of the operative treatment of Achilles tendon rupture. Clin Orthop Rel Res 201:80–83, 1985.

49. Persson A, Wedmark T. The treatment of total rupture of the Achilles tendon by plaster immobilisation. Int Orthop 3:149–152, 1979.

50. Percy E. The surgical treatment of ruptured tendo-Achilles. Am J Sports Med 6:132–136, 1978.

51. Quenu J, Stoianovitch S. Les ruptures du tendon d'Achille. Rev Chir Paris 67:647–678, 1929.

52. Shields C, Kerlan R, Jobe F, et al. The Cybex II evaluation of surgically repaired Achilles tendon ruptures. Am J Sports Med 6:369–372, 1978.

53. Carden DG. Rupture of the calcaneal tendon. J Bone Joint Surg Br 69:416–20, 1987.

54. Lynn TA. Repair of the torn Achilles tendon using the plantaris tendon as a reinforcing membrane. J Bone Joint Surg Am 48:268–272, 1966.

55. Carter JR, Fowler PJ. Functional postoperative treatment of Achilles tendon repairs. Am J Sports Med 20:459, 1992.

56. Solveborn S, Moberg A. Immediate free ankle motion after surgical repair of Achilles tendon ruptures. Am J Sports Med 22:607–610, 1994.

57. Ma G, Griffith T. Percutaneous repair of closed rupture of the Achilles tendon. Clin Orthop 128:247–255, 1977.

58. Bradley J, Tibone J. Percutaneous and open surgical repairs of Achilles tendon ruptures. Am J Sports Med 18:188–195, 1990.

59. Fitzgibbons R, Hefferon J, Hil J. Percutaneous Achilles tendon repair. Am J Sports Med 21:724–727, 1993.

60. Hockenbury R, Johns JC. A biomechanical and in vitro comparison of open versus percutaneous repair of tendo Achillis. Foot Ankle 11:67–72, 1990.

61. Barnes MJ, Hardy AE. Delayed reconstruction of the calcaneal tendon. J Bone Joint Surg Br 68:121–124, 1986.

62. Conway AM, Dorner RW. Regeneration of resected calcaneal tendon in the rabbit. Anat Rec 1958:43–49, 1967.

63. Keene J, Lash E, Fisher D, DeSmet A. Magnetic resonance imaging of Achilles tendon ruptures. Am J Sports Med 17:333–337, 1989.

64. Allenmark C. Partial Achilles tendon tears. Clin Sports Med 11:759, 1992.
65. Ljungquist R. Subcutaneous partial rupture of the Achilles tendon. Acta Orthop Scand 113:10–86, 1968.
66. Teuffer AP. Traumatic rupture of the Achilles tendon: reconstruction by transplant and graft of the peroneus brevis. Orthop Clin North Am 5:89–93, 1974.
67. Mann RA, Holmes GB, et al. Chronic rupture of the Achilles tendon: a new technique of repair. J Bone Joint Surg Am 73:214–218, 1991.
68. Wapner KL, Pavlock GS, Hecht PJ, et al. Repair of chronic Achilles tendon rupture with flexor hallucis longus tendon transfer. Foot Ankle 14:443–449, 1993.
69. Bugg EI, Boyd BM. Repair of neglected rupture or laceration of the Achilles tendon. Clin Orthop 56:73–75, 1968.
70. Abraham E, Pancovich, AM. Neglected rupture of the Achilles tendon: treatment by a V-Y tendinous flap. J Bone Joint Surg Am 57:253–255, 1975.
71. Leitner A, Voigt C, Rahmanzadeh R. Treatment of extensive aseptic defects in old Achilles tendon ruptures. Foot Ankle 13:176–180, 1992.
72. Howard CB, Winston I, Bell W, Jenkins DRH. Late repair of the calcaneal tendon with carbon fibre. J Bone Joint Surg Br 66:206–208, 1984.
73. Parsons JR, Weiss AB, Schenk RS, et al. Long term follow up of Achilles tendon repair with polymer-carbon fiber composite. Foot Ankle 9:179–184, 1989.
74. Ozaki J, Fujik J, Sugimoto K, Tamai J. Reconstruction of neglected Achilles tendon rupture with Marlix mesh. Clin Orthop 238:204–208, 1989.
75. Williams J. Achilles tendon injuries in sport. Sports Med 3:114–135, 1986.
76. Lennox D, Wang G, McCue F, Stamp W. The operative treatment of Achilles tendon injuries. Clin Orthop Rel Res 148:152–155, 1980.
77. Gabel S, Manoli A. Neglected rupture of the Achilles tendon. Foot Ankle 15:512–517, 1994.
78. Wills C, Washburn S, Caiozzo V, Prietto C. Achilles tendon rupture: a review of the literature comparing surgical versus nonsurgical treatment. Clin Orthop Rel Res 207:156–163, 1986.

33 Physical Therapy for Ankle and Rearfoot Disorders

Michael Levinson

The primary goals of any rehabilitation program are to return the patient to normal function as quickly and safely as possible and to avoid recurrence of the injury. Each patient has individual goals and progresses individually. This progression should be guided by the patient's symptoms and the clinician's evaluation and continuous re-evaluation.

A thorough history is important to any evaluation before rehabilitation. Many disorders of the ankle and rearfoot are related to an overuse during a particular activity. Changes in activities, intensity of training, footwear, and poor mechanics are often contributing factors to foot and ankle disease. For example, a runner who suddenly increases mileage or incorporates more hills into a training program may be susceptible to certain disorders.

Objective evaluation should include edema, crepitus, point tenderness, atrophy, range of motion (active and passive), and strength deficits. Resistive motions are helpful with certain musculotendinous diseases. In addition, the clinician must evaluate the structural alignment of the foot and ankle for any varus or valgus deformity at both the forefoot and rearfoot. Gait should be evaluated closely. Both hyperpronation and hypopronation can predispose the patient to various disorders. Finally, the patient must be evaluated for any abnormality of deficits at the hip and knee. When treating the foot and ankle, one must view it in relation to the entire kinetic chain. Any lack of proximal flexibility or strength may predispose the patient to a foot or ankle disorder. Any deviation in hip or tibial rotation or loss of proximal muscle flexibility, such as hamstrings, iliopsoas, or hip rotators, may change the biomechanics of the foot and ankle.

In following a progressive treatment plan for all foot and ankle disorders, the initial goal is to reduce the patient's symptoms. This is accomplished by avoiding or limiting the causative activity. It is important to educate the patient regarding this point. The patient must be aware that pain, inflammation, and swelling are indications of excessive activity, and cautious progression through this initial phase will actually allow a more aggressive path later. Various modalities, such as cryotherapy, ultrasonography, electrical stimulation, whirlpool, phonophoresis, and iontophoresis, are used for these symptoms. However, it must be noted that these modalities are not a substitute for addressing the underlying causes of the disorder. These should be used in conjunction with exercise to return the patient to function.

Normal joint range of motion and flexibility must be restored within the healing parameters of the structures involved. Selective flexibility deficits are common in many foot and ankle disorders. A common finding is tightness of the gastrocnemius-soleus complex and Achilles tendon. This can result in several biomechanical flaws that are discussed more specifically later. Restoring flexibility should be a gradual process. Stretching should always be performed in a pain-free range of motion. Stretching should be done several times a day and preferably while the patient's muscles are warm. The idea is to not overstretch the muscle. Each stretch should be held for approximately 15 to 30 seconds.

Restoring function to the foot and ankle also includes restoring normal strength and proprioception. Strengthening is also progressed according to the patient's symptoms. Depending on the evaluation, simple active range of motion or pain-free isometrics may be initiated to prevent atrophy. As the patient becomes less symptomatic, isotonic strengthening may be incorporated into the program. Weights, tubing, elastic resistance, or manual resistance may be used for isotonic training. As with stretching, these exercises should be performed within a pain-free range of motion.

Eccentric muscular activity appears to play a significant role at the foot and ankle during most activities. Therefore, an eccentric component should be included at some point. However, caution should be used because this type of exercise may tend to increase the onset of muscle soreness.

As an adequate strength base is established, the strengthening program may be advanced to more functional, multijoint activities to restore normal neuromuscular function. Exercises performed on a balance board such as a BAPS (biomechanical ankle platform system) board (Fig. 33–1) will help strengthen the foot and ankle in a more functional position and help to restore proprioceptive awareness.

While rehabilitating, it is also important to maintain the patient's cardiovascular status and prevent deconditioning. Often, stationary cycling, swimming, or upper body ergometry provide alternative means of conditioning while the patient is rehabilitating a foot or ankle injury. It has also been my experience that the active patient benefits

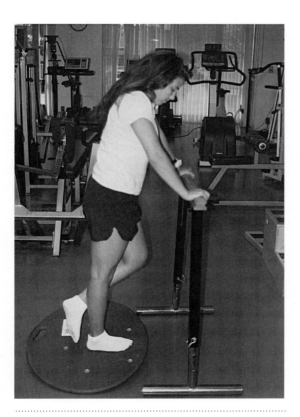

Figure 33–1. BAPS board.

from incorporating a nonexacerbating exercise program.

Finally, the patient must be educated to avoid recurrence of injury. This includes providing a home exercise program that will maintain the strength and flexibility of the foot and ankle. Changes may need to be made in a patient's training program or simply in activities of daily living. Education regarding footwear may also be a factor.

The focus of this chapter is to describe rehabilitation principles for the most common ankle and rearfoot disorders. All the previous principles should be incorporated into the treatment plan. Regardless of the disorder, each plan should follow a rational, functional progression based on current research. Each patient should be progressed individually based on the clinician's continuous re-evaluation and the patient's individual goals.

ANKLE SPRAIN

Studies have documented the great prevalence of ankle sprains in the athletic population.[1–3] Despite the frequency of this injury, there remains significant variation in the treatment plans. The goal of the rehabilitation program is to restore normal dynamic stability to the ankle while allowing the injured tissues to heal adequately. Inadequate treatment of the ankle sprain can result in decreased strength of the dynamic stabilizers and proprioceptive deficits.[4, 5] Failure to restore normal neuromuscular function may lead to chronic instability and ensuing degenerative changes.

When creating a treatment plan, several factors determine the rate and course of progression for each individual patient. First, the clinician must be aware of the mechanism of injury and the structures involved. The most common injury is the inversion sprain, involving the lateral ankle ligaments, and this section focuses on that injury. Second, the severity of the injury must be taken into account. To ensure a full return to activity, injured tissues must be allowed to heal optimally. Third, the patient's history may be a factor. The patient with a history of chronic ankle instability may present with degenerative changes that will dictate greater caution in the treatment plan.

Successful comprehensive rehabilitation

of the ankle sprain should include several important elements: early reduction of edema, early controlled motion, early controlled weight bearing, and restoration of normal neuromuscular function. The key aspects of restoring normal neuromuscular function appear to be retraining proprioceptive awareness and restoring normal peroneal strength. It has been hypothesized that trauma to the ankle may have an adverse effect on the joint and muscle mechanoreceptors, thus leading to deafferentation of the joint.[6, 7] Glencross and Thornton theorized that loss of position sense is attributed to muscle spindle damage caused by overstretch.[8] Their study demonstrated deficits in ability to replicate actively passive ankle and foot proprioception in sprained ankles. Konradsen and Ravn found a prolonged peroneal reaction to inversion stress with chronic instability of the ankle.[9] Most recently, Lofvenberg and others found a significantly longer muscular reaction time to sudden angular displacement with chronic lateral instability.[10]

These concepts provide rationale for incorporating certain types of exercise into the rehabilitation program. Initially, closed-chain activities should make up a large component of the program. Closed-chain activities, which are performed with the distal aspect of the limb fixed, contribute in several positive ways. Most ankle sprains will occur in a closed chain (i.e., with the foot on the ground). By performing closed-chain exercises, that patient is more closely simulating the neuromuscular activity during which a sprain will occur. In restoring normal function, it is important to facilitate the joint receptors in a weight-bearing position. In addition, these exercises provide compressive forces that promote joint stability.[11] Second, an eccentric component should be included in strengthening the peroneals, because most ankle sprains include inversion. The reaction of the peroneals eccentrically may assist in preventing excessive eversion. Finally, a speed component must be incorporated into the program. Many ankle sprains will involve inversion at high velocities. After building a strength base, activities should progress from low speed to higher speeds.

Rehabilitation for the ankle sprain may be classified into several progressive phases. Each phase has its own specific goals and guidelines, and advancement to the next phase should be based on specific criteria. As with any rehabilitation program, each patient should progress through these phases individually.

Acute Phase

The goals of the acute phase are to control pain and spasm, reduce edema, and begin to restore range of motion while protecting the joint and allowing optimal soft tissue healing. It is important to educate the patient regarding awareness and respect of symptoms. Although it is impossible to control the patient's activities of daily living completely, modifying these activities will enable the patient to advance from the acute phase more rapidly. Early reduction of edema is perhaps the most significant factor in rapid recovery of the ankle sprain. Besides improving patient comfort, decreasing edema will allow weight bearing to progress more rapidly. In addition, as mentioned, there is evidence that edema, by stretching the joint capsule, may affect the function of the mechanoreceptors, thus compromising the proprioceptive awareness of the joint even further.

A combination of elevation, cryotherapy, and compression is used to reduce edema. Sims in 1986 studied the effects of positioning on edema of the ankle and demonstrated a significant decrease in volume in those with their lower extremities elevated.[12] The use of cryotherapy in the control and reduction of edema has been well documented. Weston and colleagues demonstrated immediate and sustained vasoconstriction with cold pack application after inversion sprains.[13] Ice may be used not only in the acute phase but throughout all phases of rehabilitation to prevent edema and inflammation.

Compression in conjunction with cryotherapy will assist in reduction of edema during this phase. Several commercial devices are available that apply compression using air or cold water. An Ace wrap may be used to provide compression and may be combined with taping to provide support with weight bearing. In addition, a U-shaped felt or foam rubber pad around the lateral malleolus may be used to apply focal compression to the lateral ligamentous region. Wilkerson found that focal compression to the lateral ankle appears to speed recovery time.[14] The rationale for this is that edema is forced from an area that may mechanically interfere with normal ankle function and is dispersed away from the injury site, thus enhancing removal of the fluid by the lymphatic system.[14, 15]

Electrical stimulation may be used to aid in edema reduction. By producing a current strong enough to cause muscle contraction, a mechanical pump is created to remove excess fluid by squeezing the vessels and milking the fluids out of the area.[16]

The trend in rehabilitation today is toward early controlled motion and early progressive weight bearing. Again, symptoms such as pain, spasm, and persistent edema must be monitored carefully. Any increase in symptoms must alert the clinician to modify the progression. Several studies support the concept that early mobilization increases the rate of recovery and return to activity.[6, 16, 17] Early controlled motion appears to stimulate healing and have a positive effect on ligament strength.[18–20] With this in mind, active and active assistive range-of-motion exercises may be initiated within a pain-free range. Range-of-motion exercises may be progressed from simple plane motions to multiplanar motions. Inversion range is limited to allow optimal healing of the lateral ligaments. If symptoms allow, range of motion on a balance board may be initiated while sitting to provide early proprioceptive training (Fig. 33–2). Finally, towel stretches should be initiated to maintain flexibility of the Achilles tendon (Fig. 33–3).

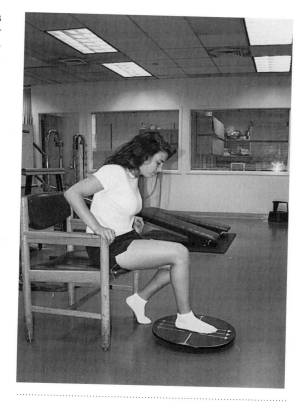

Figure 33–2. Seated balance board.

Early progressive weight bearing is allowed within the patient's tolerance. Crutches may be used initially until the patient is able to ambulate comfortably and safely without them. Taping or the use of an orthosis is used to provide support and

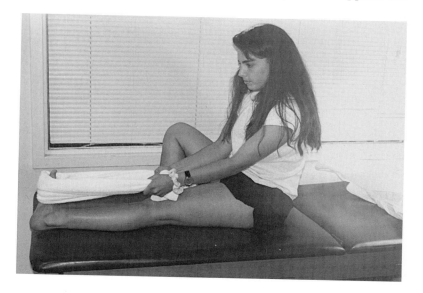

Figure 33–3. Towel stretch for Achilles tendon.

limit the amount of inversion and eversion. Early progressive weight bearing may provide several positive effects. First, proprioceptive loss is limited. Second, muscular atrophy is reduced. Finally, it provides an active muscular pump to mobilize fluids and assist in edema reduction.

Intermediate Phase

The goals of this phase are to restore full ankle range of motion and flexibility, begin to restore strength and proprioception, and normalize the patient's gait pattern. Isotonics for plantar flexion and dorsiflexion may be initiated using manual resistance with rubber tubing. Inversion and eversion strengthening may begin isometrically and advanced to isotonics depending on the patient's symptoms (Fig. 33–4). However, inversion range should continue to be limited to prevent excessive stress to lateral ligaments. As muscular strength increases, multiplanar resistive exercises may be incorporated. Stationary cycling is incorporated to begin to restore the patient's cardiovascular function. Resistance is progressed according to the patient's symptoms. When available, hydrotherapy may be used during this phase. Underwater ambulation may be useful for the patient who is having difficulty making the transition to full weight bearing or normalizing gait. As the patient's pain, inflammation, and edema subside, functional, closed-chain activities may be

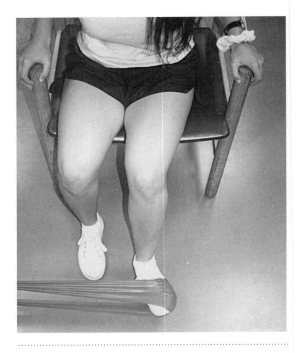

Figure 33–4. Eversion strengthening.

advanced. These may be advanced from bilateral activities to unilateral activities as symptoms allow. These may include the use of a leg press, BAPS board, step-up exercises, squats, and contralateral hip exercises (Figs. 33–5 to 33-8). Gastrocnemius-soleus strengthening may be advanced to standing calf raises as strength improves (Fig. 33–9). Retroambulation on a treadmill

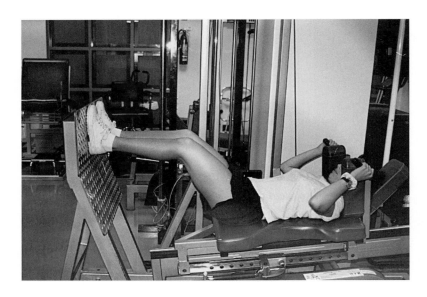

Figure 33–5. Leg press.

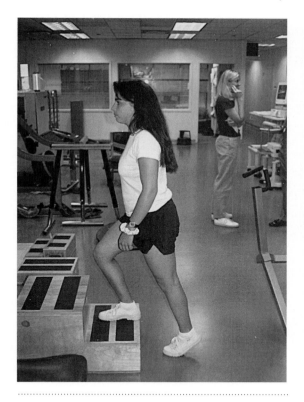

Figure 33–6. Step-ups.

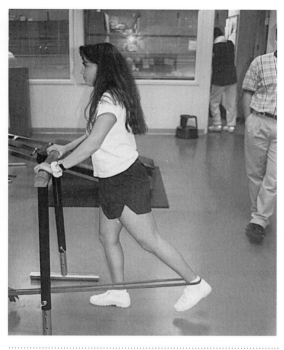

Figure 33–8. Contralateral hip exercises.

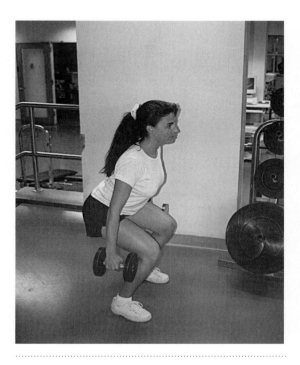

Figure 33–7. Squats.

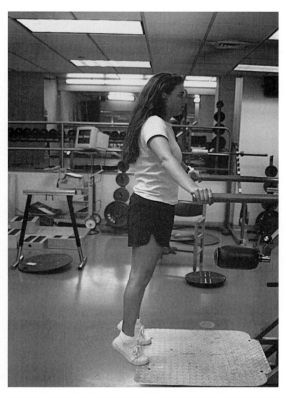

Figure 33–9. Calf raises.

may also be incorporated to increase calf strength (Fig. 33–10). All of these activities should progress by degree of difficulty according to the clinician's continuous re-evaluation of the patient's functional status and symptoms. Finally, normal flexibility, especially for the Achilles tendon, should be restored. Stretching may be advanced from a non–weight-bearing to a weight-bearing position. A standing wall stretch or a slant board may be used (Fig. 33–11).

Late Phase

The goals of this phase are to restore normal neuromuscular function and prepare the patient to return to activity. The patient should have normal range of motion, a good strength base, and good muscular flexibility. In addition, the patient should be without pain or edema. Isotonic strengthening of all ankle musculature is progressed with emphasis on eccentric peroneal strengthening. Resistive strengthening should be contin-

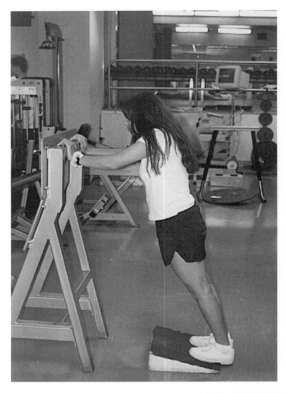

Figure 33–11. Stretch using slant board.

ued until there are no deficits when compared with the noninvolved ankle.

Functional activities should be progressed to include a speed component. Backward running against elastic resistance such as Sportscord can be incorporated (Fig. 33–12). This may be progressed to lateral running and eventually performing an alternating crossover drill (a carioca) using the same resistance. The Fitter or Euroglide are also used to reproduce the lateral stresses to the ankle that may be encountered in many activities (Fig. 33–13).

Cardiovascular training may also be advanced, with more emphasis on closed-chain activities. Equipment such as stepping or stair-climbing machines can be used to restore the patient's fitness level (Fig. 33–14). Caution should be taken to avoid any type of overuse syndrome. Maintaining normal muscular flexibility should not be overlooked throughout this phase.

Return to Activity

This phase is highly variable and is dependent on the patient's individual goals. Obvi-

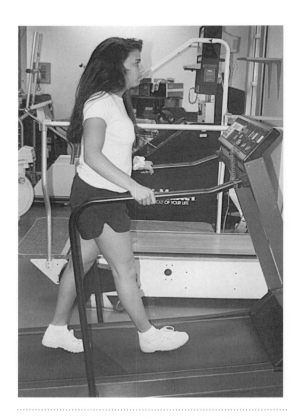

Figure 33–10. Treadmill retroambulation (patient walking backwards).

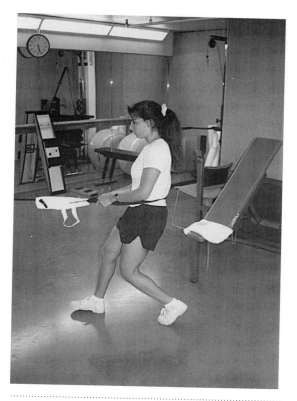

Figure 33–12. Backward running using elastic resistance.

plyometric program may be incorporated. However, the program should be activity specific and be progressed from straight-ahead running and retrorunning to lateral running and eventually a carioca drill. From this progression, more functional specific drills may be added, such as figure-eight running, pivoting, and jumping.

The final aspect to be addressed is that of external support. This remains a widely controversial concept. In recent years, numerous studies have attempted to demonstrate the usefulness of taping, orthoses, or high-top shoes[21–26] for ankle stability. At this point, there appears to be no clear-cut consensus. Taping is still commonly used on all levels of organized sport. However, there is evidence of loosening and loss of restriction after activity.[21, 23] In addition, for the recreational athlete, taping on a regular basis may prove to be a costly and difficult task. Studies have shown various orthoses to restrict inversion and eversion motion after exercise.[22, 26] One concern in the athletic population has been impairment of performance when wearing an orthosis. Studies, however, have shown no effect on performance.[27, 28] To this point, there appears to be no general consensus regarding external support.

ously, the competitive athlete will have different functional needs than the relatively sedentary patient. For the athletic population, this phase would be used to make the transition to a particular patient's sport. A

ACHILLES TENDINITIS

Achilles tendinitis is quite common in running and jumping sports.[29, 30] In addition, dancers and gymnasts who perform many

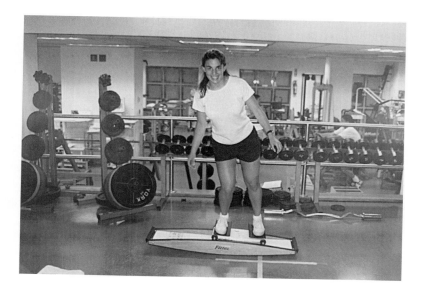

Figure 33–13. Fitter.

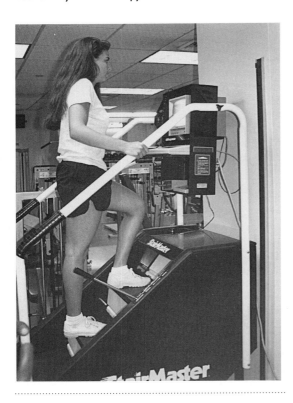

Figure 33–14. Stairmaster.

joint. Training errors may lead to tendinitis. Recent increases in running mileage or jumping activities can contribute to the cause. Increase in hill running may predispose the patient to Achilles tendinitis.

Initially, treatment will focus on the reduction of pain and inflammation. Ice and ultrasonography are the most frequently used modalities. In addition, phonophoresis may be used to introduce an anti-inflammatory locally in a noninvasive manner.[15] As the patient becomes less symptomatic, friction massage may be used to separate adhesions and scar tissue in the tendon. Caution should be used in that this is often quite uncomfortable for the patient. A heel pad may be used to relieve tension to the tendon.

Flexibility must then be restored to the Achilles tendon and gastrocnemius-soleus complex. Initially, a non-weight-bearing stretch may be done, using a towel or a strap. As always, the stretch should be performed within a pain-free range of motion. The stretching may be progressed to weight bearing using a slant board or performing a standing wall stretch. The stretching should be performed with the knee in both exten-

activities in plantar-flexed positions, thus creating tightness of the tendon, are also susceptible. This structure, which is the common tendon of the gastrocnemius and soleus, twists laterally as it descends and has an area of reduced vascularity approximately 2 to 6 cm proximal to its insertion at the calcaneus.[31] These anatomic features have been theorized to contribute to the cause.

Lack of flexibility can predispose the individual to Achilles tendinitis. Schepsis and Leach found most chronic cases to be associated with decreased passive dorsiflexion.[32] With a shortened Achilles tendon, there is a greater strain on the tendon throughout a particular range of motion.[31] In addition, loss of dorsiflexion can also create excessive pronation at the subtalar joint. This has been shown to pull the tendon medially and result in a "whipping effect" at push-off.[33] Excessive pronation may be caused by other flexibility deficits or variations in foot or tibial alignment. On the other hand, a cavus foot alignment may also contribute because there is a greater stress through the tendon as a result of hypomobility of the subtalar

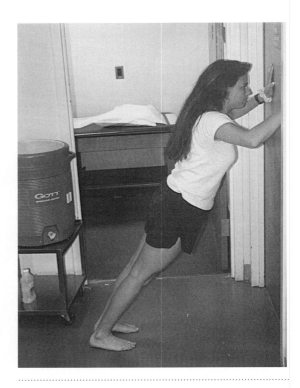

Figure 33–15. Standing stretch.

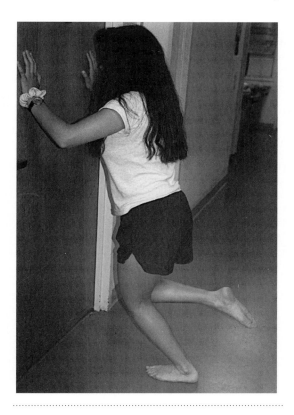

Figure 33–16. Standing stretch with knee flexion.

sion and flexion so as to include both the gastrocnemius and soleus muscles (Figs. 33–15 and 33–16). Flexibility of the hamstrings must also be addressed because tightness can also result in excessive subta-

lar pronation. During this period of reducing symptoms and restoring flexibility, the aggravating activity must be replaced by an alternative cardiovascular activity. Often stationary cycling with low resistance may be an adequate substitute and provide a good warm-up before stretching.

Strengthening should be initiated when the patient is relatively asymptomatic. Initially, tubing or TheraBand can be used for resistance in a non-weight-bearing position (Fig. 33–17). As the patient progresses, calf raises and resistive seated calf raises for the soleus muscle are incorporated. Resistance is increased as tolerated. Eccentric calf strengthening should become a significant portion of the program because eccentric activity of the gastrocnemius-soleus complex tends to place the highest stress on the Achilles tendon.[34] When walking or running, a large component of the muscular activity is eccentric. The injured lower extremity can be challenged by performing a bilateral calf raise and then lowering the body with only the injured calf. More functional activities can be added as tolerated, using a BAPS board or elastic resistance. Retrowalking at a 10% grade on a treadmill has been shown to increase the muscular activity of the calf musculature.[35] As strength and flexibility become adequate, training can be advanced to more strenuous activities to the calf, such as stepping and climbing machines (Fig. 33–18).

When returning to normal activity, modifications may have to be made in training

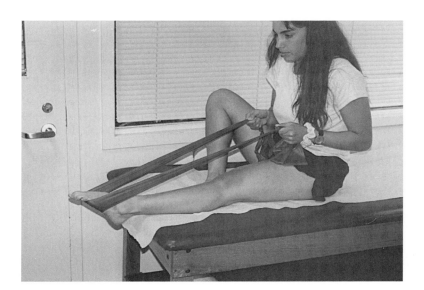

Figure 33–17. Calf strengthening with elastic resistance.

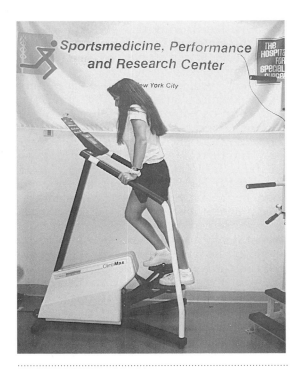

Figure 33–18. ClimbMAX.

routines. Hill running must be modified or avoided. The patient must be educated as to avoiding the need to work through pain and inflammation. Orthotics are often used for the patient who pronates excessively. Footwear should be chosen correctly. Rearfoot control is important. A firm heel counter is adequate. Sole flexibility is important to allow metatarsophalangeal (MTP) extension, so the lever arm from the forefoot to the ankle is not lengthened excessively.[36]

PLANTAR FASCIITIS

The plantar fascia is a dense, multilayered fibrous connective tissue that helps support the longitudinal arch of the foot. Individuals taking part in activities involving a great deal of running or jumping are at higher risk for this disorder. Dancers who perform many activities in extremes of ankle dorsiflexion are also susceptible. The mechanism by which the plantar fascia provides support has been described as a windlass or bowstring effect. As the toes are dorsiflexed, the plantar fascia is tightened and the longitudinal arch elevated.[37]

The onset of pain is generally gradual and insidious. Often the patient presents with localized pain at the medial distal heel or medial arch. This pain may become more diffuse as the condition progresses. The patient often complains of increased pain on taking the first steps in the morning. This is most likely a result of the tissues contracting overnight and then being overstretched on initial weight bearing. The pain is generally lessened when wearing a shoe.

As always, it is important for the clinician to understand the underlying causes of the disorder, and in the case of plantar fasciitis it is often multidimensional. Certain biomechanical factors may predispose the individual to injury. Kwong and colleagues showed that pronation will increase the tensile stress to the plantar fascia.[38] On the other hand, a cavus foot will have less ability to dissipate forces from heel strike to midstance because of lack of pronation.[38] This also will increase stress to the plantar fascia. Certain posterior muscle deficits may contribute to the disorder. Kibler and others found significant deficits in plantar flexion strength and dorsiflexion range of motion in runners with plantar fasciitis.[39] They hypothesized that the tight posterior structures create a valgus heel position at heel strike and push-off, restricting supination and dorsiflexion. They also indicated that the weak plantar flexors increased tensile loading on the muscle and ligament attachments.

Finally, other factors, such as recent weight gain, increase in training, or change of footwear, may contribute. In general, any combination of these factors may contribute to the plantar fascia assuming a greater amount of force than it can accommodate.

The initial goals of the treatment plan are to reduce the pain and inflammation and begin to restore flexibility. Various modalities such as ice, phonophoresis, iontophoresis, or whirlpool may be used to treat local pain and inflammation. As the patient becomes less symptomatic, deep friction massage can be used. The patient should be given a period of active rest, avoiding the aggravating activity. Stationary cycling or swimming may provide substitute cardiovascular training until symptoms subside. Flexibility for the posterior calf musculature should be initiated within a pain-free range. Stretching with the knee both extended for the gastrocnemius and flexed to include the soleus should be initiated in a non-weight-bearing position using a towel or strap. As the patient becomes less symptomatic, weight-bearing stretching using a wall stretch or a slant board may begin. Stretching should be performed several times a day, preferably when the patient is warmed up. Stretching of the plantar fascia may be accomplished by dorsiflexion of MTP joints. Hunter advocated the use of rolling the arch over a rolling pin.[40] Range of motion of the first MTP joint should be specifically addressed. Creighton and Olson found a decrease in range of motion of the first MTP joint in runners with plantar fasciitis.[41] A lack of dorsiflexion of this joint may compromise the windlass effect of the plantar fascia. In those severely limited, joint mobilization techniques may be used. Jaivin and Ferkel advocated the use of night splints to increase flexibility of the gastrocnemius-soleus complex and the plantar fascia to reduce morning stiffness and pain.[42] However, I have not used this method in this treatment. In addition, taping of the longitudinal arch may provide some pain relief for the patient while ambulating.

As symptoms become less acute, strengthening of the gastrocnemius-soleus complex should be initiated. Tubing or other elastic resistance can be used to begin plantar strengthening. Once again, the exercises should be performed with both a flexed and extended knee to include the entire complex. Strengthening of the intrinsic foot musculature should be included because these muscles will assist in supporting the longitudinal arch. This may be accomplished by having the patient roll up a towel with the plantar aspect of the toes while seated (Fig. 33–19). As strength improves, a BAPS board may be used to strengthen these muscles in a weight-bearing position.

When returning the patient to activity, modifications may need to be made in athletic activities. Cross-training, as opposed to simply distance running, may prevent recurrence of the injury. Orthotics may help, depending on the mechanism of injury. Several authors advocated the use of orthotics in those patients who hyperpronate to reduce the tension in the longitudinal arch.[38, 40, 43] In addition, heel pads or heel cups can be used to share the absorption function of the plantar fascia.

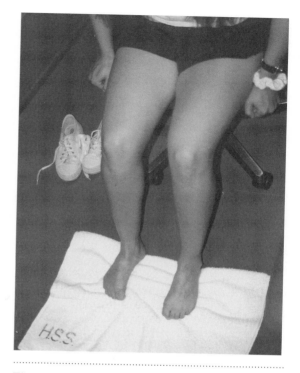

Figure 33–19. Towel roll for intrinsic strengthening.

POSTERIOR SHIN SPLINTS

The term *shin splints* refers to a general group of overuse syndromes affecting the lower leg. Pain results from tendon or periosteal inflammation. Medial tibial stress syndrome is another term used in the literature.[44] There is no specific cause for this syndrome; rather, a variety of factors may contribute. This syndrome is very common in runners and in athletes in sports that require sudden stops. Poor conditioning, inadequate footwear, biomechanical abnormalities, and improper training techniques may all be contributing factors. Runners who train on banked surfaces are often susceptible.

Excessive pronation of the subtalar joint is often a cause of this posterior medial leg pain. With increased pronation, there is greater stress to the posterior medial musculature as it attempts to stabilize the foot. Tibialis posterior tendinitis is commonly a cause of this pain. A strong invertor and plantar flexor, the muscle functions to control subtalar pronation and tibial internal rotation at heel strike and then reverses its function during stance.[45] Any planovalgus alignment may predispose someone to this injury. Clinically, the patient may present with difficulty standing on toes. There may be pain or swelling posterior to the medial malleolus or near the insertion at the navicular. Resistance to inversion and plantar flexion may produce pain. Often there will be a deficit in dorsiflexion range, because tightness of the gastrocnemius-soleus complex and Achilles tendon can cause the patient to pronate excessively.

Another mechanism of injury may be related to running pattern. Cibulka and colleagues theorized that a lack of heel strike or forefoot contact running may have a possible relationship with posterior medial shin splints.[46] The rationale given for this relationship included higher ground reaction forces, insufficient subtalar pronation for reducing ground reaction forces, and increased activity of the plantar flexors throughout the stance phase.

Treatment, as with any inflammatory condition, begins with reduction of symptoms. Local modalities such as ultrasonography, phonophoresis, and ice are used for pain, edema, and inflammation. During this initial phase, the patient's activity is modified to avoid symptom exacerbation. Stationary cycling often provides an alternative cardiovascular activity. Stretching of the gastrocnemius-soleus complex should be initiated in a pain-free range. If the pain is quite acute, the stretching may begin in a non-weight-bearing manner using a towel or a strap. As symptoms subside, the stretching may be advanced to weight bearing. In addition, any proximal flexibility deficits, such as hamstring, hip rotators, or flexors should be addressed, because they can also lead to foot and ankle pathomechanics.

For the patient who pronates excessively, a medial posted orthosis or medial heel wedge can be used. A slight heel lift may also be helpful in reducing stress to the posterior musculature. Taping of the longitudinal arch is another possibility.

As symptoms are reduced, strengthening for all ankle musculature should be initiated. Resistive exercises may be performed in isolated patterns. Caution should be observed when initiating inversion strengthening so as to not aggravate the tibialis posterior tendon. As ankle strength improves, multiplanar activities should be incorporated into the program. Foot intrinsic

strengthening may assist in supporting the longitudinal arch if excessive pronation is a factor. Eccentric training of the calf musculature and tibialis posterior should be included. Functional closed-chain activities previously mentioned in this chapter should be included to prepare the patient to return to activity.

In returning to activity, patient education is of extreme importance. Cross-training is often encouraged to avoid recurrence of injury. Changes in training programs may be helpful. Runners are often encouraged to limit hill training or avoid banked surfaces. Changes in running style may have to be considered. Proper footwear must also be encouraged. Finally, the patient must have a proper home exercise program to continue to maintain adequate strength and flexibility.

SUMMARY

1. Each rehabilitation program should be individualized and based on the patient's history, clinical evaluation, and goals.

2. The rate of progression is guided by symptoms such as pain, inflammation, and edema.

3. Modalities are an important adjunct for treatment of symptoms; however, they should never replace treatment and correction of the underlying cause.

4. Biomechanical abnormalities and strength or flexibility deficits must be addressed not only at the foot and ankle but also at the lower leg, knee, and hip.

5. Eccentric muscle activity appears to play a significant role at the foot and ankle during all functional activities. This should be accounted for in the treatment plan.

6. Before returning to activity, corrections should be made in footwear, training error, or biomechanics so as to avoid recurrence. Patient education as to precautions, activity modifications, and home exercise programs to maintain strength and flexibility is of extreme importance.

REFERENCES

1. Jackson DW, Ashley RL, Powell JW. Ankle sprains in young athletes. Clin Orthop 101:201, 1974.
2. Mack RP. Ankle injuries in athletics. Clin Sports Med 1:71, 1982.
3. Garrick JG. The frequency of injury, mechanism of injury and epidemiology of ankle sprains. Am J Sports Med 5:241, 1977.

4. Hamilton WG. Sprained ankles in ballet dancers. Foot Ankle 3:99, 1982.

5. Brand RL, Black HM, Cox JS. The natural history of inadequately treated ankle sprains. Am J Sports Med 5:248, 1977.

6. Freeman MAR. Treatment of ruptures of lateral ligaments of the ankle. J Bone Joint Surg Br 47:661, 1965.

7. Freeman MAR, Dean MRE, Hanham IWF. The etiology and prevention of functional instability of the foot. J Bone Joint Surg Br 47:678, 1965.

8. Glencross D, Thornton E. Position sense following joint injury. J Sports Med Phys Fitness 21:23, 1981.

9. Konradsen L, Ravn JB. Ankle instability caused by prolonged peroneal reaction time. Acta Orthop Scand 51:399, 1990.

10. Lofvenberg R, Karrholm J, Gunnevi S, et al. Prolonged reaction time in patients with chronic lateral instability of the ankle. Am J Sports Med 23:414, 1995.

11. Tippett SR: Closed chain exercise. Orthop Phys Ther Clin North Am 1:253, 1992.

12. Sims D. Effects of positioning on ankle edema. J Orthop Sports Phys Ther 8:30, 1986.

13. Weston M, Taber C, Casagranda L, et al. Change in local blood volume during cold gel pack application to traumatized ankles. J Orthop Sports Phys Ther 19:197, 1994.

14. Wilkerson GB. Treatment of ankle sprains with external compression and early mobilization. Phys Sports Med 13:83, 1985.

15. Kolb P, Denegar C. Traumatic edema and the lymphatic system. Athl Train 18:339, 1983.

16. Strakey C. Therapeutic Modalities for Athletic Trainers. Philadelphia: F. A. Davis, 1983.

17. Konradsen L, Holmer P, Sondergaard L. Early mobilizing treatment for grade III ankle ligament injuries. Foot Ankle 12:69, 1991.

18. Eiff MP, Smith TZ, Smith GE. Early mobilization versus immobilization in the treatment of lateral ankle sprains. Am J Sports Med 22:83, 1994.

19. Gamble JG, Edwards CC, Max SR. Enzymatic adaptation in ligaments during immobilization. Am J Sports Med 12:221–228, 1984.

20. Tipton CM, Matthes RD, Maynard JA, et al. The influence of physical activity on ligaments and tendons. Med Sci Sports Exerc 7:165, 1975.

21. Gross MT, Lapp AK, Davis JM. Comparison of Swede-O-Universal ankle support and Aircast Sport-stirrup orthoses and ankle tape in restricting eversion-inversion before and after exercise. J Orthop Sports Phys 13:11, 1991.

22. Gross MT, Ballard CL, Mears HG, et al. Comparison of Don Joy Ankle Ligament protector and Aircast Sport-stirrup orthoses in restricting foot and ankle motion before and after exercise. J Orthop Sports Phys 16:60, 1992.

23. Greene TA, Wight CR. A comparative support evaluation of three ankle orthoses before, during, and after exercise. J Orthop Sports Phys 11:453, 1990.

24. Shapiro MS, Kabo JM, Mitchell PW, et al. Ankle sprain prophylaxis: an analysis of the stabilizing effects of braces and tape. Am J Sports Med 22:78, 1994.

25. Ashton-Miller JA, Ottoviani RA, Hutchinson C, et al. What best protects the inverted weightbearing ankle against further inversion? Evertor muscle strength compares favorably with shoe height, athletic tape, and three orthoses. Am J Sports Med 24:800, 1996.

26. Thonnard JL, Bragard D, Willems PA, et al. Stability of the braced ankle: a biomechanical investigation. Am J Sports Med 24:356, 1996.

27. Pienkowski D, McMorrow M, Shapiro R, et al. The effect of ankle stabilizers on athletic performance: a randomized prospective study. Am J Sports Med 23:757, 1995.

28. MacKean LC, Bell G, Burnham RS. Prophylactic ankle bracing vs. taping: effects on functional performance in female basketball players. J Orthop Sports Phys 22:77, 1995.

29. Clement DB, Taunton JE, Smart GW, et al. A survey of overuse running injuries. Phys Sports Med 9:47, 1981.

30. James S, Bates B, Ostering L. Injuries to runners. Am J Sports Med 6:40, 1978.

31. Curwin S, Stanish W. Tendinitis: its etiology and treatment. Lexington, MA: Collamore Press, D.C. Heath, 1984.

32. Schepsis AA, Leach RE. Surgical management of Achilles tendinitis. Am J Sports Med 15:308, 1987.

33. Clement D, Taunton J, Smart G. Achilles tendinitis and peritendinitis: etiology and treatment. Am J Sports Med 12:174, 1984.

34. Stanish W, Rubinovich R, Curwin S. Eccentric exercise in chronic tendinitis. Clin Orthop 208:65, 1986.

35. Cipriani DJ, Armstrong CW, Gaul S. Backward walking at three levels of treadmill inclination: an electromyographic and kinematic analysis. J Orthop Sports Phys 22:95, 1995.

36. Reynolds NL, Worrell TW. Chronic Achilles peritendinitis: etiology, pathophysiology, and treatment. J Orthop Sports Phys 13:171, 1991.

37. Hicks JH. The mechanics of the foot. J Anat 88:25, 1984.

38. Kwong PK, Kay D, Voner RT. Planar fasciitis: mechanics and pathomechanics of treatment. Clin Sports Med 7:119, 1988.

39. Kibler BW, Goldberg C, Chandler JT. Functional biomechanical deficits in running athletes with plantar fasciitis. Am J Sports Med 19:66, 1991.

40. Hunter S. Rehabilitation of foot injuries. In Prentiss WE, ed. Rehabilitation Techniques in Sports Medicine, ed 2. St. Louis: Mosby–Year Book, 1994, p. 450.

41. Creighton DS, Olson VL. Evaluation of range of motion of the first metatarsophalangeal joint in runners with plantar fasciitis. J Orthop Sports Phys 8:357, 1987.

42. Jaivin JS, Ferkel RD. Ankle and foot injuries. In Fu FH, Stone DA, eds. Sports Injuries: Mechanisms, Prevention, Treatment. Baltimore, MD: Williams & Wilkins, 1994, p. 997.

43. Gross ML, Davlin LB, Evanski PM. Effectiveness of orthotic shoe inserts in the long distance runner. Am J Sports Med 19:409, 1991.

44. Mubarak SJ, Gould RN, Lee YF, et al. The medial tibial stress syndrome (a cause of shin splints). Am J Sports Med 10:201, 1982.

45. Mulligan E. Lower leg, ankle, and foot rehabilitation. In Andrews JR, Harrelson GL, ed. Physical Rehabilitation of the Injured Athlete. Philadelphia: W. B. Saunders, 1991, p. 197.

46. Cibulka MT, Sinacore DR, Mueller MJ. Shine splints and forefoot contact running: a case report. J Orthop Sports Phys 20:98, 1994.

34 Orthotic Therapy in the Treatment of Heel, Achilles Tendon, and Ankle Injuries

Ellen Sobel

Mark A. Caselli

Rock G. Positano

The aim of this chapter is to present current orthotic and prosthetic treatment modalities for rearfoot and ankle disorders. The basic deformities of the rearfoot and ankle are described briefly, and orthotic therapy is discussed. Because plantar fasciitis is the most common cause of rearfoot pain, this condition is used as the prototype rearfoot condition, and several of the orthotics devices are introduced under this condition.

PLANTAR FASCIITIS AND HEEL PAIN: ORTHOTIC-SHOE THERAPY

Plantar heel pain is the most common foot problem seen in an office setting.[1, 2] Plantar fasciitis is by far the most common cause of plantar heel pain.[3–6] Other frequent causes of heel pain include nerve entrapment, fat pad atrophy, stress fracture of the calcaneus, and plantar fascia rupture.[2] Less commonly, tarsal tunnel syndrome, sciatica, bone and soft tissue tumors, infection, inflammatory arthritis, gout, and sarcoidosis have all been reported to cause heel pain.

The plantar fat pad is composed of hard, fibrous septa, which creates an optimal capacity for shock absorption.[2] The plantar fascia supports the longitudinal arch and is under constant strain during walking and standing. Precipitating factors leading to plantar fasciitis include overuse injuries, hyperpronated foot, cavus foot, aging with degenerative changes, and systemic disorders such as inflammatory arthritis.[7] The classic history of plantar fasciitis is marked by the insidious onset of sharp pain at the fascial insertion on the plantar surface of the anteromedial calcaneus. Arch fatigue and generalized soreness are present on the sole of the foot. The pain is usually more severe when the patient first arises, eases some after walking awhile, and returns at the end of the day. During the initial stages of exercise, the symptoms are more pronounced, easing as exercise continues. This alteration reflects the degree of stiffness and contracture in the plantar fascia.

Palpation typically reveals heel tenderness anteromedially at the origin of the plantar fascia on the medial calcaneal tubercle. However, the pain can be present along the entire length of the plantar fascia. Tenderness over the distal and midportion of the plantar fascia suggests the less common distal plantar fasciitis. If the entire heel is tender, a stress fracture, calcaneal apophysitis (Sever's disease) in a child, or possibly a bone tumor should be considered. Pain under the fat pad in older patients suggests fat pad atrophy.[8] Elderly patients who have acute heel pain should be evaluated for a stress fracture of the calcaneus resulting from severe generalized osteopenia.[9]

Heel Pads and Cushions

Heel cushions provide a first line of relief for plantar fasciitis. Heel cushions provide extra shock absorption in the heel area. They help absorb the shock of heel strike in walking and running (Fig. 34–1). Heel pads are generally constructed of polyvinyl chloride, silicone, leather, polyethylene foams like Plastizote, and thermoplastics.

Soft heel cups cushion and contain the fat pad[10] and are effective for a plantar calcaneal bursitis or plantar heel spur syndrome (see Fig. 34–1). In patients with heel pain from fat pad atrophy, hard plastic heel cups (M-F Athletic company, Cranston, RI) (Fig. 34–1) are sometimes effective in positioning the heel pad underneath the calcaneus, restoring the natural cushioning and compressibility.[11, 12] The Anti-Shox heel cra-

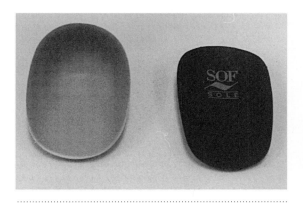

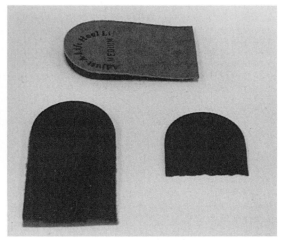

Figure 34–1. M-F Heel Protector (M-F Athletic Company, Cranston, RI) shown on the left and a soft heel pad on the right.

Figure 34–3. Variety of heel lifts cut to different lengths.

dle (Apex Foot Health Industries, Inc, South Hackensack, NJ) is made from a firm, open cell polymer and is designed to cup the heel, providing both shock absorption and support. The SofSpot Viscoheel (Bauerfeind, Germany) is a silicone heel cushion that has a built-in area of softer durometer especially designed to disperse weight around the plantar medial tubercle of the calcaneus (Fig. 34–2). Sometimes a heel lift is helpful to shift pressure to the forefoot (Fig. 34–3). A heel lift in the shoe should be no thicker than one-quarter inch.

Custom and Prefabricated Foot Orthoses

Excessive pronation lowers the arch and puts tensile strain on the plantar fascia. Similarly, weight bearing on the high arched foot often places the plantar fascia under tension. An orthosis is defined as one of a variety of devices that is used inside the shoe to provide support, increase shock absorption, or influence foot position.[13] An orthosis includes dynamic insoles, heel cushions, prefabricated commercial foot orthoses, and custom foot orthoses. An orthosis reduces arch strain associated with plantar fasciitis. Dynamic insole orthoses can be constructed from Spenco (Spenco Medical Corp, Waco, TX), which is a closed-cell neoprene impregnated with nitrogen bubbles. Prefabricated foot orthoses are commercially available in a wide variety of styles (Fig. 34–4). Premade orthoses are adequate for many athletes with plantar fasciitis and are significantly less expensive than custom-made orthoses (Fig. 34–5).

A custom-made orthosis is fabricated from a negative plaster impression of the patient's foot. The orthosis is composed of the shell, a layer of material next to the foot, and the posting, the material that fills

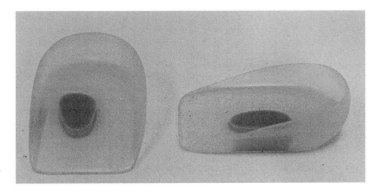

Figure 34–2. Viscoelastic silicone soft heel cushions.

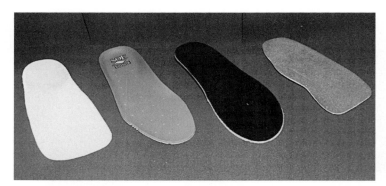

Figure 34–4. Various prefabricated foot orthoses.

in the space between the shell and the shoe. Additional materials such as metatarsal pads can be added to the device to customize it further. Some have referred to this as the Total Contact Insert.[13, 14] In podiatry, this same orthosis is called the Root Functional Foot Orthosis.[15] A custom-made foot orthosis may be required for the more severe athletic and foot injury. Custom foot orthoses can be made of leather (Fig. 34–6) or plastic (Fig. 34–7). Leather has the advantage of comfort and ease of orthotic adjustments and is able to absorb 30% of its weight before it feels wet.[16] A whale pad design and deep heel seat leather orthosis is well suited for the treatment of painful heel as a result of plantar fasciitis (Fig. 34–8). A custom device is more important for the cavus foot type than for the hyper-pronated foot, which will generally improve with a well-constructed prefabricated orthosis.

University of California Biomechanics Laboratory Orthosis

The University of California Biomechanics Laboratory (UCBL) orthosis was originally designed to maintain a flexible paralytic valgus foot deformity in the corrected position.[17] However, since then it has been extensively used to treat flexible flatfoot, plantar fasciitis, and calcaneal spurs.[18–20] Recently, the UCBL orthosis with medial posting has been successfully used to treat posterior tibial tendon dysfunction.[21] The UCBL is casted in a semi–weight-bearing

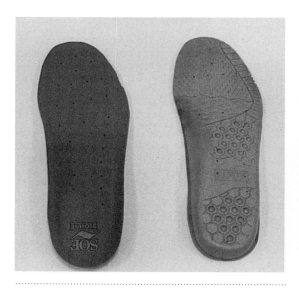

Figure 34–5. Prefabricated foot orthoses made of polyvinylurethane.

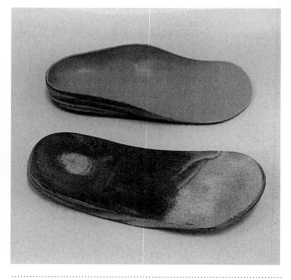

Figure 34–6. Custom-made leather foot orthosis with high medial and lateral flange, deep heel seat, and cork and latex (rubber butter) sole.

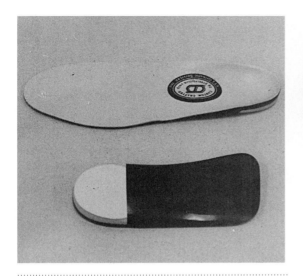

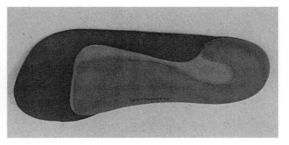

Figure 34–8. Leather orthosis with whale pad shell design.

Figure 34–7. Custom-made plastic foot orthoses. Top orthosis has full-length cover over the thermoplastic orthotic shell. Bottom orthosis is left uncovered and ends proximal to the metatarsal heads.

position.[15, 17, 20] The device elevates the arch by holding the foot in a position of forefoot adduction and hindfoot inversion (Fig. 34–9). It must be worn with a large shoe, either a running sneaker or Blucher oxford. We have found that many adults do not tolerate the high flanges on the device. Heel stabilizers serve the same function as the UCBL (Fig. 34–10).

Posterior Splint

The posterior night splint has been widely used most recently for treatment of plantar fasciitis[22–27] and is a classic treatment for Achilles tendinitis[28] (Fig. 34–11). In 11 of 14 patients, recalcitrant plantar fasciitis was resolved with the use of a night splint.[23] The purpose of the splint is to stretch the Achilles tendon and plantar fascia. The splint is an ankle-foot orthosis (AFO) positioned in about 5° of dorsiflexion worn only at night (Fig. 34–12). This device prevents contractures of the Achilles tendon and plantar fascia that occur as a result of the plantar-flexed posture of the foot during sleep. The posterior splint has been traditionally used in the lower extremity after trauma to the foot and ankle. Tone-reducing night splints are used to prevent contractures in individuals with neuromuscular disease and in patients confined to bedrest. A splint can also be used to maintain ankle position after a variety of surgical procedures.

The posterior splint can be fabricated from plaster or is available commercially as the Universal Plantar Fasciitis Orthosis

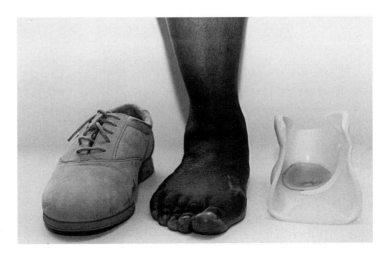

Figure 34–9. University of California Biomechanics Laboratory orthosis with high flanges.

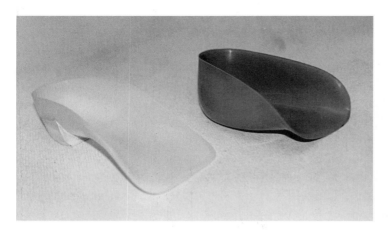

Figure 34–10. *Left*, University of California Biomechanics Laboratory orthosis. *Right*, Helfet heel stabilizer.

(Orthomerica Products, CA) (see Fig. 34–12). The splint that is used for immobilization of the foot and ankle must fit the extremity well and maintain the desired position once it has been applied.

Plaster or Fiberglas can be used to make a posterior splint.[29] In fabricating the splint, the patient lies prone with a stockinette initially placed on the leg. Five to six layers of 6-inch plaster splints or three to four layers of Fiberglas are molded to the lower extremity from the toes up to behind the knee. An extra 2 inches should be allowed when measuring with the dry splints because the splint shrinks after immersion. Overlapping side splint stirrups are added. The side stirrups add strength to the cast and prevent it from failing in plantar flexion. The splint is not free standing because it is a cast and will not stay on the extremity without some mechanism to bind it on, such as an Ace bandage or straps. The entire splint is held in place with a circular Ace bandage, which can also be dipped in water to help with

molding. The plaster cast bivalved may be used as a posterior splint.

POSTERIOR TIBIAL TENDINITIS: ORTHOTIC-SHOE THERAPY

The posterior tibial muscle, because of the distance of its tendon from the subtalar joint axis, is the most powerful inverter of the foot.[30] The causes of posterior tibial tendinitis include overuse of the pronated foot, trauma, and degeneration as a result of rheumatic diseases. There is an association between posterior tibial tendinitis and the pes planovalgus foot type.[31] Insertional posterior tibial tendinitis is associated with an

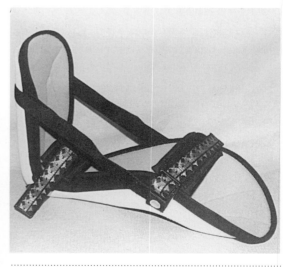

Figure 34–12. Universal plantar fasciitis orthosis (Orthomerica, Oakland, CA) used to treat plantar fasciitis.

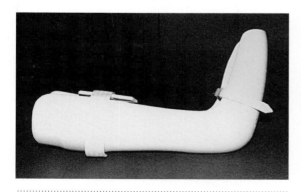

Figure 34–11. Posterior night splint.

accessory navicular bone, which clinically can be detected as a bony prominence anterior and inferior to the medial malleolus.[32] Symptoms of posterior tibial tendinitis include pain in the medial aspect of the hindfoot aggravated by weight bearing. There is tenderness, thickening, and swelling from the navicular to the medial malleolus and along the course of the tendon. The pain is aggravated by active inversion and passive dorsiflexion and eversion, which stretches the tendon. Diagnosis is confirmed by the "too-many-toes" sign or the inability to perform a single heel rise on the affected foot.[33]

During the acute period of posterior tibial tenosynovitis, there is acute medial pain and swelling. Mechanical therapy at this time might include immobilization for 6 to 8 weeks and an ankle stirrup brace.[34] During the more chronic phases of the condition, while the foot is still flexible, a foot orthosis may be appropriate. The purpose of the foot orthosis for posterior tibial tendinitis is support of the flattened arch.[33] Prefabricated or custom-made orthoses may be effective. A rearfoot varus heel post added to the orthosis will also supinate the foot. Features added to the shoe may include a medial heel and sole wedge, a firm medial

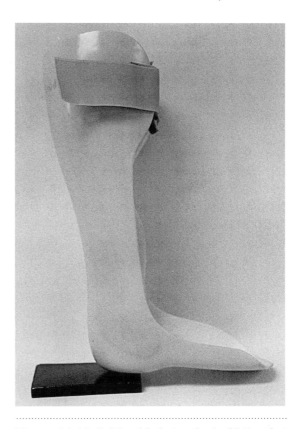

Figure 34–14. Solid ankle-foot orthosis. Notice that anterior trim lines encase the ankle and are cut anterior to the malleoli.

heel counter, or a medial flare. A hinged ankle foot orthosis may also be used at this time (Fig. 34–13). The advanced and chronic stage of posterior tibial tendon dysfunction consists of a rigid flatfoot with a valgus hind foot. At this time, it may be necessary to fit the patient with a solid AFO (Fig. 34–14).

PERONEAL TENDINITIS: ORTHOTIC-SHOE THERAPY

The peroneal tendons are the major lateral tendons of the ankle. They function as strong everters and relatively weak plantar flexors. They are the primary lateral dynamic stabilizers of the ankle joint.[35] Peroneal tendinitis results in pain in the lateral aspect of the rearfoot and ankle. Tenderness is present along the course of the peroneal tendon from the base of the fifth metatarsal where the peroneus brevis inserts to the posterior aspect of the lateral malleolus. Ac-

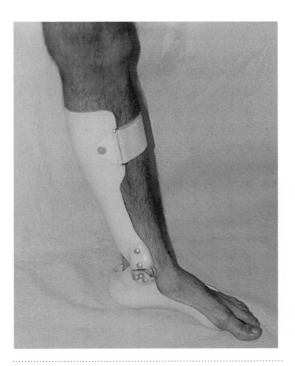

Figure 34–13. Articulated ankle-foot orthosis.

tive eversion and passive inversion stretching of the tendon will elicit pain. The foot orthosis used to treat peroneal tendinitis must reduce pressure on the peroneal tendon and decrease excessive supination.[13] Lateral support in the midfoot and hindfoot will perform this function (Fig. 34–15). This may consist of a valgus post on the forefoot and rearfoot. Shoe corrections include any type of lateral build-up, among them a lateral float and lateral buttressing.

REARFOOT DEFORMITIES AND INJURIES

Tenderness in the posterior aspect of the heel may be associated with insertional Achilles tendinitis, calcaneal bursitis (superficial), and retrocalcaneal bursitis (deep).[36] Achilles bursitis and insertional tendinitis occur from repetitive irritation during running and walking.[36, 37] The problem tends to occur in older individuals. There may be an associated Haglund's deformity over the bony prominence of the posterior calcaneal tuberosity. The main symptoms consist of tenderness in the retrocalcaneal space anterior to the Achilles tendon. Crepitance occurs with dorsiflexion and plantar flexion of the ankle if the Achilles tendon is involved.

Achilles peritendinitis, defined as an inflammation of the peritendon of the tendo-Achilles, is the most common injury in runners and is a common jumping injury.[38] Clinically, tenderness in peritendinitis remains in the same position when the foot is moved up and down because the tendon sheath does not move.[32] Males, obese individuals, dancers, and those with cavus feet,

flatfeet, and a tight heel cord are more prone to Achilles tendinitis. The pain in Achilles tendinitis or peritendinitis generally occurs 2 to 6 cm proximal to the Achilles tendon insertion, a relatively avascular area of the Achilles tendon. Achilles tendinitis or peritendinitis is often associated with decreased range of motion caused by the inflammation.[39]

Haglund's deformity is a prominent posterosuperior calcaneal tuberosity. Irritation of the prominent bone results in bursitis and Achilles tendinitis.[40] The disorder is more common in cavus feet and in those with a varus heel. Adolescent girls first wearing high heels with stiff rigid heel counters are prone to this problem. Ice skaters wearing ice skates with rigid heel counters are also likely to encounter this posterior heel problem. The symptoms include pain and swelling of the posterior heel made worse by exercise. There is tenderness and thickening of the overlying skin and signs of localized inflammation. The orthotic and shoe therapy consists of staying away from high-heeled shoes, wearing shoes with cutout heels, or padding the heel counter of the shoe with a soft material such as moleskin.

The purpose of the orthoses for Achilles tendinitis and other posterior heel problems is to reduce tension on the Achilles tendon. For Achilles tendinitis, the classic treatment is a 1/4-inch heel lift to reduce tension on the Achilles tendon (see Fig. 34–3). The heel lift can be made of felt, dense foam, PPT, or leather. If there is excessive pronation associated with the Achilles tendinitis, an orthosis with a deep heel cup with varus posting may stabilize the heel and reduce strain on the Achilles tendon. A specialized AFO with a posterior heel cutout might be

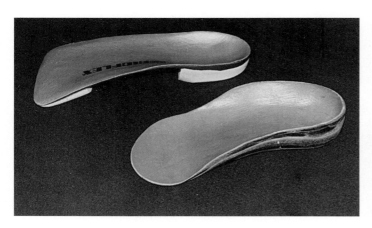

Figure 34–15. *Bottom,* foot orthosis, made of leather, has high lateral flange and is indicated for peroneal tendon problems to increase lateral stabilization. *Top,* foot orthosis has extrinsic rear foot and forefoot varus posting, which might be helpful for posterior tibial tendon dysfunction.

used in the treatment of a very tender rearfoot from a Haglund's deformity, Achilles tendon rupture, or posterior heel ulcer (Fig. 34–16).

ANKLE SPRAIN AND INSTABILITY

Ligamentous ankle injuries comprise the most common acute disorder seen in sport.[41] Ankle injuries comprise 12% of all injuries seen in emergency departments.[42] Ankle sprains account for 15% of all sports injuries.[42] The lateral ankle is affected in 85% of ankle injuries; the typical mechanism of injury is inversion.[43] Inversion stress results in mild to severe sprains of the anterior talofibular, calcaneal fibular, and infrequently the posterior talofibular lateral collateral ligaments of the ankle. Medial ankle sprains are most common in tackle football.[44] It may be an isolated injury, or it may be associated with interosseous sprains or severe lateral ankle injuries. Deltoid ligament injuries are most commonly caused by valgus or external rotation forces. Sprains of the deltoid ligament tend to heal quite

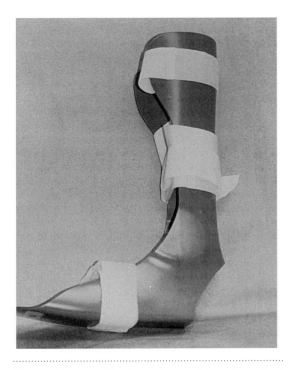

Figure 34–16. Ankle-foot orthosis with posterior heel cutout.

well with conservative management and require no special diagnosis or treatment.

Examination of the sprained ankle most often reveals swelling and tenderness to palpation over the anterior talofibular ligament. Ecchymoses may or may not be present. Routine radiographs are not helpful in diagnosing the extent of ligament damage.[45]

Generally, ankle sprains are categorized into grades. A grade I sprain is defined as an injury in which some of the fibers in the ligament are stretched, but the ligament itself remains intact with no evidence of laxity. Treatment includes rest, protected weight bearing, compression dressing, air casts, Unna boots, and adhesive strapping. Grade II sprains involve partial tear of the fibers of the calcaneal fibular (CF) ligament and anterior talofibular ligament (ATF) with mild laxity but generally good stability. Immobilization is necessary as with grade I sprain, followed by rehabilitation with peroneal strengthening and proprioceptive exercises. Grade III sprains involve a complete tear of the ATF ligaments and CF ligaments, resulting in a grossly unstable ankle. Surgical treatment offers the best results in these cases.

The acute treatment phase for a sprained ankle begins at the onset of injury and lasts for approximately 5 days. Early treatment consists of rest, ice, compression, and elevation (RICE). The subacute treatment phase lasts from 5 days to 6 weeks.[46] Ankle bracing and exercises should be instituted during the subacute phase. Finally, foot orthoses might be considered for long-term use to prevent future ankle injuries.

ANKLE BRACES AND SHOE THERAPY FOR ANKLE INSTABILITY

The modern ankle braces prevent inversion and eversion but allow plantar flexion and dorsiflexion of the ankle.[47] A heel lock may provide subtalar support (Fig. 34–17). Stirrup braces are used mainly for inversion or eversion injuries. The Aircast stirrup is the original ankle brace (Fig. 34–18). It has molded sides to approximate the ankle. The inner stirrup support system is an adjustable air cell mechanism with two compartments that allow for graduated compression from inferior to superior and prevent slipping of the air cushion from around the

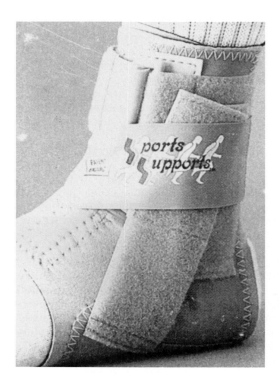

Figure 34–17. Commercial ankle brace with heel lock wraps around the ankle and ties with Velcro closures.

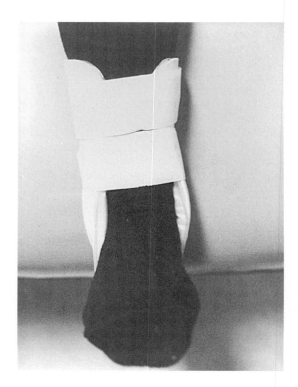

Figure 34–18. Air stirrup ankle brace.

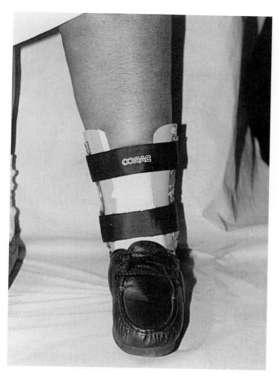

Figure 34–19. Darco air gel ankle brace.

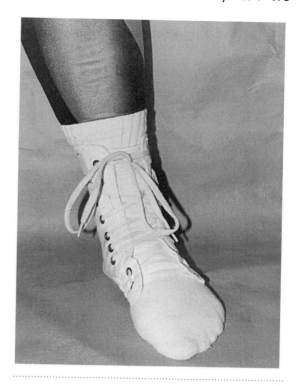

Figure 34–20. Laced canvas ankle brace.

malleoli. The air cells are lined with a compressible foam. The straps used to secure the stirrup are wide and comfortable. The DarcoGel stirrup brace applies pressure and cold to the ankle with unique gel pack inserts (Fig. 34–19). It is helpful for chronic problems. The hinged ankle brace has a stirrup with a hinge at the malleoli level for greater comfort and function. The Sure Step stirrup brace (Joint Solution, Tustin, CA) has hinges that can be locked to provide more stability than does casting in grade III sprains. The foot plate helps maintain arch support and a subtalar joint neutral position. Full ankle support braces lace up and can be made entirely of fabric (Fig. 34–20). The laced canvas ankle orthosis provides excellent mediolateral support. In the subacute phase, when swelling has been reduced, the canvas brace fits comfortably inside the shoe. The Swede-0-1200 ankle orthosis is a lace-up brace with vertical struts on the side for added support and medial lateral stability (Figs. 34–20 and 34–21). The patient with arthritic involvement of the ankle or major joints of the foot may

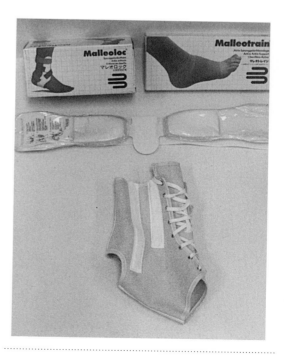

Figure 34–21. Vertical struts on the laced ankle brace offer mediolateral ankle support. Aircast shown in middle. Malleoloc ankle brace on top.

do well with an immobilizing AFO (Fig. 34–22).

The shoe for a patient with ankle instability might have an outflared lateral heel; that is, the heel should be broadened laterally to provide an outrigger effect, making it more difficult to turn over on the ankle. Lateral buttressing and a valgus wedge may also have this same effect. High-top shoes provide maximum ankle stability.

FOOT ORTHOSES FOR THE SPRAINED ANKLE

Individuals with a cavus foot are more prone to lateral ankle inversion sprains. Theoretically, the rigid forefoot valgus forces the hindfoot into inversion when the patient bears weight, stressing the lateral ankle.[48] An orthosis will ease stress on the ankle by balancing the forefoot and stabilizing the rearfoot with 0° hindfoot post and extrinsic forefoot valgus tip posting.[49] Individuals with cavus feet and frequent ankle sprains can also be prescribed orthoses with full-foot valgus posting. The supramalleolar orthosis (Fig. 34–23) provides sufficient me-

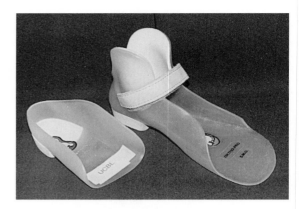

Figure 34–23. *Right*, supramalleolar orthosis; *left*, University of California Biomechanics Laboratory orthosis.

diolateral stability for some patients without having the posterior shell go all the way up the leg. It is frequently used in children with neuromuscular disease.[50, 51]

PREFABRICATED WALKING CAST

The Controlled Ankle Motion (CAM) Walker (Orthomedics, Pasadena, CA) (Fig. 34–24) or one of its many commercial equivalents is commonly used for injuries to the rearfoot and ankle. It can also be used postoperatively after foot surgery and tendon repair. It is sometimes used after a plaster cast has been removed or even instead of a plaster cast after surgery or for immobilization of fractures (Fig. 34–25). It provides the necessary stability while allowing easy donning and doffing for physical therapy sessions, washing, and sleeping. A rocker sole (Fig. 34–26) or ankle joints (Fig. 34–27) may be added to facilitate ambulation.

Diabetic patients with pain, deformity, and insensitivity as a result of neurotrophic osteoarthropathy of the foot frequently benefit from various types of bracing.[52] The patient who has Charcot involvement of the ankle or tarsal joints may require unweighting of the rearfoot with a patellar tendon-bearing orthosis (PTBO) (Fig. 34–28). The prefabricated below-knee walking brace can sometimes be substituted for cast treatment of neuropathic ulcers and immobilization of the Charcot foot in diabetic patients (Fig. 34–29).[53]

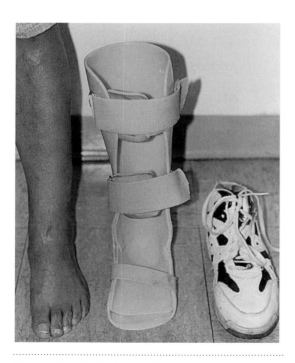

Figure 34–22. Patient with traumatic arthritis resulting from an ankle fracture, wearing solid ankle-foot orthosis with low quarter running shoe.

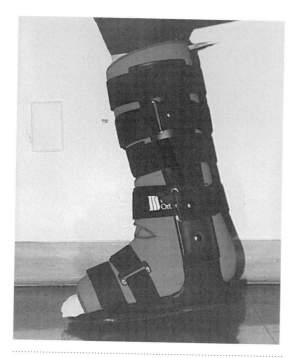

Figure 34–24. Controlled ankle motion (CAM) prefabricated walking brace.

ANKLE-FOOT ORTHOSIS

An AFO is a brace, fabricated of metal (Fig. 34–30) or plastic (Fig. 34–31), that is used to control foot and ankle problems.[54–56] Se-

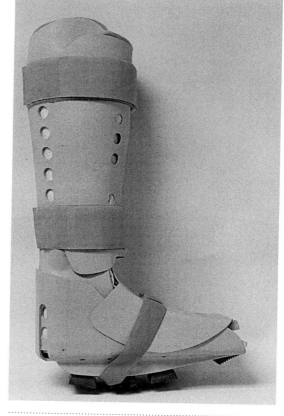

Figure 34–26. Prefabricated walking brace with rocker sole.

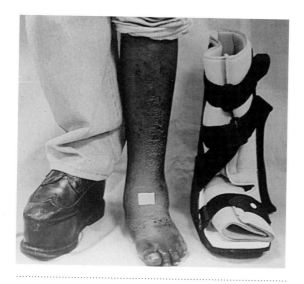

Figure 34–25. Prefabricated walking brace used to treat Lisfranc's fracture dislocation in a diabetic male with Charcot's foot.

vere lateral ankle instability as well as ankle and rearfoot fractures may require total immobilization and stability that only an AFO can provide. The double upright AFO consists of two metal uprights connected to a metal or plastic calf band (see Fig. 34–30). The distal end of each upright is connected to a shoe stirrup through an intervening ankle-level orthotic joint. The stirrup is riveted directly into the sole of the shoe under the anterior section of the heel and connects the shoe with the upright. This device is used mostly by patients with neuromuscular problems and is not used often for sports injuries to the foot and ankle. Plastic AFOs (see Fig. 34–31) have now largely replaced the metal AFO; the most common materials are polypropylene and laminated plastics. The plastic orthosis consists of a calf shell and a foot plate with a Velcro strap calf band closure. There are three plastic AFO designs: the posterior leaf

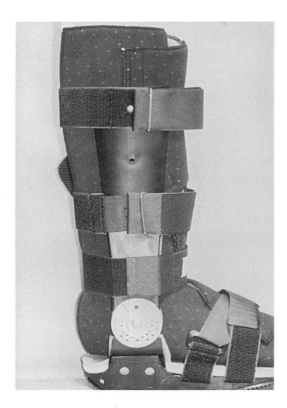

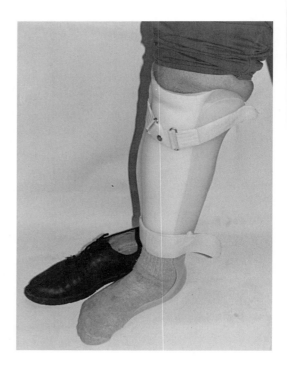

Figure 34–27. Prefabricated walking brace with articulated ankle.

Figure 34–28. Patellar tendon bearing orthosis for a patient with calcaneal fracture.

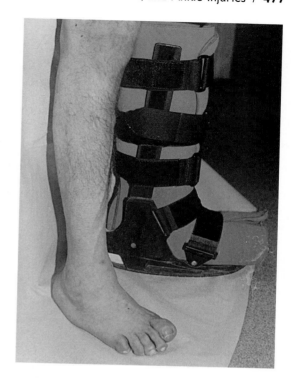

Figure 34–29. Prefabricated walking brace worn by a patient with diabetic Charcot's foot.

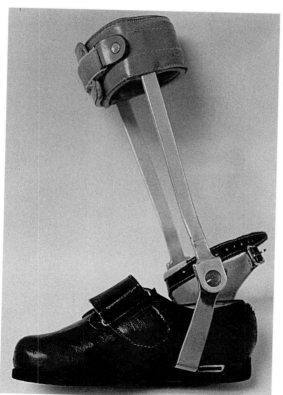

Figure 34–30. Double upright metal ankle-foot orthosis. Notice the split stirrup with metal opening in the heel of the shoe. This orthosis can be worn with more than one shoe.

spring (PLS) orthosis (see Fig. 34–31), the solid AFO (see Figs. 34–14 and 34–22), and the articulated AFO (Fig. 34–13). The PLS orthosis is indicated for peripheral nerve injuries resulting in a flaccid drop foot in which all that is needed is toe clearance during swing phase. It provides minimal mediolateral stability and may control mild spasticity. The rigid solid AFO restricts all motion at the ankle and is useful for traumatic arthritis of the ankle or other conditions in which complete immobilization of the ankle is required. It is also indicated for control of severe spasticity and is, therefore, useful in stroke patients. The articulated AFO is a plastic brace with joints at the ankle (see Fig. 34–13). It is useful for tone reduction for spastic conditions or injuries to the foot and ankle when increased motion of the ankle joint is desirable.

The PTBO has a pretibial component in which the patient rests the upper leg and knee when ambulating (Fig. 34–32; see also Fig. 34–28). In this way, the PTBO can unweight a painful leg and rearfoot. Patients are trained to walk by sinking their weight into the pretibial shell, and the weight is transferred down the uprights to the floor,

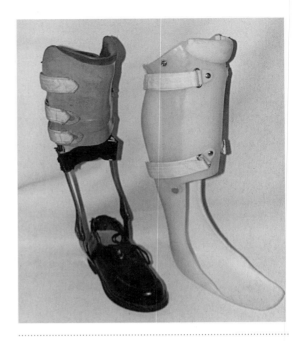

Figure 34–32. The patellar tendon bearing orthosis (PTBO) may be fabricated as a double upright metal orthosis *(left)* or as a plastic shoe insert–type orthosis *(right)*.

bypassing the leg and the rearfoot. When patients are trained to walk properly with the PTBO, it has been found to reduce weight bearing on the leg and rearfoot up to 60%.[57] The PTBO is indicated for patients with fractures of the leg and rearfoot and to unweight a painful diabetic Charcot rearfoot. It comes in metal and plastic varieties and must be constructed with a solid ankle to work properly.[58, 59]

REFERENCES

1. Dale SJ, David DJ, Sykes TF. Effective approaches to common foot complaints. Patient Care 31:158, 1997.
2. Pfeffer GB, Baxter DE, Graves S, et al. Symposium: the management of plantar heel pain. Contemp Orthop 32:357, 1996.
3. Duddy RK, Duggan RJ, Visser HJ, et al. Diagnosis, treatment, and rehabilitation of injuries to the lower leg and foot. Clin Sport Med 8:861, 1989.
4. Mitchetti ML, Jacobs SA. Calcaneal heel spurs: etiology, treatment and a new surgical approach. J Foot Surg 22:234, 1983.
5. Graham CE. Painful heel syndrome: rationale of diagnosis and treatment. Foot Ankle 3:261, 1983.
6. LeMelle DP, Kisilewicz P, Janis LR. Chronic plantar fascial inflammation and fibrosis. Clin Podiatr Med Surg 7:385, 1990.
7. Batt ME, Tanji JL. Management options for plantar fasciitis. Phys Sport Med 23:77, 1995.

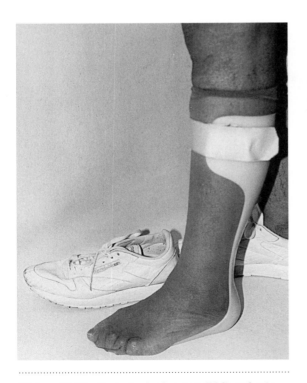

Figure 34–31. Posterior leaf spring (PLS) orthosis.

8. Shapiro SL. Heel pain management starts with correct differential diagnosis. Biomechanics 4:25, 1997.
9. Karpman RR. Foot problems in the geriatric patient. Clin Orthop Rel Res 316:59, 1995.
10. Karr SD. Subcalcaneal heel pain. Orthop Clin North Am 25:161, 1994.
11. Snook GA, Chrisman OD. The management of subcalcaneal pain. Clin Orthop 82:163, 1972.
12. Jorgensen U, Bojsen-Moller F. Shock absorbency of factors in the shoe-heel with special focus on role of the heel pad. Foot Ankle 9:294, 1989.
13. Janisse DJ. Indications and Prescriptions for Orthoses in Sports. Orth Clin North Am 25:95–107, 1994.
14. Riegler HF. Orthotic devices for the foot. Orthop Rev 16:293, 1987.
15. Sobel E, Levitz SJ. Reappraisal of the negative impression cast and the subtalar joint neutral position. J Am Podiatr Med Assoc 87:32, 1997.
16. Pribut S. Leather as an orthotic material. Biomechanics 4:61, 1997.
17. Henderson WH, Campbell JW. UC-BL insert casting and fabrication. Bull Pros Res 10:149, 1971.
18. Campbell JW, Inman VT. Treatment of plantar fasciitis and calcaneal spurs with the UC-BL shoe insert. Orthot Pros 31:23, 1977.
19. Bowman GD. New concepts in orthotic management of the adult hyperpronated foot: preliminary findings. J Pros Orthot 9:77, 1997.
20. Sobel E, Levitz SJ, Jones LS. Orthotic variants. J Am Podiatr Med Assoc 87:23, 1997.
21. Chao W, Wapner KL, Lee TH, et al. Nonoperative management of posterior tibial tendon dysfunction. Foot Ankle 17:736, 1996.
22. Mizel MS, Marymoont JV, Trepman E. Treatment of plantar fasciitis with a night splint and shoe modification consisting of a steel shank and anterior rocker bottom. Foot Ankle 17:732, 1996.
23. Wapner KL, Sharkey PF. The use of night splints for treatment of recalcitrant plantar fasciitis. Foot Ankle 12:135, 1991.
24. Batt BE, Tanji JL, Skattum N. Plantar fasciitis: a prospective randomized clinical trial of the tension night splint. Clin J Sport Med 6:158, 1996.
25. Pezzullo DJ. Using night splints in the treatment of plantar fasciitis in the athlete. J Sport Rehabil 2:287, 1993.
26. Ryan J. Use of posterior night splints in the treatment of plantar fasciitis. Am Fam Phys 52:891, 1995.
27. Jimenez AL, Goecker RM. Night splints: conservative management of plantar fasciitis. Biomechanics 4:29, 1997.
28. Subotnick S. Achilles and peroneal tendon injuries in the athlete. Clin Podiatr Med Surg 14:447, 1997.
29. Giorgini RJ, Sobel E. Postoperative immobilization and rehabilitation. Podiatry Management 16:61, 1997.
30. Duchenne GBA. Physiology of Motion. Philadelphia: W. B. Saunders, 1949.
31. Williams R. Chronic nonspecific tendosynovitis of the tibialis posterior. J Bone Joint Surg Br 45:512, 1963.
32. Gellman R, Burns S. Walking aches and running pains. Prim Care 23:263, 1996.
33. Lin SS, Lee TH, Chao W, et al. Nonoperative treatment of patients with posterior tibial tendinitis. Foot Ankle Clin 1:261, 1996.
34. Myerson M. Adult required flatfoot deformity: treatment of dysfunction of the posterior tibial tendon. J Bone Joint Surg Am 78:780, 1996.
35. Scheller AD, Kasser JR, Quigley TB. Tendon injuries about the ankle. Clin Sport Med 2:631, 1983.
36. Nork SE, Coughlin RR. How to examine a foot and what to do with a bunion. Prim Care 23:281, 1996.
37. Gerken AP, McGarvey WC, Baxter DE. Insertional Achilles tendinitis. Foot Ankle Clin 1:237, 1996.
38. Rogers BS, Leach RE. Achilles tendinitis. Foot Ankle Clin 1:249, 1996.
39. Haddad SL, Myerson MS. Managing Achilles tendon disorders. Biomechanics 3:23, 1996.
40. Stephens MM. Heel pain, shoes, exertion, and Haglund's deformity. Phys Sport Med 20:87, 1992.
41. Mascaro TB, Swanson LE. Rehabilitation of the foot and ankle. Orthop Clin North Am 25:147, 1994.
42. Rubin A, Sallis R. Evaluation and diagnosis of ankle injuries. Am Fam Phys 54:1609, 1996.
43. Garrick JG, Schelkun PH. Managing ankle sprains: keys to preserving motion and strength. Phys Sport Med 25:56, 1997.
44. Lindenfeld TN. The differentiation and treatment of ankle sprains. Orthopedics 11:203, 1988.
45. Boruta PM, Bishop JO, Braly WG, et al. Acute lateral ankle ligament injuries: a literature review. Foot Ankle 11:107, 1990.
46. Geiringer SR. Management of the athletic ankle sprain: from acute injury to rehabilitation. Biomechanics 4:25, 1997.
47. Gallagher SP. Which ankle brace is right for your patient? Biomechanics 3:35, 1996.
48. Nesbitt L. A practical guide to prescribing orthoses. Phys Sport Med 20:76, 1992.
49. Subotnick SI. Foot orthoses: an update. Phys Sport Med 11:103, 1983.
50. Hylton NM. Postural and functional impact of dynamic AFO's and FO's in a pediatric population. J Pros Orthot 2:40, 1989.
51. Shamp JK. Neurophysiologic orthotic designs in the treatment of central nervous system disorders. J Pros Orthot 2:14, 1989.
52. Rubin G, Cohen E, Rzonca EC. Prostheses and orthoses for the foot and ankle. In Frykberg RG, ed. The High Risk Foot in Diabetes Mellitus. New York: Churchill Livingstone, 1991, pp. 463–486.
53. Brodsky JW. Outpatient diagnosis and care of the diabetic foot. In Heckman JD, ed. Instructional Course Lectures: Volume 42. Rosemont, IL: American Association of Orthopedic Surgeons, 1993, pp. 121–139.
54. Sobel E. The ankle foot orthosis and its uses in the podiatric practice. Podiatr Management 16:68, 1997.
55. Rubin G, Cohen E. Prostheses and orthoses for the foot and ankle. Clin Podiatr Med Surg 5:695, 1988.
56. Cohen-Sobel E. Advances in foot prosthetics. In Kominsky SJ, ed. Advances in Podiatric Medicine and Surgery, vol 1. St. Louis: Mosby–Year Book, 1995, pp. 213–294.
57. Lehmann JF, Warren CG. Ischial and patellar-tendon weight-bearing braces: function, design, adjustment, and training. Bull Prosthet Res 10:6, 1973.
58. Cohen-Sobel E, Caselli MA, Rizzuto J. Prosthetic management of a Chopart amputation variant. J Am Podiatr Med Assoc 84:505, 1994.
59. Rubin G, Staros A, Cohen-Sobel E. Letter to the editor. Foot Ankle 15:46, 1994.

Index